Evidence-Based Geriatric Nursing
Protocols for Best Practice

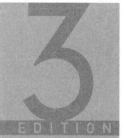

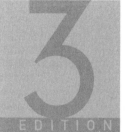

Evidence-Based
Geriatric Nursing
Protocols for
Best Practice

Editors

Elizabeth Capezuti, PhD, RN, FAAN

DeAnne Zwicker, MS, APRN, BC

Mathy Mezey, EdD, RN, FAAN

Terry Fulmer, PhD, RN, FAAN

Associate Editor

Deanna Gray-Miceli, DNSc, APRN, FAANP

Managing Editor

Malvina Kluger

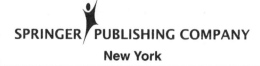

SPRINGER PUBLISHING COMPANY

New York

Springer Publishing Company, LLC
11 West 42nd Street
New York, NY 10036
www.springerpub.com

Acquisitions Editor: Sally J. Barhydt
Managing Editor: Mary Ann McLaughlin
Production Editor: Tenea Johnson
Cover design: Mimi Flow
Composition: Aptara Inc.

08   09   10/5   4   3

Library of Congress Cataloging-in-Publication Data

Evidence-based geriatric nursing protocols for best practice / Elizabeth Capezuti... [et al.], editors.—3rd ed.
    p. ; cm.
  Rev. ed. of: Geriatric nursing protocols for best practice / Mathy Mezey... [et al.], editors. 2nd ed. © 2003.
  Includes bibliographical references and index.
  ISBN 978-0-8261-1103-6 (hardback)
  1. Geriatric nursing.   2. Nursing care plans.   3. Evidence-based nursing.   I. Capezuti, Liz.   II. Geriatric nursing protocols for best practice.
  [DNLM: 1. Geriatric Nursing—methods.   2. Nursing Care.   3. Aged.
4. Evidence-Based Medicine.   5. Nursing Assessment. WY 152 E93 2007]
RC954.G465 2007
618.97'0231—dc22   2007029671

Printed in the United States of America by Bang Printing.

About the Editors

Elizabeth Capezuti, PhD, RN, ARNP-BC, FAAN, is an Associate Professor at New York University College of Nursing. She also serves as Co-director for The Hartford Institute for Geriatric Nursing at New York University, where she directs the Nurses Improving Care for Health System Elders (NICHE) and the Geriatric Nursing Research Scholars programs. Dr. Capezuti received her doctoral degree in nursing from the University of Pennsylvania in 1995 and is a nationally certified Geriatric Nurse Practitioner. She was also on the faculty of the University of Pennsylvania School of Nursing from 1984 through 2000, where she received the 1995 Provost's Award for Distinguished Teaching. From 2000 to 2003, she held the Independence Foundation Wesley Woods Chair in Gerontologic Nursing at Emory University. Dr. Capezuti's program of research focuses on the development and testing of interventions aimed at improving care of frail older adults. Findings from her research have been used to draft both state legislation and federal regulations related to nursing home care. She serves on several national boards and has been a consultant to the Hospital Bed Safety Workgroup of the U.S. Food and Drug Administration and the Center for Medicare and Medicaid Services. Dr. Capezuti has published extensively in the areas of fall prevention, restraint and side-rail elimination, elder mistreatment, and legal liability issues. She is a Fellow of the American Academy of Nursing, the Gerontological Society of America, the American Association of Nurse Practitioners, and the New York Academy of Medicine.

DeAnne Zwicker, MS, APRN, BC, is an ANCC certified adult primary care and geriatric nurse practitioner. She is currently a Senior Advisor for The Hartford Institute for Geriatric Nursing at New York University's College of Nursing and a doctoral student at Drexel University in Philadelphia. She was managing editor and coauthor of two chapters in *Geriatric Nursing Protocols for Best Practice,* 2nd Edition (awarded Geriatric Book of the Year, 2003, by *American Journal of Nursing*) and editor of The Hartford Institute's on-line Gerontologic Nursing Certification Review Course. Her clinical practice includes being a Clinical Services Manager for a managed-care company that provides nurse practitioners in long-term care and clinical faculty at NYU Division of Nursing in the advanced-practice adult and geriatric nurse practitioner programs. Ms. Zwicker has been a registered nurse for more than 30 years in acute care, including medical ICU, oncology, and general medicine. She has been a nurse practitioner for 15 years with extensive clinical experience working in adult primary care and with geriatric populations in multiple settings, including long-term care, primary care, subacute care, and rehabilitation.

Mathy Mezey, EdD, RN, FAAN, received her undergraduate and graduate education at Columbia University. She worked as a public health nurse and at Jacobi Hospital in New York City. Dr. Mezey taught at Lehman College of the City University of New York. For 10 years, she was a professor at the University of Pennsylvania School of Nursing, where she directed the geriatric nurse practitioner program and the Robert Wood Johnson Foundation Teaching Nursing Home Program. Since 1991, she has been a professor at New York University College of Nursing. In 1996, Dr. Mezey assumed the position of Director of The Hartford Institute for Geriatric Nursing at NYU.

Dr. Mezey has authored 10 books and has more than 60 publications that focus on the preparation of baccalaureate and advanced practice nurses to care for older adults, nursing practice with older adults, and bioethical issues that affect decisions at the end of life. A Member of the American Academy of Nursing, Dr. Mezey is Editor for the Springer Series in Geriatric Nursing and Co-Editor of the Springer publication, *The Encyclopedia of Elder Care.* Her current research and writing focus on quality of care for older people in hospitals and long-term care.

Dr. Mezey is a Fellow in the American Academy of Nursing and the Gerontological Society of America, sits on the Board of the Visiting Nurse Service of New York, and is Trustee Emeritus, Columbia University.

Terry Fulmer, PhD, RN, FAAN, is The Erline Perkins McGriff Professor and Dean of the College of Nursing at New York University. She received her bachelor's degree from Skidmore College, her master's and doctoral degrees from Boston College, and her Geriatric Nurse Practitioner Post-Master's Certificate from New York University. Dr. Fulmer's program of research focuses on acute care of the elderly and, specifically, elder abuse and neglect. She served on the National Research Council's panel to review risk and prevalence of elder abuse and neglect and has published widely on this topic. She has received the status of Fellow in the American Academy of Nursing, the Gerontological Society of America, and the New York Academy of Medicine. She is a member of the National Committee for Quality Assurance geriatric measurement assessment panel and the Veteran's Administration Geriatrics and Gerontology Advisory Committee. She completed a Brookdale National Fellowship and is a Distinguished Practitioner of the National Academies of Practice. Dr. Fulmer was the first nurse to be elected to the board of the American Geriatrics Society and the first nurse to serve as the president of the Gerontological Society of America.

Deanna Gray-Miceli, DNSc, APRN, FAANP, is consultant to New York University-Hartford Institute for Geriatric Nursing (HIGN) and Project Director for the HIGN/American Association of Colleges of Nursing–sponsored grant, *Preparing Nursing Students to Care for Older Adults: Enhancing Gerontology in Senior-Level Undergraduate Courses, The G-NEC Experience,* and an Adjunct Assistant Professor of Nursing at the University of Pennsylvania School of Nursing. As a nationally certified gerontological nurse practitioner for more than 2 decades, Dr. Gray-Miceli has devoted her clinical and research interests to evaluation and care of older adults who fall. In the mid-1990s, she founded and directed the first academic nurse-managed Fall Assessment and Prevention

Program in the country, housed at a school of medicine. In 2001, she completed a doctoral degree, focusing her dissertation research on the "Lived experience and meaning of a serious fall to older adults." In 2002, Dr. Gray-Miceli was awarded a Post-Doctoral Scholarship by The John A. Hartford Building Academic Geriatric Nursing Capacity Program, working with faculty mentors from the School of Nursing and School of Medicine at the University of Pennsylvania. Dr. Gray-Miceli's program of research includes the development, validation, and feasibility for Registered Nurses to use a post-fall assessment tool for older adults in nursing homes. The tool is capable of detecting reasons for fall events by clinical staff.

For the past 4 years, Dr. Gray-Miceli has been an invited consultant to a state department of health for statewide fall prevention initiatives including development of programs and services for older adults. Several health care provider and professional initiatives directed at fall prevention in clinical practice settings have also been launched. In 2006, she was an invited reviewer to the State and Territorial Injury Prevention Directors Association (STIPDA), Injury Surveillance Workgroup on Falls [ISWF] Report: Consensus Recommendations for Surveillance of Falls and Fall-Related Injuries, and contributed to ECRI's book "Fall Prevention Strategies in Health Care Settings" and national webinar educational series on fall prevention. Dr. Gray-Miceli has published more than 25 refereed journal articles and 10 book chapters, authored a book titled "Falls Toolkit," and presented more than 25 papers or posters at national and local scientific meetings mostly related to falls in older adults. She is a Fellow of the American Academy of Nurse Practitioners and the Gerontological Society of America.

Malvina Kluger, BA, is Senior Administrator of The Hartford Institute at the New York University College of Nursing. In this role, she plans, implements, and manages various initiatives, primarily in nursing education and policy. She has been editor of The Hartford Institute newsletter *Nursing Counts*, and her background includes research and family services social work.

Contributors

Elaine J. Amella, PhD, APRN, BC, FAAN
Associate Dean for Research & Evaluation, College of Nursing
Medical University of South Carolina
Charleston, South Carolina

Jacqueline M. Arena, BS, BSN, RN
Fairfield University, School of Nursing
Fairfield, Connecticut

Elizabeth A. Ayello, PhD, RN, APRN, BC, CWOCN, FAPWCA, FAAN
President, Ayello, Harris, & Associates, Inc.
Clinical Associate Editor, *Advances in Skin & Wound Care*
Faculty, Excelsior College, School of Nursing
Executive Editor, *Journal of World Council of Enterostomal Therapists*

Michele C. Balas, PhD, RN, CCRN, CRNP, BC
2005–2007 Building Academic Geriatric Nursing Capacity Hartford–Atlantic Fellow
University of Pennsylvania, School of Nursing
Philadelphia, Pennsylvania

Christine Bradway, PhD, CRNP
Assistant Professor of Gerontological Nursing & 2005–2007 John A. Hartford Foundation
    Building Academic Geriatric Nursing Capacity Fellow
University of Pennsylvania, School of Nursing
Philadelphia, Pennsylvania

Tom Braes, RN, MSN, PhDCan
Centre for Health Services and Nursing Research
Katholieke Universiteit
Leuven, Belgium
And
Department of Internal Medicine, Division of Geriatric Medicine
University Hospitals of Leuven, Belgium

Pamela Z. Cacchione, PhD, RN, BCGNP
Associate Professor
Saint Louis University, Doisy College of Health Sciences
St. Louis, Missouri

Colleen M. Casey, BS, RN, CCRN
Predoctoral Scholar
2005–2007 John A. Hartford Foundation Building Academic Geriatric Nursing Capacity
Oregon Health & Science University
Portland, Oregon

Eileen R. Chasens, RN, DSN
Assistant Professor
University of Pittsburgh
Pittsburgh, Pennsylvania

Deborah A. Chyun, PhD, RN, FAHA
Associate Professor and Director, Adult Advanced Practice Nursing Specialty
Yale University School of Nursing
New Haven, Connecticut

Valerie T. Cotter, MSN, CRNP, FAANP
Program Director, Adult Health and Gerontology Nurse Practitioner Programs
University of Pennsylvania, School of Nursing
Philadelphia, Pennsylvania

Jessica Shank Coviello, MSN, APRN
Yale University School of Nursing
New Haven, Connecticut

Rose Ann DiMaria-Ghalili, PhD, RN, CNSN
Associate Professor
West Virginia University, School of Nursing
Morgantown, West Virginia

Annemarie Dowling-Castronovo, RN, MA-GNP
Doctoral Candidate
Rutgers, The State University of New Jersey
College of Nursing
Newark, New Jersey

Kathleen Fletcher, RN, MSN, APRN-BC, GNP, FAAN
Director Senior Services
Assistant Professor of Nursing
University of Virginia Health System
Charlottesville, Virginia

Marquis D. Foreman, PhD, RN, FAAN
Professor and Associate Dean for Nursing Science Studies
University of Illinois at Chicago, College of Nursing
Chicago, Illinois

Deborah C. Francis, MSN, APRN, BC
Geriatric Clinical Nurse Specialist
Kaiser Permanente Medical Center
South Sacramento, California

Terry Fulmer, PhD, RN, FAAN
Dean and The Erline Perkins McGriff Professor
New York University, College of Nursing
New York City, New York

Deanna Gray-Miceli, DNSc, APRN, FAANP
Geriatric Consultant, The Hartford Institute for Geriatric Nursing
New York University, College of Nursing
New York City, New York
And
Adjunct Assistant Professor
University of Pennsylvania, School of Nursing
Philadelphia, Pennsylvania
And
Fall Prevention Consultant to a State Department of Health

Barbara L. Halliday, RN, MSN
Clinical Nurse Specialist
Department of Nursing
MetroHealth Medical Center
Cleveland, Ohio

Mary Beth Happ, PhD, RN
Associate Professor
University of Pittsburgh, School of Nursing and Center for Bioethics and Health Law
And
Adjunct Associate Professor
University of Pennsylvania, School of Nursing

Theresa A. Harvath, PhD, RN, CNS
Associate Professor and Director, Advanced Practice Gerontology
Oregon Health & Science University, School of Nursing
Portland, Oregon

Ann L. Horgas, RN, PhD, FGSA, FAAN
Associate Professor and Associate Dean for Research
University of Florida, College of Nursing
Gainesville, FLorida

Susan Kaplan Jacobs, MLS, MA, RN, AHIP
Associate Curator, Health Sciences Librarian
Elmer Holmes Bobst Library, New York University
New York City, New York

Denise M. Kresevic, RN, PhD
Geriatric Nurse Practitioner/Researcher
Louis Stokes Cleveland MAMC
University Hospitals of Cleveland
Case Western Reserve University
Cleveland, Ohio

Lenore H. Kurlowicz, PhD, RN, CS, FAAN
Assistant Professor of Geropsychiatric Nursing
University of Pennsylvania, School of Nursing
Philadelphia, Pennsylvania

Rona F. Levin, PhD, RN
Professor
Pace University, Lienhard School of Nursing
And
Visiting Faculty
Visiting Nurse Service of New York
New York City, New York

Janet C. Mentes, PhD, APRN, BC
Assistant Professor
University of California Los Angeles, School of Nursing
Los Angeles, California

Deborah C. Messecar, PhD, MPH, RN, CNS
Associate Professor
Oregon Health & Science University, School of Nursing
Portland, Oregon

Koen Milisen, RN, PhD
Associate Professor
Center for Health Services and Nursing Research
Katholieke Universiteit
Leuven, Belgium

Lorraine C. Mion, PhD, RN, FAAN
Director, Nursing Research and Geriatric Nursing
Department of Nursing
MetroHealth Medical Center
Cleveland, Ohio

Ethel L. Mitty, EdD, RN
Adjunct Clinical Professor of Nursing
New York University, College of Nursing
New York City, New York

Madeline Naegle, APRN-BC, PhD, FAAN
Professor and Director, WHO Collaborating Center
New York University, College of Nursing
New York City, New York

Linda J. O'Connor, MSN, RNC, APRN-BC
Clinical Nurse Manager, Medical Services
The Mount Sinai Medical Center
New York City, New York

Janine Overcash, PhD, ARNP, BC
Assistant Professor
University of South Florida
Tampa, Florida

Lenard L. Parisi, RN, MA, CPHQ, FNAHQ
Vice President, Quality Management/Performance Improvement
Metropolitan Jewish Health System
Brooklyn, New York

Linda Farber Post, JD, MA, BSN
Director of Bioethics
Hackensack University Medical Center
Hackensack, New Jersey

Gloria C. Ramsey, JD, RN
Associate Professor, Graduate School of Nursing
Assistant Research Professor, School of Medicine
Director, Community Outreach and Information Dissemination
Center for Health Disparities Research and Education
Uniformed Services, University of the Health Sciences
Bethesda, Maryland

Satinderpal K. Sandhu, MD
Assistant Professor
Department of Family Practice/Geriatrics
MetroHealth Medical Center
And
Case Western Reserve University School of Medicine
Cleveland, Ohio

R. Gary Sibbald, BSc, MD, FRCPC (Med) (Derm), MEd
Professor of Public Health Sciences and Medicine
Director of Wound Healing Clinic, The New Women's College Hospital
Director of Medical Education at Women's College Hospital
President-Elect of World Union of Wound Healing Societies
Toronto, Canada

Joanne K. Singleton, PhD, APRN, BC, FNAP
Professor & Co-Director, Institute for Healthy Aging
Pace University, Lienhard School of Nursing
New York City, New York

Constance M. Smith. PhD, RN
Wilmington, Delaware

Dorothy F. Tullmann, PhD, RN
Assistant Professor
University of Virginia, School of Nursing
Charlottesville, Virginia

Mary Grace Umlauf, RN, PhD, FAAN
Professor
University of Alabama, School of Nursing
Birmingham, Alabama

Meredith Wallace, PhD, APRN
Associate Professor
Yale University School of Nursing
New Haven, Connecticut

Laura L. Williams, MSN, CRNP
Doctoral Student
University of Alabama, School of Nursing
Birmingham, Alabama

Saunjoo L. Yoon, PhD, RN
Assistant Professor
University of Florida, College of Nursing
Gainesville, Florida

DeAnne Zwicker, MS, APRN, BC
Content Editor *GeroNurseOnline* &
Senior Advisor for Special Projects
The Hartford Institute for Geriatric Nursing
New York University, College of Nursing
New York City, NY

Foreword

In the context of an aging population, use of services by the elderly throughout the health care system continues to grow, particularly among those aged 85 years and older. According to 2004 national survey data, 38% of hospital discharges are people aged 65 years and older (Russo & Elixhauser, 2003). Simultaneously, dramatic advances in prevention, treatment, and control of numerous chronic diseases and related illnesses have led to greatly increased complexity of care for older adults in today's modern health care systems. Consequently, substantial challenges for nursing care have emerged as treatment side effects from medications, surgical procedures, and the hazards of hospitalization conspire to threaten quality of life among older adults during the acute phase of care. A growing base of evidence confirms the pivotal role that bedside nurses play in influencing health trajectories among older adults, particularly in the acute-care setting (Fitzpatrick, Salinas, O'Connor, Callahan & White, 2004; Mezey, Boltz, Esterson, & Mitty, 2005).

Concurrent with the growth in number of frail older adults in health care settings, the scientific basis for care of the elderly has strengthened considerably. New strategies for the synthesis and dissemination of this knowledge base for care have made scientific findings more broadly available to clinicians, administrators, patients, and family members and their advocates, raising expectations for care.

To effectively care for today's older adults, therefore, nurses must integrate knowledge of care for acutely ill patients with the emerging science base of how patterns of chronic, co-morbid conditions affect presentation of illness and how to anticipate and treat geriatric syndromes. Nurses are charged with doing this while eliciting and honoring patient preferences for various care options and being mindful of how family and informal caregivers are involved in care. Meeting this care standard would be a tall order under any circumstances, but it becomes particularly challenging during a time of nursing shortage. Increased utilization of paraprofessional nursing staff, for example, underscores the need for standardized approaches to care that nurses can use with caregivers from diverse educational and cultural backgrounds.

Evidence-Based Geriatric Nursing Protocols for Best Practice, now in its third edition, is a timely addition to the resources nurses and health care organizations need to address the specialized-care needs of older adults throughout the continuum of care. Editors Elizabeth Capezuti, DeAnne Zwicker, Mathy Mezey, and Terry Fulmer have engaged some of the top clinician–scientists in the country to frame, acquire, appraise, and synthesize the best evidence for care of the most prevalent clinical problems and syndromes faced by older adults when they are ill. Expanding on prior success with earlier editions of this book and with the innovative geriatric nursing care portal, www.ConsultGeriRN.org, this edition offers updated and refined sections on previously featured topics such as advance directives. A key refinement to the protocols is making an explicit link between the guideline recommendations and the supporting evidence. Several new protocols critically needed for effective nursing care of the elderly, such as protocols for dehydration prevention, recognition, and treatment, have been added. Each section includes a model case study to demonstrate application of the evidence and protocol.

The update and expansion of these protocols have important implications for nurses at every level of practice. Bedside-care nurses now can have ready access to preappraised scientific evidence, accompanied by practical implementation strategies on which to base practice as they confront growing numbers of frail older adults in their care. Members of nursing practice councils, nurse managers, and nurse executives now have an explicit, graded scientific basis for standardizing care practices at the unit level, which should, in turn, assist in forecasting needed staffing and services and development or refinement of systems of care that are "older adult-friendly." Nursing faculty will find the protocols and evidence summary a useful guide for prioritizing curriculum improvements, and the protocols also serve as a source for identifying gaps in our knowledge base that require new empirical studies. The greatest beneficiaries of these new practice protocols, however, will be the older adults and their family members who stand to benefit from the greater consistency in care and improved outcomes from care based on the best evidence that is tempered with the expertise of advanced clinician–scholars.

Eleanor S. McConnell, RN, PhD, APRN, BC
Associate Professor & Director, Gerontological Nursing Specialty;
Clinical Nurse Specialist, Durham Veterans Administration Medical Center,
Geriatric Research, Education, and Clinical Center
Durham, North Carolina

References

Fitzpatrick, J., Salinas, T. K., O'Connor, L. J., Callahan, B., & White, M. T. (2004). Nursing care quality initiative for hospitalized elders and their families. *Journal of Nursing Care Quality, 19*(2), 156–161.

Mezey, M., Boltz, M., Esterson, J., & Mitty, E. (2005). Evolving models of geriatric nursing care. *Geriatric Nursing, 26*(1), 11–15.

Russo, C. A., & Elixhauser, A. (2003). *Hospitalizations in the elderly population, 2003.* Statistical Brief #6. May 2006. Rockville, MD: Agency for Healthcare Research and Quality. Retrieved February 5, 2007, from http://www.hcup-us.ahrq.gov/reports/statbriefs/sb6.pdf

Preface

As an experienced nursing leader in the hospital arena and with a specialty focus on older persons in our society, I can attest that this third edition holds the promise of bringing yet another level of depth and sophistication to understanding the best practices for assessment, interventions, and anticipated outcomes in our care of older adults.

Health care in our nation, in particular, is becoming increasingly complex. This complexity is also occurring at a time when the number of those older than 65 years of age will soon be the vast majority of our population. Providers of care, both professional and our highly invested public, search daily for the best way to address and manage the multiple levels of care challenges that our older population faces. Third-party payers make decisions about the appropriateness of care seemingly without regard to the efficacy of the treatment modality or interventions but rather based on the short-term cost-effectiveness. Hospital stays are shorter—and rightfully so in light of the higher risk for infection and other complications in our nation's facilities. The push toward subacute care, intermediate-care units, long-term care, and assisted-living settings makes decision making about care problems even more difficult and imperative. Providers of care increasingly try to sort out the alternatives available for these issues, often without the time required to recall or find the best evidence-based approach. Recognition that quality care is generally also the most cost-effective requires use of the evidence that produces the best outcomes.

The nation's "baby-boomers" are driving ever higher levels of expectation for the best possible care for their parents, loved ones, and themselves. The Internet is the vehicle for providing access to more information than most of us have the time and capacity to absorb. That this text draws upon the valuable resources of GeroNurseOnline.org is testament to the usefulness of this mode of information. Therefore, it is critical that those of us who are perceived as experts help our fellow professionals and the educated public to find what really *is* evidenced based.

The dynamic of evidenced-based practice is an ever-changing area of knowledge synthesis and contextual analysis. It is to the editors' credit that Stetler et al. and the Melnyk & Fineout-Overholt models of evidence ranking were not only selected as the framework for this edition but also that the chapter authors are required to reference the formal Level of Evidence (see chapter 1 on the AGREE rationale) within the text to provide that distinction and reinforcement of the models. Such referencing establishes the current state of the evidence, lends reliability to the recommendations, sets forth potential areas of inquiry for research, and demonstrates contemporary sound practice. Using evidence-based practice compels the provider to set aside biases, dispel and destroy sacred cows, and exercise critical thinking at every step.

Evidence-Based Geriatric Nursing Protocols for Best Practice is intended to bring the most current evidence-based protocols known to experts in geriatric nursing to the audience of students, both graduate and undergraduate; practitioners at the staff level, from novice to expert; clinicians in specialty roles (i.e., educators, care managers, and advanced practice nurses); and nursing leaders of all levels. The content recognizes that nursing is a cognitive discipline and gives professionals the tools to use. As with any text, the value is in the use and implementation of the protocols to improve the care of older persons. That challenge is clear to those of us in practice, service, and education. We owe a debt of gratitude to the many authors and the editors for bringing this work to us.

Susan Bowar-Ferres, PhD, RN, CNAA-BC
Senior Vice President & Chief Nursing Officer
New York University Hospitals Center
New York City, New York

Introduction

Older adults are overwhelmingly the majority of hospitalized patients and are by far the most complicated patients to care for in the acute-care setting. They suffer from multiple complex medical problems, take multiple medications, are the most vulnerable to iatrogenic events, experience prolonged hospital stays, and are more likely to die in the hospital (versus the community or other setting). Acute-care nurses have an enormous responsibility when providing care to older adults in this rapidly changing health care environment with increasing regulatory requirements and short staffing. Even though older persons are our fastest growing segment in the United States, most nursing programs, like medical programs, are just now incorporating geriatrics into the curriculum. Many of those unfamiliar with geriatrics might ask: What's so different about old people? Don't they have the same diagnoses as younger adults, like diabetes, hypertension, and heart disease? The answer to those questions is yes, they do have the same diseases; however, physiological changes that occur with aging, multiple coexisting medical problems, and multiple medications place older adults at significantly higher risk for complications, including death, while hospitalized. The nurse armed with information on the unique ways in which older adults present with subtle signs and symptoms may actually avert complications. Additionally, the nurse equipped with knowledge about and skill in proactive assessment and interventions may actually prevent these complications in the first place.

As in the previous second edition (titled *Geriatric Nursing Protocols for Best Practice* and honored as *American Journal of Nursing* Geriatric Book of the Year in 2003), we present assessment and interventions for common geriatric syndromes. Geriatric syndromes are increasingly recognized as being related to preventable iatrogenic complications, or those that occur as a direct result of medical and nursing care, causing serious adverse outcomes in older patients (see chapter 11, *Iatrogenesis*). We are also very happy to present 13 new topics and several new expert contributors in this edition. Many of these topics have been updated from the protocols that appear on the Web site of The Hartford Institute for Geriatric Nursing at NYU (www.ConsultGeriRN.org). The new topics in this edition are as follows:

- Dementia
- Nutrition in Aging
- Managing Oral Hydration in Older Adults
- Oral Health Care
- Age-Related Changes in Health
- Sensory Changes

- Iatrogenesis: The Nurse's Role in Preventing Patient Harm
- Family Caregiving for Older Adults
- Comprehensive Assessment and Management of the Critically Ill Older Adult
- Fluid Overload: Identifying and Managing Heart Failure Patients at Risk for Hospital Readmission
- Cancer and the Older Patient: Assessment and Intervention Strategies for the Acute-Care Nurse
- Issues Regarding Sexuality in Older Adults
- Substance Abuse

In this third edition of *Evidence-Based Geriatric Nursing Protocols for Best Practice*, we provide guidelines that are developed by experts on the topics of each chapter and are based on best available evidence. A systematic method, the AGREE Appraisal Process (see AGREE Collaboration, 2001; Levin, in press; Singleton & Levin, in press), was used to evaluate the protocols in the second edition and identify a process to help us improve validity of the book's content. This systematic process, described in chapter 1, was developed to retrieve and evaluate the level of evidence of key references related to specific assessment and management strategies in each chapter. The purpose of determining the best available evidence was to answer the clinical questions posed. The chapter authors rated the levels of evidence based on the work of Stetler et al. (1998) and Melnyk and Fineout-Overholt (2005). Chapter 1, *Developing and Evaluating Clinical Practice Guidelines: A Systematic Approach,* details the process of how the clinical practice guidelines were developed and how they complied with the AGREE items for rigor of development (AGREE Collaboration, 2001). This chapter, written by leaders in the field of evidence-based practice in the United States, will likely be the most important chapter reference for understanding the rating of the levels of evidence. Most of the protocols reflect assessment and intervention strategies for acute care recommended by expert authors who have reviewed the evidence using this process; the evidence provided may come from all levels of care and may not have been specifically tested in the hospital setting.

How to Best Use This Book

The standard nursing approach was used as a guideline for the outline of each topic as deemed appropriate by the chapter author(s) providing overview and background information on the topic, evidence-based assessment and intervention strategies, and a topic-specific case study with discussion. The text of the chapter provides the context and detailed evidence for the protocol; the tabular protocol is not intended to be used in isolation from the text. We recommend that readers consider the following when reading the chapters:

- Review the objectives to ascertain what is to be achieved by reviewing the chapter.
- Review the text noting level of evidence that supports the content, with Level I being the highest (i.e., Systematic Review/Meta-analysis) and

Level VI the lowest (i.e., Expert opinion) and refer to chapter 1, Figure 1.2, for definitions of Level of Evidence to understand the quantitative evidence that supports each recommendation. Keep in mind that it is virtually impossible to have evidence for all assessments and interventions, which *does not* mean it is not to be used as an intervention. Many interventions that have been successfully used for years have not been quantitatively researched but are well known to be effective to experts in the field of geriatrics.

- Review the protocols and keep in mind that they reflect assessment and intervention strategies for acute care recommended by experts who have reviewed the evidence. This evidence is from all levels of care (e.g., community, primary care, long-term care), not necessarily the hospital setting, and should be applied to the unique needs of individual patients.
- The focus should always be patient-centered, which considers many other factors specific to the individual.
- Review the case study and discussion in each topic, which provides a more real-life, practical manner in which the protocol may be applied in clinical practice.
- Resources in each chapter provide easy access to tools discussed in the chapter and to link readers with organizations that provide ongoing, up-to-date information and resources on the topic.
- An appendix provides additional geriatric-specific resources for readers that can be applied to all topics.

Although this book refers to *Evidence-Based Geriatric Nursing Protocols for Best Practice,* the text may be used by educators for geriatric nursing courses and advance practice nurses and by many others, including interdisciplinary team members, nursing-home and other staff educators, social workers, dieticians, physician assistants, and physicians. Many interventions that are proactively identified by nurses can make a significant difference in improving outcomes, but nurses cannot provide for the complex needs of older adults in isolation. Research has shown that interdisciplinary teams have dramatically improved geriatric patient care and outcomes, as indicated in the Institute of Medicine (IOM) report: communication and collaboration are vital to ensure appropriate exchange of information and care coordination whereas lack of communication is considered a major contributor to iatrogenic complications (IOM, 2001). Caring for older adults as the baby-boomer population continues to "age in" will be an ultimate challenge in health care. Each of us must work together and be committed to provide a culture of safety that vulnerable older adults need in order to receive the safest evidence-based clinical care with optimal outcomes.

We would like to thank the following for their involvement, support, and leadership during the production of this book:

- all of the expert contributors for this third edition
- those nursing experts who participated in the Nurse Competence in Aging project and contributed chapters to GeroNurseOnline, many of which were the impetus for new topics added to this edition
- the institutions that supported faculty and geriatric clinicians participating as contributors of the evidence-based protocols

- those who provided valuable contributions in the first and second editions and their ongoing geriatric research
- faculty and clinicians involved in the project of the American Association of Colleges of Nursing to develop geriatric content for upper-division baccalaureate nursing programs
- Springer Publishing Company for its continuing support of quality geriatric nursing publications
- Nurses Improving Care for Health System Elders (NICHE) Hospitals, which bring many of these protocols to the bedside and serve as leaders in ensuring geriatric nursing best practices (see Dedication and Acknowledgments)

Elizabeth Capezuti
DeAnne Zwicker
Mathy Mezey
Terry Fulmer

Acknowledgement

The editors would like to thank Susan Kaplan Jacobs and Rona Levin for their involvement, support, and leadership during the production of this book.

References

AGREE Collaboration (2001). *Appraisal of guidelines research and evaluation, AGREE instrument.* Retrieved November 21, 2006, from http://www.agreecollaboration.org/instrument/

Institute of Medicine (2001). Crossing the quality chasm: A new health system for the 21st century. Washington, DC: National Academy Press.

Levin, R. (2007). Evidence-based practice: A guide to negotiate the clinical practice guideline maze. *Research and Theory in Nursing Practice, 11,* 5–9.

Melnyck, B. M., & Fineout-Overholt, E. (2005). *Evidence-based practice in healthcare.* Philadelphia: Lippincott.

Singleton, J. K., & Levin, R. F. (In press). Strategies for learning evidence-based practice: Critically appraising clinical practice guidelines. *Journal of Nursing Education.*

Stetler, C. B., Morsi, D., Rucki, S., Broughton, S., Corrigan, B., Fitzgerald, J., et al. (1998). Utilization-focused integrative reviews in a nursing service. *Applied Nursing Research, 11,* 195–206.

Dedication and Acknowledgments

Evidence-Based Geriatric Nursing Protocols for Best Practice, 3rd Edition, is dedicated to all hospitals participating in the Nurses Improving Care for Health System Elders (NICHE) program for their commitment to providing quality care for older adults. This edition is also dedicated to the Specialty Nursing Associations participating in the Nurse Competence in Aging (NCA) project (affiliated with GeroNurseOnline and The Hartford Institute for Geriatric Nursing) who have added geriatric-specific content to their Web sites. We thank all of you for your recognition and support for improving the outcomes of older adults. Following is a list of the NICHE Hospitals and Specialty Nursing Associations.

NICHE Hospitals

(As of May 2007)

Arizona

Tucson Medical Center, Tucson

California

California Pacific Medical Center, San Francisco
Eisenhower Medical Center, Rancho Mirage
John Muir Medical Center–Walnut Creek Campus
Pomerado Hospital, Poway
Palomar Pomerado Medical Center, Escondido
St. Joseph Hospital, Orange
UCSF Medical Center at Parnassus, San Francisco

Colorado

Boulder Community Hospital, Boulder
North Colorado Medical Center, Greeley

Connecticut

Bridgeport Hospital, Bridgeport
Greenwich Hospital, Greenwich
Hartford Hospital, Hartford
Stamford Hospital, Stamford
Yale–New Haven Hospital, New Haven

Delaware

Bayhealth Medical Center, Dover
Christiana Care Health System, Wilmington
Christiana Hospital
Wilmington Hospital
Riverside Transitional Care Facility
Christiana Care VNA

Florida

Boca Raton Community Hospital, Boca Raton
Florida Hospital Medical Center, Orlando
Lakeland Regional Medical Center, Lakeland
Morton Plant Hospital, Clearwater
Mease Dunedin Hospital, Clearwater
Sarasota Memorial Hospital, Sarasota

Georgia

Piedmont Hospital, Atlanta

Hawaii

Kaiser Permanente, Honolulu

Idaho

Kootenai Medical Services, Coeur d'Alene

Illinois

Edward Hospital, Naperville
Memorial Medical Center, Springfield
Northwest Community Hospital, Arlington Heights
OSF Saint Anthony Medical Center, Rockford
OSF Saint Francis Medical Center, Peoria
Resurrection Health Care, Saint Joseph Hospital, Chicago
Rush North Shore Medical Center, Skokie
Sarah Bush Lincoln Health Center, Mattoon
Swedish Covenant Hospital, Chicago

Indiana

Schneck Medical Center, Seymour
Wishard Hospital, Indianapolis

Iowa

Mercy Medical Center, Des Moines
Mercy Medical Center, Sioux City
Mercy Medical Center North Iowa, Mason City
Palo Alto County Health Services, Emmetsburg
University of Iowa Hospitals and Clinics, Iowa City

Kentucky

University of Kentucky Hospital, Lexington

Louisiana

Ochsner Clinic Foundation, New Orleans
Tenet Health Center, Memorial Medical Center, New Orleans

Maine

Maine Medical Center, Portland

Maryland

Baltimore–Washington Medical Center
Greater Baltimore Medical Center, Glen Burnie
Maryland General Hospital, Baltimore

Massachusetts

Addison Gilbert Hospital, Gloucester
Beth Israel Deaconess Medical Center, Boston
Dana Farber Cancer Institute, Boston
Jewish Geriatric Services, Longmeadow
Massachusetts General Hospital, Boston
Newton Wellesley Hospital, Newton
Spaulding Rehabilitation Hospital, Boston
Tewksbury Hospital, Tewksbury

Michigan

Blodgett Memorial Medical Center
Bronson Methodist Hospital, Kalamazoo
Chelsea Community Hospital, Chelsea
Detroit Receiving Hospital, Detroit
Huron Valley–Sinai Hospital, Detroit
Metro Health Hospital, Grand Rapids
Oakwood Healthcare System, Dearborn
Sinai–Grace Hospital, Detroit
Spectrum Health, Grand Rapids, Grand Rapids
St. John's Hospital and Medical Center, Detroit
Saint Joseph Hospital, Apple Valley
St. Joseph Mercy–Oakland, Pontiac
W. A. Foote Memorial Hospital, Jackson
William Beaumont Hospital, Royal Oak

Minnesota

Allina Unity, Fridley
Fairview University Medical Center, Minneapolis
Mayo Clinic Health System, Rochester
North Memorial Medical Center, Robbinsdale

Nebraska

Nebraska Methodist Hospital, Omaha

Missouri

Saint Joseph Health Center, Kansas City
Phelps County Regional Medical Center, Rolla

New Hampshire

Dartmouth Hitchcock Medical Center, Lebanon
Frisbie Memorial Hospital, Rochester
Saint Joseph Hospital, Nashua

New Jersey

Chilton Memorial Hospital, Pompton Plains
Englewood Hospital and Medical Center, Englewood
Meridian Health System, Jersey Shore Medical Center, Neptune
Meridian Health System, Medical Center of Ocean County, Brick Township
Meridian Health System, Riverview Medical Center, Red Bank
Newark Beth Israel Medical Center, Newark
Raritan Bay Medical Center, Perth Amboy
Robert Wood Johnson University Hospital, New Brunswick
Robert Wood Johnson University Hospital at Rahway
Saint Clare's Health System
Saint Clare's Sussex
Saint Clare's Dover General
Saint Clare's Denville
Saint Clare's Boonton
Franciscan Oaks Continuing Care Retirement Community/Saint Francis
Residential Community, Denville
Saint Joseph's Regional Medical Center, Patterson
Saint Peter's University Hospital, New Brunswick
The Valley Hospital, Ridgewood
Trinitas Hospital, Elizabeth
Union Hospital, Union

New York

Benedictine Hospital, Kingston
Crouse Hospital, Syracuse
Geneva General Hospital (Finger Lakes Health), Geneva
Highland Hospital (Strong Health)/UR School of Nursing, Rochester
The Highlands at Brighton (Strong Health)/UR School of Nursing, Rochester
The Highlands Living Center (Strong Health)/UR School of Nursing
Kaledia Health, Buffalo General Hospital Site, Buffalo
King's County Hospital, New York City
Long Island Jewish (LIJ) Medical Center, New Hyde Park
Memorial Sloan-Kettering Cancer Center, New York City
Mount Sinai Medical Center, New York City
New York Hospital Medical Center of Queens, Flushing

New York Presbyterian Hospital–The Allen Pavilion, New York
NYU Downtown Hospital, New York City
NYU Medical Center, Tisch Hospital, New York City
North Shore University Hospital (NSUH) at Forest Hills, Forest Hills
NSUH at Glen Cove, Glen Cove
NSUH LIJ: Huntington Hospital, Huntington
NSUH at Manhasset
Rochester General Hospital, Rochester
Schervier Nursing Care Center, New York City
Soldiers & Sailors Memorial Hospital (Finger Lakes Health), Penn Yan
Strong Memorial Hospital (Strong Health)/UR School of Nursing, Rochester
The Mount Sinai Hospital of Queens
Unity Hospital, Rochester

North Carolina

Duke Health Raleigh Hospital, Durham
Duke University Medical Center, Durham
Forsyth Medical Center, Winston-Salem
Gaston Memorial Hospital, Gastonia
Mission Hospitals, Asheville
Moses Cone Health System, Greensboro
University of North Carolina Hospitals, Chapel Hill
Wake Forest University Baptist Medical Center, Winston-Salem

North Dakota

Saint Alexius Medical Center, Bismarck

Ohio

Akron General Medical Center, Akron, Ohio
Bethesda North Hospital, Cincinnati
Metro Health Medical Center, Cleveland
Premiere Health Partners, Good Samaritan Hospital, Dayton
Premiere Health Partners, Miami Valley Hospital, Dayton
Southwest General Hospital, Middleburg Heights
The Cleveland Clinic Foundation, Cleveland
The Cleveland Clinic Health System, Euclid Hospital, Euclid
University Hospitals Case Medical Center, Cleveland
University Hospitals Geneva Medical Center, Geneva

Oklahoma

Jane Phillips Medical Center, Bartlesville
Oklahoma State University Medical Center, Tulsa
Saint Francis Hospital, Tulsa

Oregon

Legacy Good Samaritan Hospital & Medical Center, Portland
Oregon Health Science University Hospital, Portland
Peace Health, Sacred Heart Medical Center, Eugene

Providence Milwaukee Hospital, Milwaukee
Providence Portland Medical Center, Portland
Providence St. Vincent Medical Center, Portland
Rogue Valley Medical Center, Medford
Three Community Hospital and Medical Center, Grant Pass

Pennsylvania

Abington Memorial Hospital, Abington
Community Medical Center, Scranton
Crozer Keystone Health System, Crozer Chester, Upland
Crozer Keystone Health System, Delaware County Hospital, Drexel Hill
Crozer Keystone Health System, Springfield Hospital, Springfield
Crozer Keystone Health System, Taylor Hospital, Ridley Park
Moses Taylor Hospital, Scranton
Suburban General Hospital, Pittsburgh

Rhode Island

The Miriam Hospital, Providence
Rhode Island Hospital, Providence
Roger Williams Medical Center, Providence

South Dakota

Sioux Valley Hospital USD Medical Center, Sioux Falls

Tennessee

Blount Memorial Center, Maryville, TN
Baptist Memorial Hospital–Memphis
Covenant Health: Fort Sanders Loudon Medical Center, Loudon
Covenant Health: Fort Sanders Regional Medical Center, Knoxville
Covenant Health: Fort Sanders Regional Parkwest Hospitals, Knoxville
Methodist Extended Care Hospital, Memphis
Vanderbilt Medical Center, Nashville

Texas

Rolling Plains Memorial Hospital, Sweetwater
St. Luke Episcopal Hospital, Houston
The Methodist Hospital, Houston
University of Texas Medical Branch, Galveston
University of Texas Health Center, Tyler

Vermont

Fletcher Allen Health Care, Colchester
Rutland Regional Medical Center, Rutland

Virginia

Bon Secours DePaul Medical Center, Norfolk
Inova Fairfax Hospital, Falls Church
University of Virginia Health System, Charlottesville

Washington

Overlake Hospital Medical Center, Bellevue
Virginia Mason Medical Center, Seattle

West Virginia

Cabell-Huntington Hospital, Huntington

Wisconsin

Aurora Health Care, St. Luke's South Shore Hospital, Cudahy
Aurora Sinai Medical Center, Milwaukee
Meriter Health Services, Madison
University of Wisconsin Hospital and Clinics, Madison
Waukesha Memorial Hospital, Waukesha
Wheaton Franciscan Healthcare–Elmbrook Memorial Hospital
Wheaton Franciscan Healthcare–Marian Franciscan Center
Wheaton Franciscan Healthcare–St. Francis Hospital
Wheaton Franciscan Healthcare–St. Joseph

CANADA

Calgary District Health Authority

Foothills Medical Centre, Calgary, Alberta
Peter Lougheed Hospital, Calgary, Alberta
Rockyview Hospital, Calgary, Alberta

Cape Breton District Health Authority, Nova Scotia

Cape Breton Regional Hospital
Glace Bay Health Care Facility
New Waterford Consolidated Hospital
Northside General Hospital
Victoria County Memorial Hospital
Sacred Heart Community Health Centre
Inverness Consolidated Memorial
Buchanan Memorial Community Health Centre

New Brunswick

River Valley Health, Fredericton
Saint Joseph's Hospital, St. John
Stan Cassidy Centre for Rehabilitation, Fredericton

Ontario

Mount Sinai Hospital, Toronto

Winnipeg District Health Authority

Deer Lodge Centre
Grace General Hospital
Health Sciences Centre

Riverview Health Centre
Seven Oaks General Hospital
St. Boniface General Hospital
Victoria General Hospital

THE NETHERLANDS
University Medical Center at Nymegen

NCA-AFFILIATED SPECIALTY ORGANIZATONS WITH GERIATRIC CON-
TENT

(As of May 2007)
Academy of Medical-Surgical Nurses (AMSN)   www.medsurgnurse.org
American Holistic Nurses Association (AHNA)   www.ahna.org
American Nephrology Nurses' Association (ANNA)   www.annanurse.org
American Organization of Nurse Executives (AONE)   www.aone.org
American Radiological Nurses Association (ARNA)   www.arna.net
Asian American/Pacific Islander Nurses Association (AAPINA)   http://aapina.
    org
Association of Nurses in AIDS Care (ANAC)   www.anacnet.org
Assoc. of Women's Health, Obstetric, and Neonatal Nurses (AWHONN)   www.
    awhonn.org
Dermatology Nurses' Association (DNA)   www.dnanurse.org
Emergency Nurses Association (ENA)   www.ena.org
Hospice and Palliative Nurses Association (HPNA)   www.hpna.org
National Association of Clinical Nurse Specialists (NACNS)   www.nacns.org
National Association of Nurse Massage Therapists (NANMT)   www.nanmt.org
National Nursing Staff Development Organization (NNSDO)   www.nnsdo.org/
National Student Nurses' Association (NSNA)   www.nsna.org
Philippine Nurses Association of America (PNAA)   www.philippinenursesaa.
    org/
Preventive Cardiovascular Nurses Association (PCNA)   www.pcna.net
Society of Otorhinolaryngology and Head-Neck Nurses (SOHN)
    www.sohnnurse.com

Contents

Evidence-Based
Geriatric Nursing
Protocols for
Best Practice

3

Developing and Evaluating Clinical Practice Guidelines: A Systematic Approach

1

Rona F. Levin
Joanne K. Singleton
Susan Kaplan Jacobs

Clinical decision making that is grounded in the best available evidence is essential to promote patient safety and quality health care outcomes. With the knowledge base for geriatric nursing rapidly expanding, assessing geriatric clinical practice guidelines for their validity and incorporation of the best available evidence is critical to the safety and outcomes of care. In the second edition of this book, Lucas and Fulmer (2003) challenged geriatric nurses to take the lead in the assessment of geriatric clinical practice guidelines (CPGs), recognizing that in the absence of best evidence, guidelines and protocols have little value for clinical decision making.

The purpose of this chapter is to describe the process that was used to create the third edition of *Evidence-Based Geriatric Nursing Protocols for Best Practice*. In previous editions of this book, each chapter author individually gathered and synthesized evidence on a particular topic and then developed a "Nursing

Standard of Practice Protocol" based on that evidence. There was no standard process or specific criteria for protocol development nor was there any indication of the "level of evidence" of each source cited in the chapter (i.e., the evidence base for the protocol). In this third edition, the process previously used to develop the geriatric nursing protocols has been enhanced. This chapter is a guide to understanding how the geriatric nursing protocols in this third edition were developed and describes how to use the process to guide the assessment and/or development and updating of practice protocols in any area of nursing practice.

Definition of Terms

Evidence-based practice (EBP) is a framework for clinical practice that integrates the best available scientific evidence with the expertise of the clinician and with patients' preferences and values to make decisions about health care (Levin & Feldman, 2006; Sackett, Straus, Richardson, Rosenberg, & Haynes, 2000). Health care professionals often use the terms *recommendations, guidelines,* and *protocols* interchangeably but they are not synonymous.

A recommendation is a suggestion for practice, not necessarily sanctioned by a formal, expert group. A clinical practice guideline is an "official recommendation" or suggested approach to diagnose and manage a broad health condition (e.g., heart failure, smoking cessation, or pain management). A protocol is a more detailed guide for approaching a clinical problem or health condition and is tailored to a specific practice situation. For example, guidelines for falls prevention recommend developing a protocol for toileting elderly, sedated, or confused patients. The specific practices or protocol each agency implements, however, is agency-specific. The validity of any of these practice guides can vary depending on the type and the level of evidence on which they are based. Using standard criteria to develop or refine CPGs or protocols assures reliability of their content. Standardization gives both nurses, who use the guideline/protocol, and patients, who receive care based on the guideline/protocol, assurance that the geriatric content and practice recommendations are based on the best evidence.

In contrast to these practice guides, "standards of practice" are not specific or necessarily evidence-based; rather, they are a generally accepted, formal, published framework for practice. As an example, the American Nurses' Association document, *Nursing: Scope and Standards of Practice* (2003), contains a standard regarding nurses' accountability for making of a patient's health status. The standard is a general statement. A protocol, on the other hand, may specify the assessment tool(s) to use in that assessment—for example, an instrument to predict pressure-ulcer risk.

The *AGREE* Instrument

The AGREE instrument (*Instrument for Appraisal of Guidelines for Research & Evaluation*, http://www.agreecollaboration.org/), created and evaluated by international guideline developers and researchers for use by the National Health

1.1

Rigor of development.

Item 8. Systematic methods were used to search for evidence.

Item 9. The criteria for selecting the evidence are clearly described.

Item 10. The methods used for formulating the recommendations are clearly described.

Item 11. The health benefits, side effects and risks have been considered in formulating the recommendations.

Item 12. There is an explicit link between the recommendations and the supporting evidence.

Item 13. The guideline has been externally reviewed by experts prior to its publication.

Item 14. A procedure for updating the guideline is provided.

AGREE Collaboration. (2001). *Appraisal of Guidelines Research and Evaluation, AGREE Instrument.* Retrieved November 21, 2006 from the World Wide Web:

http://www.agreecollaboration.org/instrument/.

Services (AGREE Collaboration, 2001), was initially supported by the United Kingdom National Health Services Management Executive and later by the European Union (Cluzeau, Littlejohns, Grimshaw, Feder, & Moran, 1999).

Released in its final and current form in 2001, the purpose of the AGREE instrument is to provide standard criteria with which to appraise CPGs. This appraisal includes evaluation of the methods used to develop the CPG, assessment of the validity of the recommendations made in the guideline, and consideration of factors related to the use of the CPG in practice. Although the AGREE instrument was created to critically appraise CPGs, the process and criteria can also be applied to the development and evaluation of clinical practice protocols. Thus, the AGREE instrument has been expanded for that purpose to standardize the creation and revision of the geriatric nursing practice protocols in this book.

The AGREE instrument has six quality domains: scope and purpose, stakeholder involvement, rigor of development, clarity and presentation, application, and editorial independence. A total of 23 items divided among the domains are rated on a four-point Likert scale from "strongly disagree" to "strongly agree." Appraisers evaluate how well the guideline they are assessing meets the criteria (i.e., items) of the six quality domains. For example, when evaluating the rigor of development, appraisers rate seven items (Figure 1.1). The reliability of the AGREE instrument is increased when each guideline is appraised by more than one appraiser. Each of the six domains receives an individual domain score and, based on these scores, the appraiser subjectively assesses the overall quality of a guideline.

The rigor of development section of the AGREE instrument provides standards for literature-searching and documenting the databases and terms searched. Adhering to these criteria to find and use the best available evidence on a clinical question is critical to the validity of geriatric nursing protocols and ultimately to patient safety and outcomes of care.

Published guidelines can be appraised using the AGREE instrument as discussed previously. In the process of guideline development, however, the clinician is faced with the added responsibility of appraising all available evidence for its quality and relevance. In other words, how well does the available evidence support recommended clinical practices? The clinician needs to be able to support or defend the inclusion of each recommendation in the protocol based on its level of evidence. To do so, the guideline must reflect a systematic, structured approach to find and assess the available evidence.

Levels of Evidence

Levels of evidence are a schema for understanding the value of the information presented to the clinical topic or question under review. Among the many schema available, there are commonalities in their hierarchical structure, often represented by a pyramid or "publishing wedge" (Haynes, 2005; McKibbon, Eady, & Marks, 1999, p. 8). The highest level of evidence is at the top of a pyramid and is characterized by the increased relevance of the evidence to the clinical setting (Duke University Medical Library, 2005). Authors in this book rated levels of evidence based on the work of Stetler et al. (1998) and Melnyk and Fineout-Overholt (2005) (Figure 1.2). A Level I evidence rating is given to evidence obtained from synthesized sources: systematic reviews, which can either be meta-analyses or structured integrative reviews of evidence, and CPGs based on Level I evidence. Evidence rated Level II derives from a single experimental study or randomized controlled trial (RCT). A quasi-experimental study such as a nonrandomized controlled single group pre-post test time series or matched case-controlled study is considered Level III evidence. Level IV evidence is a nonexperimental study, such as correlational descriptive research or case-controlled studies. A case report systematically obtained and of verifiable quality or program evaluation data are rated as Level V. Level VI evidence consists of the opinions of respected authorities based on their clinical experience or the opinions of an expert committee, including their interpretation of nonresearch-based information. This level also includes regulatory or legal opinions. Level I evidence is considered the strongest level of evidence.

The Search for Evidence Process

Locating the best evidence in the published research is dependent on framing a focused, searchable clinical question. The PICO format—an acronym for population, intervention (or occurrence or risk factor), comparison (or control), and outcome—can frame an effective literature search (Glasziou, Del Mar, & Salisbury, 2003). One example of an answerable clinical question asked in this book is: "What is the effectiveness of **restraints** in reducing the occurrence of **falls** in patients **65 years of age and older**?" In this question, the population

1.2

Levels of quantitative evidence.

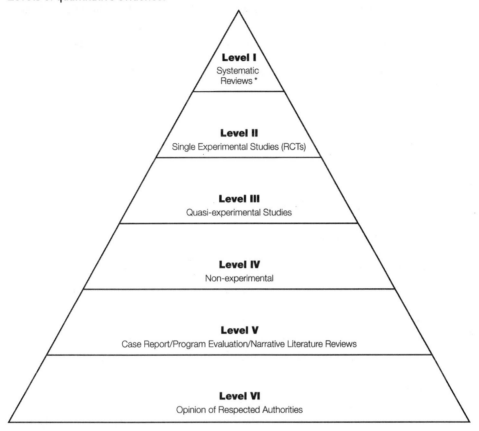

Level I
Systematic
Reviews *

Level II
Single Experimental Studies (RCTs)

Level III
Quasi-experimental Studies

Level IV
Non-experimental

Level V
Case Report/Program Evaluation/Narrative Literature Reviews

Level VI
Opinion of Respected Authorities

* Systematic Reviews (integrative/Meta-analyses/CPG's based on systematic reviews)
Adapted from: Melnyk & Fineout-Overholt, 2005; Stetler, Morsi, Rucki, Broughton, Corrigan, Fitzgerald, et al., 1998

is patients 65 years of age and older, the intervention is use of restraints, the implied control or comparison is no restraints, and the outcome is falls.

Not every nurse, whether he or she is a clinical practitioner, educator, or administrator, has proficient database-search skills to find the best evidence on a clinical topic. Many nurses report that limited access to resources, gaps in information, literacy skills, and—most of all—a lack of time are barriers to "readiness" for EBP (Pravikoff, Tanner, & Pierce, 2005). For the third edition of this book, the editors enlisted the assistance of the New York University Health Sciences librarian to ensure a standardized and efficient approach to collecting evidence on clinical topics. A literature search was conducted to find the best available evidence for each clinical question addressed in the book. With the framework of the evidence pyramid as a model (see Figure 1.2), the results were rated for level of evidence and sent to the respective chapter author(s) to provide possible substantiation for the nursing practice protocol being developed.

1.3

Search steps used in finding the evidence base for geriatric nursing protocols for the question:
"What is the effectiveness of restraints in reducing the occurrence of falls in patients 65 years
of age and older?"

1. Select a database (Cochrane Database of Systematic Reviews, CINAHL, MEDLINE...)

2. Translate the terms of the question into the controlled vocabulary of the database. For

example: Falls maps to "Accidental Falls"

3. Apply categorical limits for publication type, year, and age groups

   For example:

   Limit to age group "Aged, 65 and over"

   Limit to publication years 2001–2006

   Limit to publication type: "systematic review or meta analysis"

4. Consider other databases, e.g. PsycINFO

5. Evaluate search results; expand or narrow search terms; repeat from Step 2 as needed.

In addition to rating each literature citation as to its level of evidence, each citation was given a general classification, coded as "Risks," "Assessment," "Prevention," "Management," "Evaluation/Follow-up," or "Comprehensive." The citations were organized in a searchable database for later retrieval and output to chapter authors. All authors had to review the evidence and decide on its quality and relevance for inclusion in their chapter or protocol. They had the option, of course, to reject or not use the evidence provided as a result of the search or to dispute the applied level of evidence.

Developing a Search Strategy

Development of a search strategy to capture best evidence begins with database selection and translation of search terms into the controlled vocabulary of the database, if possible. Figure 1.3 details the search strategy used to find the best evidence. In descending order of importance, the three major databases for finding the best primary evidence for most clinical nursing questions are the Cochrane Database of Systematic Reviews, Cumulative Index to Nursing and Allied Health Literature (CINAHL), and Medline or PubMed. In addition, the PsycINFO database was used to ensure capture of relevant evidence in the psychology and behavioral sciences literature for many of the topics. Synthesis sources such as UpToDate® and BMJ Clinical Evidence and abstract journals such as *Evidence Based Nursing* supplemented the initial searches. Searching of other specialty databases may have to be warranted depending on the clinical question.

1.4

An example of a coded literature citation supplied to protocol author.

REF ID: 1661

Level I: Systematic Reviews

Topic 2: Prevention

Gillespie, L. D., Gillespie, W. J., Robertson, M. C., Lamb, S. E., Cumming, R. G., & Rowe, B.

H. (2006). Interventions for preventing falls in elderly people. *The Cochrane Library*, (1).

It bears noting that the database architecture can be exploited to limit the search to articles tagged with the publication type "meta-analysis" in Medline or "systematic review" in CINAHL. Filtering by standard age groups such as "65 and over" is another standard categorical limit for narrowing for relevance. A literature search retrieves the initial citations that begin to provide evidence. Appraisal of the initial literature retrieved may lead the searcher to other cited articles, triggering new ideas for expanding or narrowing the literature search with related descriptors or terms in the article abstract. Using the previous example, a search of the CINAHL database on "falls" and physical restraints in the elderly may ultimately lead the searcher to explore the broader area of patient safety or the related area of side rails. The process of discovery is iterative, not linear. There is no single path to locating best evidence.

An additional feature of this third edition is inclusion of the level and type of evidence for each citation, which can then be applicable to a recommendation for practice (Figure 1.4). This type of standardized approach ensures that this book contains protocols and recommendations for use with geriatric patients and their families that are based on the best available evidence.

Conclusion

The systematic process used for finding, retrieving, and disseminating the best evidence for the third edition of *Evidence-Based Geriatric Nursing Protocols for Best Practice* is a model both for nursing education and clinical practice. Translating nursing research into practice requires competency in information literacy: the ability to gather evidence, critically appraise, and discern the context of a research article. Best evidence was defined as published research, which met the highest level of evidence according to availability. The authors of each chapter, however, had the responsibility of evaluating the quality of the evidence. The AGREE instrument was the standard for the process of evidence-searching and evidence-utilization in chapter and protocol development. The protocols contained in this edition have been refined, revised, and/or developed by the authors using the best available research evidence as a foundation, with the ultimate goal of improving patient safety and outcomes.

References

AGREE Collaboration (2001). *Appraisal of guidelines research and evaluation, AGREE instrument.* Retrieved November 21, 2006, from http://www.agreecollaboration.org/instrument/

American Nurses Association (2003). *Nursing: Scope and standards of practice.* Maryland: Author.

Cluzeau, F. A., Littlejohns, P., Grimshaw, J. M., Feder, G., & Moran, S. E. (1999). Development and application of a generic methodology to assess the quality of clinical practice guidelines. *International Journal of Quality Health Care, 11*(1), 21–28.

Duke University Medical Library (2005). *Evidence pyramid.* Retrieved November 3, 2006, from http://www.mclibrary.duke.edu/subject/ebm/searching/ebmresources.pdf

Glasziou, P., Del Mar, C., & Salisbury, J. (2003). *Evidence-based medicine workbook.* London: BMJ.

Haynes, R. B. (2005). Of studies, summaries, synopses, and systems: The "4S" evolution of services for finding current best evidence. *Evidence Based Nursing, 8*(1), 4–6.

Levin, R. F., & Feldman, H. R. (2006). Teaching evidence-based practice in nursing: A guide for academic and clinical settings. New York: Springer Publishing Company.

Lucas, J. A., & Fulmer, T. (2003). Evaluating clinical practice guidelines: A best practice. In M. Mezey, T. Fulmer, & I. Abraham (Eds.), *Geriatric nursing protocols for best practice* (2nd ed.). New York: Springer Publishing Company.

McKibbon, A., Eady, A., & Marks, S. (1999). *PDQ: Evidence-based principles and practice.* Hamilton, Ontario: B. C. Decker, Inc.

Melnyk, B. M., & Fineout-Overholt, E. (2005). *Evidence-based practice in nursing & healthcare: A guide to best practice* (p. 10). Philadelphia: Lippincott.

Pravikoff, D. S., Tanner, A. B., & Pierce, S. T. (2005). Readiness of U.S. nurses for evidence-based practice: Many don't understand or value research and have had little or no training to help them find evidence on which to base their practice. *American Journal of Nursing, 105*(9), 40–52.

Rich, E. R., & Newland, J. A. (2006). Creating clinical protocols with an Apgar of 10. In R. F. Levin & H. R. Feldman (Eds.), *Teaching evidence-based practice in nursing: A guide for academic and clinical settings.* New York: Springer Publishing Company.

Sackett, D. L., Straus, S. E., Richardson, W. S., Rosenberg, W., & Haynes, R. B. (2000). *Evidence-based medicine: How to teach and practice EBM* (2nd ed.). Edinburgh, Scotland: Churchill Livingston.

Stetler, C. B., Morsi, D., Rucki, S., Broughton, S., Corrigan, B., Fitzgerald, J., et al. (1998). Utilization-focused integrative reviews in a nursing service. *Applied Nursing Research, 11*(4), 195–206.

Measuring Performance, Improving Quality

2

Lenard L. Parisi

Educational Objectives

After completion of this chapter, the reader will be able to:

1. discuss key components of the definition of quality as outlined by the Institute of Medicine (IOM)

2. describe three challenges of measuring quality of care

3. delineate three strategies for addressing the challenges of measuring quality

4. list three characteristics of a good performance measure

Nadzam and Abraham (2003) state that "The main objective of implementing best practice protocols for geriatric nursing is to stimulate nurses to practice with greater knowledge and skill, and thus improve the quality of care to older adults." Although improved patient care and safety is certainly a goal, providers also need to focus on the implementation of evidence-based practice (EBP) and improving outcomes of care. The implementation of evidenced-based nursing practice as a means to providing safe, quality patient care, and positive outcomes is well supported in the literature. However, to ensure that protocols are implemented correctly, as is true with the delivery of all nursing care, it is essential to evaluate the care provided. Outcomes of care are gaining increased attention and will be of particular interest to providers as the health care industry continues to move toward a "pay-for-performance" reimbursement model.

The improvement of care and clinical outcomes—or, as it is commonly known, Performance Improvement—requires a defined, organized approach. Improvement efforts are typically guided by the IOM's Quality Assessment (measurement) and Performance Improvement (process improvement) model. Some well-known models or approaches for improving care and processes include Plan-Do-Study-Act (PDSA) (Institute for Health Care Improvement, see http://www.ihi.org/ihi) and Six Sigma (see http://www.motorola.com/motorolauniversity.jsp). These methodologies are simply an organized approach to defining improvement priorities, collecting data, analyzing the data, making sound recommendations for process improvement, implementing identified changes, and then reevaluating the measures. Through Performance Improvement, standards of care (e.g., Nurses Improving Care for Healthsystem Elders [NICHE, www.nicheprogram.org] protocols, in this case) are identified, evaluated, analyzed for variances, and improved. The goal is to standardize and improve patient care and outcomes. "Improvements in quality of patient care occur through restructuring, redesigning and innovating processes. For these changes to occur, nursing professionals need to be supported by a structure that provides a vision for continuous improvement (CI), empowers them to make changes, and delivers ongoing and reliable outcomes information" (Johnson, Hallsey, Meredith, & Warden, 2006).

From the beginning of the NICHE project in the early 1990s (for an overview, see Fulmer et al., 2002), the NICHE team has struggled with the following questions: How can we measure whether the combination of models of care, staff education and development, and organizational change leads to improvements in patient care? How can we provide hospitals and health systems committed to improving their nursing care to older adults with guidance and frameworks, let alone tools for measuring the quality of geriatric care? In turn, these questions generated many other questions: Is it possible to measure quality? Can we identify direct indicators of quality? Or do we have to rely on indirect indicators (e.g., if 30-day readmissions of patients older than the age of 65 drop, can we reasonably state that this reflects an improvement in the quality of care)? What factors may influence our desired quality outcomes, whether these are unrelated factors (e.g., the pressure to reduce length of stay) or related factors (e.g., the severity of illness)? How can we design evaluation programs that enable us to measure quality without adding more burden (of data collection, of taking time away from direct nursing care)? No doubt, the results from evaluation programs should be useful at the "local" level. Would it be helpful, though, to have results that are comparable across clinical settings (i.e., within the same hospital or health system) and across institutions (i.e., as quality benchmarking tools)? Many of these questions remain unanswered today, although the focus on defining practice through an evidence-based approach is becoming the standard. Defining outcomes for internal and external reporting is expected as is the improvement of processes required to deliver safe, affordable, quality patient care.

This chapter provides guidance in the selection, development, and use of performance measures to monitor quality of care as a springboard to Performance Improvement initiatives. Following a definition of quality of care, the chapter identifies several challenges in the measurement of quality. The concept of performance measures as the evaluation link between care delivery and quality improvement is introduced. Next, the chapter offers practical advice on what and how to measure (Fulmer et al., 2002). It also describes external comparative databases sponsored by the Center for Medicare Services (CMS) and other quality-improvement organizations. It concludes with a description of the challenge to selecting performance measures.

It is important to reaffirm two key principles for the purposes of evaluating nursing care in this context. First, at the management level, it is indispensable to measure the quality of geriatric nursing care; however, doing so must help those who actually provide care (i.e., nurses) and must impact those who receive care (i.e., elderly patients). Second, measuring quality of care is not the end goal; rather, it is done to enable the continuous use of quality-of-care information to improve patient care.

Quality Health Care Defined

It is not uncommon to begin a discussion of quality-related topics without reflecting on one's own values and beliefs surrounding quality health care. Many have tried to define the concept; however, like the old cliché, "beauty is in the eye of the beholder," so is our own perception of quality. Health care consumers and providers alike are often asked, what does quality mean to you? The response typically varies and includes answers such as a safe health care experience, receiving correct medications, receiving medications in a timely manner, a pain-free procedure or postoperative experience, compliance with regulation, accessibility to services, effectiveness of treatments and medications, efficiency of services, good communication among providers, and a caring environment. These are important attributes to remember when discussing the provision of care with clients and patients.

The IOM defines quality of care as "the degree to which health services for individuals and populations increase[s] the likelihood of desired health outcomes and are consistent with current professional knowledge" (Kohn, Corrigan, & Donaldson, 2000). This definition does not tell us what quality is but rather what quality should achieve. This definition also does not say that quality exists if certain conditions are met (e.g., a ratio of x falls to y elderly orthopedic surgery patients; a 30-day readmission rate of z). Instead, it emphasizes that the likelihood of achieving desired levels of care is what matters. In other words, quality is not a matter of reaching something but rather the challenge, over and over, of improving the odds of reaching the desired level of outcomes. Thus, the definition implies the cyclical and longitudinal nature of quality: What we achieve today must guide us as to what to do tomorrow—better and better, over and over, the focus being on improving processes while demonstrating sustained improvement.

The IOM definition stresses the framework within which to conceptualize quality: knowledge. The best knowledge to have is research evidence—preferably from randomized clinical trials (i.e., experimental studies)—yet without ignoring the relevance of less rigorous studies (i.e., nonrandomized studies, epidemiological investigations, descriptive studies, even case studies). Realistically, in nursing we have limited evidence to guide the care of older adults. Therefore, professional consensus among clinical and research experts is a critical factor in determining quality. Furthermore, knowledge is needed at three levels: to achieve quality, we need to know what to do (knowledge about best practice), we need to know how to do it (knowledge about behavioral skills), and we need to know what outcomes to achieve (knowledge about best outcomes).

The IOM definition of quality of care contains several other important elements. "Health services" focuses the definition on the care itself. Granted, the quality of care provided is determined by such factors as knowledgeable professionals, good technology, and efficient organizations, yet these are not the focus of quality measurement. Rather, the definition implies a challenge to health care organizations: The system should be organized in such a way that knowledge-based care is provided and that its effects can be measured. This brings us to the "desired health outcomes" element of the definition. Quality is not an attribute (as in "My hospital is in the top 100 hospitals in the United States as ranked by *U.S. News & World Report*") but rather an ability (as in "Only x% of our elderly surgical patients go into acute confusion; of those who do, y% return to normal cognitive function within z hours after onset").

In the IOM definition, *degree* implies that quality occurs on a continuum from unacceptable to excellent. The clinical consequences are on a continuum as well. If the care is of unacceptable quality, the likelihood that we will achieve the desired outcomes is nil. In fact, we probably will achieve outcomes that are the opposite of what are desired. As the care moves up the scale toward excellent, the more likely the desired outcomes will be achieved. *Degree* also implies quantification. Although it helps to be able to talk to colleagues about, say, unacceptable, poor, average, good, or excellent care, these terms should be anchored by a measurement system. Such systems enable us to interpret what, for instance, poor care is by providing us with a range of numbers that correspond to *poor*. In turn, these numbers can provide us with a reference point for improving care to the level of average: We measure care again, looking at whether the numbers have improved, then checking whether these numbers fall in the range defined as *average*. Likewise, if we see a worsening of scores, we will be able to conclude whether we have gone from, say, good to average. The term *individuals and populations* underscores that quality of care is reflected in the outcomes of one patient and in the outcomes of a set of patients. It focuses our attention on providing quality care to individuals while aiming to raise the level of care provided to populations of patients.

In summary, the IOM definition of quality of care forces us to think about quality in relative and dynamic rather than absolute and static terms. Quality of care is not a state of being but rather a process of becoming. Quality is and should be measurable, using performance measures: "a quantitative tool that provides an indication of an organization's performance in relation to a specified process or outcome" (Schyve & Nadzam, 1998).

Quality improvement is a process of attaining ever better levels of care in parallel with advances in knowledge and technology. It strives toward increasing the likelihood that certain outcomes will be achieved. This is the professional responsibility of those who are charged with providing care (i.e., clinicians, managers, and their organizations). On the other hand, consumers of health care (i.e., patients, but also purchasers, payors, regulators, and accreditors) are much less concerned with the processes in place, as with the results of those processes.

Clinical Outcomes and Publicly Reported Quality Measures

Although it is important to evaluate clinical practices and processes, it is equally important to evaluate and improve outcomes of care. Clinical-outcome indicators are receiving unprecedented attention within the health care industry from providers, payors, and consumers alike. Regulatory and accrediting bodies review outcome indicators to evaluate the care provided by the organization prior to and during surveys and to evaluate clinical and related processes. Organizations are expected to use outcome data to identify and prioritize the processes that support clinical care and demonstrate an attempt to improve performance. Providers may use outcomes data to support best practices by benchmarking their results with similar organizations. The benchmarking process is supported through publicly reported outcomes data at the national and state levels. National reporting occurs on the CMS Web site, where consumers and providers alike may access information and compare hospitals, home-care agencies, and nursing homes. For example, the Web sites http://www.hospitalcompare.hhs.gov, http://www.medicare.gov/NHCompare, and http://www.medicare.gov/HHCompare list outcome indicators relative to the specific service or delivery model. Consumers may use those Web sites to select organizations and compare outcomes, one against another, to aid in their selection of a facility or service. These Web sites also serve as a resource for providers to benchmark their outcomes against those of another organization. Outcomes data also become increasingly important to providers as the industry shifts toward a "pay-for-performance" model.

In a pay-for-performance model, practitioners are reimbursed for achieved quality-of-care outcomes. Currently, the CMS has several pay-for-performance initiatives (see http://www.cms.hhs.gov/apps/media/press/release.asp?Counter =1,343 for details). The Hospital Quality Initiative is part of the U.S. Department of Health and Human Services' broader national quality initiative that focuses on an initial set of 10 quality measures by linking reporting of those measures to the payments the hospitals receive for each discharge. The purpose of the Premier Hospital Quality Incentive Demonstration is to improve the quality of inpatient care for Medicare beneficiaries by giving financial incentives to almost 300 hospitals for high quality. The Physician Group Practice Demonstration, mandated by the Medicare, Medicaid, and SCHIP Benefits Improvement and Protection Act of 2000 (BIPA), is the first pay-for-performance initiative for physicians under the Medicare program (BIPA, 2000). The Medicare Care Management Performance Demonstration (Medicare Modernization Act [MMA] section 649), modeled on the "bridges to excellence" program, is a 3-year pay-for-performance demonstration with physicians to promote the adoption and use of health information technology to improve the quality of patient care for chronically ill Medicare patients. The Medicare Health Care Quality Demonstration (MMA section 646), mandated by section 646 of the MMA, will be a 5-year demonstration program under which projects enhance quality by improving patient safety, reducing variations in utilization by appropriate use of evidence-based care and best practice guidelines, encouraging shared decision making, and using culturally and ethnically appropriate care.

Measuring Quality of Care

Schyve and Nadzam (1998) identified several challenges to measuring quality. First, the suggestion that quality of care is in the eye of the beholder points to the different interests of multiple users. This issue encompasses both measurement and communication challenges. Measurement and analysis methods must generate information about the quality of care that meets the needs of different stakeholders. In addition, the results must be communicated in ways that meet these different needs. Second, we must have good and generally accepted tools for measuring quality. Thus, user groups must come together in their conceptualization of quality care so that relevant health care measures can be identified and standardized. A common language of measurement must be developed, grounded in a shared perspective on quality that is cohesive across yet meets the needs of various user groups. Third, once the measurement systems are in place, data must be collected. This translates into resource demands and logistical issues as to who is to report, record, collect, and manage data. Fourth, data must be analyzed in statistically appropriate ways. This is not just a matter of using the right statistical methods; it is more important that user groups must agree on a framework for analyzing quality data to interpret the results. Fifth, health care environments are complex and dynamic in nature. There are differences across health care environments, between types of provider organizations, and within organizations. Furthermore, changes in health care occur frequently, such as the movement of care from one setting to another and the introduction of new technology. Finding common denominators is a major challenge.

Addressing the Challenges

These challenges are not insurmountable. However, making a commitment to quality care entails a commitment to putting the processes and systems in place to measure quality through performance measures and to report quality-of-care results. This commitment applies as much to a quality-improvement initiative on a nursing unit as it does to a corporate commitment by a large health care system. In other words, once an organization decides to pursue excellence (i.e., quality), it must accept measurement and reporting and overcome the various challenges. Let us examine how this could be done in a clinical setting.

McGlynn and Asch (1998) offer several strategies for addressing the challenges to measuring quality. First, the various user groups must identify and balance competing perspectives. This is a process of giving and taking: proposing highly clinical measures (e.g., number of pressure ulcers) but also providing more general data (e.g., use of restraints). It is a process of asking and responding: asking management for monthly statistics on medication errors but also agreeing to provide management with the necessary documentation of why physical restraints have been used for some patients. Second, there must be an accountability framework. Committing to quality care implies that nurses assume several responsibilities and are willing to be held accountable for each of them: (1) providing the best possible care to older patients, (2) examining their own geriatric nursing knowledge and practice, (3) seeking ways to improve it,

(4) agreeing to evaluation of their practice, and (5) responding to needs for improvement. Third, there must be objectivity in the evaluation of quality. This requires setting and adopting explicit criteria for judging performance, then building the evaluation process on these criteria. Nurses, their colleagues, and their managers need to reach consensus on how performance will be measured and what will be considered excellent (and good, average, etc.) performance. Fourth, once these indicators have been identified, nurses need to select a subset of indicators for routine reporting. Indicators should give a reliable snapshot of the team's care to older patients. Fifth, it is critical to separate as much as possible the use of indicators for evaluating patient care and the use of these indicators for financial or nonfinancial incentives. Should the team be cost-conscious? Yes, but cost should not influence any clinical judgment as to what is best for patients. Finally, nurses in the clinical setting must plan how to collect the data. At the institutional level, this may be facilitated by information systems that allow performance measurement and reporting. Ideally, point-of-care documentation will also provide the data necessary for a systematic and goal-directed quality-improvement program, thus eliminating separate data abstraction and collection activities.

The success of a quality-improvement program in geriatric nursing care (and the ability to overcome many of the challenges) hinges on the decision as to what to measure. We know that good performance measures must be objective, that data collection must be easy and as burdenless as possible, that statistical analysis must be guided by principles and placed within a framework, and that communication of results must be targeted toward different user groups. Conceivably, we could try to measure every possible aspect of care; realistically, however, the planning for this will never reach the implementation stage. Instead, nurses need to establish priorities by asking these questions: Based on our clinical expertise, what is critical for us to know? What aspects of our care to older patients are high risk or high volume? What parts of our elder care are problem-prone either because we have experienced difficulties in the past or because we can anticipate problems due to the lack of knowledge or resources? What clinical indicators would be of interest to other user groups: patients, the general public, management, payors, accreditors, and practitioners? Throughout this prioritization process, nurses should keep asking themselves: What questions are we trying to answer and for whom?

Measuring Performance-Selecting Quality Indicators

The correct selection of performance measures or quality indicators is a crucial step in evaluating nursing care and is based on two important factors: frequency and volume. Clearly, high-volume practices or frequent processes require focused attention—to ensure that the care is being delivered according to protocol or processes are functioning as designed. Problem-prone or high risk processes would also warrant a review because these are processes with inherent risk to patients or variances in implementing the process. The selection of indicators must also be consistent with organizational goals for improvement. This provides buy-in from practitioners as well as administration when reporting and identifying opportunities for improvement. Performance measures (i.e., indicators) must be based on either a standard of care, policy, procedure, or protocol. These documents, or standards of care, define practice and expectations in the clinical setting and, therefore, determine the criteria for the monitoring tool. The measurement of these standards simply reflects adherence to or implementation of these standards. Once it is decided what to measure, nurses in the clinical geriatric practice setting face the task of deciding how to measure performance. There are two possibilities: Either the appropriate measure (indicator) already exists or a new performance measure must be developed. Either way, there are a number of requirements of a good performance measure that will need to be applied.

Although indicators used to monitor patient care and performance do not need to be subject to the rigors of research, it is imperative that they reflect some of the attributes necessary to make relevant statements about the care. The measure and its output need to focus on improvement, not merely the description of something. It is not helpful to have a very accurate measure that just tells the status of a given dimension of practice. Instead, the measure needs to inform about current quality levels and relate them to previous and future quality levels. It needs to be able to compute improvements or declines in quality over time so that we can plan for the future. For example, to have a measure that only tells the number of medication errors in the past month would not be helpful. Instead, a measure that tells what types of medication errors were made, perhaps even with a severity rating indicated, compares this to medication errors made during the previous months and shows in numbers and graphs the changes over time that will enable us to do the necessary root-cause analysis to prevent more medication errors in the future.

Performance measures need to be clearly defined, including the terms used, the data elements collected, and the calculation steps employed. Establishing the definition prior to implementing the monitoring activity allows for precise data collection. It also facilitates benchmarking with other organizations, when the data elements are similarly defined and the data-collection methodologies are consistent. Imagine that we want to monitor falls on the unit. The initial questions would be: What is considered a fall? Does the patient have to be on the floor? Does a patient slumping against the wall or onto a table while trying to prevent himself or herself from falling to the floor constitute a fall? Is a fall due to physical weakness or orthostatic hypotension treated the same as a fall due to tripping over an obstacle? The next question would be: Over what time period are falls measured: a week, a fortnight, a month, a quarter, a year? The time frame is not a matter of convenience but rather of accuracy. To be able to monitor falls accurately, we need to identify a time frame that will capture enough events to be meaningful and interpretable from a quality improvement point of view. External indicator definitions, such as those defined for use in the National Database of Nursing Quality Indicators, provide guidance for both the indicator definition and the data-collection methodology for *nursing-sensitive indicators*. The nursing-sensitive indicators reflect the structure, process, and outcomes of nursing care. The *structure* of nursing care is indicated by the supply of nursing staff, the skill level of the nursing staff, and the education and certification of nursing staff. *Process* indicators measure aspects of nursing care such as assessment, intervention, and RN job satisfaction. Patient *outcomes* are determined to be either nursing-sensitive indicators, which improve if there is a greater quantity or quality of nursing care (e.g., pressure ulcers, falls, IV infiltrations) or those that are not considered nursing-sensitive (e.g., frequency of primary C-sections, cardiac failure) (for details, see http://www.nursingquality.org/FAQPage.aspx#1). Several nursing organizations across the country participate in data collection and submission, which allows for a robust data base and excellent benchmarking opportunities.

Additional indicator attributes include validity, sensitivity, and specificity. *Validity* refers to whether the measure "actually measures what it purports to measure" (Wilson, 1989). *Sensitivity* and *specificity* refer to the ability of the measure to capture all true cases of the event being measured, and only true cases. We want to ensure that a performance measure identifies true cases as true, and false cases as false, and does not identify a true case as false or a false case as true. Sensitivity of a performance measure is the likelihood of a positive test when a condition is present. Lack of sensitivity is expressed as false-positives—that is, the indicator calculates a condition as present when in fact it is not. Specificity refers to the likelihood of a negative test when a condition is not present. False-negatives reflect lack of specificity: The indicators calculate that a condition is not present when in fact it is. Consider the case of depression and the recommendation in chapter 5 to use the Geriatric Depression Scale, in which a score of 11 or greater is indicative of depression. How robust is this cutoff score of 11? What is the likelihood that someone with a score of 9 or 10 (i.e., negative for depression) might actually be depressed (i.e., false-negative)? Similarly, what is the likelihood that a patient with a score of 13 would not be depressed (i.e., false-positive)?

Reliability means that results are reproducible; that is, the indicator measures the same attribute consistently across the same patients and across time. Reliability begins with a precise definition and specification, as described previously. A measure is reliable if different people calculate the same rate for the same patient sample. The core issue of reliability is measurement error, or the difference between the actual phenomenon and its measurement: The greater the difference, the less reliable the performance measure. For example, suppose that we want to focus on pain management in elderly patients with end-stage cancer. One way of measuring pain would be to ask patients to rate their pain as none, a little, some, quite a bit, or a lot. An alternative approach would be to administer a visual analog scale, a 10-point line on which patients indicate their pain levels. Yet another approach would be to ask the pharmacy to produce monthly reports of analgesic use by type and dose. Generally speaking, the more subjective the scoring or measurement, the less reliable it will be. If all these measures were of equal reliability, they would yield the same result. The concept of reliability, particularly inter-rate reliability, becomes increasingly important to consider in those situations in which data collection is assigned to several staff members. It is important to review the data-collection methodology and the instrument in detail to avoid different approaches by the various people collecting the data.

Several of the examples given previously imply the criterion of interpretability. A performance measure must be interpretable; that is, it must convey a result that can be linked to the quality of clinical care. First, the quantitative output of a performance measure must be scaled in such a way that users can interpret it. For example, a scale that starts with 0 as the lowest possible level and ends with 100 is much easier to interpret than a scale that starts with 13.325 and has no upper boundary except infinity. Second, we should be able to place the number within a context. Suppose we are working in a hemodialysis center that serves a large proportion of end-stage renal disease (ESRD) patients older than the age of 60—the group least likely to be fit for a kidney transplant yet with several years of life expectancy remaining. We know that virtually all ESRD patients develop anemia (i.e., Hb less than 11 g/dL), which in turn impacts their activities of daily living (ADL) and independent activities of daily living (IADL) performance. In collaboration with the nephrologists, we initiate a systematic program of anemia monitoring and management, relying in part on published best practice guidelines. We want to achieve the best practice guideline of 85% of all patients having hemoglobin levels equal to or greater than 11 g/dL. We should be able to succeed because the central laboratory provides us with Hb levels, which allows us to calculate the percentage of patients at Hb of 11 g/dL or greater.

The concept of risk-adjusted performance measures or outcome indicators is an important one. Some patients are sicker than others, some have more co-morbidities, some are older and frailer. No doubt, we could come up with many more risk variables that influence how patients respond to nursing care. Good performance measures consider this differential risk. They create a "level playing field" by adjusting quality indicators on the basis of the (risk for) severity of illness of the patients. It would not be fair to the health care team if the patients on the unit are a lot sicker than those on the unit a floor above. The team is at greater risk for having lower quality outcomes, not because they provide inferior care but because the patients are a lot sicker and are at greater risk for a compromised response to the care provided. The sicker patients are more demanding in terms of care and ultimately less likely to achieve the same outcomes as less ill patients. Performance measures must be easy to collect. The many examples cited previously also refer to the importance of using performance measures for which data are readily available, can be retrieved from existing sources, or can be collected with little burden. The goal is to gather good data quickly without running the risk of having "quick and dirty" data.

We begin the process of deciding how to measure by reviewing existing measures. There is no need to "reinvent the wheel" especially if good measures are out there. Nurses should review the literature, check with national organizations, and consult with colleagues. Yet, we should not blindly adopt existing measures; instead, we need to subject them to a thorough review using the characteristics identified previously. Also, health care organizations that have adopted these measures can offer their experience.

It may be that after an exhaustive search, we cannot find measures that meet the various requirements outlined herein. We decide instead to develop our own in-house measure. Following are some important guidelines:

1. *Zero in on the population to be measured.* If we are measuring an undesirable event, we must determine the group at risk for experiencing that event, then limit the denominator population to that group. If we are measuring a desirable event or process, we must identify the group that should experience the event or receive the process. Where do problems tend to occur? What

variables of this problem are within our control? If some are not within our control, how can we zero in even more on the target population? In other words, we exclude patients from the population when good reason exists to do so (e.g., those allergic to the medication being measured).

2. *Define terms.* This is a painstaking but essential effort. It is better to measure 80% of an issue with 100% accuracy than 100% of an issue with 80% accuracy.

3. *Identify and define the data elements and allowable values required to calculate the measure.* This is another painstaking but essential effort. The 80%/100% rule applies here as well.

4. *Test the data-collection process.* Once we have a prototype of a measure ready, we must examine how easy or difficult it is to get all the required data.

Implementing the Quality Assessment and Performance-Improvement Program

Successful Performance Improvement programs require an organizational commitment to implementation of the Performance Improvement processes and principles outlined in this chapter. Consequently, this commitment requires a defined, organized approach that most organizations embrace and define in the form of a written plan. The plan outlines the approach that the organization uses to improve care and safety for its patients. There are several important elements that must be addressed to implement the Performance Improvement program effectively. The scope of service, which addresses the types of patients and care that is rendered, provides direction on the selection of performance measures. An authority and responsibility statement in the document defines who is able to implement the quality program and make decisions that will affect its implementation. Finally, it is important to define the committee structure used to effectively analyze and communicate improvement efforts to the organization.

The success of the Performance Improvement program is highly dependent on a well-defined structure and appropriate selection of performance measures. The following is a list of issues that, if not addressed, may negatively impact the success of the quality program:

- *Lack of focus*: a measure that tries to track too many criteria at the same time or is too complicated to administer, interpret, or use for quality monitoring and improvement
- *Wrong type of measure*: a measure that calculates indicators the wrong way (e.g., uses rates when ratios are more appropriate; uses a continuous scale rather than a discrete scale; measures a process, when the outcome is measurable and of greater interest)
- *Unclear definitions*: a measure that is too broad or too vague in its scope and definitions (e.g., population is too heterogeneous, no risk adjustment, unclear data elements, poorly defined values)
- *Too much work*: a measure that requires too much clinician time to generate the data or too much manual chart abstraction

■ *Reinventing the wheel*: a measure that is a reinvention rather than an improvement of a performance measure
■ *Events not under control*: measure focuses on a process or outcome that is out of the organization's (or the unit's) control to improve
■ *Trying to do research rather than quality improvement*: data collection and analysis are done for the sake of research rather than for improvement of nursing care and the health and well-being of the patients
■ *Poor communication of results*: the format of communication does not target and enable change
■ *Uninterpretable and underused*: uninterpretable results are of little relevance to improving geriatric nursing care

In summary, the success of the Quality Assessment Performance Improvement Program's ability to measure, evaluate, and improve the quality of nursing care to health-system elders is in the planning. First, define the scope of services provided and those to be monitored and improved. Second, identify performance measures that are reflective of the care provided. Indicators may be developed internally or obtained from external sources of outcomes and data-collection methodologies. Third, analyze the data, pulling together the right people to evaluate processes, make recommendations, and improve care. Finally, it is important to communicate findings across the organization and celebrate success.

Acknowledgment

I would like to acknowledge the exceptional work of Deborah M. Nadzam and Ivo L. Abraham, who wrote the original chapter in the previous edition of this book.

Website Resources

http://www.hospitalcompare.hhs.gov
http://www.medicare.gov/NHCompare
http://www.medicare.gov/HHCompare

References

Benefits Improvement and Protection Act of 2000 (BIPA). Retrieved from www.hhs.gov/apps/media/press/release.asp?counter=1343
Fulmer, T., Mezey, M., Bottrell, M., Abraham, I. L., Sazant, J., Grossmann, C., et al. (2002). Nurses improving care for health system elders (NICHE): Using outcomes and benchmarks for evidence-based practice. *Geriatric Nursing, 23*, 121–127.
Johnson, K., Hallsey, D., Meredith, R. L., & Warden, E. (2006). A nurse-driven system for improving patient quality outcomes. *Journal of Nursing Care Quality, 21*(2),168–175.
Kohn, L. T., Corrigan, J. M., & Donaldson, M. S. (Eds.) (2000). *To err is human: Building a safer health system* (p. 222). Washington, DC: National Academy Press.
McGlynn, E. A., & Asch, S. M. (1998). Developing a clinical performance measure. *American Journal of Preventative Medicine, 14*(35), 14–21.

Mezey, M., Fulmer, T., & Abraham, I. L. (2003). *Geriatric nursing protocols for best practice* (2nd. ed.). New York: Springer Publishing Company.

Nadzam, D. M., & Abraham, I. L. (2003). Measuring performance, improving quality. In M. Mezey, T. Fulmer, & I. L. Abraham. (Eds.), *Geriatric nursing protocols for best practice* (2nd ed., pp. 15–30). New York: Springer Publishing Company.

Schyve, P. M., & Nadzam, D. M. (1998). Performance measurement in healthcare. *Journal of Strategic Performance Measurement, 2*(4), 34–42.

Wilson, H. S. (1989). Research in nursing (2nd ed., p. 355). Reading, MA: Addison-Wesley.

Additional Readings

Bowling, A. (1997). *Measuring health: A review of quality of life measurement scales* (2nd ed.) Philadelphia, PA: Open University Press.

Bryant, L. L., Floersch, N., Richard, A. A., & Schlenker, R. E. (2004). Measuring healthcare outcomes to improve quality of care across post-acute care provider settings. *Journal of Nursing Home Quality, 19*(4), 368–376.

Coopey, M., Nix, N. P., & Clancy, C. M. (2006). Translating research into evidence-based nursing practice and evaluating effectiveness. *Journal of Nursing Home Quality, 21*(3), 195–202.

Hart, S., Bergquist, S., Gajewski, B., & Dunton, N. (2006). Reliability testing of the National Database of Nursing Quality Indicators pressure ulcer indicator. *Journal of Nursing Home Quality, 21*(3), 256–265.

Lageson, C. (2004). Quality focus of the first-line nurse manager and relationship to unit outcomes. *Journal of Nursing Home Quality, 19*(4), 336–342.

Soo Hoo, W., & Parisi, L. L. (2005). Nursing informatics approach to analyzing staffing effectiveness indicators. *Journal of Nursing Care Quality, 20*(3), 215–219.

Assessment of Function

3

Denise M. Kresevic

Educational Objectives

On completion of this chapter, the reader should be able to:

1. identify physical functioning as an important clinical indicator of health/illness, response to treatment, and need for services for older adults

2. describe common components of standardized functional assessment instruments

3. identify unique challenges to gathering information from older adults regarding functional assessments

4. describe common nursing care strategies to restore, maintain, and promote functional health in older adults

Overview

Physical functioning is a dynamic process of interaction between individuals and their environments. The process is influenced by motivation, physical capacity, illness, cognitive ability, and the external environment including social supports. Functional assessments serve as the common language of health for patients, family members, and health care providers of older adults. The ability to manage day-to-day activities such as eating, bathing, ambulating, managing money, and keeping track of medications serves as the foundation of safe, independent functioning for all adults.

For a description of Evidence Levels cited in this chapter, see chapter 1, Evaluating Clinical Practice Guidelines, page 4.

The consequences of not assessing for change in status are significant. Acute changes in functional ability often signal an acute illness and increased need for assistance to maintain safety. These changes have important implications for nursing care across settings but especially during hospitalization. The ability to assess functional status is a critical nursing competency to accurately assess normal aging changes, illness, and disability and to develop an individualized care plan for continuity of care across settings. The failure to assess function can lead to increased decline including severe malnutrition and falls, resulting in the need for institutional care as well as a decrease in quality of life.

Background

The ability to manage day-to-day rather than the absence of disease or age is the cornerstone of health for older adults. Function includes the ability to carry out activities of daily living (ADLs) such as bathing, dressing, and toileting, as well as managing medications and walking. As individuals age or become ill, they may require assistance to accomplish these activities independently. It is estimated that between 20% and 40% of all older adults experience functional decline during hospitalization (Landefeld, Palmer, Kresevic, Fortinsky, & Kowa, 1995 [Level II]). Whereas the exact cause of the decline is often a combination of factors including acute illness, it can be due in part to environmental factors of hospitalization that may be prevented or ameliorated by skilled nursing care (McCusker, Kakuma, & Abrahamowicz, 2002 [Level I]). In fact, hospitalization provides a unique opportunity to assess function, plan for services, and promote "successful aging."

Common risk factors for functional decline include injuries, acute illness, medication side effects, depression, malnutrition, and decreased mobility from the use of physical restraints due to associated iatrogenic complications such as incontinence, falls, and pressure sores (Creditor, 1993 [Level VI]). In one randomized clinical trial of hospitalized elders, the daily nursing assessment of ability to perform bathing, dressing, grooming, toileting, transferring, and ambulation during routine nursing care yielded information necessary for maintenance of function in self-care activities (Landefeld et al., 1995 [Level II]).

This chapter addresses the goals and the need for functional assessment of older adults in acute care, and it provides a clinical practice protocol to guide nurses in the functional assessment of older adults (Box 3.1).

Assessment of Function

Assessment of function includes an ongoing systematic process of identifying the older person's physical abilities and need for help. Functional assessment also provides the opportunity to identify individual strengths and measures of "successful aging." This information is especially important for nurses in planning and evaluating care. Functional capacity may be assessed by self- or proxy report and direct observation of actual performance. Nurses are in a pivotal position in all care settings to assess elders' functional status by direct observation

		3.1	Functional Assessment of Older Adults	

Dimension	Assessment Parameter	Standardized Instrument	Nursing Strategy

ADLs
  Bathing
  Dressing
  Eating
  Toileting
  Hygiene
  Transferring
	Self-report of patient, surrogate report
	Observation during hospitalization
		Katz ADL (Katz et al., 1963)
		Situation Test (Skurla, Rogers, & Sunderland, 1988) (Lowenstein et al., 1989; Kurianski & Gurland, 1976)
			Orient to environment
			Encourage active participation while in hospital
			Range of motion exercises
			Encourage to be out of bed
			Consult PT/OT for strengthening

Mobility
  Balance: sitting; standing
  Gait steadiness
  Turns
	Self-, surrogate report
	Observation
		Get up and Go test (Mathias, Nayak, & Isaacs, 1986)	Ambulate daily
			PT/OT consult
			Mobility aids
			Community referrals

IADL's
  Housework
  Finances
  Driving
  Shopping
  Meal preparation
  Reading
  Medication adherence
  Aware of current events
  Hobbies
  Employment
  Volunteer work
	Self-, surrogate report (able to balance check book), no traffic violations	DAFS (Karagiozis et al., 1989)
		Lawton IADL (Lawton & Brody, 1969; Gurland et al., 1994)
			Able to find hospital room
			Community referrals for transportation
			Meals on Wheels
			Orders hospital meals from menu
			OT consult for simulating kitchen evaluation
			Reads newspaper
			Can read pill bottles
			Family home care
			Nurse to fill pill bottles

ADLs = activities of daily living; IADLs = instrumental activities of daily living; PT/OT = physical therapist/occupational therapist

during routine care and through information gathered from the individual patient, the patient's family, and any other long-term caregivers.

Including critical components of functional assessments into routine assessments in the acute care setting can provide (1) baseline functional capacity and recent changes in level of independence indicating possible illness, especially infections; (2) baseline information to benchmark patients' response to treatment as they move along the continuum from acute care to rehabilitation or from acute to subacute care (e.g., following a new stroke or hip-replacement surgery); (3) information regarding care needs and eligibility for services, including safety needs, physical therapy needs, and posthospitalization needs; and (4) information on quality of care. The ongoing use of a standardized functional assessment instrument promotes systematic communication of patients' health status between care settings and allows units to compare their level of care with other units in the facility and to measure outcomes of care (see Table 3.1) (Campbell, Seymour, Primrose, & ACME-plus Project, 2004 [Level I]).

Although gathering information about functional status is a critical indicator of quality care in geriatrics, it is not always a task easily accomplished and requires significant time, skill, and knowledge. Older persons often present to the care setting with multiple medical conditions resulting in fatigue and pain. In addition, sensory aging changes, particularly vision and hearing, can threaten the accuracy of responses. Ideally, information regarding functional status should be elicited as part of the routine history of older adults and incorporated in daily-care routines of all caregivers. In addition, comprehensive assessment of function provides an opportunity to teach patients and families about normal aging and indicators of pathology.

Assessment Instruments

Systematic gathering of information on ADLs including bathing, dressing, and ambulating, as well as using a telephone, taking medications, and managing finances, can be accomplished by the use of standardized instruments. The use of standardized instruments serves to ensure inclusive assessments, the ability to communicate in a common language, and the ability to benchmark information over time. Several instruments have been developed over the years to measure function. Although all measure components of function, the decision of which instrument should be used depends on the primary purpose of the assessment and the institutional preferences and resources. No single instrument will meet the needs of all care settings. Each should be carefully evaluated for primary purpose of assessment and care setting priorities (Kane & Kane, 2000 [Level VI]). Beginning in the 1950s, Dr. Sidney Katz began studying the pattern of return to function in patients following hip fracture. He and his colleagues identified a constellation of ADLs including bathing, dressing, transferring, toileting, continence, and feeding that described outcomes of rehabilitation and prognosis of older adults (Katz, Ford, Moscokowitz, Jackson, & Jaffe, 1963 [Level I]). Since that time, the Katz Index of Independence in Activities of Living has been used widely to assess function of elders in all settings, including during hospitalization (Mezey, Rauckhorst, & Stokes, 1993 [Level VI]).

Originally, the scale was proposed as an observation tool with scoring ranging from 1 to 3, indicating independent ability, limited assistance, and extensive assistance for each activity. Over time, the instrument has evolved into a dichotomized tool, independent versus dependent ability in each task (Kane & Kane, 2000 [Level VI]). It has established reliability (i.e., 0.94–0.97) and is easy to use either as an observational or self-reported measure (Kane & Kane, 2000

[Level VI]). The Katz ADL index is easily incorporated into history and physical assessment flowsheets and takes little time to complete. Older adults are evaluated according to levels of independence.

Similarly, the Barthel Index of Instrumental Activities of Daily Living (IADLs) was originally developed in the 1950s in an effort to measure improvements in independent functioning related to persons with neuromuscular disorders and their ability to function within a specific environment. This measure of physical function often relies on patient or proxy report. Scores range from 0, indicating total dependence on caregivers, to 100, indicating self-care for all activities. High reliability coefficients have been reported (i.e., 0.95–0.96) (Kane & Kane, 2000 [Level VI]).

The Barthel index for physical functioning includes bathing, grooming, continence, stair-climbing, and the ability to propel a wheelchair (Mahoney & Barthel, 1965 [Level III]; Mezey et al., 1993 [Level VI]). This instrument has been useful in rehabilitation settings to monitor improvements over time. The Barthel instrument allows differentiation among task performance, including amount of help and amount of time needed to accomplish each task.

In addition to self-care in ADLs measured by Katz or Barthel tools, additional instruments to measure more complex physical function, called IADLs, have also been proposed to include in a comprehensive assessment of function in older adults. The majority of these instruments assess the individual's function relative to the environment. Common IADL skills have been identified and include using a telephone, shopping, meal preparation, housekeeping, laundry, medication administration, transportation, and money management (Kane & Kane, 2000 [Level VI]). Whereas assessment of ADL provides useful information for nursing care needs during and after hospitalization, IADL information helps target information critical for planning posthospital care needs. Common instruments used to measure IADLs include the Lawton IADL scale, the Older Americans Resource and Services (OARS–IADL) scale, and the Direct Assessment of Functional Abilities (DAFA) scale. Perhaps the most widely used IADL instrument for hospitalized older adults is the Lawton scale, which assesses eight items and is scored from a total possible score of 8, indicating independent self-care, to 0, indicating dependence in all areas. Reliability coefficients have been reported to be 0.96 for men and 0.93 for women (Kane & Kane, 2000 [Level VI]).

The OARS instrument for physical function is similar in scope of measurement to the Katz scale, including bathing, dressing, grooming, and continence (Burton, Damon, Dillinger, Erickson, & Peterson, 1978 [Level III]; Kane & Kane, 2000 [Level VI]). However, unlike the Katz instrument, which uses caregiver observation, the OARS instrument relies on self-report. Self-reports of capacity may be less valid than observations of performance, with some older adults overestimating or underestimating actual capacity (Kidd et al., 1995 [Level III]).

The Functional Independence Measure (FIM™) was designed to assess "the burden of care" in six areas: self-care, transfers, sphincter control, locomotion, communication, and social cognition. This instrument has been used to assess outcomes of patients with orthopedic and neurologic conditions. Information may be gathered by telephone, mail, self-report, or proxy report using the appropriate version. Each item is scored from 1 to 7, with 1 indicating a need for total assistance and 7 completely independent in a timely and safe manner

(Kane & Kane, 2000 [Level VI]). (See www.ConsultGeriRN.org for assessment instruments and the Resources section of this chapter.)

Assessment of function in individuals with dementia provides a unique challenge. A recently developed instrument, the DAFA, is a 10-item observational measure of IADLs useful in assessing function in the presence of dementia (Karagiozis, Gray, Sacco, Shapiro, & Dawas, 1998 [Level III]). The assessment of IADLs, including the ability to prepare meals and administer medications safely, may not be observed during an acute hospitalization, although assessment of capacity in these domains has important implications for planning posthospitalization services. Regardless of the instrument used, basic ADL and IADL function should be assessed for each patient, including capacity for dressing, eating, transferring, toileting, hygiene, ambulation, and medication adherence (see chapter 12, *Reducing Adverse Drug Events*). Appropriate assessment instruments should be readily available on the acute care unit for easy accessibility and reference and/or incorporated into routine documentation instruments for history, daily assessment, and discharge planning. To adequately assess function, sensory capacity and cognitive capacity must be established. Environmental adaptations such as magnifying glasses or amplifiers may be necessary to ensure accurate assessment and should be accessible to nursing staff.

Direct Assessment of Patient

Although nurses often rely on reports of patients and family members about physical functioning and capacity for ADLs and IADLs, direct observation provides strong support for current capacity versus past ability.

Functional assessments are constantly conducted by nurses every time they notice that a patient can no longer pick up a fork or has difficulty walking. A comprehensive functional assessment leads to more than simply noticing a change in activity or ability, however. In a systematic manner, nurses need to assess the ability of a patient to perform ADLs in the context of the patient's baseline functional status and hospitalization status.

While assessing functional status, the patient should be made as comfortable as possible, with frequent rest periods allowed. Adaptive aids, such as glasses and hearing aids, should be applied. Often, family members accompany an older person and can assist in answering questions regarding function. It is important for patients and family members to understand that baseline functional levels as well as recent changes in function need to be reported. Many older adults may be reluctant to report decline in function, fearing that such reports will threaten their autonomy and independent living.

Occasionally, the history given in a physical exam may reveal clues to further assess function. Muscle weakness and atrophy of legs may indicate lack of ability to safely ambulate independently. Temporal muscle wasting may indicate moderate to severe malnutrition resulting from inability to shop, prepare, and adequately consume sufficient calories. Hand contractures indicative of arthritis or cerebral vascular accidents alert the nurse to assess performance versus self-report of ability to open pill bottles, dial a telephone, or write checks. General appearance, including hair, teeth, fingernails, condition of clothing, and clean and dry versus urine-soaked undergarments, may give rise to information on bathing, dressing, continence, and ability to do laundry.

Specific Functional Assessments

Ambulation

Inherent in ADL and IADL ability is the capacity to walk, a critical parameter for functional assessment. Early assessment of this function is important for nurses in the hospital to ensure safety and prevent falls and injuries (see chapter 9, *Preventing Falls in Acute Care*). The ability to safely ambulate is contingent on the ability to transfer, propel forward, and pivot with sufficient strength and balance. Ambulation is a critical skill necessary for self-care in the hospital and posthospital discharge. It is also a sensitive indicator of acute health changes. Therefore, the ability to ambulate should not be assessed only by self- or proxy report but also by direct observation.

Some instruments used to assess ambulation, balance, and gait are sensitive measures of mobility (Applegate, Blass, & Franklin, 1990 [Level IV]); however, they are also complex and time-consuming to use. Direct observation of an individual's ability to get out of bed, sit in a chair, assume a standing position, and steadily walk a short distance–with or without assistive devices–is important to ensure safety in ADL capacity (Applegate et al., 1990 [Level IV]; Cress et al., 1995).

An efficient performance-based measure of ambulation, balance, and gait that can be observed during routine care during hospitalization is the "Get Up and Go" test (Applegate et al., 1990 [Level IV]). To do a Get Up and Go test, patients can be observed sitting in a chair, standing, walking, and pivoting. Performance is scored from 1, indicating normal balance and steady gait, to 5, severely abnormal, indicating clear evidence of a falls risk (Kane & Kane, 2000 [Level VI]). Although this bedside physical performance measure of ambulation is easy to do, it does yield significant subjectivity in scoring that may be enhanced by timing the tasks (Kane & Kane, 2000 [Level VI]).

Direct observation of transfer and ambulation should include an assessment of speed of performance, hesitancy, stumbling, swaying, grabbing for support, or unsafe maneuvers such as sitting too close to the edge of a chair or dizziness while pivoting (Tinetti & Ginter, 1988 [Level I]). The Get Up and Go test can be used by nurses for ambulation assessments during routine daily activities of older individuals (Applegate et al., 1990 [Level IV]). Assessment of unsafe transfers or ambulation indicates the need to begin immediate restorative therapies to prevent injuries and falls. Care should reflect attention to environmental designs, including walking paths free of clutter, rails and rest areas, and care routines that encourage daily ambulation as opposed to bedrest and immobility (Creditor, 1993 [Level VI]).

Sensory Capacity

Evaluation of the potential impact of sensory changes on the performance of ADLs is often underestimated. A simple test for functional vision is to have older adults read a headline from the newspaper. A moderate impairment can be noted if only the headline can be read (Tinetti & Ginter, 1988 [Level I]). Another way to assess vision is to have older persons read prescription bottles. Functional assessment of safe medication administration use includes the ability to read pill bottles and repeat directions for use and side effects for when to contact a health care provider. Glasses should be available with clean lenses. Inability to read raises questions of literacy, undiagnosed vision difficulties, and safety for medication administration. Often overlooked is the number of older people who may not be able to read but are too embarrassed to reveal that information. In fact, as part of routine care, older adults should be encouraged to actively participate each day in learning about medications. In addition, at the time of discharge, nurses need to verify patient and family knowledge and skills regarding medications. This may include discussing medications as well as directly observing older adults open pill bottles and identify correct pills.

Hearing ability is essential to function and cognition. Individuals with decreased hearing may be inaccurately labeled as cognitively impaired. Hearing aids may not have been sent to the hospital with the elder. The family should obtain these aids. Hearing acuity may be validated by asking patients to identify the sound of a ticking watch. The "whisper test" may also be used. This is performed by whispering 10 words while standing 6 inches away from the individual. Inability to repeat 5 of the 10 words indicates a need for further assessment of hearing acuity. Occlusion of the external ear canal by cerumen may be found on visualization, an easily treatable problem in decreased hearing acuity (Mathias, Nayak, & Isaacs, 1986 [Level VI]). Individuals with hearing deficits, detected as part of a bedside assessment, should be referred for additional assessment and treatment. Amplifier devices may be useful and are an inexpensive item to stock on nursing units in hospitals.

Cognitive Capacity

Cognitive function is a major factor in a person's functional capacity. Baseline cognitive function is important to assess. However, such assessments most often initially rely on information provided by family members because acute illness may be clinically manifested as acute confusional states and does not reflect baseline cognitive function (Kurianski & Gurland, 1976 [Level VI]). Nurses can assess components of cognitive function (including attention, language, and memory) during interviews and routine care, although anxiety and illness may be complicating factors. Observations to assess cognitive function during hospitalization may include the ability to call the nurse for help; ordering food from a menu; using the telephone; and following directions for activity, turning, and bathing (Kresevic et al., 1998 [Level VI]). Fluctuating attention may indicate an acute, reversible impairment (i.e., delirium) or temporary reactions to hospitalization. An acute change in cognition should be evaluated immediately for a potentially life-threatening, reversible medical condition (see chapter 7, *Delirium: Prevention, Early Recognition, and Treatment*).

Cause of Functional Decline

All instances of functional decline should also be assessed for an underlying reversible cause such as acute illness. In the presence of acute illness (e.g., urinary tract infection, pneumonia, or recovery after surgery), impaired ADLs are expected to return to baseline with appropriate care and rehabilitation as the illness resolves. Comprehensive musculoskeletal or neurologic examination, laboratory tests, or referral for a therapeutic trial of physical or occupational therapy may be needed.

Nursing Strategies to Prevent Functional Decline

Functional ability is a sensitive indicator of health in older adults. The need for assistance with ADLs is an important nursing assessment that assists with care planning in the hospital as well as for posthospitals care needs. Sudden loss of function, including the ability to ambulate, is the hallmark of acute illness in older adults. Whereas recovery from illness may be associated with improvements in function, early nursing interventions to address care needs, refer to therapy, and modify environments of care are all interventions that ensure safety and decrease further loss of function. Therefore, all nurses must be skilled at incorporating a comprehensive functional assessment into all patient-care assessments. Nurses need to be knowledgeable and skilled in assessment of function, adapting supportive environments, and providing geriatric sensitive care to prevent functional decline. Geriatric sensitive care incorporates strategies to prevent bedrest and encourage exercise and ambulation, to ensure adequate nutrition, and to encourage ongoing communication among all team members. Such care is essential to maximizing safe independent functioning of hospitalized older adults.

Use of Assessment Information

Knowledge of ADLs and IADLs, including shopping, housework, finances, food preparation, medication administration, and transportation, is an important part of providing individual nursing care for comprehensive discharge planning (Woolf, 1990 [Level VI]). In summary, for older people, the evaluation of function represents the cornerstone of good nursing care and affords a sound baseline by which to provide information essential to planning for continued care across settings.

Case Study and Discussion

Mrs. Hope, a 74-year-old retired night nurse and recent widow, is admitted to the hospital from her physician's office. Her admitting diagnosis is pneumonia, dehydration, and weakness. She is accompanied by her daughter. Her past medical history is significant for hypertension and COPD. She is extremely hard of hearing but has refused to wear her hearing aide. She smokes approximately 10 cigarettes a day, which she has done for more than 50 years. Her daughter admits that lately Mrs. Hope has been forgetting her pills. She has also been losing weight despite a good appetite and intake. Laboratory values indicate anemia with a very low hematocrit. A chest CT scan reveals inoperable lung cancer and a bone scan indicates metastatic bone disease.

While on the unit, Mrs. Hope prefers to sleep in the recliner, saying she is most comfortable there and prefers to nap during the day. Despite intravenous fluids, oxygen therapy, occupational therapy for energy conservation, and round-the-clock acetaminophen for "aches and pains," Mrs. Hope continues to be weak and need assistance with daily bathing and ambulation. She is able to communicate well using an amplifier, after her ears are cleaned for wax. She is assessed by the multidisciplinary care team during the next several days. At the family conference, the staff shares Mrs. Hope's poor medical prognosis, declining ADLs, concerns for safety and comfort, and available community services including hospice care. Mrs. Hope, her daughter, and the care team all collaborate to plan for Mrs. Hope to be discharged to her daughter's home with hospice care.

This case study indicates the need to assess baseline function, changes in function, and trajectory of function following acute care. Assessment in this case used components from several standardized functional assessment instruments and incorporated them into existing care routines. The case relies on individual preferences and resources as well as the functional level. Despite the level of function this case strives to maintain and enhance physical functioning within the current care setting within a context of safety.

Acknowledgment

This chapter was supported by a grant from The John A. Hartford Foundation.

Resources

Several Resources are now Available to Guide Adoption of Evidenced-Based Nursing Interventions to Enhance Function in Older Adults.

AHRQ Clinical Practice Guidelines, 1996. Accessed October 2006. http://www.ahrq.gov/clinic/cpgonline.htm

Joanna Briggs Best Practice, McGill University Web site. Accessed October 2006. http://www.muhc-ebn.mcgill.ca/ http://www.muhc-ebn.mcgill.ca/EBN_tools.htm

National Quality Forum Web site. Accessed October 2006. http://www.qualityforum.org/nursing/defult.htm

Registered Nurses Association of Ontario (RNAO)/NGC, 2005, McGill University.Web site. Accessed October 2006. http://www.muhc-ebn.mcgill.ca/EBN_tools.htm

Geriatric Protocols - University of Iowa www.nursing.uiowa.edu/centers/gnirc/protocols.htm

Box 3.1

Nursing Standard of Practice Protocol: Assessment of Function in Acute Care

GOAL: The following nursing care protocol was designed to help bedside nurses to monitor function in elders, to prevent decline, and to maintain the function of elders during acute hospitalization.

OBJECTIVE: The goal of nursing care is to maximize physical functioning, prevent or minimize decline in ADL function, and plan for future care needs.

I. BACKGROUND

A. Functional status of individuals describes the capacity and performance of safe ADLs and IADLs (Applegate et al., 1990 [Level IV]; Kane & Kane, 2000 [Level VI]; Katz et al., 1963 [Level I]; Lawton & Brody, 1969 [Level IV]) and is a sensitive indicator of health or illness in elders and therefore a critical nursing assessment (Byles, 2000 [Level I]; Campbell, et al., 2004 [Level I]; Kresevic & Holder, 1998 [Level VI]; Mezey, et al., 1993 [Level VI]).

B. Some functional decline may be prevented or ameliorated with prompt and aggressive nursing intervention (e.g., ambulation, toileting schedules, enhanced communication, adaptive equipment, and attention to medications and dosages) (Bates-Jensen et al., 2004 [Level V]; Counsell et al., 2000 [Level II]; Landefeld et al., 1995 [Level II]; Palmer, Counsell, & Landefeld, 1998 [Level I]).

C. Some functional decline may occur progressively and is not reversible. This decline often accompanies chronic and terminal disease states such as degenerative joint disease, Parkinson's disease, dementia, heart failure, and cancer (Hirsch, 1990 [Level IV]).

D. Functional status is influenced by physiological aging changes, acute and chronic illness, and adaptation to the physical environment. Functional decline is often the initial symptom of acute illness such as infections (e.g., pneumonia and urinary tract infection). These declines are usually reversible and require medical evaluation (Applegate et al., 1990 [Level IV]; Sager & Rudberg, 1998 [Level II]). Functional status is contingent on motivation, cognition, and sensory capacity, including vision and hearing (Pearson, 2000 [Level VI]).

E. Risk factors for functional decline include injuries, acute illness, medication side effects, pain, depression, malnutrition, decreased mobility, prolonged bedrest (including the use of physical restraints), prolonged use of Foley catheters, and changes in environment or routines (Counsell et al., 2000 [Level II]; Creditor, 1993 [Level VI]; Landefeld et al., 1995 [Level II]).

F. Additional complications of functional decline include loss of independence, falls, incontinence, malnutrition, decreased socialization, and increased risk for long-term institutionalization and depression (Covinsky et al., 1998 [Level II]; Creditor, 1993 [Level VI]; Landefeld et al., 1995 [Level II]). (See related chapters.)

G. Recovery of function can also be a measure of return to health, such as for those individuals recovering from exacerbations of cardiovascular or respiratory diseases and acute infections, recovering from joint replacement surgery, or new strokes (Katz et al., 1963 [Level I]).

H. Functional status evaluation assists in planning future care needs posthospitalization, such as short-term skilled care and home care (Graf, 2006 [Level V]; Landefeld et al., 1995 [Level II]).

I. Physical environments of care with attention to the special needs of older adults serve to maintain and enhance function (i.e., chairs with arms, elevated toilet seat, levers versus doorknobs, enhanced lighting) (Kresevic & Holder, 1998 [Level VI]; Landefeld et al., 1995 [Level II]).

II. ASSESSMENT PARAMETERS

A. Comprehensive functional assessment of elders includes independent performance of basic ADLs, social activities, or IADLs; the assistance needed to accomplish these tasks; and sensory ability, cognition, and capacity to ambulate. (Campbell et al., 2004 [Level I]; Doran et al., 2006 [Level VI]; Freedman, Martin, & Schoeni, 2002 [Level I]; Kane & Kane, 2000 [Level VI]; Katz et al., 1963 [Level I]; Lawton & Brody, 1969 [Level IV]; Lightbody & Baldwin, 2002 [Level VI]; McCusker, Kakuma, & Abramowicz, 2002 [Level I]; Tinetti & Ginter, 1988 [Level I]).

1. Basic ADLs
   a. Bathing
   b. Dressing
   c. Grooming
   d. Eating
   e. Continence
   f. Transferring

2. IADLs
   a. Meal preparation
   b. Shopping
   c. Medication administration
   d. Housework
   e. Transportation
   f. Accounting

3. Mobility
   a. Ambulation
   b. Pivoting

B. Elderly patients may view their health in terms of how well they can function rather than in terms of disease alone. Strengths should be emphasized as well as needs for assistance (Dopp & Jeste, 2006 [Level I]; Pearson, 2000 [Level VI]).

C. The clinician should document baseline functional status and recent or progressive decline in function (Graf, 2006 [Level V]).

D. Function should be assessed over time to validate capacity, decline, or progress (Applegate, 1990 [Level VI]; Callahan et al., 2002 [Level VI]; Kane & Kane, 2000 [Level VI]).

E. Standard instruments selected to assess function should be efficient to administer and easy to interpret. They should provide useful practical information for clinicians and be incorporated into routine history taking and daily assessments (Kane & Kane, 2000 [Level VI]; Kresevic & Holder, 1998 [Level VI]). (See Function topic at www.ConsultGeriRN.org for tools.)

F. Interdisciplinary communication regarding functional status, changes, and expected trajectory should be part of all care settings (Counsell et al., 2000 [Level II]; Kresevic & Holder, 1998 [Level VI]; Landefeld et al., 1995 [Level II]).

G. Multidisciplinary team conferences including patient and family whenever possible (Covinsky et al., 1998 [Level II]; Kresevic & Holder, 1998 [Level VI]).

III. CARE STRATEGIES

A. Strategies to maximize functional status and to prevent decline:
1. Maintain individual's daily routine. Help to maintain physical, cognitive, and social function through physical activity and socialization. Encourage ambulation, allow flexible visitation including pets, and encourage reading of the newspaper (Kresevic & Holder, 1998 [Level VI]; Landefeld et al., 1995 [Level II]).
2. Educate elders, family, and formal caregivers on the value of independent functioning and the consequences of functional decline (Graf, 2006 [Level V]; Kresevic & Holder, 1998 [Level VI]; Vass, Avlund, Lauridsen, & Hendriksen, 2005 [Level II]).
   a. Physiological and psychological value of independent functioning.
   b. Reversible functional decline associated with acute illness (Hirsch, 1990 [Level VI]; Sager & Rudberg, 1998 [Level II]).
   c. Strategies to prevent functional decline: exercise, nutrition, pain management, and socialization (Kresevic & Holder, 1998 [Level VI]; Landefeld et al., 1995 [Level II]; Siegler, Glick, & Lee, 2002; Tucker et al., 2004 [Level VI]).
   d. Sources of assistance to manage decline.
3. Encourage activity, including routine exercise, range of motion, and ambulation to maintain activity, flexibility, and function

(Counsell et al., 2000 [Level II]; Landefeld et al., 1995 [Level II]; Pedersen & Saltin, 2006 [Level I]).

4. Minimize bedrest (Bates-Jensen et al., 2004 [Level VI]; Covinsky et al., 1998 [Level II]; Landefeld et al., 1995 [Level II]; Kresevic & Holder, 1998 [Level VI]).

5. Explore alternatives to physical-restraints use (Covinsky et al., 1998 [Level II]; Kresevic & Holder, 1998 [Level VI]). (See chapter 22, *Physical Restraints and Side Rails in Acute and Critical Care Settings: Legal, Ethical, and Practice Issues.*)

6. Judiciously use medications, especially psychoactive medications, in geriatric dosages (Inouye, 1998 [Level III]). (See chapter 12, *Reducing Adverse Drug Events.*)

7. Assess and treat for pain (Covinsky et al., 1998 [Level II]).

8. Design environments with handrails, wide doorways, raised toilet seats, shower seats, enhanced lighting, low beds, and chairs of various types and height (Kresevic et al., 1998 [Level VI], Cunningham & Michael, 2004 [Level I]).

9. Help individuals regain baseline function after acute illnesses by using exercise, physical therapy consultation, nutrition, and coaching (Conn, Minor, Burks, Rantz, & Pomeroy, 2003 [Level I]); Engberg, Serika, McDowell, Weber, & Brodak, 2002 [Level II]; Forbes, 2005 [Level VI]; Hodgkinson, Evans, & Wood, 2003 [Level I]; Kresevic et al., 1998 [Level V]).

10. Obtain assessment for physical and occupational therapies needed to help regain function (Covinsky et al., 1998 [Level II]).

B. Strategies to help older individuals cope with functional decline

1. Help older adults and family members determine realistic functional capacity with interdisciplinary consultation (Kresevic & Holder, 1998 [Level VI]).

2. Provide caregiver education and support for families of individuals when decline cannot be ameliorated despite nursing and rehabilitative efforts (Graf, 2006 [Level V]).

3. Carefully document all intervention strategies and patient response (Graf, 2006 [Level V]).

4. Provide information to caregivers on causes of functional decline related to acute and chronic conditions (Covinsky et al., 1998 [Level II]).

5. Provide education to address safety care needs for falls, injuries, and common complications. Short-term skilled care for physical therapy may be needed; long-term care settings may be required to ensure safety (Covinsky et al., 1998 [Level II]).

6. Provide sufficient protein and caloric intake to ensure adequate intake and prevent further decline. Liberalize diet to include personal preferences (Edington et al., 2004 [Level II]; Landefeld et al., 1995 [Level II]).

7. Provide caregiver support community services, such as home care, nursing, and physical and occupational therapy services to

manage functional decline (Covinsky et al., 1998 [Level II]; Graf, 2006 [Level V]).

IV. EXPECTED OUTCOMES

A. Patients can:
1. Maintain safe level of ADLs and ambulation.
2. Make necessary adaptations to maintain safety and independence, including assistive devices and environmental adaptations.
3. Strive to attain highest quality of life despite functional level.

B. Providers can demonstrate:
1. Increased assessment, identification, and management of patients susceptible to or experiencing functional decline. Routine assessment of functional capacity despite level of care.
2. Ongoing documentation and communication of capacity, interventions, goals, and outcomes.
3. Competence in preventive and restorative strategies for function.
4. Competence in assessing safe environments of care that foster safe independent function.

C. Institution will experience:
1. System-wide incorporation of functional assessment.
2. A reduction in incidence and prevalence of functional decline.
3. A decrease in morbidity and mortality rates associated with functional decline.
4. Reduction in the use of physical restraints, prolonged bedrest, Foley catheters.
5. Decreased incidence of delirium.
6. An increase in prevalence of patients who leave hospital with baseline or improved functional status.
7. Decreased readmission rate.
8. Increased early utilization of rehabilitative services (i.e., occupational and physical therapy).
9. Support of institutional policies and programs that promote function.
10. Evidence of geriatric-sensitive physical-care environments that facilitate safe independent function, such as caregiver educational efforts and walking programs.
11. Evidence of continued interdisciplinary assessments, care planning, and evaluation of care related to function.

VII. RELEVENT PRACTICE GUIDELINES

Several resources are now available to guide adoption of evidenced-based nursing interventions to enhance function in older adults.

A. AHRQ Clinical Practice Guidelines, 1996. Accessed October 2006. http://www.ahrq.gov/clinic/cpgonline.htm

B. Joanna Briggs Best Practice, McGill University Web site. Accessed October 2006. http://www.muhc-ebn.mcgill.ca/

C. Joanna Briggs Best Practice, McGill University Web site. Accessed October 2006. http://www.muhc-ebn.mcgill.ca/EBN_tools.htm

D. National Quality Forum Web site. Accessed October 2006. http://www.qualityforum.org/nursing/defult.htm

E. Registered Nurses Association of Ontario (RNAO)/NGC, 2005, McGill University Web site. Accessed October 2006. http://www.muhc-ebn.mcgill.ca/EBN_tools.htm

F. Geriatric Protocols - University of Iowa www.nursing.uiowa.edu/centers/gnirc/protocols.htm

References

Applegate, W. B., Blass, J., & Franklin, T. (1990). Instruments for the functional assessment of older patients. *New England Journal of Medicine, 322,* 1207–1214. Evidence Level IV: Nonexperimental Study.

Bates-Jensen, B. M., Alessi, C. A., Cadogan, M., Levy-Storms, L., Jorge, J., Yoshil, J., et al. (2004). The minimum data set bedfast quality indicators: Differences in nursing homes. *Nursing Research, 53,* 260–272. Evidence Level V: Program Evaluation.

Burton, R. M., Damon, W. W., Dillinger, D. C., Erickson, D. J., & Peterson, D. W. (1978). Nursing home rest and care: An investigation of alternatives. In E. Pfeiffer (Ed.), *Multidimensional functional assessment: The DARS methodology.* Durham, NC: Duke Center for Study of Aging Human Development. Evidence Level III: Quasi-experimental Study.

Byles, J. E. (2000). A thorough going over: Evidence for health assessments for older persons. *Australian & New Zealand Journal of Public Health, 24,* 117–123. Evidence Level I: Systematic Review.

Callahan, E. H., Thomas, D. C., Goldhirsh, S. L., & Leipzig, R. M. (2002). Geriatric hospital medicine. *Medical Clinics of North America, 86*(4), 707–729. Evidence Level VI: Expert Opinion.

Campbell, S. E., Seymour, D. G., Primrose, W. R., & ACME-plus Project (2004). A systematic literature review of factors affecting outcomes in older medical patients admitted to hospital. *Age and Ageing, 33,* 110–115. Evidence Level I: Systematic Review.

Conn, V. S., Minor, M. A., Burks, K. J., Rantz, M. J., & Pomeroy, S. H. (2003). Integrative review of physical activity intervention research with aging adults. *Journal of the American Geriatrics Society, 51*(80), 1159–1168. Evidence Level I: Systematic Review.

Counsell, S. R., Holder, C. M., Liebenauer, L. L., Palmer, R. M., Fortinsky, R. H., Kresevic, D. M., et al. (2000). Effects of a multicomponent intervention on functional outcomes and process of care of hospitalized older patients: A randomized controlled trial of Acute Care for Elders (ACE) in a community hospital. *Journal of the American Geriatric Society, 48*(12), 1572–1581. Evidence Level II: Individual Experimental Study.

Covinsky, K. E., Palmer, R. M., Kresevic, D. M., Kahana, E., Counsell, S. R., Fortinsky, R. H., et al. (1998). Improving functional outcome in older patients. *Joint Commission Journal on Quality Improvement, 24*(2), 63–76. Evidence Level II: Individual Experimental Study.

Creditor, M. C. (1993). Hazards of hospitalization of elderly. *Annals of Internal Medicine, 118,* 219–223. Evidence Level VI: Expert Opinion.

Cress, M. E., Schectman, K. B., Mulrow, C. D., Fiatarone, M. A., Gerety, M. B., & Buchner, D. M. (1995). Relationship between physical performance and self-perceived physical function. *Journal of the American Geriatric Society, 43,* 93–101.

Cunningham, G. O., & Michael, Y. L. (2004). Concepts guiding the study of the impact of the built environment on physical activity for older adults: A review of the literature. *American Journal of Health Promotion, 18*(6), 435–443. Evidence Level I: Systematic Review.

Dopp, C. A., & Jeste, D. V. (2006). Definitions and predictors of successful aging: A comprehensive review of larger quantitative studies. *American Journal of Geriatric Psychiatry, 14*(1), 6–20. Evidence Level I: Systematic Review.

Doran, D. M., Harrison, M. B., Laschinger, H. S., Hiredes, J. P., Rukholm, F., Sudabum S., et al. (2006). Nursing-sensitive outcomes data collection in acute care and long term care settings. *Nursing Research, 55*(2 Supp.), S75–S81. Evidence Level VI: Expert Opinion.

Edington, J., Barnes, R., Bryan, F., Dupree, E., Frost, G., Hickson, M., et al. (2004). A prospective randomized controlled trial of nutritional supplementation in malnourished elderly in the community: Clinical and health economic outcomes. *Clinical Nutrition, 23*(2), 195–204. Evidence Level II: Individual Experimental Study.

Engberg, S., Serika, S. M., McDowell, B. J., Weber, E., & Brodak, I. (2002). Effectiveness of prompted voiding in treating urinary incontinence in cognitively impaired homebound older adults. *Journal of Wound, Ostomy & Continence Nursing, 29*(5), 252–265. Evidence Level II: Individual Experimental Study.

Forbes, D. A. (2005). An educational programme for primary healthcare providers improved functional ability in older people living in the community. *Evidenced Based Nursing, 8,* 122. Evidence Level VI: Expert Opinion.

Freedman, V. A., Martin, L. G., & Schoeni, R. F. (2002). Recent trends in disability and functioning among older adults in the United States: A systematic review. *Journal of the American Medical Association, 288*(24), 3137–3146. Evidence Level I: Systematic Review.

Graf, C. (2006). Functional decline in hospitalized older adults. *American Journal of Nursing, 106*(1), 58–67. Evidence Level V: Narrative Review.

Gurland, B. J., Cross, I., Chen, C., Wilder, D. E., Pine, Z. M., Lantigua, R. A., et al. (1994). A new performance test of adaptive cognitive functioning: The medication management (MM) test. *International Journal of Geriatric Psychiatry, 9,* 875–885. Evidence Level VI: Expert Opinion.

Hirsch, C. H. (1990). The natural history of functional morbidity in hospitalized older patients. *Journal of the American Geriatrics Society, 38,* 1296–1303. Evidence Level IV: Nonexperimental Study.

Hodgkinson, B., Evans, D., & Wood, J. (2003). Maintaining oral hydration in older adults: A systematic review. *International Journal of Nursing Practice, 9*(3), S19–S28. Evidence Level I: Systematic Review.

Inouye, S. R. (1998). Does delirium contribute to poor hospital outcomes? A three-site epidemiological study. *Journal of General Internal Medicine, 13,* 234–242. Evidence Level III: Quasi-experimental Study.

Kane, R. A., & Kane, R. L. (2000). *Assessing older persons: Measures, meaning, and practical applications.* New York: Oxford. Evidence Level VI: Expert Opinion.

Karagiozis, H., Gray, S., Sacco, J., Shapiro, M., & Dawas, C. (1998). The Direct Assessment of Functional Abilities (DAFA): A comparison to an indirect measure of instrumental activities of daily living. *Gerontologist, 38,* 113–121. Evidence Level III: Quasi-experimental Study.

Katz, S., Ford, A. B., Moscokowitz, R. W., Jackson, B. A., & Jaffe, M. W. (1963). Studies of illness and the aged: The index of ADL. A standardized measure of biological and psychosocial function. *Journal of the American Medical Association, 185,* 914–919. Evidence Level I: Systematic Review.

Kidd, D., Stewart, G., Baldry, J., Johnson, J., Rossiter, D., Petruckevitch, A., et al. (1995). The Functional Independence Measure: A comparative validity and reliability study. *Disability and Rehabilitation, 17,* 10–14. Evidence Level III: Quasi-experimental study.

Kresevic, D., Counsel, S., Covinsky, K., Palmer, R., Landefeld, C. S., Holder, C., et al. (1998). A patient-centered model of acute care for elders. *Nursing Clinics of North America, 3,* 515–527. Evidence Level VI: Expert Opinion.

Kresevic, D., & Holder, C. (1998). Interdisciplinary care. *Clinics in Geriatric Medicine, 14,* 787–798. Evidence Level VI: Expert Opinion.

Kurianski, J., & Gurland, B. (1976). The performance test of activities of daily living. *International Journal of Aging and Human Development, 7,* 343–352. Evidence Level VI: Expert Opinion.

Landefeld, C. S., Palmer, R. M., Kresevic, D. M., Fortinsky, R. I., & Kowa, J. (1995). A randomized trial of care in a hospital medical unit especially designed to improve the functional outcomes of acutely ill older patients. *New England Journal of Medicine, 332,* 1338–1344. Evidence Level II: Individual Experimental Study.

Lawton, M. P., & Brody, E. M. (1969). Assessment of older people: Self-maintaining and instrumental activities of daily living. *Gerontologist, 9,* 179–186. Evidence Level IV: Nonexperimental Study.

Lightbody, E., & Baldwin, R. (2002). Inpatient geriatric evaluation and management did not reduce mortality but reduced functional decline. *Evidenced Based Mental Health, 5,* 109. Evidence Level VI: Expert Opinion.

Lowenstein, D. A., Amigo, E., Duara, R., Guterman, A., Hurwitz, D., Berkowitz, N., et al. (1989). A new scale for the assessment of functional status in Alzheimer's disease and related disorders. *Journal of Gerontology, 44,* 114–121.

Mahoney, F. L., & Barthel, D. W. (1965). Functional evaluation: The Barthel index. *Maryland State Medical Journal, 14,* 61–65. Evidence Level III: Quasi-experimental Study.

Mathias, S., Nayak, U. S., & Isaacs, B. (1986). Balance in elderly patients: The "Get Up and Go" test. *Archives of Physical and Medical Rehabilitation, 67,* 387–389. Evidence Level VI: Expert Opinion.

McCusker, J., Kakuma, R., & Abrahamowicz, M. (2002). Predictors of functional hospitalized elderly patients: A systematic review. *Journals of Gerontology. Series A: Biological Sciences and Medical Sciences, 57A,* M569–M577. Evidence Level I: Systematic Review.

Mezey, M. D., Rauckhorst, L. H., & Stokes, S. A. (1993). *Health assessment of the older individual.* New York: Springer Publishing Company. Evidence Level VI: Expert Opinion.

Palmer, R. M., Counsell, S., & Landefeld, C. S. (1998). Clinical interventions trials: The ACE Unit. *Clinical Geriatric Medicine, 14,* 831–849. Evidence Level I: Systematic Review.

Pearson, V. I. (2000). Assessment of function in older adults. In R. I. Kane & R. A. Kane (Eds.), *Assessing older persons: Measures, meanings and practical applications* (pp. 17–34). New York: Oxford University Press. Evidence Level VI: Expert Opinion.

Pedersen, B. K., & Saltin, B. (2006). Evidence for prescribing exercise as therapy in chronic disease. *Scandinavian Journal of Medicine & Science in Sports, 16* (Supp. I), 3–63. Evidence Level I: Systematic Review.

Sager, M., & Rudberg, M. M. (1998). Functional decline associated with hospitalization for acute illnesses. *Clinics in Geriatric Medicine, 14,* 669–679. Evidence Level II: Individual Experimental Study.

Siegler, E. L., Glick, D., & Lee, J. (2002). Optimal staffing for acute care of the elderly (ACE) units. *Geriatric Nursing, 23*(3), 152–155. Evidence Level VI: Expert Opinion.

Skurla, E., Rogers, J. C., & Sunderland, T. (1988). Direct assessment of activities of daily living in Alzheimer's disease: A controlled study. *Journal of the American Geriatrics Society, 36,* 97–103.

Tinetti, M. E., & Ginter, S. F. (1988). Identify mobility dysfunctions in elderly patients: Standard neuromuscular examination or direct assessment? *Journal of the American Medical Association, 259,* 1190–1193. Evidence Level I: Meta-analysis.

Tucker, D. M., Molsberger, S. C. & Clark; A. (2004). Walking and wellness: A collaborative program to maintain mobility in hospitalized older adults. *Geriatric Nursing, 25,* 242–245.

Vass, M., Avlund, K., Lauridsen, J., & Hendriksen, C. (2005). Feasible model for prevention of functional decline in older people: Municipality-randomized controlled trial. *Journal of the American Geriatrics Society, 53*(4), 563–568. Evidence Level II: Individual Experimental Study.

Woolf, S. H. (1990). Screening for hearing impairment. In R. B. Goldbloom & R. S. Lawrence (Eds.), *Preventing disease: Beyond the rhetoric* (pp. 331–346). New York: Springer-Verlag. Evidence Level VI: Expert Opinion.

Assessing Cognitive Function

4

Tom Braes
Koen Milisen
Marquis D. Foreman

Educational Objectives

On completion of this chapter, the reader should be able to:

1. discuss the importance of assessing cognitive function

2. describe the goals of assessing cognitive function

3. compare and contrast the clinical features of delirium, dementia, and depression

4. incorporate the assessment of cognitive function into daily practice

Overview

Cognitive functioning comprises perception, memory, and thinking—the processes by which a person perceives, recognizes, registers, stores, and uses information (Foreman & Vermeersch, 2004 [Level I]). Cognitive functioning can be affected, positively and negatively, by illness and its treatment. Consequently, assessing an individual's cognitive functioning is paramount for identifying the presence of specific pathological conditions, such as dementia and delirium; for monitoring the effectiveness of various health interventions; and for

For a description of Evidence Levels cited in this chapter, see chapter 1,
Developing and Evaluating Clinical Practice Guidelines, page 4.

determining an individual's readiness to learn and ability to make decisions (Foreman & Vermeersch, 2004 [Level I]). Despite the importance of assessment, physicians and nurses routinely fail to assess an individual's cognitive functioning (Foreman & Milisen, 2004 [Level I]). This has profoundly serious consequences that include the failure to detect a potentially correctable condition of cognitive impairment and death (Inouye, Foreman, Mion, Katz, & Cooney, 2001 [Level IV]) — outcomes that could be prevented or minimized by early recognition of their existence afforded by the routine assessment of cognitive functioning (Foreman & Milisen, 2004 [Level I]). More important, given that nurses tend to have the most frequent and longest duration of contact with individuals seeking health care, they are instrumental for the early recognition of impairment and monitoring of cognitive functioning (Milisen, Braes, Fick, & Foreman, 2006 [Level VI]).

Background and Statement of Problem

Declines in cognitive functioning are a hallmark of aging (McEvoy, 2001 [Level VI]); however, most declines in cognition with aging are not pathological. Examples of nonpathological changes include a diminished ability to learn complex information, a delayed response time, and minor loss of recent memory; declines are especially evident with complex tasks or with those requiring multiple steps for completion (McEvoy, 2001 [Level VI]).

Pathological conditions of cognitive impairment that are prevalent with aging include delirium, dementia, and depression (Table 4.1 compares the clinical features among delirium, dementia, and depression. See also chapter 6, *Dementia,* and chapter 7, *Delirium*). There are protocols to prevent and treat delirium and protocols to slow the progression of decline with dementia; however, these opportunities exist only when and if these conditions are detected early, and the possibility of early detection exists only when cognitive function is assessed systematically (Chow & MacLean, 2001 [Level I]; Registered Nurse Association of Ontario [RNAO], 2003 [Level I]). Without systematic assessment, these pathological conditions go unchecked, and the individuals with these conditions face much greater accelerated and long-term cognitive and functional decline and death (Fick, Agostini, & Inouye, 2002 [Level I]; Fick & Foreman, 2000 [Level IV]; Hopkins & Jackson, 2006 [Level IV]; Lang et al., 2006 [Level IV]). Health care providers report greater frustration and job stress in caring for these individuals (Milisen et al., 2004 [Level IV]), and the cost of providing care to these individuals is much greater (Milbrandt et al., 2004 [Level IV]).

Despite these profoundly negative consequences for the afflicted individuals and their families, as well as for their care providers, nurses and physicians fail to assess cognitive function (Ely et al., 2004 [Level IV]; Foreman & Milisen, 2004 [Level I]; Inouye et al., 2001 [Level IV]). Yet, it is clear that the assessment of cognitive function is the first and most crucial step in a cascade of strategies to prevent, reverse, halt, or minimize cognitive decline (Chow & MacLean, 2001 [Level I]; RNAO, 2003 [Level I]). Thus, the purpose of this chapter is to provide a best practice protocol for the assessment of cognitive function, see Box 4.1.

A Comparison of the Clinical Features of Delirium, Dementia, and Depression

Clinical Feature	Delirium	Dementia	Depression
Onset	Sudden/abrupt; depends on cause; often at twilight	Insidious/slow and often unrecognized; depends on cause	Coincides with major life changes; often abrupt but can be gradual
Course	Short; diurnal fluctuations in symptoms; worse at night, in darkness, and on awakening	Long, no diurnal effects, symptoms progressive yet relatively stable over time, may see deficits with increased stress	Diurnal effects, typically worse in the morning; situational fluctuations in symptoms but less than with delirium
Progression	Abrupt	Slow but uneven	Variable; rapid or slow but generally even
Duration	Hours to less than 1 month; longer if unrecognized and untreated	Months to years	At least 6 weeks, can be several months to years
Consciousness	Disturbed	Clear	Clear
Alertness	Fluctuates from stuporous to hypervigilant	Generally normal	Normal
Attention	Inattentive, easily distractible and may have difficulty shifting attention from one focus to another	Generally normal	Minimal impairment but is distractible
Orientation	Generally impaired; disoriented to time and place, should not be disoriented to person	Generally normal	Selective disorientation
Memory	Recent and immediate impaired; unable to recall events of hospitalization and current illness; forgetful, unable to recall instructions	Recent and remote impaired	Selective or "patchy" impairment, "islands" of intact memory, evaluation often difficult due to low motivation

4.1 A Comparison of the Clinical Features of Delirium, Dementia, and Depression

Clinical Feature	Delirium	Dementia	Depression
Thinking	Disorganized; rambling, irrelevant and incoherent conversation; unclear or illogical flow of ideas	Difficulty with abstraction, thoughts impoverished; judgment impaired; words difficult to find	Intact but with themes of hopelessness, helplessness, or self-deprecation
Perception	Perceptual disturbances such as illusions and visual and auditory hallucinations; misperceptions of common people and objects	Misperceptions usually absent	Intact; delusions and hallucinations absent except in severe cases
Psychomotor behavior	Variable; hypoactive, hyperactive, and mixed	Normal, may have apraxia	Variable; psychomotor retardation or agitation
Associated features	Variable affective changes; symptoms of autonomic hypo-hyper-arousal	Affect tends to be superficial, inappropriate, and labile; attempts to conceal deficits in intellect; personality changes, aphasia, agnosia may be present; lacks insight	Affect depressed; dysphoric mood, exaggerated and detailed complaints; preoccupied with personal thoughts; insight present; verbal elaboration; somatic complaints; poor hygiene; and neglect of self
Assessment	Distracted from task; fails to remember instructions, frequent errors without notice	Failings highlighted by family, frequent "near miss" answers, struggles with test, great effort to find an appropriate reply, frequent requests for feedback on performance	Failings highlighted by individual; frequent "don't know" answers, little effort; frequently gives up; indifferent toward test; does not care or attempt to find answer

Source: Adapted from Foreman et al. (2003). Assessing cognitive functioning. In M. Mezey et al., *Geriatric nursing protocols for best practice* (2nd ed., pp. 102–103). New York: Springer Publishing Company.

Assessment of Cognitive Functioning

Reasons for Assessing Cognitive Functioning

As mentioned previously, there are several reasons or purposes for assessing an individual's cognitive functioning, described as follows.

Screening is conducted to determine the presence or absence of impairment. Information obtained in screening can be useful for determining whether the individual is cognitively impaired; however, bedside screening methods such as those described herein (e.g., Mini-Mental State Examination [MMSE] and Mini-Cog) are not useful in and of themselves for diagnosing specific pathological conditions of impairment such as delirium or dementia. Screening is also an important element in determining an individual's readiness to learn and capacity to consent (Assessing Care of Vulnerable Elders [ACOVE] Investigators, 2001 [Level I]). As a result, screening activities enable the early detection of impairment that affords the opportunity to determine the nature of the impairment. That is, is the impairment delirium, dementia, or depression, or possibly one superimposed on another? Only through early detection can treatment be initiated promptly and accurately to either reverse, halt, or slow the progression of impairment (Chow & MacLean, 2001 [Level I]; RNAO, 2003 [Level I]).

Monitoring is conducted to track cognitive function over time as a means for following the progression or regression of impairment, especially in response to treatment (ACOVE Investigators, 2001 [Level I]; RNAO, 2003 [Level I]).

How to Assess Cognitive Functioning

For assessing cognitive functioning, Folstein's MMSE (Folstein, Folstein, & McHugh, 1975 [Level IV]) is the most frequently recommended instrument (British Geriatrics Society, 2005 [Level I]; Brodaty, Low, Gibson, & Burns, 2006 [Level I]; Fletcher, 2007 [Level VI]; Michaud et al., 2007 [Level I]; Milisen et al., 2006 [Level VI]; O'Keefe, Mulkerrin, Nayeem, Varughese, & Pillay., 2005 [Level IV]; RNAO, 2003 [Level I]; Scottish Intercollegiate Guidelines Network, 2005 [Level I]; Tullman, Mion, Fletcher, & Foreman, 2007 [Level VI]). The MMSE has been the most commonly used screening instrument for cognitive functioning for more than 25 years because it is brief, it consists of 11 items and takes about 7 to 10 minutes to complete, and it is easy to use. It is composed of items assessing orientation, attention, memory, concentration, language, and constructional ability (Tombaugh & McIntyre, 1992 [Level I]). Each question is scored as either correct or incorrect; the total score ranges from 0 to 30 and reflects the number of correct responses. A score of less than 24 is considered evidence of impaired cognition (Tombaugh & McIntyre, 1992 [Level I]).

Although considered the best available method for screening for impairment, the performance on the MMSE is significantly influenced by education (individuals with less than an eighth-grade education commit more errors), language (individuals for whom English is not their primary language commit more errors), verbal ability (the MMSE can only be used with individuals who can respond verbally to questioning), and age (older people do less well) (Tombaugh & McIntyre, 1992 [Level I]). Others contend that the MMSE takes too long to administer (Borson, Scanlan, Watanabe, Tu, & Lessig, 2005 [Level IV]). Despite these limitations, it remains the most frequently recommended and most commonly used tool to assess cognitive functioning.

To minimize the limitations of the MMSE while maximizing practical aspects of assessing cognitive function, the Mini-Cog was developed (Borson, Scanlan, Brush, Vitaliano, & Dokmak, 2000 [Level IV]). The aim was to have a brief screening test that required no equipment and little training to use while not being negatively influenced by age, education, or language (Borson et al., 2000 [Level IV]; Borson et al., 2005 [Level IV]). The Mini-Cog is a four-item screening test consisting of a three-item recall similar to the MMSE and a clock-drawing item. For the three-item recall, the individual is asked to listen to three unrelated words, repeat them, and, finally, remember them for later. The individual is then asked to draw the face of a clock, number the clock face, and place the hands on the clock face to indicate a specific time, such as 10:20. The individual is then asked to recall the three items he or she was previously instructed to remember. Each item correctly recalled receives 1 point for a total of 3 points; a correctly drawn clock face receives 2 points, for a total score of 5 (Borson et al., 2000 [Level IV]). If any error is made in drawing the clock, no points are assigned.

Since its initial development in 2000, the Mini-Cog has been used with various samples of people from different cultural, educational, age, and language backgrounds. In a recent systematic review, it was reported that the Mini-Cog was suitable for the routine screening for cognitive impairment (Brodaty et al., 2006 [Level I]); even more recently, it was found to predict the development of in-hospital delirium (Alagiakrishnan et al., 2007 [Level IV]).

The fact that most practice guidelines and systematic reviews recommend the use of the MMSE for systematic screening of cognitive functioning does not necessarily mean it is the best instrument for this purpose. Using it is beneficial, but studies in which the performance of the MMSE and the Mini-Cog are compared in the same subjects have demonstrated the Mini-Cog to be more accurate while less influenced by age, education, and language (Brodaty et al., 2006 [Level I]). Moreover, the Mini-Cog takes about half the time to administer and score than the MMSE, making the practical value of the Mini-Cog greater than the MMSE. However, more research is needed on this topic (Brodaty et al., 2006 [Level I]).

Both the MMSE and the Mini-Cog are classified as simple bedside cognitive screens. This means that they are both qualified for determining the presence or absence of cognitive impairment; however, neither is capable of indicating whether the impairment is delirium, dementia, or depression. If the results of this cognitive assessment or screening indicate that the individuals are impaired, further evaluation is necessary to confirm a diagnosis of dementia, depression, delirium, or some other health problem (Brodaty et al., 2006 [Level I]). One example of a diagnostic instrument is the Confusion Assessment Method (Inouye et al., 1990 [Level IV]) for diagnosing delirium; other instruments useful for diagnosing dementia and delirium and these diagnostic instruments are discussed in greater detail in chapters 6, *Dementia* and 7, *Delirium: Prevention, Early Recognition, and Treatment*.

When to Assess Cognitive Functioning

When and how frequently to assess cognitive functioning, using either the MMSE or Mini-Cog, is in part a function of the purpose for the assessment, the condition of the patient, and the results of prior or current testing. Recommendations for the systematic assessment of cognition using standardized and validated tools include the following:

- On admission to and discharge from an institutional care setting (ACOVE Investigators, 2001 [Level I]; British Geriatric Society, 2005 [Level I])
- On transfer from one care setting to another (ACOVE Investigators, 2001 [Level I])
- During hospitalization, every 8 to 12 hours throughout hospitalization (http://www.icudelirium.org/delirium)
- As follow-up to hospital care, within 6 weeks of discharge (ACOVE Investigators, 2001 [Level I])
- Before making important health care decisions as an adjunct to determining an individual's capacity to consent (ACOVE Investigators, 2001 [Level I])
- On the first visit to a new care provider (ACOVE Investigators, 2001 [Level I])
- Following major changes in pharmacotherapy (ACOVE Investigators, 2001 [Level I])
- With behavior that is unusual for the individual and/or inappropriate to the situation (Foreman & Vermeersch, 2004 [Level I])

It also is recommended that formal cognitive testing, with either the MMSE or Mini-Cog, be supplemented with information from intimate others (Cole et al., 2002 [Level II]; RNAO, 2003 [Level I]) and from naturally occurring observations and conversations (Foreman et al., 2003 [Level VI]). One method for obtaining information from intimate others (Cole et al., 2002 [Level II]) is through the use of the Informant Questionnaire on Cognitive Decline in the Elderly (IQCDE) (Jorm, 1994 [Level IV]). Obtaining information from intimate others about an individual's cognitive functioning assists in determining the duration of impairment necessary for determining whether the impairment is delirium or dementia (see chapters 6, *Dementia* and 7, *Delirium: Prevention, Early Recognition, and Treatment*). However, naturally occurring observations and conversations during everyday nursing care activities in which it becomes apparent that an individual is inattentive and responding unusually or inappropriately to conversation or questioning may be the first indication of the need to assess the individual's cognitive functioning.

Cautions for Assessing Cognitive Functioning

When assessing cognitive functioning, various characteristics of the physical assessment environment should be considered to ensure that the results of the assessment accurately reflect the individual's abilities and not extraneous factors. Overall, the ideal assessment environment should maximize the comfort and privacy of both the assessor and the individual. With respect to the individual, the environment should enhance performance by maximizing the individual's ability to participate in the assessment process (Dellasega, 1998 [Level VI]). To accomplish this, the room should be well lit and of comfortable ambient temperature so that neither participant is distracted from the cognitive task. Lighting must be balanced to be sufficient for the individual to adequately see the examination materials while not being so bright as to create glare. Also, the assessment environment should be free from distractions that can result from extraneous noise, scattered assessment materials, or brightly colored and/or patterned clothing and flashy jewelry on the assessor (Lezak, Howieson, & Loring, 2004 [Level VI]).

Regarding the interpersonal environment, it will be vital to prepare the individual for the assessment; explaining what will take place and how long it will take reduces anxiety and creates an emotionally nonthreatening environment and a safe individual–assessor relationship (Engberg & McDowell, 1999 [Level VI]). Performing the assessment in the presence of others should be avoided when possible because the other individual may be distracting. If the other is a significant intimate relative, additional problems arise. For example, when the individual fails to respond or responds in error, significant others have been known to provide the answer or to make comments such as, "Now, you know the answer to that" or "Now, you know that's wrong." In most instances, the presence of another only heightens anxiety. Rarely does the presence of another facilitate the performance of an individual on cognitive assessment. Older adults are especially sensitive to any insinuation that they may have some "memory problem"; therefore, the dilemma for the assessor is to stress the importance of the assessment while taking care not to increase the individual's anxiety. It is important to create an environment in which the individual is motivated to perform and to perform well while not being overly anxious and, therefore, perform poorly. Similarly, it can be counterproductive to describe the assessment as consisting of "simple," "silly," or "stupid" questions. Such explanations tend to diminish motivation to perform and only heighten anxiety when errors are committed. Anxiety also is heightened following a series of failures on assessment.

Various characteristics of the assessor and individual should also be considered. The assessment of cognitive functioning can be perceived by the individual as intrusive, intimidating, fatiguing, and offensive—characteristics that can seriously and negatively affect performance. Consequently, Lezak et al. (2004 [Level VI]) recommend an initial period to establish rapport with the individual. This period also allows a determination of the individual's capacity for assessment. For example, this period can be used to establish whether the individual has any special problems that could influence testing or its interpretation (e.g., sensory decrements). With elderly individuals who may have some decrements in sensory abilities, the assessor can improve the examinee's ability to perform through simple methods. For example, if the individual has any degree of hearing impairment, taking a position across from the assessor or a little to the side may enhance hearing. In this position, the individual can readily use the assessor's nonverbal communication as well as read the assessor's lips. Both strategies improve communication and therefore assessment. Sitting or standing a little to the side of the ear with the better auditory function of the individual also improves better hearing. Positioning also is important relative to lighting and glare.

When selecting the most suitable moment for assessing an individual's cognitive status, one should generally avoid periods immediately on awakening from sleep (wait at least 30 minutes), immediately before and after meals, immediately before and after medical diagnostic or therapeutic procedures, and when the individual is in pain or is uncomfortable. By avoiding these periods, performance is more likely to reflect the individual's cognitive abilities (Foreman et al., 2003 [Level VI]).

Case Study and Discussion

Mrs. O. is a 79-year-old retired nurse who lives at home with her husband, who is physically frail. Mrs. O. was diagnosed with probable Alzheimer's disease approximately 3 years ago. In addition, she has Type II diabetes that is generally well controlled on Actoplus (i.e., pioglitazone hydrochloride and metformin hydrochloride). She and her husband are able to remain living in their own home because of help from their children, neighbors, friends, and a monthly visit from a home health nurse. Mrs. O. is quite mobile but recently has begun to wander at times. Her husband reports that she seems more confused in the past few days and has fallen twice since yesterday. There is evidence of minor physical injury, which Mrs. O. insists is "nothing." Her husband also is concerned that she has not been taking her Actoplus as prescribed; although she has been eating okay, he is concerned that she has not been drinking enough. Because of these concerns, he calls the home health nurse to come and evaluate the situation because he is concerned that his wife may need urgent attention. [Mr. O.'s concerns are real and the call to the home health nurse is appropriate.]

When the nurse arrives, she assesses Mrs. O., including her cognitive functioning. The results of her assessment with the MMSE indicate that Mrs. O.'s cognitive functioning has deteriorated significantly since the nurse's visit 2 weeks ago. Mrs. O. is more disoriented to time and place, is more easily distracted, her conversation is disorganized, and she has greater difficulty following commands and remembering simple objects. She scored 18 out of 30 on the MMSE 2 weeks ago, which is usual for her, but now scores 12 out of 30. In talking with the husband, the nurse learns that these changes occurred in the past 2 days. The nurse suspects delirium, as evidenced by the sudden and dramatic decline in Mrs. O.'s cognitive abilities. The nurse thinks that Mrs. O. may be severely dehydrated because her diabetes is no longer controlled and is concerned about impending hyperosmolar, nonketotic coma. The nurse seeks an emergency admission to the local hospital for further diagnostic work to determine the cause for her suspected delirium; is she hyperglycemic and dehydrated? [The nurse's suspected diagnosis is certainly a health emergency warranting further diagnostic workup to confirm a diagnosis of delirium and the identification of the underlying causes.]

Mrs. O. is admitted with a diagnosis of mental-status changes. On admission to the hospital, the nurse describes Mrs. O. as "cooperative, lying quietly in bed, but being slow to respond." Being short staffed that day and given Mrs. O.'s history of dementia, the hospital nurse decides that the husband is being overprotective and that these changes are merely a worsening of her dementia and nothing new. The nurse moves on to other patients and more "important" patient-care concerns. A couple of hours later, the nurse goes back to check on Mrs. O., only to find her obtunded, unresponsive to physical stimuli, hypotensive, and tachycardic. The nurse calls a code, but Mrs. O. fails to respond and dies. [What went wrong here? It is likely that the assessment performed by the home health nurse was not transmitted to the nurse in the hospital. Thus, vital information was missing, and the nurse in the hospital was working at a disadvantage.] In addition, it is not uncommon for health care providers to assume that an older person's confusion is a result of either age or an exacerbation of an underlying dementia or both (Fick & Foreman, 2000 [Level IV]). However, this is an erroneous assumption and, in this case, dangerous because the undetected worsening of Mrs. O.'s cognitive impairment resulted in lack of treatment of the underlying hyperglycemia and severe dehydration, leading to her eventual death. The cascade of mortal events could have been prevented with detection of the impairment, diagnosis of delirium, and prompt treatment of the underlying cause.

Summary and Conclusions

The determination of an individual's cognitive status is critical in the process and outcomes of illness and its treatment. Being competent in the assessment of cognitive functioning requires (1) knowledge and skill as they relate to the performance of the assessment of cognitive functioning, (2) sensitivity to the issues that can negatively bias the results and interpretation of this assessment, (3) accurate and comprehensive documentation of the assessment, and (4) the incorporation of the results of the assessment in the development of the individual's plan of care.

Resources

Recommended Instruments for Assessing Cognitive Functioning

Mini-Mental State (Tombaugh & McIntyre, 1992 [Level I]). Retrieved March 9, 2007, from http://www.minimental.com

Mini-Cog (Borson et al., 2000 [Level IV]; Borodaty et al., 2006 [Level I]).

Additional On-Line Information About Cognition in Older Persons

http://www.ConsultGeriRN.org/index.cfm?section_id=31&geriatric_topic_id=11& subsection_id=77&page_id=166&tab=2. Anonymous; last updated January 2005. Normal aging changes. Normal changes with aging of the various body systems, including cognitive functioning, are reviewed in this document.

Additional On-Line Information About Assessing Cognitive Functioning

The Iowa Index of Geriatric Assessment Tools (IIGAT). Retrieved March 9, 2007, from http://fm.iowa.uiowa.edu/fmi/xsl/iigat/index.xsl

"Try This," a series of tips on various aspects of assessing and caring for older adults sponsored by The Hartford Institute for Geriatric Nursing at New York University College of Nursing. Retrieved March 9, 2007, from http://www.ConsultGeriRN.org/publications/trythis/

The Registered Nurse Association of Ontario Best Practice Guideline for *Screening for Delirium, Dementia and Depression in Older Adults.* Retrieved March 9, 2007, from http://rnao.org/Page.asp?PageID=924&ContentID=818

The U.S. Preventive Services Task Force recommendations for *Screening for Dementia.* Retrieved March 9, 2007, from http:www.ahrq.gov/clinic/cps3dix. htm

Recommendations for the early detection of dementia from The American Academy of Neurology. Retrieved March 9, 2007, from http://aan.com/professionals/practice/guideline/index.cfm?a=0&fc=1

Geriatric Toolkits. Retrieved March 9, 2007, from http://www.gericareonline.net/tools/index.html

An Interactive Software Toolkit for the Comprehensive Geriatric Assessment. Retrieved March 9, 2007, from http://www.contexio.com/englishversion.htm

The Health Service/Technology Assess Text Service of the National Library of Medicine provides full text documents of information for making health decisions. Retrieved March 9, 2007, from http://hstat.nlm.nih.gov/hg/Hquest

The National Guideline Clearinghouse. http://www.guideline.gov

Treating delirium: A quick reference guide, by the American Psychiatric Association. Retrieved March 9, 2007, from http://www.psych.org/psych_pract/treatg/pg/prac_guide.cfm

British Geriatrics Society *Guidelines for the prevention, diagnosis, and management of delirium in older people in hospital.* Retrieved March 9, 2007, from http://www.bgs.org.uk/publications/Publications%20Downloads/Delirium-2006.DOC

Delirium & Cognitive Impairment Study Group (2006). *Brain dysfunction in critically ill patients.* Retrieved March 9, 2007, from http://www.icudelirium.org/delirium/

European Delirium Association Web site. Retrieved March 9, 2007, from http://www.europeandeliriumassociation.com

Assessing care of vulnerable elders (ACOVE). Retrieved March 9, 2007, from http://www.rand.org or: http://www.acove.com

Box 4.1

Nursing Standard of Practice Protocol: Assessing Cognitive Functioning

I. GOAL: The goals of cognitive assessment include:
- A. To determine an individual's cognitive abilities.
- B. To recognize early the presence of an impairment in cognitive functioning.
- C. To monitor an individual's cognitive response to various treatments.

II. OVERVIEW

- A. Undetected impairment in cognition is associated with greater morbidity and mortality (Inouye et al., 2001 [Level IV]).
- B. Assessing cognitive function is the foundation for early detection and prompt treatment of impairment (ACOVE Investigators, 2001 [Level I]).

III. BACKGROUND AND STATEMENT OF PROBLEM

A. Definition of cognitive functioning includes the processes by which an individual perceives, registers, stores, retrieves, and uses information.

B. Conditions in which cognitive functioning is impaired:

1. *The Dementias* (e.g., Alzheimer's or vascular) are a syndrome of cognitive deterioration that involves memory impairment and a disturbance in at least one other cognitive function (e.g., aphasia, apraxia, or agnosia) that results in changes in function and behavior (APA, 2000).

2. *Delirium* is a disturbance of consciousness with impaired attention and disorganized thinking that develops rapidly. Evidence of an underlying physiologic or medical condition is generally present (APA, 2000).

3. *Depression* is a syndrome of either depressed mood or loss of interest or pleasure in most activities of the day. These symptoms represent a change from usual functioning for the individual and have been present for at least 2 weeks (APA, 2000).

IV. ASSESSMENT OF COGNITIVE FUNCTION

A. Reasons/Purposes of Assessment

1. Screening: to determine the absence or presence of impairment (Foreman et al., 2003 [Level VI]).

2. Monitoring: to track cognitive status over time, especially response to treatment (Foreman et al., 2003 [Level VI]).

B. How to Assess Cognitive Function

1. Mini-Mental State Examination (Folstein et al., 1975 [Level IV]) can be used to screen for or monitor cognitive function instrument; however, performance on the MMSE is adversely influenced by education, age, language, and verbal ability. The MMSE also is criticized for taking too long to administer and score.

2. Mini-Cog (Borson et al., 2000 [Level IV]) also can be used to screen and monitor cognitive function; is not adversely influenced by age, language, and education; and it takes about half as much time to administer and score as the MMSE.

3. IQCDE is useful to supplement testing with the MMSE or Mini-Cog because it is useful to determine onset, duration, and functional impact of the cognitive impairment. Information from intimate others can be obtained by using the Informant Questionnaire on Cognitive Decline in the Elderly (IQCDE) (Jorm, 1994 [Level IV]).

4. Naturally occurring interactions: Observations and conversations during naturally occurring care interactions can be the impetus for additional screening/monitoring of cognitive function with the MMSE or Mini-Cog (Foreman et al., 2003 [Level VI]).

C. When to Assess Cognitive Function
   1. On admission to and discharge from an institutional care setting (ACOVE Investigators, 2001 [Level I]; British Geriatric Society, 2005 [Level I]).
   2. On transfer from one care setting to another (ACOVE Investigators, 2001 [Level I]).
   3. During hospitalization, every 8 to 12 hours throughout hospitalization (http://www.icudelirium.org/delirium).
   4. As follow-up to hospital care, within 6 weeks of discharge (ACOVE Investigators, 2001 [Level I]).
   5. Before making important health care decisions as an adjunct to determining an individual's capacity to consent (ACOVE Investigators, 2001 [Level I]).
   6. On the first visit to a new care provider (ACOVE Investigators, 2001 [Level I]).
   7. Following major changes in pharmacotherapy (ACOVE Investigators, 2001 [Level I]).
   8. With behavior that is unusual for the individual and/or inappropriate to the situation (Foreman & Vermeersch, 2004 [Level I]).
D. Cautions for Assessing Cognitive Function
   1. Physical environment (Dellasega, 1998 [Level VI]).
      a. Comfortable ambient temperature.
      b. Adequate lighting (i.e., not glaring).
      c. Free of distractions (e.g., should be conducted in the absence of others and other activities).
      d. Position self to maximize individual's sensory abilities.
   2. Interpersonal environment (Engberg & McDowell, 1999 [Level VI]).
      a. Prepare individual for assessment.
      b. Initiate assessment within nonthreatening conversation.
      c. Let individual set pace of assessment.
      d. Be emotionally nonthreatening.
   3. Timing of assessment (Foreman et al., 2003 [Level VI]).
      a. Select time of assessment to reflect actual cognitive abilities of the individual.
      b. Avoid the following times:
         i. Immediately on awakening from sleep; wait at least 30 minutes.
         ii. Immediately before and after meals.
         iii. Immediately before and after medical diagnostic or therapeutic procedures.
         iv. In the presence of pain or discomfort.

V. EVALUATION/EXPECTED OUTCOMES

A. Patient
   1. Is assessed at recommended time points.

2. Any impairment detected early.
3. Care tailored to appropriately address cognitive status/impairment.
4. Satisfaction with care improved.
B. Health Care Provider
1. Competent to assess cognitive function.
2. Able to differentiate among delirium, dementia, and depression.
3. Uses standardized cognitive assessment protocol.
4. Satisfaction with care improved.
C. Institution
1. Improved documentation of cognitive assessments.
2. Impairments in cognitive function identified promptly and accurately.
3. Improved referral to appropriate advanced providers (e.g., geriatricians, geriatric nurse practitioners) for additional assessment and treatment recommendations.
4. Decreased overall costs of care.

VI. FOLLOW-UP MONITORING

A. Provider competence in the assessment of cognitive function.
B. Consistent and appropriate documentation of cognitive assessment.
C. Consistent and appropriate care and follow-up in instances of impairment.
D. Timely and appropriate referral for diagnostic and treatment recommendations.

VII. RELEVANT PRACTICE GUIDELINES

A. The Registered Nurse Association of Ontario Best Practice Guideline for *Screening for Delirium, Dementia and Depression in Older Adults*. Retrieved March 9, 2007, from http://rnao.org/Page.asp?PageID=924&ContentID=818
B. The U.S. Preventive Services Task Force recommendations for *Screening for Dementia*. Retrieved March 9, 2007, from http:www.ahrq.gov/clinic/cps3dix.htm
C. Recommendations for the early detection of dementia from The American Academy of Neurology. Retrieved March 9, 2007, from http://aan.com/professionals/practice/guideline/index.cfm?a=0&fc=1.
D. The National Guideline Clearinghouse. http://www.guideline.gov.

References

ACOVE Investigators (2001). ACOVE quality indicators. *Annals of Internal Medicine, 135*, 653–667. Evidence Level I: Systematic Review.
Alagiakrishnan, K., Marrie, T., Rolfson, D., Coke, W., Camicioli, R., Duggan, D., et al. (2007). Simple cognitive testing (Mini-Cog) predicts in-hospital delirium in the elderly [letter].

Journal of the American Geriatrics Society, 55, 314–316. Evidence Level IV: Nonexperimental Study.

American Psychiatric Association (2000). *Diagnostic and statistical manual of mental disorders* (4th ed., text revision). Washington, DC: Author.

Borson, S., Scanlan, J. M., Brush, M., Vitaliano, P., & Dokmak, A. (2000). The Mini-Cog: A cognitive 'vital signs' measure for dementia screening in multi-lingual elderly. *International Journal of Geriatric Psychiatry, 15*, 1021–1027. Evidence Level IV: Nonexperimental Study.

Borson, S., Scanlan, J. M., Watanabe, J., Tu, S., & Lessig, M. (2005). Simplifying detection of cognitive impairment: Comparison of the Mini-Cog and Mini-Mental State Examination in a multiethnic sample. *Journal of the American Geriatrics Society, 53*, 871–874. Evidence Level IV: Nonexperimental Study.

British Geriatrics Society (2005). Guidelines for the prevention, diagnosis, and management of delirium in older people in hospital. Retrieved March 9, 2007, from http://www.bgs.org.uk/publications/Publications%20Downloads/Delirium-2006.DOC. Evidence Level I: Systematic Review.

Brodaty, H., Low, L. F., Gibson, L., & Burns, K. (2006). What is the best dementia screening instrument for general practitioners to use? *American Journal of Geriatric Psychiatry, 14*, 391–400. Evidence Level I: Systematic Review.

Chow, T. W., & MacLean, C. H. (2001). Quality indicators for dementia in vulnerable community-dwelling and hospitalized elders. *Annals of Internal Medicine, 135*, 668–676. Evidence Level I: Systematic Review.

Cole, M. G., McCusker, J., Bellavance, F., Primeau, F. J., Bailey, R. F., Bonnycastle, M. J., et al. (2002). Systematic detection and multidisciplinary care of delirium in older medical inpatients: A randomized trial. *Canadian Medical Association Journal, 167*, 753–759. Evidence Level II: Single Experimental Study.

Delirium and Cognitive Impairment Study Group (2006). *Brain dysfunction in critically ill patients*. Retrieved March 9, 2007, from http://www.icudelirium.org/delirium

Dellasega, C. (1998). Assessment of cognition in the elderly: Pieces of a complex puzzle. *Nursing Clinics of North America, 33*, 395–405. Evidence Level VI: Expert Opinion.

Ely, E. W., Stephens, R. K., Jackson, J. C., Thomason, J. W. W., Truman, B., Gordon, S., et al. (2004). Current opinions regarding the importance, diagnosis, and management of delirium in the intensive care unit: A survey of 912 healthcare professionals. *Critical Care Medicine, 32*, 106–112. Evidence Level IV: Nonexperimental Study.

Engberg, S. J., & McDowell, J. (1999). Comprehensive geriatric assessment. In J. T. Stone, J. F. Wyman, & S. A. Salisbury (Eds.), *Clinical gerontological nursing: A guide to advanced practice* (2nd ed., pp. 63–85). Philadelphia: Saunders. Evidence Level VI: Expert Opinion.

Fick, D. M., Agostini, J. V., & Inouye, S. K. (2002). Delirium superimposed on dementia: A systematic review. *Journal of the American Geriatrics Society, 50*, 1723–1732. Evidence Level I: Systematic Review.

Fick, D. M., & Foreman, M. D. (2000). Consequences of not recognizing delirium superimposed on dementia in hospitalized elderly individuals. *Journal of Gerontological Nursing, 26*, 30–40. Evidence Level IV: Nonexperimental Study.

Fletcher, K. (2007). Dementia. In E. Capezuti, D. Zwicker, M. Mezey, & T. Fulmer (Eds.), *Evidence-based geriatric nursing protocols* (3rd ed., chap. 6). New York: Springer Publishing Company. Evidence Level VI: Expert Opinion.

Folstein, M. F., Folstein, S. E., & McHugh, P. R. (1975). "Mini-Mental State": A practical method for grading the cognitive state of patients for the clinician. *Journal of Psychiatric Research, 12*, 189–198. Evidence Level IV: Nonexperimental Study.

Foreman, M. D., Fletcher, K., Mion, L. C., & Trygstad, L. (2003). Assessing cognitive function. In M. Mezey, T. Fulmer, & I. Abraham (Eds.), & D. Zwicker (Managing Ed.), *Geriatric nursing protocols for best practice* (2nd ed., pp. 99–115). New York: Springer Publishing Company. Evidence Level VI: Expert Opinion.

Foreman, M. D., & Milisen, K. (2004). Improving recognition of delirium in the elderly. *Primary Psychiatry, 11*, 46–50. Evidence Level I: Systematic Review.

Foreman, M. D., & Vermeersch, P. E. H. (2004). Measuring cognitive status. In M. Frank-Stromborg & S. J. Olsen (Eds.), *Instruments of clinical health-care research* (3rd ed., pp. 100–127). Sudbury, MA: Jones and Bartlett. Evidence Level I: Systematic Review.

Han, L., Cole, M., Bellavance, F., McCusker, J., & Primeau, F. (2000). Tracking cognitive decline in Alzheimer's disease using the Mini-Mental State Examination: A meta-analysis. *International Psychogeriatrics, 12*, 231–247. Evidence Level I: Systematic Review.

Hopkins, R. O., & Jackson, J. C. (2006). Assessing neurocognitive outcomes after critical illness: Are delirium and long-term cognitive impairments related? *Current Opinion in Critical Care, 12,* 388–394. Evidence Level IV: Nonexperimental Study.

Inouye, S. K., Foreman, M. D., Mion, L. C., Katz, K. H., & Cooney, L. M., Jr. (2001). Nurses' recognition of delirium and its symptoms: Comparison of nurse and researcher ratings. *Archives of Internal Medicine, 161,* 2467–2473. Evidence Level IV: Nonexperimental Study.

Inouye, S. K., Van Dyck, C. H., Alessi, C. A., Balkin, S., Siegel, A. P., & Horwitz, P. I. (1990). Clarifying confusion: The Confusion Assessment Method. A new method for detecting delirium. *Annals of Internal Medicine, 113,* 941–948. Evidence Level IV: Nonexperimental Study.

Jorm, A. (1994). A short form of the Informant Questionnaire on Cognitive Decline in the Elderly (IQCODE): Development and cross-validation. *Psychological Medicine, 24,* 145–153. Evidence Level IV: Nonexperimental Study.

Lang, P. O., Heitz, D., Hedelin, G., Drame, M., Jovenin, N., Ankri, J., et al. (2006). Early markers of prolonged hospital stays in older people: A prospective, multicenter study of 908 inpatients in French acute hospitals. *Journal of the American Geriatrics Society, 54,* 1031–1039. Evidence Level IV: Nonexperimental Study.

Lezak, M. D., Howieson, D. B., & Loring, D. W. (2004). *Neuropsychological assessment,* 4th ed. New York: Oxford University Press. Evidence Level VI: Expert Opinion.

McEvoy, C. L. (2001). Cognitive changes in aging. In M. D. Mezey (Ed.), *The encyclopedia of elder care* (pp. 139–141). New York: Springer Publishing Company. Evidence Level VI: Expert Opinion.

Michaud, L., Bula, C., Berney, A., Camus, V., Voellinger, R., Stiefel, F., et al. (2007). Delirium: Guidelines for general hospitals. *Journal of Psychosomatic Research, 62,* 371–383. Evidence Level I: Systematic Review.

Milbrandt, E. B., Deppen, S., Harrison, P. L., Shintani, A. K., Speroff, T., Stiles, R. A., et al. (2004). Costs associated with delirium in mechanically ventilated patients. *Critical Care Medicine, 32,* 955–962. Evidence Level IV: Nonexperimental Study.

Milisen, K., Braes, T., Fick, D. M., & Foreman, M. D. (2006). Cognitive assessment and differentiating the 3 Ds (dementia, depression, delirium). *Nursing Clinics of North America, 1,* 1–22. Evidence Level VI: Expert Opinion.

Milisen, K., Cremers, S., Foreman, M. D., Vandevelde, E., Haspeslagh, M., DeGeest, S., et al. (2004). The Strain of Care for Delirium Index: A new instrument to assess nurses' strain in caring for patients with delirium. *International Journal of Nursing Studies, 41,* 775–783. Evidence Level IV: Nonexperimental Study.

O'Keefe, S. T., Mulkerrin, E. C., Nayeem, K., Varughese, M., & Pillay, I. (2005). Use of serial Mini-Mental State Examinations to diagnose and monitor delirium in elderly hospital patients. *Journal of the American Geriatrics Society, 53,* 867–870. Evidence Level IV: Nonexperimental Study.

Peterson, R. C., Stevens, J. C., Ganguli, M., Tangalos, E. G., Cummings, J. L., & DeKosky, S. T. (2001). Practice parameters: Early detection of dementia: Mild cognitive impairment (an evidence-based review). Report of the Quality Standards Subcommittee of the American Academy of Neurology. *Neurology, 56,* 1133–1142. Evidence Level I: Systematic Review.

Registered Nurse Association of Ontario (RNAO) (2003). *Screening for Delirium, Dementia and Depression in Older Adults.* Retrieved March 9, 2007, from http://rnao.org/Page.asp?PageID=924&ContentID=818

Scottish Intercollegiate Guidelines Network (2005). Management of patients with dementia: A national clinical guideline. Retrieved March 9, 2007, from http://www.guideline.gov/summary/summary.aspx?doc_id=8809&nbr=4855. Evidence Level I: Systematic Review.

Tombaugh, T. N., & McIntyre, N. J. (1992). The Mini-Mental State Examination: A comprehensive review. *Journal of the American Geriatrics Society, 40,* 922–935. Evidence Level I: Systematic Review.

Tullman, D. F., Mion, L. C., Fletcher, K., & Foreman, M. D. (2007). Delirium: Prevention, early recognition, and treatment. In E. Capezuti, D. Zwicker, M. Mezey, T. Fulmer (Eds.), *Evidence-based geriatric nursing protocols* (3rd ed., chap. 6). New York: Springer Publishing Company. Evidence Level VI: Expert Opinion.

U.S. Preventive Services Task Force (2003). Screening for dementia: Recommendation and rationale. *Annals of Internal Medicine, 138,* 925–926. Evidence Level I: Systematic Review.

Depression

5

Lenore H. Kurlowicz
Theresa A. Harvath

Educational Objectives

On completion of this chapter, the reader will be able to:

1. discuss the consequences of late-life depression

2. discuss the major risk factors for late-life depression

3. identify the core competencies of a systematic nursing assessment for depression with older adults

4. identify nursing strategies for older adults with depression

Depression in Older Adults

Contrary to popular belief, depression is not a normal part of aging. Rather, depression is a medical disorder that causes suffering for patients and their families, interferes with a person's ability to function, exacerbates coexisting medical illnesses, and increases utilization of health services (Lebowitz, 1996). Despite the efficacious treatments available for late-life depression, many older adults lack access to adequate resources; barriers in the health care reimbursement system are particular challenges for low-income and ethnic minority

For a description of Evidence Levels cited in this chapter, see chapter 1, Developing and Evaluating Clinical Practice Guidelines, page 4.

elders (Charney et al., 2003). In a comprehensive review of research on the prevalence of depression in later life, Hybels & Blazer (2003) found that although major depressive disorders are not prevalent in late life (1% to 5%), the prevalence of clinically significant depressive symptoms is high. What is more, these depressive symptoms are associated with higher morbidity and mortality rates in older adults (Bagulho, 2002 [Level V]; Lyness et al., 2007 [Level IV]).

The rates of depressive symptoms vary, depending on the population of older adults: community-dwelling older adults (3% to 26%), primary care (10%), hospitalized elders (23%), and nursing home residents (16% to 30%) (Hybels & Blazer, 2003). Certain subgroups have higher levels of depressive symptoms, particularly those with more severe or chronic disabling conditions, such as those older adults in acute- and long term care settings. Depression also frequently coexists with dementia, specifically Alzheimer's disease, with prevalence rates ranging from 22% to 54% (Zubenko et al., 2003). Cognitive impairment may be a secondary symptom of depression or depression may be the result of dementia (Blazer, 2002; Blazer, 2003 [both Level VI]). The prevalence of major depression has been increasing in those born more recently; therefore, it can be expected that the prevalence of depression in older adults will increase in the years to come.

Late-life depression occurs within a context of medical illnesses, disability, cognitive dysfunction, and psychosocial adversity frequently impeding timely recognition and treatment of depression, with subsequent unnecessary morbidity and death (Bagulho, 2002 [Level V]; Lyness et al., 2007 [Level IV]). A substantial number of older patients encountered by nurses will have clinically relevant depressive symptoms. Nurses remain at the front line in the early recognition of depression and the facilitation of older patients' access to mental-health care. This chapter presents an overview of depression in older patients, with emphasis on age-related assessment considerations, clinical decision making, and nursing-intervention strategies for older adults with depression. A standard of practice protocol for use by nurses in practice settings also is presented.

What Is Depression?

In the broadest sense, depression is defined as a syndrome consisting of a constellation of affective, cognitive, and somatic or physiological manifestations (National Institute of Health [NIH] Consensus Development Panel, 1992 [Level II]). Depression may range in severity from mild symptoms to more severe forms, both of which can persist over longer periods with negative consequences for the older patient. Suicidal ideation, psychotic features (especially delusional thinking), and excessive somatic concerns frequently accompany more severe depression (NIH Consensus Development Panel, 1992 [Level II]). Symptoms of anxiety may also coexist with depression in many older adults (Cassidy, Lauderdale, & Sheikh, 2005 [Level III]; DeLuca et al., 2005 [Level IV]). In fact, comorbid anxiety and depression have been associated with more severe symptoms, decreases in memory, poorer treatment outcomes (Deluca et al., 2005 [Level IV]; Lenze et al., 2001), and increased rates of suicidal ideation (Sareen et al. [Level IV], 2005).

Major Depression

The *Diagnostic and Statistical Manual of Mental Disorders* (*DSM-IV-TR*) (American Psychiatric Association, 2000 [Level VI]) lists criteria for the diagnosis of major depressive disorder, the most severe form of depression. These criteria are frequently used as the standard by which older patients' depressive symptoms are assessed in clinical settings (American Psychiatric Association, 2000 [Level VI]). Five criteria from a list of nine must be present nearly every day during the same 2-week period and must represent a change from previous functioning: (1) depressed, sad, or irritable mood; (2) anhedonia or diminished pleasure in usually pleasurable people or activities; (3) feelings of worthlessness, self-reproach, or excessive guilt; (4) difficulty with thinking or diminished concentration; (5) suicidal thinking or attempts; (6) fatigue and loss of energy; (7) changes in appetite and weight; (8) disturbed sleep; and (9) psychomotor agitation or retardation. For this diagnosis, at least one of the five symptoms must include either depressed mood, by the patient's subjective account or observation of others, or markedly diminished pleasure in almost all people or activities. Concurrent medical conditions are frequently present in older patients and should not preclude a diagnosis of depression; indeed, there is a high incidence of medical co-morbidity.

Major depression, as defined by the *DSM-IV-TR*, seems to be as common among older as younger cohorts. However, older adults may more readily report somatic or physical symptoms than depressed mood (Pfaff & Almeida, 2005 [Level IV]). The somatic or physical symptoms of depression, however, are often difficult to distinguish from somatic or physical symptoms associated with acute or chronic physical illness, especially in hospitalized older patients, or the somatic symptoms that are part of common aging processes (Kurlowicz, 1994). For instance, disturbed sleep may be associated with chronic lung disease or congestive heart failure. Diminished energy or increased lethargy may be caused by an acute metabolic disturbance or drug response. Therefore, a challenge for nurses in acute care hospitals and other clinical settings is to not overlook or disregard somatic or physical complaints while also "looking beyond" such complaints to assess the full spectrum of depressive symptoms in older patients. In older adults with acute medical illnesses, somatic symptoms that persist may indicate a more serious depression, despite treatment of the underlying medical illness or discontinuance of a depressogenic medication (Kurlowicz, 1994). Older patients may link their somatic or physical complaints as the cause of their depressed mood or anhedonia. Depression may also be expressed through repetitive verbalizations (e.g., calling out for help) or agitated vocalizations (e.g., screaming, yelling, or shouting), repetitive questions, expressions of unrealistic fears (e.g., fear of abandonment, being left alone), repetitive statements that something bad will happen, repetitive health-related concerns, and verbal and/or physical aggression (Cohen-Mansfield, Werner, & Marx, 1990).

Minor Depression

Depressive symptoms that do not meet standard criteria for a specific depressive disorder are highly prevalent (15% to 25%) in older adults. These symptoms are clinically significant and warrant treatment (Bagulho, 2002 [Level V]; Lyness et al., 2007) [Level IV]. Such depressive symptoms have been variously referred to in the literature as *minor depression*, *subsyndromal depression*, *dysthymic depression*, *subclinical depression*, *elevated depressive symptoms*, and *mild depression*. The *DSM-IV-TR* also lists criteria for the diagnosis of *minor depressive disorder* and includes episodes of at least 2 weeks of depressive symptoms but with fewer than the five criteria required for major depressive disorder. Minor depression is two to four times as common as major depression in older adults, is associated with increased risk of subsequent major depression and greater use of health services, and has a negative impact on physical and social functioning and quality of life (Bagulho, 2002 [Level V]; Gaynes, Burns, Tweed, & Erickson, 2002 [Level III]; Lyness et al., 2007 [Level IV]).

Course of Depression

Depression can occur for the first time in late life or it can be part of a long-standing affective or mood disorder with onset in earlier years. Hospitalized older medical patients with depression are also more likely to have had previous depression and experience higher rates of mortality than older patients without depression (von Ammon Cavanaugh, Furlanetto, Creech, & Powell, 2001 [Level III]). As in younger people, the course of depression in older adults is characterized by exacerbations, remissions, and chronicity (NIH Consensus Development Panel, 1992 [Level I]). Therefore, a wait-and-see approach with regard to treatment is not recommended.

Depression in Late Life Is Serious

Depression is associated with serious negative consequences for older adults, especially for frail older patients, such as those recovering from a severe medical illness or those in nursing homes. Consequences of depression include heightened pain and disability, delayed recovery from medical illness or surgery, worsening of medical symptoms, risk of physical illness, increased health care utilization, alcoholism, cognitive impairment, worsening social impairment, protein-calorie subnutrition, and increased rates of suicide and nonsuicide-related death (Bagulho, 2002 [Level V]; von Ammon Cavanaugh et al., 2001 [Level III]). The "amplification" hypothesis proposed by Katz, Streim, and Parmelee (1994) stated that depression can "turn up the volume" on several aspects of physical, psychosocial, and behavioral functioning in older patients, ultimately accelerating the course of medical illness. Indeed, a recent study by Gaynes et al. (2002 [Level III]) found that major depression and co-morbid medical conditions interacted to adversely affect health-related quality of life in older adults. For older nursing home residents, depression is also associated with poor adjustment to the nursing home, resistance to daily care, treatment refusal, inability to participate in activities, and further social isolation (Achterberg et al., 2003 [Level IV]).

Mortality by suicide is higher among older persons with depression than among their counterparts without depression (Juurlink, Herrmann, Szalai, Kopp, & Redelmeier, 2004 [Level IV]). Rates of suicide among older adults (i.e., 15 to 20 per 100,000) are the highest of any age group and even exceed rates among adolescents (McKeown, Cuffe, & Schulz, 2006 [Level V]). This is in large part due to the fact that White men older than age 85 are at greatest risk for suicide, where rates of suicide are estimated to be 80 to 113 per 100,000 (Erlangsen, Vach, & Jeune, [Level IV] 2005 [Level III]). In the oldest old (i.e., 80 years or older), men and women have higher suicide rates than nonhospitalized older adults in the same age range; this age group has significantly higher rates of hospitalization than younger cohorts; and three or more medical diagnoses are associated with increased suicide risk (Erlangsen et al., 2005 [Level III]).

Depressive symptoms, perceived health status, sleep quality, and absence of confidant predict late-life suicide (Turvey et al., 2002 [Level IV]). Whereas physical illness and functional impairment increase risk for suicide in older adults, it appears that this relationship is strengthened by co-morbid depression (Conwell, Duberstein, & Caine, 2002 [Level VI]). Disruption of social support (Conwell et al., 2002 [Level VI]), family conflict, and loneliness (Waern, Rubenowitz, & Wilhelmson, 2003 [Level V]) are also significantly associated with suicide in late life. Treatment of depression rapidly decreases suicidal ideation in older adults (Bruce et al., 2004 [Level II]; Szanto, Mulsant, Houck, Dew, & Reynolds, 2003 [Level V]). However, elders in higher risk groups (i.e., male, older) need a significantly longer response time to demonstrate a decrease in suicidal ideation (Szanto et al., 2003 [Level V]).

Studies have also shown that contact between suicidal older adults and their primary-care provider is common (Luoma, Martin, & Pearson, 2002 [Level V]). Almost half of older suicide victims have seen their primary-care provider within 1 month of committing suicide (Luoma et al., 2002 [Level V]), and 20% have seen a mental-health provider. Most of the suicidal patients experienced their first episode of major depression, which was only moderately severe, yet the depressive symptoms went unrecognized and untreated. Older adults with clinically significant depressive symptomatology present with physical rather than psychological symptoms, including patients who, when asked, admitted having suicidal ideation (Pfaff & Almeida, 2005 [Level IV]).

Although the risk for suicide increases with advancing age (Hybels & Blazer, 2003), a growing body of evidence suggests that depression is also associated with higher rates of nonsuicide mortality in older adults (Schulz, Drayer, & Rollman, 2002). Depression can also influence decision-making capacity and may be the cause of indirect life-threatening behavior such as refusal of food, medications, or other treatments in older persons (McDade-Montez, Christensen, Cvengros, & Lawton, 2006; Stapleton, Nielsen, Engelberg, Patrick, & Curtis, 2005). These observations suggest that accurate diagnosis and treatment of depression in older patients may reduce the mortality rate in this population. It is in the clinical setting, therefore, that screening procedures and assessment protocols have the most direct impact.

Depression in Late Life Is Misunderstood

Despite its prevalence, associated negative outcomes, and good treatment response, depression in older adults is highly under-recognized, misdiagnosed, and subsequently under-treated. According to a report by the Administration on Aging (2001), less than 3% of older adults receive treatment from mental-health professionals. Use of mental-health services is lower for older adults than any other age group (Administration on Aging, 2001). Barriers to care for older adults with depression exist at many levels. In particular, some older adults refuse to seek help because of perceived stigma of mental illness.

Others may simply accept their feelings of profound sadness without realizing they are clinically depressed. Recognition of depression also is frequently obscured by anxiety and/or the various somatic or dementia-like symptoms manifest in older patients with depression, or because patient or providers believe that it is a "normal" response to medical illness, hospitalization, relocation to a nursing home, or other stressful life events. However, depression—major or minor—is not a necessary or normative consequence of life adversity (Snowdon, 2001). When depression occurs after an adverse life event, it represents pathology that should be treated.

Treatment for Late-Life Depression Works

The goals of treating depression in older patients are to decrease depressive symptoms, reduce relapse and recurrence, improve functioning and quality of life, improve medical health, and reduce mortality and health care costs. Depression in older patients can be effectively treated using either pharmacotherapy or psychosocial therapies, or both (Blazer, 2002; Blazer, 2003; Mackin & Arean, 2005 [all Level VI]). If recognized, the treatment response for depression is good: 60% to 80% of older adults remain relapse-free with medication maintenance for 6 to 18 months (NIH Consensus Development Panel, 1992 [Level I]). In addition, treatment of depression improves pain and functional outcomes in older adults (Lin et al., 2003 [Level II]). Recurrence of depression is a serious problem and has been associated with reduced responsiveness to treatment and higher rates of cognitive and functional decline (Driscoll et al., 2005 [Level IV]). When compared to younger patients, older adults demonstrate comparable treatment response rates; however, they tend to have higher rates of relapse following treatment (Mitchell & Subramaniam, 2005 [Level I]). Therefore, continuation of treatment to prevent early relapse and longer-term maintenance treatment to prevent later occurrences is important. Even in those patients with depression who have a co-morbid medical illness or dementia, treatment response can be good (Iosifescu, 2007 [Level V]). Depressed older patients who have mild cognitive impairment are at greater risk for developing dementia if their depression goes untreated (Modrego & Ferrandez, 2004 [Level IV]).

Cause and Risk Factors

Several biologic and psychosocial causes for late-life depression have been proposed. Genetic factors or heredity seem to play more of a role when older adults have had depression throughout their life (Blazer & Hybels, 2005 [Level VI]). Additional biologic causes proposed for late-life depression include neurotransmitter or "chemical messenger" imbalance or dysregulation of endocrine function (Blazer, 2002; Blazer, 2003 [both Level VI]). Neuroanatomic correlates, cerebrovascular disease, brain metabolism alterations, gross brain disease, and the presence of apolipoprotein E have also been etiologically linked to late-life depression (Butters et al., 2003 [Level IV]). Possible psychosocial causes for depression in older adults include cognitive distortions, stressful life events (especially loss), chronic stress, low self-efficacy expectations (Blazer, 2002; Blazer, 2003; Blazer & Hybels, 2005 [all Level VI]), and a history of alcohol abuse (Hasin & Grant, 2002 [Level III]) (see chapter 29, *Substance Abuse*).

The social and demographic risk factors for depression in older adults include female sex, unmarried status (particularly widowed), stressful life events, and the absence of a supportive social network (NIH Consensus Development Panel, 1992 [Level I]). It is interesting that in a meta-analysis of the impact of negative life events on depression in older adults, Kraaij, Arensman, and Spinhoven (2002 [Level I]) found that although specific negative life events (e.g., death of significant others, illness in self or spouse, or negative relationship events) were moderately associated with increases in depression, the total number of negative life events and daily hassles had the strongest relationships to depression in older adults. The stress associated with family caregiving has been repeatedly associated with higher rates of depression in older caregivers (Pinquart & Sorensen, 2004 [Level I]). In particular, caring for an older adult with dementia has been associated with higher rates of depression than other caregiving situations (Pinquart & Sorensen, 2004 [Level I]). This suggests that clinicians should pay close attention to the accumulation of negative life events and daily hassles when developing programs and targeting interventions to mitigate depression in an older adult who is at risk for developing depression.

In older adults, there is additional emphasis on the co-occurrence of specific physical conditions such as stroke, cancer, dementia, arthritis, hip-fracture surgery, myocardial infarction, chronic obstructive pulmonary disease, and Parkinson's disease. Medical co-morbidity is the hallmark of depression in older patients, and this factor represents a major difference from depression in younger populations (Alexopoulos, Schultz, & Lebowitz, 2005 [Level VI]). In an evidence-based review, Cole (2005 [Level I]) found that disability, older age, new medical diagnosis, and poor health status were among the most robust and consistent of all correlates of depression among older medical patients. Those with functional disabilities, especially those with new functional loss, are also at risk. For example, co-morbid depression is common in older patients with hip fractures (Holmes & House, 2000 [Level I]; see table 5.1).

Major depressive disorder has been found to be twice as common in community-dwelling older adults compared to primary-care settings (Bruce et al., 2002 [Level VI]). In a systematic review and meta-analysis, Cole and Dendukuuri (2003 [Level I]) found that depression in community-dwelling older adults was associated with bereavement, sleep disturbance, disability, prior depression, and female gender. Other significant factors included poor health status, poor self-perceived health, and new medical illness with disability (Cole, 2005; Cole & Dendukuuri, 2003 [both Level I]).

Depression Among Minority Older Adults

Rates of depression among minority older adults are not well understood. Beals and colleagues (2005 [Level IV]) found that the rates of major depressive episodes among older American Indians were 30% of the national average. In a review, Kales and Mellow (2006 [Level VI]) found lower rates of depression and higher rates of psychotic diagnoses among African American older adults. Williams and colleagues (2007 [Level IV]) found that when African American and Caribbean Blacks experience a major depressive disorder, it is usually untreated, more severe, and more disabling than for non-Hispanic Whites. Furthermore, significant disparities exist in the quality of mental-health services received by minority older adults (Virnig et al., 2004 [Level IV]). A

5.1 Physical Illnesses Associated with Depression in Older Patients Alexopoulos et al., 2005 [Level VI]; Cole, 2005 [Level I]; Holmes & House, 2000 [Level I]

Metabolic disturbances
- Dehydration
- Azotemia, uremia
- Acid-base disturbances
- Hypoxia
- Hyponatremia and hypernatremia
- Hypoglycemia and hyperglycemia
- Hypocalcemia and hypercalcemia

Endocrine disorders
- Hypothyroidism and hyperthyroidism
- Hyperparathyroidism
- Diabetes mellitus
- Cushing's Disease
- Addison's Disease

Infections
- Viral
  - Pneumonia
  - Encephalitis
- Bacterial
- Pneumonia
- Urinary tract
- Meningitis
- Endocarditis
- Other
  - Tuberculosis
  - Brucellosis
  - Fungal meningitis
  - Neurosyphilis

Cardiovascular disorders
- Congestive heart failure
- Myocardial infarction, angina

Pulmonary disorders
- Chronic obstructive lung disease
- Malignancy

5.1 **(continued)**

Gastrointestinal disorders
- Malignancy (especially pancreatic)
- Irritable bowel
- Other organic causes of chronic abdominal pain, ulcer, diverticulosis
- Hepatitis

Genitourinary disorders
- Urinary incontinence

Musculoskeletal disorders
- Degenerative arthritis

Osteoporosis with vertebral compression or hip fractures
- Polymyalgia rheumatica
- Paget's disease

Neurologic disorders
- Cerebrovascular disease
- Transient ischemic attacks
- Stroke
- Dementia (all types)
- Intracranial mass
- Primary or metastatic tumors
- Parkinson's disease

Other Illness
- Anemia (of any cause)
- Vitamin deficiencies
- Hematologic or other systemic malignancy

Immune Disorders

study of Medicare-plus enrollees revealed that minority older adults received substantially less follow-up for mental-health problems following hospitalization (Virnig et al., 2004 [Level IV]).

Although misdiagnosis and subsequent inappropriate treatment can lead to poor health outcomes for minority older adults (Kales & Mellow, 2006 [Level VI]), it is not clear that "simple" bias alone can explain the disparities in depression management that exist. For example, Beals and colleagues (2005 [Level IV]) point out that differences in the social construction of depressive experiences may confound the measurement of depression in ethnic older adults. Older American Indians may be reluctant to endorse symptoms of depression because cultural norms associate these complaints with weakness (Beals et al., 2005 [Level IV]). In a thoughtful analysis of health disparities, Cooper and colleagues (2006 [Level VI]) explored the complex interactions and relationships between patients and providers that frame the context in which disparities can occur. They point out that many historical, cultural, and class-related factors can influence the development of therapeutic relationships between providers and patients. Until more research clarifies the symptom pattern of late-life depression in minority populations, it is important that clinicians be open to atypical presentations of depression that warrant closer scrutiny.

Assessment of Depression in Older Adults

Box 5.1 presents a standard of practice protocol for depression in older adults that emphasizes a systematic assessment guide for early recognition of depression by nurses in hospitals and other clinical settings. Early recognition of depression is enhanced by targeting high risk groups of older adults for assessment methods that are routine, standardized, and systematic, by use of both a depression-screening tool and individualized depression assessment or interview (Piven, 2001 [Level VI]).

Depression-Screening Tool

Nursing assessment of depression in older patients can be facilitated by the use of a screening tool designed to detect symptoms of depression. Several depression-screening tools have been developed for use with older adults. In a systematic review, Watson and Pignone (2003 [Level I]) evaluated the accuracy of different depression-screening tools. They found that the Geriatric Depression Scale-Short Form (GDS-SF) (Sheikh & Yesavage, 1986), the Center for Epidemiological Studies Depression Scale (CES-D) (Radloff, 1977), and the SELFCARE(D) (Banerjee, Shamash, MacDonald, & Mann, 1998) were the most accurate screening tools to detect major depression as well as subsyndromal depressive symptoms (Watson & Pignone, 2003 [Level I]).

The GDS-SF is a 15-item self-report depression screening tool that is frequently used in a variety of clinical settings. This scale has been validated and used extensively with older adults, including those who are mentally ill, mild to moderately cognitively impaired, or institutionalized. It has a brief yes/no response format and takes approximately 5 minutes to complete. The GDS-SF contains few somatic items that may be potentially confounded with symptoms caused by a medical illness. A GDS-SF score of 11 or greater is almost always indicative of depression, and a score of 6 to 9 indicates possible depression warranting further evaluation (Sheikh & Yesavage, 1986). The GDS-SF is not a substitute for an individualized assessment or a diagnostic interview by a mental-health professional but is a useful screening tool to identify an elderly patient's depression. Because many older adults do not present with obvious depressive symptoms (Pfaff & Almeida, 2005 [Level IV]), it is important that screening for depression among older adults is incorporated into routine health assessments.

Individualized Assessment and Interview

Central to the individualized depression assessment and interview is a focused assessment of the full spectrum of symptoms (nine) for major depression as delineated by the *DSM-IV-TR* (American Psychiatric Association, 2000 [Level VI]). Furthermore, patients should be asked directly and specifically if they have been having suicidal ideation—that is, thoughts that life is not worth living—or if they have been contemplating or have attempted suicide. The number of symptoms, type, duration, frequency, and patterns of depressive symptoms, as well as a change from the patient's normal mood of functioning, should be noted. Additional components of the individualized depression assessment include evidence of psychotic thinking (especially delusional thoughts), anniversary dates of previous losses or nodal/stressful events, previous coping style (specifically alcohol or other substance abuse), relationship changes, physical health changes, a history of depression or other psychiatric illness that required some form of treatment, a general loss and crises inventory, and any concurrent life stressors. Subsequent questioning of the family or caregiver is recommended to obtain further information about the elder's verbal and nonverbal expressions of depression.

Differentiation of Medical or Iatrogenic Causes of Depression

Once depressive symptoms are recognized, medical and drug-related causes should be explored. As part of the initial assessment of depression in the older patient, it is important to obtain and review the medical history and physical and/or neurological examinations. Key laboratory tests also should be obtained and/or reviewed and include thyroid-stimulating hormone levels, chemistry screen, complete blood count, and medication levels, if needed. An electrocardiogram, serum B12, urinalysis, and serum folate also should be considered to assess for coexisting medical conditions. These conditions may contribute to depression or might complicate treatment of the depression (Alexopoulos, Katz, Reynolds, Carpenter, & Docherty, 2001 [Level VI]; see Table 5.2). In medically ill older patients, who frequently have multiple medical diagnoses and are prescribed multiple medications, these "organic" factors in the cause of depression are a major issue in nursing assessment. In collaboration with the patient's physician, efforts should be directed toward treatment, correction, or stabilization of associated metabolic or systemic conditions. When medically feasible, depressogenic medications should be eliminated, minimized, or substituted with those that are less depressogenic (Dhondt et al., 1999 [Level IV]). Even when an underlying medical condition or medication is contributing to the depression, treatment of that condition or discontinuation or substitution of the offending agent alone is often not sufficient to resolve the depression, and antidepressant medication is often needed.

Antihypertensives
- Reserpine
- Methyldopa
- Propranolol
- Clonidine
- Hydralazine
- Guanethidine
- Diuretics*

Narcotic analgesics
- Narcotic
- Morphine
- Codeine
- Meperidine
- Pentazocine
- Propoxphene

Nonnarcotic analgesic
- Indomethacin

Antiparkinsonian agents
- L–Dopa

Antimicrobials
- Sulfonamides
- Isoniazid

Cardiovascular agents
- Digitalis
- Lidocaine+

Hypoglycemic agents+
- Steroids
- Corticosteroids
- Estrogens

Others
- Cimetidine
- Cancer chemotherapeutic agents

*By causing dehydration or electrolyte imbalance.
+Toxicity.
++By causing hypoglycemia.

Clinical Decision Making and Treatment

Regardless of the setting, older patients who exhibit the number of symptoms indicative of a major depression, specifically suicidal thoughts or psychosis, and who score *above* the established cutoff score for depression on a depression-screening tool (e.g., 5 on the GDS-SF) should be referred for comprehensive psychosocial services (i.e., psychiatric liaison nurses, geropsychiatric advanced practice nurses, social workers, psychiatrists, psychologists, clergy) psychiatric evaluation. Older patients with less severe depressive symptoms without suicidal thoughts or psychosis but who also score above the cutoff score on the depression screening tool (e.g., 5 on the GDS-SF) should be referred to available psychosocial services (i.e., psychiatric liaison nurses, geropsychiatric advanced practice nurses, social workers, psychiatrists, psychologists, clergy) for psychotherapy or other psychosocial therapies, as well as to determine whether medication for depression is warranted. Older adults at risk for depression may benefit from brief interventions that prevent the development of depression (Cole & Dendukuuri, 2004 [Level I]).

The two major categories of treatment for depression in older adults are biologic therapies (e.g., pharmacotherapy and electroconvulsive therapy) and psychosocial therapies (e.g., psychotherapies such as cognitive-behavioral, interpersonal, and brief psychodynamic) in both individual and group formats. A compelling body of evidence supports the efficacy of both treatment modalities for older adults with depression (Arean & Cook, 2002 [Level VI]; Hollon et al., 2005 [Level VI]). Marital and family therapy may also be beneficial in treating older adults with depression, especially older spouses engaged in caregiving (Buckwalter et al., 1999; Gitlin et al., 2003 [both Level IV]).

Several studies support the use of an interdisciplinary geriatric assessment team for late-life depression. These teams improve physical functioning in older adults with major depressive disorder (Callahan et al., 2005 [Level II]) and effectively reduce the depressive symptoms in community-dwelling older adults (age 70+ years) who were at risk for hospitalization (Boult et al., 2001 [Level II]). Ethnic minority elders experience improved treatment of depression when treated by an interdisciplinary treatment team (Arean et al., 2005 [Level VI]). Similarly, patients with multiple co-morbid medical conditions responde positively to an interdisciplinary approach to depression management (Harpole et al., 2005; Unutzer et al., 2002 [both Level II]). Although older adults with co-morbid anxiety disorders took longer to respond to treatment, they experience greater reductions in depression when treated by an interdisciplinary team than similar patients receiving usual primary care (Hegel et al., 2005 [Level II]).

In the past, tricyclic antidepressants (TCAs) were often contraindicated in older adults because of the anticholinergic side-effect profile (Mottram, Wilson, & Strobl, 2006 [Level I]). More recently, however, there has been a dramatic increase in the development and testing of different pharmacological agents used to treat depression in older adults. The most common classes of these newer medications include the Selective Serotonin Reuptake Inhibitors (SSRIs), Serotonin-Norepinephrine Reuptake Inhibitors (SNRIs), and TCA-related medications. These agents work selectively on neurotransmitters in the brain to alleviate depression. When the SSRIs are compared to other classes of antidepressants to treat late-life depression (e.g., SNRIs, TCAs, TCA-related medications), they have similar treatment efficacy (Salzman, Wong, & Wright, 2002 [Level V]; Shanmugham, Karp, Drayer, Reynolds, & Alexopoulos, 2005 [Level VI]). However, SSRIs and SNRIs generally pose a lower treatment risk for older adults with depression (Shanmugham et al., 2005 [Level VI]). Still, in a systematic review of the literature, Wilson and Mottram (2004 [Level I]) found that although SSRIs are generally well tolerated in the elderly, a significant minority of older adults experiences serious side effects, including nausea, vomiting, dizziness, and drowsiness. TCA-related drugs may be an effective alternative for older adults who cannot tolerate SSRIs (Wilson & Mottram, 2004 [Level I]).

The type and severity of depressive symptoms influence the type of treatment approach. In general, more severe depression, especially with suicidal thoughts or psychosis, requires intensive psychiatric treatment, including hospitalization, medication with an antidepressant or antipsychotic drug, electroconvulsive therapy, and intensive psychosocial support (Blazer, 2002; Blazer, 2003 [both Level VI]). Less severe depression without suicidal thoughts or psychosis may require treatment with psychotherapy or medication, often on an outpatient basis. Collectively, these data also suggest that patients who have depression complicated by multiple medical and psychiatric co-morbidities may benefit from a referral to an interdisciplinary treatment team with specific expertise in geropsychiatry.

Individualized Nursing Interventions

Psychosocial and behavioral nursing interventions can be incorporated into the plan of care, based on the patient's individualized need. Provision of safety precautions for patients with suicidal thinking is a priority. In acute medical settings, patients may require transfer to the psychiatric service when suicidal risk is high and staffing is not adequate to provide continuous observation of the patient. In outpatient settings, continuous surveillance of the patient should be provided while an emergency psychiatric evaluation and disposition is obtained.

Promotion of nutrition, elimination, sleep/rest patterns, physical comfort, and pain control have been recommended specifically for depressed medically ill older patients (Voyer & Martin, 2003 [Level VI]). Relaxation strategies should be offered to relieve anxiety as an adjunct to pain management. Nursing interventions should also focus on enhancement of the elder's physical function through structured and regular activity and exercise; referral to physical, occupational, and recreational therapies; and the development of a daily activity schedule (Barbour & Blumenthal, 2005 [Level VI]). Enhancement of social support is also an important function of the nurse. This may be done by identifying, mobilizing, or designating a support person such as family, a confidant, friends, volunteers or other hospital resources, a church member, support groups, patient or peer visitors, and particularly by accessing appropriate clergy for spiritual support.

Nurses should maximize an older adult's autonomy, personal control, self-efficacy, and decision making about clinical care, daily schedules, and personal routines (Lawton, Moss, Winter, & Hoffman, 2002 [Level IV]). The use of a graded task assignment where a larger goal or task is subdivided into several smaller steps can be helpful in enhancing function, assuring successful experiences, and building elderly patients' confidence in their performance of various activities (Arean & Cook, 2002 [Level VII]). Participation in regular, predictable, pleasant activities can result in more positive mood changes for elderly patients with depression (Koenig, 1991 [Level VI]). A pleasant-events inventory, elicited from the patient, can be used to incorporate pleasurable activities into an older patient's daily schedule (Koenig, 1991 [Level VI]). Music therapy customized to the patient's preference also is recommended to reduce depressive symptoms (Siedliecki & Good, 2006 [Level IV]).

Pleasant reminiscences can enhance self-esteem and sometimes alleviate a depressed mood (Hsieh & Wang, 2003 [Level I]). In systematic reviews of the literature, reminiscence therapy was also found to significantly reduce depression in older adults (Bohlmeijer, Smit, & Cuijpers, 2003 [Level I]; Hsieh & Wang, 2003 [Level I]; Mackin & Arean, 2005 [Level VI]). Nursing interventions to encourage reminiscence include asking patients directly about their past or by linking events in history with a patient's life experience. The use of photographs, old magazines, scrapbooks, and other objects can also stimulate discussion. Nurses should provide emotional support to depressed older patients by providing empathetic, supportive listening; encouraging patients to express their feelings in a focused manner on issues such as grief or role transition; providing supportive adaptive coping strategies; identifying and reinforcing strengths and capabilities; maintaining privacy and respect; and instilling hope.

Older patients should be closely monitored for therapeutic response to and potential side effects of antidepressant medication in order to assess whether dose adjustment may be warranted. Although, in general, it is necessary to start antidepressant medication at low doses in older patients, it is also necessary to ensure that older adults with persistent depressive symptoms receive adequate treatment (American Association of Geriatric Psychiatry, 1992; Buffum & Buffum, 2005 [both Level VI]). In particular, it is important to increase the patient's and family's awareness of the symptoms as part of a depression that is treatable and not the person's fault as a result of personal inadequacies.

Case Study and Discussion

Ray Stimson is an 87-year-old man with multiple medical problems. He has a history of coronary artery disease (CAD) and had triple bypass surgery 4 years ago. He also has hypertension and Type II diabetes and is hard of hearing. He was admitted to the hospital for surgical repair of a hip fracture following a fall in his home. Mr. Stimson is widowed (11 months) and has two adult children who do not live locally. Prior to his fall, he was living independently in the community; however, his children were growing increasingly concerned about his safety. Following surgery, Mr. Stimson was irritable and resisted efforts by the nursing staff to participate in self-care activities (e.g., walking, bathing). They often found him laying stoically in bed, staring into space. The nurses also observed that he was occasionally confused and would ask about his deceased wife.

A subsequent referral to the geropsychiatric consultation liaison nurse revealed that Mr. Stimson was experiencing a great deal of postoperative pain that was not well treated on his current medicine regimen. Nursing staff had charted concerns that his opiod analgesic was contributing to his mental confusion. The geropsychiatric evaluation also revealed that Mr. Stimson had been growing increasingly depressed over the past few months and was still actively grieving the loss of his wife of 62 years. As his health had failed and his independent living was threatened, he admitted he had contemplated suicide, stating, "Life is just not worth living anymore." Further assessment revealed that he did not have a specific plan in mind and admitted that he didn't really think that was a solution to his problems, but that he couldn't see that he had many options.

The liaison nurse worked with the medical team to develop a more aggressive plan for pain management. She also arranged for a family conference to discuss discharge-planning issues. During the family conference, the liaison nurse spoke to Mr. Stimson's children about long-term planning. She explained how important it was for Mr. Stimson to participate in any placement decisions they may be contemplating and to have a sense of control. Although his children were able to express their reservations and concerns about safety, they agreed to explore kinds of community support services that could be activated to help support their father in his own home for as long as possible.

Mr. Stimson was able to participate in rehabilitation and gained enough strength to return to his home. Arrangements were made for follow-up with mental-health services. He was started on an antidepressant medication and agreed to participate in the senior lunch program twice a week to increase the opportunity for socialization. Several months after his discharge, Mr. Stimson reported that he still missed his wife terribly and that he still was lonely at times. However, he had developed some friendships at the senior center and was getting out one or two times each week. His children called more often and had, for the time being, stopped sending him brochures for assisted-living facilities. He acknowledged that he may need to move to a more supervised setting in the future, but for now, he was content to stay in the home where he had many pleasant memories to keep him company.

Conclusion

Depression significantly threatens the personal integrity and "experience of life" of older adults. Depression is often reversible with prompt and appropriate treatment. Early recognition can be enhanced by the use of a standardized protocol that outlines a systematic method for depression assessment. Early identification of depressed intervention and successful treatment demonstrates to society that depression is the most treatable mental problem in late life. As Blazer (1989) stated, "When there is depression, hope remains."

Resources

Depression Screening Tools

Geriatric Depression Scale–Short Form (GDS–SF):

Sheikh, J. I., & Yesavage, J. A. (1986). Geriatric depression scale (GDS): Recent evidence and development of a shorter version. *Clinical Gerontologist, 5,* 165–173.

Center for Epidemiological Studies Depression Scale (CES-D):

Radloff, L. S. (1977). The CES-D scale: A self-report depression scale for research in the general population. *Applied Psychological Measurement, 1,* 385–401.

SELFCARE(D):

Banerjee, S., Shamash, K., MacDonald, A. J. D., & Mann, A. H. (1998). The use of SELFCARE(D) as a screening tool for depression in the clients of local authority home care services—A preliminary study. *International Journal of Geriatric Psychiatry, 13,* 695–699.

Box 5.1

Nursing Standard of Practice Protocol: Depression in Older Adults

I. BACKGROUND

A. Depression—both major depressive disorders and minor depression—is highly prevalent in community-dwelling, medically ill, and institutionalized older adults.

B. Depression is not a natural part of aging or a normal reaction to acute illness hospitalization.

C. Consequences of depression include amplification of pain and disability, delayed recovery from illness and surgery, worsening of drug side effects, excess use of health services, cognitive impairment, subnutrition, and increased suicide- and nonsuicide-related death.

D. Depression tends to be long lasting and recurrent. Therefore, a wait-and-see approach is undesirable, and immediate clinical attention is necessary. If recognized, treatment response is good.

E. Somatic symptoms may be more prominent than depressed mood in late-life depression.

F. Mixed depression and anxiety features may be evident among many older adults.

G. Recognition of depression is hindered by the coexistence of physical illness and social and economic problems common in late life. Early recognition, intervention, and referral by nurses can reduce the negative effects of depression.

*Somatic symptoms, also seen in many physical illnesses, are frequently associated with A and B; therefore, the full range of depressive symptoms should be assessed.

II. ASSESSMENT PARAMETERS

Several studies support the use of an interdisciplinary geriatric assessment team for late-life depression (Boult et al., 2005; Callahan et al., 2005; Harpole et al., 2005; Unutzer et al., 2002 [all Level II]) with the following being specific parameters of assessment:

A. Identify risk factors/high risk groups:

   1. Current alcohol /substance-use disorder (Hasin & Grant, 2002 [Level III]).
   2. Medical co-morbidity (Alexopoulos, Schulz, & Lebowitz, 2005 [Level VI]). Specific co-morbid conditions: dementia, stroke, cancer, arthritis, hip fracture, myocardial infarction, chronic obstructive pulmonary disease, and Parkinson's disease (Alexopoulos et al., 2005; Butters et al., 2003 [both Level VI]).
   3. Functional disability (especially new functional loss). Disability, older age, new medical diagnosis, and poor health status (Cole, 2005; Cole & Dendukuuri, 2003 [both Level I]).
   4. Widow/widowers (NIH, 1992 [Level I]).
   5. Older family caregivers, especially those caring for persons with dementia (Pinquart & Sorensen, 2004 [Level I]).
   6. Social isolation/absence of social support (Kraaij, Arensman, & Spinhoven, 2002; NIH, 1992 [both Level I]).
   7. Psychosocial causes for depression in older adults include cognitive distortions, stressful life events (especially loss), chronic stress, low self-efficacy expectations (Blazer, 2002 [Level VI]; Blazer, 2003 [Level VI]; Blazer & Hybels, 2005 [Level VI]; Spinhoven (2002) [Level I]).

B. Assess all at-risk groups using a standardized depression screening tool and documentation score. The GDS-SF (Sheikh & Yesavage, 1986) is recommended because it takes approximately 5 minutes to administer, has been validated and extensively used with medically ill older adults, and includes *few* somatic items that may be confounded with physical illness (Pfaff & Almeida, 2005 [Level IV]; Watson & Pignone, 2003 [Level I]).

C. Perform a *focused* depression assessment on all at-risk groups and document results. Note the number of symptoms; onset; frequency/patterns; duration (especially 2 weeks); change from normal mood, behavior, and functioning (American Psychiatric Association, 2000 [Level VI]):

   1. Depressive symptoms
   2. Depressed or irritable mood, frequent crying
   3. Loss of interest, pleasure (in family, friends, hobbies, sex)
   4. Weight loss or gain (especially loss)
   5. Sleep disturbance (especially insomnia)
   6. Fatigue/loss of energy
   7. Psychomotor slowing/agitation
   8. Diminished concentration

9. Feelings of worthlessness/guilt
10. Suicidal thoughts or attempts, hopelessness
11. Psychosis (i.e., delusional/paranoid thoughts, hallucinations)
12. History of depression, current substance abuse (especially alcohol), previous coping style
13. Recent losses or crises (e.g., death of spouse, friend, pet, retirement; anniversary dates; move to another residence, nursing home); change in physical health status, relationships, roles

D. Obtain/review medical history and physical/neurological examination (Alexopoulos et al., 2001 [Level VI]).
E. Assess for depressogenic medications (e.g., steroids, narcotics, sedative/hypnotics, benzodiazepines, antihypertensives, H2 antagonists, beta-blockers, antipsychotics, immunosuppressives, cytotoxic agents)
F. Assess for related systematic and metabolic processes that may contribute to depression or might complicate treatment of the depression (e.g., infection, anemia, hypothyroidism or hyperthyroidism, hyponatremia, hypercalcemia, hypoglycemia, congestive heart failure, kidney failure (Alexopoulos et al., 2001 [Level VI])
G. Assess for cognitive dysfunction
H. Assess level of functional ability

III. CARE PARAMETERS

A. For severe depression (i.e., GDS score 11 or greater, five to nine depressive symptoms [must include depressed mood or loss of pleasure] plus other positive responses on individualized assessment [especially suicidal thoughts or psychosis and co-morbid substance abuse], refer for psychiatric evaluation. Treatment options may include medication or cognitive-behavioral, interpersonal, or brief psychodynamic psychotherapy/counseling (individual, group, family); hospitalization; or electroconvulsive therapy (Arean & Cook, 2002; Hollon et al., 2005 [both Level VI]).
B. For less severe depression (i.e., GDS score 6 or greater, fewer than five depressive symptoms plus other positive responses on individualized assessment), refer to mental-health services for psychotherapy/counseling (see previous types), especially for specific issues identified in individualized assessment and to determine whether medication therapy may be warranted. Consider resources such as psychiatric liaison nurses, geropsychiatric advanced practice nurses, social workers, psychologists, and other community- and institution-specific mental-health services. If suicidal thoughts, psychosis, or co-morbid substance abuse is present, a referral for a comprehensive psychiatric evaluation should always be made (Arean & Cook, 2002; Hollon et al., 2005 [both Level VI]).
C. For all levels of depression, develop an *individualized* plan integrating the following nursing interventions:

1. Provide an approach to depression management (Arean et al., 2005 [Level VI]; Harpole et al., 2005 [Level II]; Hegel, 2005 [Level II]; Unutzer et al., 2002 [Level II]).
2. Institute safety precautions for suicide risk as per institutional policy (in outpatient settings, ensure continuous surveillance of the patient while obtaining an emergency psychiatric evaluation and disposition).
3. Remove or control etiologic agents:
   a. Avoid/remove/change depressogenic medications.
   b. Correct/treat metabolic/systemic disturbances.
4. Monitor and promote nutrition, elimination, sleep/rest patterns, physical comfort (especially pain control).
5. Enhance physical function (i.e., structure regular exercise/activity; refer to physical, occupational, recreational therapies); develop a daily activity schedule.
6. Enhance social support (i.e., identify/mobilize a support person(s) [e.g., family, confidant, friends, hospital resources, support groups, patient visitors]); ascertain need for spiritual support and contact appropriate clergy.
7. Maximize autonomy/personal control/self-efficacy (e.g., include patient in active participation in making daily schedules, short-term goals).
8. Identify and reinforce strengths and capabilities.
9. Structure and encourage daily participation in relaxation therapies, pleasant activities (conduct a pleasant-activity inventory), music therapy.
10. Monitor and document response to medication and other therapies; readminister depression-screening tool.
11. Provide practical assistance; assist with problem-solving.
12. Provide emotional support (i.e., empathic, supportive listening, encourage expression of feelings, hope instillation), support adaptive coping, encourage pleasant reminiscences.
13. Provide information about the physical illness and treatment(s) and about depression (i.e., that depression is common, treatable, and not the person's fault).
14. Educate about the importance of adherence to prescribed treatment regimen for depression (especially medication) to prevent recurrence; educate about *specific* antidepressant side effects due to personal inadequacies.
15. Ensure mental-health community link-up; consider psychiatric, nursing-home-care intervention.

IV. EVALUATION OF EXPECTED OUTCOMES

A. Patient:
   1. Patient safety will be maintained.

2. Patients with severe depression will be evaluated by psychiatric services.
3. Patients will report a reduction of symptoms that are indicative of depression. A reduction in the GDS score will be evident and suicidal thoughts or psychosis will resolve.
4. Patient's daily functioning will improve.

B. Health care provider:
1. Early recognition of patient at risk, referral, and interventions for depression, and documentation of outcomes will be improved.

C. Institution:
1. The number of patients identified with depression will increase.
2. The number of in-hospital suicide attempts will not increase.
3. The number of referrals to mental-health services will increase.
4. The number of referrals to psychiatric nursing-home-care services will increase.
5. Staff will receive ongoing education on depression recognition, assessment, and interventions.

V. OTHER CLINICAL PRACTICE GUIDELINES

Practice guideline for the treatment of patients with major depressive disorder. American Psychiatric Association—Medical Specialty Society, 1993 (revised 2000; reviewed 2005). 45 pages. NGC: 001831. Retrieved on June 6, 2007, from http://www.guideline.org/summary/summary.aspx?doc_id=2605&nbr=001831&string=depression.

Detection of depression in the cognitively intact older adult. University of Iowa Gerontological Nursing Interventions Research Center, Research Translation and Dissemination Core—Academic Institution, 1998 (revised 2005 May). 33 pages. NGC: 004519. Retrieved on June 6, 2007, from http://www.guideline.org/summary/summary.aspx?doc_id=8112&nbr=004519&
string=depression

Depression. American Medical Directors Association—Professional Association, 2003. 36 pages. NGC: 003520 AMDA. Retrieved on June 6, 2007, from http://www.guideline.org/summary/summary.aspx?doc_id=4952&nbr=003520&string=depression

References

Achterberg, W., Pot, A. M., Kerkstra, A., Ooms, M., Muller, M., & Ribbe, M. (2003). The effect of depression on social engagement in newly admitted Dutch nursing home residents. *The Gerontologist, 43*(2), 213–218. Evidence Level IV: Nonexperimental Study.
Administration on Aging (2001). Older adults and mental health: Issues and opportunities. Retrieved on June 6, 2007, from http://www.aoa.gov/PRESS/publications/Older-Adults-and-Mental-Health-2001.pdf

Alexopoulos, G. S., Katz, I. R., Reynolds, C. F., Carpenter, D., & Docherty, J. P. (2001). The expert consensus guidelines series: Pharmacotherapy of depressive disorders in older patients (special report). *Postgraduate Medicine*, 1–87. Evidence Level VI: Expert Opinion.

Alexopoulos, G. S., Schultz, S. K., & Lebowitz, B. D. (2005). Late-life depression: A model for medical classification. *Biological Psychiatry*, *58*, 283–289. Evidence Level VI: Expert Opinion.

American Association of Geriatric Psychiatry (1992). Position statement: Psychotherapeutic medication in nursing homes. *Journal of the American Geriatrics Society*, *40*, 946–949. Evidence Level VI: Expert Opinion.

American Psychiatric Association (2000). Diagnostic and statistical manual of mental disorders (4th ed., TR). Washington, DC: American Psychiatric Association. Evidence Level VI: Expert Opinion.

Arean, P. A., Ayalon, L., Hunkeler, E., Lin, E. H. B., Tang, L., & Harpole, L. (2005). Improving depression care for older minority patients in primary care. *Medical Care*, *43*(4), 381–390. Evidence Level VI: Expert Opinion.

Arean, P. A., & Cook, B. L. (2002). Psychotherapy and combined psychotherapy/pharmacotherapy for late-life depression. *Biological Psychiatry*, *52*(3), 293–303. Evidence Level VI: Expert Opinion.

Bagulho, F. (2002). Depression in older people. *Current Opinion in Psychiatry*, *15*(4), 417–422. Level of Evidence V: Systematic Review.

Banerjee, S., Shamash, K., Macdonald, A. J. D., & Mann, A. H. (1998). The use of SELFCARE(D) as a screening tool for depression in the clients of local authority home care services—A preliminary study. *International Journal of Geriatric Psychiatry*, *13*, 695–699.

Barbour, K. A., & Blumenthal, J. A. (2005). Exercise training and depression in older adults. *Neurobiology of Aging*, *26* (Suppl. 1), S119–S123. Evidence Level VI: Expert Opinion.

Barraclough, B. M., Bunch, J., & Nelson, B. (1974). A hundred cases of suicide: Clinical aspects. *British Journal of Psychiatry*, *125*, 355–373.

Beals, J., Manson, S. M., Whitesell, N. R., Mitchell, C. M., Novins, D. K., Simpson, S., et al. (2005). Prevalence of major depressive episode in two American Indian reservation populations: Unexpected findings with a structured interview. *American Journal of Psychiatry*, *162*, 1713–1722. Evidence Level VI: Expert Opinion.

Blazer, D. G. (1989). Depression in the elderly. *New England Journal of Medicine*, *320*, 164–166.

Blazer, D. G. (2002). *Depression in late life*. Mosby year book (3rd ed.). Level of Evidence VI: Expert Opinion.

Blazer, D. G. (2003). Depression in late life: Review and commentary. *Journals of Gerontology: Series A: Biological Sciences and Medical Sciences*, *58A*(3), 249–265. Evidence Level VI: Expert Opinion.

Blazer, D. G., & Hybels, C. F. (2005). Origins of depression in late life. *Psychological Medicine*, *35*(9), 1241–1252. Evidence Level VI: Expert Opinion.

Bohlmeijer, E., Smit, F., & Cuijpers, P. (2003). Effects of reminiscence and life review on late-life depression: A meta-analysis. *International Journal of Geriatric Psychiatry*, *18*, 1088–1094. Evidence Level I: Meta-analysis.

Boult, C., Boult, L. B., Morishita, L., Dowd, B., Kane, R. L., & Urdangarin, C. F. (2001). A randomized clinical trial of outpatient geriatric evaluation and management. *Journal of the American Geriatrics Society*, *49*, 351–359. Evidence Level II: Single Experimental Study.

Bruce, M. L., McAvay, G. J., Raue, P. J., Brown, E. L., Meyers, M.D., Keohane, D. J., et al. (2002). Major depression in elderly home health care patients. *American Journal of Psychiatry*, *159*(8), 1367–1374. Evidence Level VI: Expert Opinion.

Bruce, M. L., Ten Have, T. R., Reynolds, C. F. III, Katz, I. I., Schulberg, H. C., Mulsant, B. H., et al. (2004). Reducing suicidal ideation and depressive symptoms in depressed older primary care patients: A randomized controlled trial. *Journal of the American Medical Association*, *291*(9), 1081–1091. Evidence Level II: Randomized Controlled Trial.

Buckwalter, K. C., Gerdner, L., Kohout, F., Hall, G. R., Kelly, A., Richards, B., et al. (1999). A nursing intervention to decrease depression in family caregivers of persons with dementia. *Archives of Psychiatric Nursing*, *13*(2), 80–88. Evidence Level IV: Nonexperimental Study.

Buffum, M. D., & Buffum, J. C. (2005). Treating depression in the elderly: An update on antidepressants. *Geriatric Nursing*, *26*(3), 138–142. Evidence Level VI: Expert Opinion.

Butters, M. A., Sweet, R. A., Mulsant, B. H., Kamboh, M. I., Pollock, B. G., Begley, A. E., et al. (2003). APOE is associated with age-of-onset, but not cognitive functioning, in late-life depression. *International Journal of Geriatric Psychiatry, 18*, 1075–1081. Evidence Level IV: Nonexperimental Study.

Callahan, C. M., Kroenke, K., Counsell, S. R., Hendrie, H. C., Perkins, A. J., Katon, W. et al. (2005). Treatment of depression improves physical functioning in older adults. *Journal of the American Geriatrics Society, 53*(3), 367–373. Evidence Level II: Single Experimental Study. Evidence Level III: Quasiexperimental Study.

Cassidy, E. L., Lauderdale, S., & Sheikh, J. I. (2005). Mixed anxiety and depression in older adults: Clinical characteristics and management. *Journal of Geriatric Psychiatry and Neurology, 18*(2), 83–88.

Charney, D. S., Reynolds, C. F., III, Lewis, L., Lebowitz, B. D., Sunderland, T., Alexopoulos, G. S., et al. (2003). Depression and bipolar support alliance consensus statement on the unmet needs in diagnosis and treatment of mood disorders in late life. *Archives of General Psychiatry, 60*(7), 664–672.

Cohen-Mansfield, J., Werner, P., & Marx, M. S. (1990). Screaming in nursing home residents. *Journal of the American Geriatrics Society, 38*, 785–792.

Cole, M. G. (2005). Evidence-based review of risk factors for geriatric depression and brief preventive interventions. *Psychiatric Clinics of North America, 28*(4), 785–803. Evidence Level I: Systematic Review.

Cole, M. G., & Dendukuuri, N. (2003). Risk factors for depression among elderly community subjects: A systematic review and meta-analysis. *American Journal of Psychiatry, 160*(6), 1147–1156. Evidence Level I: Meta-analysis.

Cole, M. G., & Dendukuuri, N. (2004). The feasibility and effectiveness of brief interventions to prevent depression in older subjects: A systematic review. *International Journal of Geriatric Psychiatry, 19*(11), 1019–1025. Evidence Level I: Systematic Review.

Conwell, Y. (1994). *Suicide in the elderly*. In Schneider, L. S., Reynolds, B. D., Lebowitz, B. D., & Friedhoff, A. J. (Eds). Diagnosis and treatment of depression in late life: Results of the NIH Consensus Development Conference. Washington, DC: American Psychiatric Press. Evidence Level VI: Expert Opinion.

Conwell, Y., Duberstein, P. R., & Caine, E. D. (2002). Risk factors for suicide in later life. *Biological Psychiatry, 52*(3), 193–204. Evidence Level VI: Expert Opinion.

Cooper, L. A., Beach, M. C., Johnson, R. L., & Inui, T. S. (2006). Delving below the surface: Understanding how race and ethnicity influence relationships in health care. *Journal of General Internal Medicine, 21*, S21–S27. Evidence Level VI: Expert Opinion.

DeLuca, A. K., Lenze, E. J., Mulsant, B. H., Butters, M. A., Karp, J. F., Dew, M. A., et al. (2005). Co-morbid anxiety disorder in late-life depression: Association with memory decline over four years. *International Journal of Geriatric Psychiatry, 20*, 848–854. Evidence Level IV: Nonexperimental Study.

Dhondt, T., Derksen, P., Hooijer, C., Van Heycop Ten Ham, B., Van Gent, P. P., & Heeren, T. (1999). Depressogenic medication as an aetiological factor in major depression: An analysis in a clinical population of depressed elderly people. *International Journal of Geriatric Psychiatry, 14*, 875–881. Evidence Level IV: Nonexperimental Study.

Dreyfus, J. K. (1988). Depression assessment and interventions with medically ill frail elderly. *Journal of Gerontological Nursing, 14*, 27–36.

Driscoll, H. C., Basinski, J., Mulsanti, B. H., Butters, M. A., Dew, M. A., Houck, P. R., et al. (2005). Late-onset major depression: Clinical and treatment-response variability. *International Journal of Geriatric Psychiatry, 20*, 661–667. Evidence Level IV: Nonexperimental Study.

Erlangsen, A., Vach, W., & Jeune, B. (2005). The effect of hospitalization with medical illnesses on the suicide risk in the oldest old: A population-based register study. *Journal of the American Geriatrics Society, 53*, 771–776. Evidence Level III: Quasi-experimental Study.

Gaynes, B. N., Burns, B. J., Tweed, D. L., & Erickson, P. (2002). Depression and health-related quality of life. *The Journal of Nervous and Mental Disease, 190*(12), 799–806. Evidence Level III: Quasi-experimental Study.

Gitlin, L. N., Belle, S. H., Burgio, L. D., Czaja, S. J., Mahoney, D., Gallagher-Thompson, D., et al. (2003). Effect of multicomponent interventions on caregiver burden and depression: The REACH multisite initiative at 6-month follow-up. *Psychology & Aging, 18*(3), 361–374. Evidence Level IV: Nonexperimental Study.

Harpole, L. H., Williams, J. W. J., Olsen, M. K., Stechuchak, K. M., Oddone, E., Callahan, C. M., et al. (2005). Improving depression outcomes in older adults with co-morbid medical illness. *General Hospital Psychiatry*, *27*(1), 4–12. Evidence Level II: Single Experimental Study.

Hasin, D. S., & Grant, B. F. (2002). Major depression in 6,050 former drinkers: Association with past alcohol dependence. *Archives of General Psychiatry*, *59*, 794–800. Evidence Level III: Quasi-experimental Study.

Hegel, M. T., Unutzer, J., Tang, L., Arean, P. A., Katon, W., Noel, P. H., et al. (2005). Impact of co-morbid panic and post-traumatic stress disorder on outcomes of collaborative care for late-life depression in primary care. *American Journal of Geriatric Psychiatry*, *13*(1), 48–58. Evidence Level II: Single Experimental Study.

Hollon, S. D., Jarrett, R. B., Nierenberg, A. A., Thase, M. E., Trivedi, M., & Rush, A. J. (2005). Psychotherapy and medication in the treatment of adult and geriatric depression: Which monotherapy or combined treatment? *Journal of Clinical Psychiatry*, *66*(4), 455–468. Evidence Level VI: Expert Opinion.

Holmes, J. D., & House, A. O. (2000). Psychiatric illness in hip fracture. *Age and Ageing*, *29*(6), 537–546. Evidence Level I: Systematic Review.

Hsieh, H., & Wang, J. (2003). Effect of reminiscence therapy on depression in older adults: A systematic review. *International Journal of Nursing Studies*, *40*(4), 335–345. Evidence Level I: Systematic Review.

Hybels, C. F., & Blazer, D. G. (2003). Epidemiology of late-life mental disorders. *Clinical Geriatric Medicine*, *15*, 663–696.

Iosifescu, D.V. (2007). Treating depression in the medically ill. *Psychiatric Clinics of North America*, *30*, 77–99. Evidence Level V: Literature Review.

Juurlink, D. N., Herrmann, N., Szalai, J. P., Kopp, A., & Redelmeier, D.A. (2004). Medical illness and the risk of suicide in the elderly. *Archives of Internal Medicine*, *164*, 1179–1184. Evidence Level V: Nonexperimental Study.

Kales, H. C., & Mellow, A. M. (2006). Race and depression: Does race affect the diagnosis and treatment of late-life depression? *Geriatrics*, *61*(5), 18–21. Evidence Level VI: Expert Opinion.

Katz, I. R. (1996). On the inseparability of mental and physical health in aged persons: Lessons from depression and medical co-morbidity. *American Journal of Geriatric Psychiatry*, *4*, 1–16.

Katz, I. R., Streim, J., & Parmelee, P. (1994). Prevention of depression, recurrences, and complications in late life. *Preventive Medicine*, *23*, 743–750.

Koenig, H. G. (1991). Depressive disorders in older medical inpatients. *American Family Practice*, *44*, 1243–1250. Evidence Level VI: Expert Opinion.

Kraaij, V., Arensman, E., & Spinhoven, P. (2002). Negative life events and depression in elderly persons: A meta-analysis. *Journals of Gerontology: Series B: Psychological Sciences and Social Sciences*, *57B*(1), P87–P94. Evidence Level I: Meta-analysis.

Kurlowicz, L. H. (1994). Depression in hospitalized medically ill elders: Evolution of the concept. *Archives in Psychiatric Nursing*, *8*, 124–126.

Lawton, M. P., Moss, M. S., Winter, L., & Hoffman, C. (2002). Motivation in later life: Personal projects and well-being. *Psychology & Aging*, *17*(4), 539–547. Evidence Level IV: Nonexperimental Study.

Lebowitz, B. D. (1996). Diagnosis and treatment of depression in late life: An overview of the NIH consensus statement. *Journal of the American Geriatric Society*, *4* (Suppl. 1), S3–S6.

Lenze, E. J., Mulsant, B. H., Shear, M. K., Alexopoulos, G. S., Frank, E., & Reynolds, C. F., III (2001). Co-morbidity of depression and anxiety disorders in later life. *Depression and Anxiety*, *14*, 86–93.

Lin, E. H. B., Katon, W., Korff, M. V., Tang, L., Williams, J. W., Kroenke, K., et al. (2003). Effect of improving depression care on pain and functional outcomes among older adults with arthritis: A randomized controlled trial. *Journal of American Medical Association*, *290*(18), 2428–2434. Evidence Level II: Single Experimental Study.

Luoma, J. B., Martin, C. E., & Pearson, J. L. (2002). Contact with mental health and primary care providers before suicide: A review of the evidence. *American Journal of Psychiatry*, *159*, 909–916. Level of Evidence V: Review.

Lyness, J. M., Kim, J. H., Tang, W., Tu, X., Conwell, Y., King, D. A., et al. (2007). The clinical significance of subsyndromal depression in older primary care patients. *American Journal of Geriatric Psychiatry*, *15*(3), 214–223. Evidence Level IV: Nonexperimental Study.

Mackin, R. S., & Arean, P. A. (2005). Evidence-based psychotherapeutic interventions for geriatric depression. *Psychiatric Clinics of North America, 28*(4), 805–820. Evidence Level VI: Expert Opinion.

McDade-Montez, E. A., Christensen, A. J., Cvengros, J. A., & Lawton, W. J. (2006). The role of depression symptoms in dialysis withdrawal. *Health Psychology, 25*(2), 198–204.

McKeown, R. E., Cuffe, S. P., & Schulz, R. M. (2006). U.S. suicide rates by age group, 1970–2002: An examination of recent trends. *American Journal of Public Health, 96*(10), 1744–1751. Evidence Level V: Review.

Miller, M. (1978). Geriatric suicide: The Arizona study. *Gerontologist, 18*, 488–495.

Mitchell, A. J., & Subramaniam, H. (2005). Prognosis of depression in old age compared to middle age: A systematic review of comparative studies. *American Journal of Psychiatry, 162*(9), 1588–1601. Evidence Level I: Systematic Review.

Modrego, P. J., & Ferrandez, J. (2004). Depression in patients with mild cognitive impairment increases the risk of developing dementia of Alzheimer type: A prospective cohort study. *Archives in Neurology, 61*, 1290–1293. Evidence Level IV: Nonexperimental Study.

Mottram, P., Wilson, K., & Strobl, J. (2006). Antidepressants for depressed elderly: Review. *Cochrane Database of Systematic Reviews, 25*(1). Evidence Level I: Systematic Review.

National Institute of Health (NIH) Consensus Development Panel (1992). Diagnosis and treatment of depression in late life. *Journal of the American Medical Association, 268*, 1018–1024. Evidence Level I: Systematic Review.

Pearson, J. L., Teri, L., & Reifler, B. V. (1989). Functional status and cognitive impairment in Alzheimer's patients with and without depression. *Journal of the American Geriatric Society, 34*, 1117–1121.

Pfaff, J. J., & Almeida, O. P. (2005). Detecting suicidal ideation in older patients: Identifying risk factors within the general practice setting. *British Journal of General Practice, 55*(513), 261–262. Level of Evidence IV: Nonexperimental Study.

Pinquart, M., & Sorensen, S. (2004). Associations of caregiver stressors and uplifts with subjective well-being and depressive mood: A meta-analytic comparison. *Aging & Mental Health, 8*(5), 438–449. Evidence Level I: Systematic Review.

Piven, M. L. S. (2001). Detection of depression in the cognitive intact older adult protocol. *Journal of Gerontological Nursing, 27*(6), 8–14. Evidence Level VI: Expert Opinion.

Radloff, L. S. (1977). The CES-D scale: A self-report depression scale for research in the general population. *Applied Psychological Measurement, 1*, 385–401.

Salzman, C., Wong, E., & Wright, B. C. (2002). Drug and ECT treatment of depression in the elderly, 1996–2001: A literature review. *Biological Psychiatry, 52*(3), 265–284. Evidence Level V: Literature Review.

Sareen, J., Cox, B. J., Afifi, T. O., de Graaf, R., Asmundson, G. J., Ten Have, M., et al. (2005). Anxiety disorders and risk for suicidal ideation and suicide attempts: A population-based longitudinal study of adults. *Archives of General Psychiatry, 62*(11), 1249–1257. Evidence Level IV: Nonexperimental Study.

Schulz, R., Drayer, R. A., & Rollman, B. L. (2002). Depression as a risk factor for non-suicide mortality in the elderly. *Biological Psychiatry, 52*(3), 205–225.

Shanmugham, B., Karp, J., Drayer, R., Reynolds, C. F., III, & Alexopoulos, G. (2005). Evidence-based pharmacologic interventions for geriatric depression. *Psychiatric Clinics of North America, 28*(4), 821–835. Evidence Level VI: Expert Opinion.

Sheikh, J. I., & Yesavage, J. A. (1986). Geriatric depression scale (GDS) recent evidence and development of a shorter version. *Clinical Gerontologist, 5*, 165–173.

Siedliecki, S. L., & Good, M. (2006). Effect of music on power, pain, depression and disability. *Journal of Advanced Nursing, 54*, 553–562. Evidence Level IV: Nonexperimental Study.

Snowdon, J. (2001). Is depression more prevalent in old age? *Australian and New Zealand Journal of Psychiatry, 35*, 782–787.

Stapleton, R. D., Nielsen, E. L., Engelberg, R. A., Patrick, D. L., & Curtis, J. R. (2005). Association of depression and life-sustaining treatment. *Chest, 127*(1), 328–334.

Szanto, K., Mulsant, B. H., Houck, P., Dew, M. A., & Reynolds, C. F., III (2003). Occurrence and course of suicidality during short-term treatment of late-life depression. *Archives of General Psychiatry, 60*(6), 610–617. Evidence Level V: Nonexperimental Study.

Teri, L., & Wagner, A. (1992). Alzheimer's disease and depression. *Journal of Consultative and Clinical Psychology, 60*, 379–391.

Turvey, C. L., Conwell, Y., Jones, M. P., Phillips, C., Simonsick, E., Pearson, J. L., et al. (2002). Risk factors for late-life suicide: A prospective, community-based study. *American Journal of Geriatric Psychiatry*, *10*(4), 398–406. Level of Evidence IV: Observational.

Unutzer, J., Katon, W., Callahan, C. M., Williams, J. W. J., Hunkeler, E., Harpole, L., et al. (2002). Collaborative care management of late-life depression in the primary care setting: A randomized controlled trial. *Journal of the American Medical Association*, *288*(22), 2836–2845. Evidence Level II: Single Experimental Study.

Virnig, B., Huang, Z., Lurie, N., Musgrave, D., McBean, A. M., & Dowd, B. (2004). Does Medicare managed care provide equal treatment for mental illness across races? *Archives of General Psychiatry*, *61*, 201–205. Evidence Level IV: Nonexperimental Study.

von Ammon Cavanaugh, S., Furlanetto, L. M., Creech, S. D., & Powell, L. H. (2001). Medical illness, past depression, and present depression: A predictive triad for in-hospital mortality. *American Journal of Psychiatry*, *158*, 43–48. Evidence Level III: Quasi-experimental Study.

Voyer, P., & Martin, L. S. (2003). Improving geriatric mental health nursing care: Making a case for going beyond psychotropic medications. *International Journal of Mental Health Nursing*, *12(1)*, 11–21. Evidence Level VI: Expert Opinion.

Waern, M., Rubenowitz, E., & Wilhelmson, K. (2003). Predictors of suicide in the old elderly. *Gerontology*, *49*(5), 328–334. Level of Evidence V: Case Reports.

Watson, L. C., & Pignone, M. P. (2003). Screening accuracy for late-life depression in primary care: A systematic review. *Journal of Family Practice*, *52*(12), 956–964. Evidence Level I: Systematic Review.

Williams, D. R., Gonzalez, H. M., Neighbors, H., Nesse, R., Abelson, J. M., Sweetman, J., et al. (2007). Prevalence and distribution of major depressive disorder in African Americans, Caribbean Blacks, and non-Hispanic Whites: Results from the National Survey of American Life. *Archives in General Psychiatry*, *64*(3), 305–315. Evidence Level IV: Nonexperimental Study.

Wilson, K., & Mottram, P. (2004). A comparison of side effects of selective serotonin reuptake inhibitors and tricyclic antidepressants in older depressed patients: A meta-analysis. *International Journal of Geriatric Psychiatry*, *19*, 754–762. Evidence Level I: Meta-analysis.

Zubenko, G. A., Zubenko, W. N., McPherson, S., Spoor, E., Marin, D. B., Farlow, M. R., et al. (2003). A collaborative study of the emergence and clinical features of the major depressive syndrome of Alzheimer's Disease. *American Journal of Psychiatry*, *160*, 857–866.

Dementia

6

Kathleen Fletcher

Educational Objectives

At the completion of this chapter, the reader should be able to:

1. describe the spectrum of dementia syndromes

2. recognize the clinical features of dementia

3. discuss pharmacological and nonpharmacological approaches in the management of dementia

4. develop a nursing plan of care for an older adult with dementia

Overview

Dementia is most commonly defined as a clinical syndrome of cognitive deficits that involves both memory impairments and a disturbance in at least one other area of cognition (*DSM-IV-TR*) (American Psychiatric Association, 2000 [Level VI]). In addition to disruptions in cognition, dementia is associated with a gradual decline in function and changes in mood and behavior.

There are many causes of dementia and dementia-like presentations. Differentiating these changes early in the course of illness is important because condition-specific assessment, monitoring, and management strategies can be

For a description of Evidence Levels cited in this chapter, see chapter 1, Developing and Evaluating Clinical Practice Guidelines, page 4.

employed. Differential diagnoses among conditions that cause cognitive impairment are confounded by the fact that these conditions may coexist and disparate dementing disorders may be similarly clinically expressed.

Major goals in the clinical approach to a person presenting with cognitive impairments are identification and resolution of potentially reversible conditions (e.g., delirium), recognition and control of co-morbid conditions, and early diagnosis and management of a dementing illness. The focus of this chapter is on assessment and management of the progressive dementia syndromes.

Background and Statement of The Problem

The rapid growth of the older adult population in the United States is associated with a significant increase in the prevalence of dementia. Dementia affects about 5% of individuals 65 and older (Richie & Lovestone, 2002 [Level VI]). More than 4.5 million Americans have the most common form of dementia, Alzheimer's disease (AD), a number that is expected to triple by the middle of the 21st century (Hebert, Scheer, Bienias, Bennett, & Evans, 2003 [Level IV]).

Age is the strongest risk factor for dementia with the risk increasing to nearly 50% of individuals 85 and older (Evans et al., 1989 [Level IV]). The most common forms of progressive dementia, and discussed in this chapter, include AD, vascular dementia (VaD), and Dementia with Lewy bodies (DLB). Less common although not less significant is progressive dementia associated with Parkinson's disease, frontotemporal dementia, and the dementias associated with HIV, and Creutzfeld-Jacob disease.

AD, the most common form of dementia, accounts for more than 60% of all cases. Currently, 4 million to 5 million Americans have AD and the number is expected to increase to 13.2 million by 2050 (Hebert, Scheer, Bienias, Bennett, & Evans, 2003 [Level IV]). A chronic neurodegenerative disease, first described by Alos Alzheimer in 1907, it is characterized by neurofibrillary plaques and "tangles" in the brain. The production and accumulation of beta-amyloid peptide is increasingly recognized as key to the pathogenesis of AD (Hardy & Selkoe, 2002 [Level I]). Classic features of AD include progressive loss of memory, deterioration of language and other cognitive functions, decline in the ability to perform activities of daily living (ADLs), and changes in personality and behavior (Desai & Grossberg, 2005 [Level VI]). Mild cognitive impairment (MCI), a syndrome defined as cognitive decline greater than expected for an individual's age that minimally interferes with ADLs (Gauthier et al., 2006 [Level VI]), may be a precursor of dementia. Individuals with MCI are nearly twice as likely to die and more than three times as likely to develop AD in a 5-year period than a cohort of individuals without MCI (Bennett et al., 2002 [Level IV]).

VaD, previously known as multi-infarct dementia (MID), refers to dementia resulting from cerebrovascular disease. It is the second most common cause of dementia among older adults and represents approximately 20% of all cases of dementia in the United States (Roman, 2003a [Level VI]). Broad classifications of VaD include those attributed to multiple discrete infarctions, strategic single infarctions, diffuse subcortical white matter disease (Geldmacher, 2004 [Level VI]), and hemorrhagic lesions (Roman, 2003b [Level VI]). The diagnosis of VaD is based on the association between a cerebrovascular event and the onset of clinical features of dementia, including evidence of focal deficits, gait distur-bances, and impairments in executive function. Compared to AD, memory may not be impaired or is more mildly affected. It is not uncommon that AD and VaD pathology coexist and this, often referred to as a mixed dementia, is likely to increase as the population ages (Langa, Foster, & Larson, 2004 [Level V]).

DLB is a neurodegenerative dementia that results when Lewy bodies form in the brain. Lewy bodies are pathological aggregations of alpha-synuclein found in the cytoplasma of neurons (McKeith et al., 2003 [Level V]). Clinical fea-tures include cognitive and behavioral changes in combination with features of Parkinsonism. Disorders of executive function occur early. Hallucinations and visuospatial disturbances are prominent. Although rigidity and unsteady gait are common, tremors are not (Geldmacher, 2004 [Level VI]). Many but not all patients with Parkinson's disease develop a dementia years after the motor symptoms appear. Distinctions have been made clinically between the DLB and the dementia associated with Parkinson's disease based on the sequence of the appearance of symptoms (McKeith et al., 2005 [Level VI]).

Assessment of The Problem

Goals of Assessment

Early identification of cognitive impairment is the most important goal in assess-ment. Cognitive impairment resulting from conditions like dementia, delirium, and depression represents critically serious pathology and requires urgent as-sessment and tailored interventions. Yet, diminished or altered cognitive func-tioning is often perceived by health care professionals as a normal consequence of aging, and opportunities for timely intervention are too often missed (Milisen, Braes, Flick, & Foreman, 2006 [Level VI]). Although distinctions have been made comparing the clinical features of the common cognitive impairments associ-ated with delirium, dementia, and depression, this is difficult to do clinically because these conditions often coexist and older adults can demonstrate atypi-cal features in any of these conditions.

The second most important assessment goal is to identify a potentially re-versible primary or contributing cause of a cognitive impairment. Table 6.1 lists some of the most common causes of reversible cognitive impairment (i.e., delir-ium) in older adults; these causes are also covered in chapter 7, *Delirium: Pre-vention, Early Recognition, and Treatment.*

History Taking

Complaints from the patient or observations made by others of memory loss, problems with decision making and/or judgment, or a decline in an ADL func-tion should alert the health care professional that a progressive form of demen-tia might exist. A detailed dementia assessment and screening is important; however, the extant tools to help guide this process lack specificity and sensitiv-ity (Freund & Gravenstein, 2004 [Level VI]). There is no single comprehensive evidence-based tool that can elicit a definitive diagnosis of dementia. Suggested approaches, techniques, and tools are identified later in this chapter.

6.1 Common Causes of Reversible Cognitive Impairment (Delirium)

Metabolic disturbances
Vitamin deficiencies (B_{12}, folate)
Thyroid dysfunction
Infections
Depression
Drug-related effect
Fluid and electrolyte disorder
Hypovolemia
Hypoxia
Cerebrovascular inflammation
Brain lesions
Hydrocephalus
Pain

Collecting an accurate history is the cornerstone to the assessment process, yet this obviously is a challenge in the individual presenting with cognitive impairment. The assessment domains covered in history taking include functional, cognitive, and behavioral queries and observations. The history-taking process involves first interviewing the patient, followed perhaps by clarifying, elaborating, and validating information with the family or others familiar with the capabilities and expressions of the patient.

Functional Assessment

Because cognitive assessment can be embarrassing and/or threatening, it may be more respectful to initiate the conversation around the patient's functional domain. Asking the patient to elaborate on his or her functional abilities in ADLs as well as instrumental activities of daily living (IADLs) and eliciting any identified decline with specified chronology can provide some insight (see chapter 3, *Assessment of Function*, for the approach and tools for functional assessment).

The functional activities questionnaire (FAQ) is an informant-based measure of functional ability and has been recognized for its ability to discriminate early dementia (Pfeffer, Kurosaki, Harrah, Chance, & Filos, 1982 [Level IV]). An informant, typically the primary caregiver, is asked to rate the performance of the patient in 10 different activities. The modified Alzheimer's disease cooperative study–activities of daily living inventory (ADCS–ADL) is a specific functional tool used primarily in clinical trials to assess and monitor patients with moderate to severe AD (Galasko et al., 1997 [Level IV]). The patient's daily caregiver is asked to rate the older adult's usual performance on the more basic measures of function compared to the previous month to identify progression of functional decline.

| 6.2 | Components of Mental-Status Evaluation |

Orientation: person, place, time

Attention and concentration: ability to attend and concentrate

Memory: ability to register, recall, retain

Judgment: ability to make appropriate decisions

Executive-control functions: ability to abstract, plan, sequence, and use feedback to guide performance

Speech and language: ability to communicate ideas and receive and express a message

Presence of delusions, hallucinations

Mood and affect

Cognitive Assessment

The cognitive domain is assessed as part of a broader mental-status evaluation, the components of which are listed in Table 6.2. Whereas some of the parameters of a mental-status evaluation (e.g., memory or cognition) might be measured with a standardized tool such as the Mini-Mental State Exam (MMSE), others require specific inquiry or direct or indirect observation by the health care professional and/or caregiver. The measure of mood is totally subjective and is based on self-report status. The evaluation always provides the opportunity to identify sensory impairments (i.e., vision and hearing loss), which can further impact cognition, function, and behavior.

The "gold standard" of tools that measure cognition is the MMSE developed more than 30 years ago (Folstein, Folstein, & McHugh, 1975 [Level IV]). Used extensively in clinical trials as well as in a variety of clinical settings, it is relatively easy to administer and score and can be used to assess cognitive changes over time. The annual rate of decline on the MMSE in AD is 3.3 points annually (Han, Cole, Bellavance, McCusker, & Primeau, 2000 [Level I]). The MMSE has established validity and reliability, although concerns continue to be expressed by clinicians that it is time-consuming and in some circumstances the relevancy of selected questions has been raised. The MMSE score is strongly related to education, with high false-positive rates for those with little education, and predictive power is also significantly influenced by language (Parker & Philp, 2004 [Level VI]). It is insensitive to executive dysfunction and has been criticized for a lack of sensitivity in detecting early or mild dementia (Leifer, 2003 [Level VI]). As has been suggested with other measures of cognitive testing, the MMSE may have a cultural bias (Manley & Espino, 2004 [Level I]). Clinicians must remain aware that a high score on the MMSE does not rule out cognitive decline or the possibility of dementia, particularly in high-functioning individuals with cognitive complaints (Manning, 2004 [Level VI]). The tool is available on-line at http://www.minimental.com.

A simple and reliable measure of visual-spatial ability in dementia is the Clock Drawing Test (CDT) (Sunderland et al., 1989 [Level IV]). Scoring is based on the ability to free-hand draw the face of a clock, insert the hour numbers in the appropriate locations, and then set the hands of the clock to the time designated by the examiner. The CDT is strongly correlated with executive function (i.e., the ability to execute complex behaviors and to solve problems) and is useful in the detection of mild dementia (Royall, Mulroy, Chiodo, & Polk, 1999 [Level IV]). It also correlates moderately with driving performance because the CDT score drops as the number of driving errors increases (Freund, Gravenstein, & Ferris, 2002 [Level IV]; Freund, Gravenstein, Ferris, Burke, & Shaheen, 2005 [Level IV]). The test and instructions are available on-line at www.neurosurvival.ca/ClinicalAssistant/scales/clock_drawing_test.htm.

A clinically useful tool that combines the CDT with measures of cognition (i.e., three-word recall) is the Mini-Cognitive (Mini-Cog) test (Borson, Scanlan, Brush, Vitaliano, & Dokmak, 2000 [Level IV]). This test demonstrates a high level of sensitivity and specificity for dementia, takes less time to administer, and has less language and educational-level bias than the MMSE (Borson, Scanlan, Chen, & Ganguli, 2003 [Level IV]; Borson, Scanlan, Watanabe, Tu, & Lessig, 2005 [Level IV]). The Mini-Cog detected cognitive impairment in a community sample of a predominantly ethnic minority better than primary-care physician assessment (84% versus 41%), particularly in milder stages of the disease (Borson, Scanlan, Watanabe, Tu, & Lessig, 2006 [Level IV]). The Mini-Cog test and instructions are available on-line at http://www.hospitalmedicine.org/geriresource/toolbox/minicog.htm.

Behavioral Assessment

Behavioral changes become increasingly common as individuals progress through the stages of dementia (Volicer & Hurley, 2003 [Level V]). Regular assessment and monitoring can help identify the triggers of disruptive behavior and early manifestations of the behavior. Timely interventions that result in de-escalation of the behavior can help decrease the level of distress experienced by both the patient and the caregiver. Behavioral management can help maintain functionality and safety. Commonly demonstrated behaviors are those associated with agitation and psychosis. Asking the patient about levels of restlessness, anxiety, and irritability is important because, at times, these emotional and behavioral states occur even earlier than cognitive changes. Aggression, wandering, delusions and hallucinations, and resistance to care are manageable with pharmacological and nonpharmacological treatment options.

The Neuropsychiatric Inventory (NPI) measures frequency and severity of psychiatric symptoms and behavioral manifestations in individuals with dementias and additionally helps to distinguish the potential cause of the dementia (Cummings et al., 1994 [Level IV]). The NPI takes about 10 minutes to administer, during which the caregiver is asked screening and probing questions related to the presence and degree of behaviors such as agitation, anxiety, irritability, apathy, and disinhibition. The NPI also includes a measure of caregiver stress. A briefer questionnaire version, the NPI-Q, also has established validity (Kaufer et al., 2000 [Level IV]).

Because as many as 50% of individuals with dementia have coexisting depressive symptoms (Zubenko et al., 2003 [Level IV]), it is important to conduct an adjunctive assessment of depression. Recognizing depressive symptoms in older adults is challenging, and using an interviewer-rated instrument is recommended in addition to using clinical judgment (Onega, 2006 [Level VI]). The Geriatric Depression Scale (GDS) is a screening instrument that takes only a few minutes to administer and is discussed along with appropriate depression-management strategies in detail in chapter 5, *Depression*.

Referral of the patient to a neuropsychologist for more extensive neuropsychological testing might be indicated to provide more specific diagnostic information associated with neurodegenerative disease states and areas of brain dysfunction (Manning, 2004 [Level VI]). This kind of assessment can identify subtle cognitive impairments in higher functioning individuals, distinguish mild cognitive impairment from dementia, and provide direction and support for care providers and the family (Adelman & Daly, 2005 [Level VI]).

Physical Exam and Diagnostics

Once the functional, cognitive, and behavioral domains in progressive dementia have been established through history taking of the patient and caregiver, a thorough review of systems is undertaken followed by the physical examination. The history-taking process narrows the differential diagnosis of reversible and irreversible causes for dementia. A thorough neurological and cardiovascular examination will help to specify the etiology of a single type or combined dementia that will direct the need for laboratory and imaging tests. Cardiovascular findings such as hypertension, arrhythmias, extra heart sounds or murmurs along with focal neurological findings such as weakness and sensory deficit may favor a diagnosis of VaD; pathological reflexes, gait disorders, and abnormal cerebellar findings may be indicative of AD; and parkinsonian signs might indicate dementia associated with either Lewy bodies or Parkinson's disease (Kane, Ouslander, & Abrass, 2004 [Level VI]).

There are no specific laboratory tests for the diagnosis of progressive dementia other than those that can primarily indicate a potentially reversible or contributing cause (see Table 6.1). The American Academy of Neurology (AAN) recommends two specific laboratory tests (i.e., thyroid function and B12) in the initial evaluation of suspected dementia (Knopman et al., 2001 [Level VI]). The AAN similarly recommends that all patients with suspected dementia have a magnetic resonance imaging (MRI) study or noncontrast computed tomography (CT) as part of the initial workup. Once dementia has become clinically relevant and a cause becomes apparent, there is no further diagnostic yield afforded by imaging.

Caregiver Assessment

It is important to remember that the caregiver is a patient, too, in that they suffer as does the patient with dementia. Caregiver need and burden refer to the psychological, physical, and financial burden associated with caregiving. Caregivers are at risk for depression, physical illness, and death (Schulz & Beach, 1999 [Level IV]). The Zarit Burden Interview (ZBI) can be used to identify the degree of burden experienced by the caregiver. The ZBI is a 4-item screening followed by an additional 12 items with good reliability and validity (Bedard et al., 2001 [Level IV]). Administration of this tool to a community-dwelling caregiver can indicate the extent of impact caregiving has on the caregiver's health, social and emotional well-being, and finances. The Caregiver Strain Index (CSI) is another tool that has been used to identify families with caregiving concerns (Robinson, 1983 [Level IV]). The CSI is available on-line at http://www.ConsultGeriRN.org/publications/trythis/issue14.pdf.

Interventions and Care Strategies

There is no cure for progressive dementia. The management of individuals with dementia requires pharmacological and nonpharmacological interventions.

Pharmacological Interventions

The goals of pharmacological therapy in dementia include preserving what the disease destroys in cognitive and functional ability, minimizing what the disease imposes in the way of behavior disturbances, and slowing the progression of the disease effects brought on by the destruction of neurons (Geldmacher, 2003 [Level VI]). Nurses, regardless of whether they are the prescribers of drug therapy, need to be informed about the variety of drugs used in managing dementia and the evidence supporting the pharmacological approaches. Although there is substantial evidence that adults with mild to moderate AD (and perhaps VaD and LBD) should have drug therapy, there are no solid data in support for drug therapy into the advanced stage of the disease (Olsen, Poulsen, & Lublin, 2005 [Level I]).

Acetyl cholinesterase inhibitors are the mainstay of treatment. Four are currently available in the United States: donepezel hydrochloride (Aricept), rivistigmine tartrate (Exelon), galantamine hydrobromide (Reminyl), and tacrine hydrochloride (Tacrine)—the oldest and less favored drug due to its adverse effect and multiple daily dosing. Cognitive improvements in patients with mild to moderate AD have been shown for each of these four drugs in large double-blind randomized controlled clinical trials (Masterman, 2004 [Level VI]). These drugs also provide cognitive and behavioral improvement in other forms of progressive dementia including VaD (Del Ser et al., 2000 [Level I]) and DLB (Erkinjuntti et al., 2002 [Level VI]). With the exception of Tacrine, the acetyl cholinesterase inhibitors are safe and well tolerated; however, they may have gastrointestinal side effects (i.e., nausea, anorexia, and diarrhea). Dementia pharmacological therapy can improve the quality of life for the patient and the caregiver and delays nursing home placement (Geldmacher, 2003 [Level II]; Lopez et al., 2002 [Level III]).

Memantine (Namenda), a newer drug approved by the Federal Drug Administration (FDA) for moderate to severe dementia, has a different mechanism of action than the acetyl cholinesterase inhibitors. This N-methyl-D-aspartate receptor antagonist has neuroprotective effects that prevent excitatory neurotoxicity. Individuals with AD and VaD have improved cognition and behavior (McShane, Areosa Sastre, & Minakaran, 2006 [Level I]). Side effects of memantine, although uncommon, include diarrhea, insomnia, and agitation. Combined administration of donepezel with memantine demonstrated increased efficacy in advanced AD when compared to donepezel alone (Tariot et al., 2004 [Level II]).

Pharmacologic Therapy for Problematic Behaviors

Behavior changes are common in the mid to later stages of progressive dementia and, although nonpharmacological interventions are preferred, supplementation with a tailored drug regimen is sometimes necessary. Psychotropic medications, primarily antipsychotics, can be administered to help the individual regain control and be less disruptive—positive outcomes for the caregiver as well as the patient. Drugs must be prescribed in the lowest effective dose for the shortest amount of time (Gray, 2004 [Level VI]). The patient needs to be closely monitored for effectiveness and adverse side effects. Psychotropic medications have a high risk of adverse drug events, which are discussed in chapter 12, *Reducing Adverse Drug Events*.

Psychotropic therapy for different behaviors is always short term (i.e., 3 to 6 months). Once the target symptoms are relieved or abbreviated, then terminating therapy must be considered. Long-term psychotropic drug therapy should be considered only if the symptoms reoccur after two attempts at withdrawal (Geldmacher, 2003 [Level VI]).

Psychotic symptoms (e.g., delusions and hallucinations) frequently occur in the later stages of progressive dementia (Ropacki & Jeste, 2005 [Level I]) and are often associated with agitation and aggression (Holroyd, 2004 [Level VI]). The conventional antipsychotic haloperidol (i.e., Haldol) has been used for decades and remains the most commonly used drug for control of psychotic symptoms in individuals with dementia. A recent Cochrane Review by Lonergan, Luxenberg, and Colford (2002 [Level I]) validated the useful role of Haldol in managing aggression but did not find evidence for its role in managing agitation for patients with dementia. The side effects of conventional antipsychotics are considerable and include extrapyramidal symptoms, tardive dyskinesia, sedation, orthostatic hypotension, and falls. There is evidence from recent studies to support the use of the newer atypical antipsychotics over the conventional ones (Tariot, Profenno, & Ismail, 2004 [Level I]). Agents available on the market include risperidone, olanzapine, quetiapine, and the newest, aripiprazole. Increasingly prescribed, these drugs appear to be as equally effective as the conventionals with fewer negative effects such as Parkinsonism and tardive dysknesia (Gray, 2004 [Level VI]). Recent concerns have been raised that use of risperidone is associated with increased risk of stroke; yet, the data are not conclusive, therefore making it difficult to determine if the benefits of risperidone outweigh the risks (Carson, McDonaugh, & Peterson, 2006 [Level I]). Olanzapine, now available orally, can be most advantageous in managing an individual with dementia with a catastrophic reaction, who is resistive, combative, and at serious risk to harming self or others. Quetiapine (i.e., seroquel) is helpful in treating the hallucinations commonly occurring with agitation in DLB (Takahashi, Yoshida, Sugita, Higuchi, & Shimiqu, 2003 [Level IV]). Evidence suggests that both risperidone and olanzapine are useful in reducing aggression, but both are associated with serious adverse cardiovascular events and extrapyramidal symptoms; therefore, it should not be used routinely to treat patients with dementia unless there is considerable risk or severe distress (Ballard & Waite, 2006 [Level I]). Antipsychotic medications have been used extensively in individuals with AD and some patients can benefit from the therapy; however, the adverse effects are considerable and are no more effective than placebo when these are considered (Schneider et al., 2006 [Level II]). Additional research is needed to determine when and how to use psychotropic medications to address behaviors in individuals with dementia.

Benzodiazepines (e.g., lorazepan, oxazepan) are sometimes used to manage agitation and aggression; however, the risk-benefit ratio is often unsatisfactory. Patients with dementia are particularly sensitive to the anticholinergic effects of these drugs that can exacerbate behavioral symptoms; therefore, they should be used cautiously (Allain et al., 2000 [Level VI]). Sleep disorders can be ameliorated, for some patients, with low-dose Trazadone, which can also be helpful with depressive, psychotic, and behavioral symptoms.

Findings are equivocal in using antidepressants to treat agitated depression in dementia (Cummings, 2004 [Level VI]). Tricyclic antidepressants should be avoided because of the high anticholinergic and cardiovascular risk potential. Data from studies of selective serotonin inhibitors and mood-stabilizing anticonvulsants do not consistently support their effectiveness in agitated dementia (Lyketsos et al., 2006 [Level VI]). The narrow therapeutic window and the need for ongoing blood-level monitoring of the anticonvulsants limit the usefulness of these drugs.

Supplemental Drugs

Anti-inflammatory drugs and estrogen; herbals such as gingko; and vitamins such as B_{12}, folate, and Vitamin E—although sometimes touted and commonly used—have no proven efficacy for dementia. Dementia associated with VaD requires appropriate control of hypertension, hyperlipidemia, and aspirin therapy. Parkinsonism (rigidity), seen with DLB, may benefit from levodopa therapy.

Nonpharmacologic Strategies

Nonpharmacological strategies including those from the cognitive, behavioral, and environmental domains, in combination with staff support and education, are effective (Burgener & Twigg, 2002 [Level I]). Physical/functional, environmental, psychosocial, behavioral, and end-of-life (EOL) care interventions are discussed in this section.

Physical/Functional Interventions

Maintaining physical and functional well-being of the individual with progressive dementia facilitates independence, maintains health status, and can ease the caregiving burden. Interventions include adequate nutrition and hydration, regular exercise, maintenance of ADLs, proper rest and sleep, appropriate bowel and bladder routines, proper dental hygiene and care, and current vaccinations. Because co-morbidities are common (Lyketsos et al., 2005 [Level IV]), regular assessment, vigilant monitoring, and aggressive management of acute and chronic conditions are necessary. Vehicular driving safety might need to be examined because recent evidence indicates that individuals with mild dementia pose a risk in driving safety (Dubinsky, Stein, & Lyons, 2000 [Level VI]).

Environmental Interventions

A specialized ecological model of care, which facilitates interaction between the person and environment in a more home-like environment, has proven to be beneficial for individuals with dementia. This model affords greater privacy, encourages meaningful activities, and permits more choice than the traditional model of care. It also demonstrates that individuals with dementia experience less decline in ADLs; are more engaged with the environment; and no measurable differences are found in cognitive measures, depression, or social withdrawal (Reimer, Slaughter, Donaldson, Currie, & Eliasziw, 2004 [Level IV]).

A systematic review reported inclusive results and suggested that more research is needed with regard to the use of bright light in sleep in fostering better sleep and reducing behavior problems in dementia (Kim, Song, & Yoo, 2003 [Level I]). The use of aromatherapy to reduce disturbed behavior, promote sleep, and stimulate motivation also shows promise but needs more study (Thorgrimsen, Spector, Wiles, & Orrell, 2006 [Level I]). Manipulation of the environment (e.g., alarms, circular hallways, visual or structural barriers) to minimize wandering has not conclusively demonstrated to be effective (Peatfield, Futrell, & Cox, 2002 [Level I]).

Psychosocial Interventions

Mental and social engagement is important to the well-being of all older adults. Meaningful activity and involvement is no less important in individuals with dementia. Although the effectiveness of counseling or procedural memory stimulation is not supported in mild-stage dementia, reality orientation does appear to be effective (Bates, Boote, & Beverley, 2004 [Level I]). The evidence suggests that cognitive therapy is more beneficial than no therapy at all, but it may be patient-specific (Forbes, 2004 [Level II]). Validation therapy, based on caregiver acceptance of the reality of the person with dementia's experience, may be of value but the evidence is lacking (Neal & Briggs, 2003 [Level I]).

Recreational therapies including music and art have been explored, although the evidence to substantiate effectiveness is scanty (Gerdner, 2000 [Level VI]). Music, in particular, may have some value in reducing behavioral problems in dementia (Lou, 2001 [Level I]), but additional research is needed to demonstrate immediate and sustained benefit.

Support groups, counseling sessions, availability of a counselor, and education delay nursing home placement of those with mild to moderate AD (Mittelman, Ferris, Shulman, Steinberg, & Levin, 1996 [Level II]). Caregivers experience physical, financial, social, and emotional losses that become more pronounced over time (Bullock, 2004 [Level VI]). Teaching caregivers how to change their interactions with the person with dementia and to use problem-solving skills is effective (Burgener, Bakas, Murray, Dunahee, & Tossey, 1998 [Level II]) and can reduce caregiver burden and depression and increase their knowledge (Acton & Winter, 2002 [Level I]). Areas for caregiver education are detailed in Table 6.3.

6.3 Educating Caregivers

Information about the disease and its progression
Strategies to maintain function and independence
Preservation of cognitive and physical vitality in dementia
Maintaining a safe and comfortable environment
Giving physical and emotional care
Communicating with the individual with dementia
Managing behavioral problems
Advance planning: health care and finances
Caregiver survival tips
Building a caregiver support network

Behavioral Interventions

Behavioral and psychosocial symptoms of dementia are common with every form of progressive dementia, particularly in the moderate stage. The three most troublesome symptoms are agitation, aggression, and wandering. Problematic behaviors that occur during meals or bathing can be particularly challenging. It is important to recognize and realize that any new behavior could be a sign of an acute illness or an environmental influence. Unrecognized pain can cause disruptive behavior. Short-term use of physical restraints may be necessary, but those selected should always be the least restrictive type and used for the shortest duration of time. The Progressively Lowered Stress Threshold (PLST) is a framework to optimize function, minimize disruption, and help the caregiver (Smith, Hall, Gerdner, & Buckwalter, 2006 [Level V]). By adapting the environment and routines, interventions are designed to help the patient with dementia use his or her functional skills and minimize potentially triggering reactions. There are six essential principles of care in the PLST, as follows:

1. *Maximize safe function*: Use familiar routines, limit choices, provide rest periods, reduce stimuli when stress occurs, routinely identify and anticipate physical stressors (i.e., pain, urinary symptoms, hunger, or thirst).
2. *Provide unconditional positive regard*: Use respectful conversation, simple and understandable language, nonverbal expressions of touch.
3. *Use behaviors to gauge activity and stimulation*: Monitor for early signs of anxiety (e.g., pacing, facial grimacing) and intervene before behavior escalates.
4. *Teach caregivers to "listen" to the behaviors*: Monitor the language pattern (e.g., repetition, jargon) and behaviors (e.g., rummaging) that might be showing how the person reduces stress when needs are not being met.
5. *Modify the environment*: Assess the environment to ensure safe mobility and promote way-finding and orientation through cues.
6. *Provide ongoing assistance to the caregiver*: Assess and address the need for education and support.

Advance Planning and EOL Care Interventions

Advanced planning and providing directives for care are important in guiding the types of interventions used at the end of life and can decrease the caregiver stress in proxy decision making. Nursing homes are common sites for EOL care for people with progressive dementia; however, nationally only 51% of all nursing home residents have an advance directive (Mezey, Mitty, Bottrell, Ramsey, & Fisher, 2000 [Level VI]). As many as 90% of the 4 million Americans with dementia will be institutionalized before death (Smith, Kokmen, & O'Brien, 2000 [Level IV]), making this environment in particular an important focus for EOL care. Older adults with dementia have increased mortality rates compared to older adults without dementia (Ostbye, Hill, & Steenhuis, 1999 [Level IV]) and often die from the complication of immobility, infection, and heart disease. The end stage of AD may last as long as 2 to 3 years (Brookmeyer, Corrada, Curriero, & Kawas, 2002 [Level IV]) and frequently distressing signs and symptoms occur at this time.

Dementia itself or often-associated conditions can cause physical symptoms such as poor nutrition, urinary incontinence, skin breakdown, pain, infection, shortness of breath, fatigue, difficulty in swallowing, choking, and gurgling, in addition to the behavioral symptoms mentioned previously. There is no acceptable standard treatment for the consequences of advanced dementia and, where guidelines do exist, there is minimal to no palliative-care content. Aggressive treatments such as antibiotics, tube feedings, psychotropic drugs, and physical restraints to address problematic behaviors appear to be prevalent, although there is no substantial evidence that this approach is effective in end-stage dementia and that prognosis and life expectancy are improved by these strategies (Evers, Purohit, Perl, Khan, & Martin, 2002 [Level IV]; Finucane, Christmas, & Travis, 1999 [Level VI]). Measuring quality of care at the end of life for those with dementia poses significant challenges due to the limitations in subjective reporting and, therefore, relies on the caregiver's analysis of cues to monitor the patient's condition and experience (Volicer, Hurley, & Blasi, 2001 [Level IV]). Despite the clear recognition that significant improvements in EOL care for those with dementia is needed (Horgas & Tsai, 1998 [Level IV]; Scherder et al., 2005 [Level I]), there is a lack of systematic evidence on how to approach palliative care for this population (Sampson, Ritchie, Lai, Raven, & Blanchard, 2005 [Level I]).

Case Study and Discussion

Mrs. P. is an 85-year-old White woman brought into the primary-care clinic by her daughter for a geriatric consultation. She has a 4-year history of cognitive impairment that began with memory loss and impaired judgment and that appears to be worsening; she is now experiencing some behavioral problems. Mrs. P. is high school educated, has been widowed for 10 years, and is a retired short-order cook. She currently lives with her daughter, son-in-law (both work full time), and grandson.

Her primary-care physician completed a dementia workup at the time the symptoms appeared 4 years ago and started her on Donepezil, which was discontinued within a few days because of gastrointestinal side effects. She recently had paranoid ideation in which she accused her 15-year-old grandson of listening in on her telephone conversations and taking some money from her purse. Her daughter reports that Mrs. P. has "a short fuse" and gets agitated easily. "She called me a moron and even took a swing at me the other day when I told her she smelled bad and needed to take a shower."

Mrs. P. performs her own personal hygiene although she needs reminders and cueing at times; she is continent. She does not do any IADLs (e.g., cooking, shopping) and it was unclear if she truly was no longer capable of performing these functions or no longer had the opportunity or desire to do them. Mrs. P. reports no desire to eat and had a weight loss resulting in a change of at least three clothing sizes that has occurred slowly during the past few years. When asked about her mood, she becomes tearful and says, "I get disgusted; no one cares about me anymore." Mrs. P. says she hates to be alone and that the family "just come and goes—they never talk with me." Her MMSE score is 18/30 with deficits in memory, calculation, and ability to copy the intersecting pentagons. She scores 10/15 on the Geriatric Depression Scale (see www.ConsultGeriRN.org for the GDS scale).

Past medical history includes thyroidectomy, left cataract extraction, cholecystectomy, and hysterectomy for benign disease. Her daughter thinks that Mrs. P. may have been on antihypertensives in the past. The only medication Mrs. P. takes at present is for her thyroid, but neither she nor her daughter knew the name of the drug.

On physical exam, she is afebrile; blood pressure is 132/70, and is she is about 10 pounds below her ideal body weight. Mrs. P. is alert and cooperative and smiles at intervals during the examination. She has slight hearing loss with clear canals; no thyromegaly. The cardiovascular exam reveals no murmur, edema, or discolorations of the extremities. Pulses are strong throughout. There are no focal neurological symptoms. Gait is slow but steady. Breasts are free of masses and abdomen is soft, nontender with no organ enlargement.

A diagnosis of depression and progressive dementia of the Alzheimer's type is made and she is started on the combination of Donepezil and Mementine, both to be titrated slowly. Additional information from Mrs. P.'s primary-care physician will be consulted about her thyroid function. Antidepressant therapy may be considered at a later date. Take the initiative to do some health teaching and provide additional resource information to the family.

Depression is not uncommon in those with a progressive dementia. Severe anxiety, agitation, and aggression can occur; tearfulness and decreased appetite with weight loss may also be present (Holroyd, 2004 [Level VI]). Using the PLST model, focus on teaching the daughter to recognize triggers and prodromal signs of increasing anxiety, and intervene appropriately when anxiety and agitation occur. Emphasize strategies in each of the six PLST principles of care: maximize safe function, provide unconditional regard, use behaviors to gauge activity and stimulation, "listen" to the behaviors, modify the environment, and provide ongoing assistance to the caregiver. Emphasize using less confrontational language and behaviors in approaches and interactions with Mrs. P. Provide her with specific contact information for the geriatrician's office and for the caretaker, as well as the local and national resources available through the Alzheimer's Association (1-800-272-3900; www.alz.org) and the Alzheimer's Disease Education and Referral Center (ADEAR) (1-800-438-4380; www.alzheimers.org). Give dietary instructions and strategies to increase nutritional density, noting that additional resource information is available at the ADEAR site listed herein. Give specific medication instructions with particular emphasis on how to use the titration packet provided; further suggest the co-administration with food to reduce the likelihood of gastrointestinal side effects. Plan a follow-up telephone call for the next day and schedule a follow-up medical and health teaching appointment in 1 month to evaluate the effectiveness of the plan of care. Instruct the patient and family to call or return if new or changed behaviors or physical symptoms develop.

Summary and Conclusions

It is important that health care professionals identify cognitive impairments in older adults early and differentiate a progressive from a reversible etiology, such as delirium. Comprehensive assessment, monitoring, and pharmacological and nonpharmacological management of physical, functional, cognitive, and behavioral problems are important, both in initial identification and in the ongoing care of the individual with progressive dementia. Education and support of the family and professional caregiver are essential. It is difficult to identify clearly what constitutes quality of life for the individual with progressive dementia, which interventions enhance this quality, and how this is accomplished. Abraham, MacDonald, and Nadzam (2006 [Level VI]) note that in geriatric nursing, there is limited evidence to guide our care. It is imperative that geriatric nurses evaluate practice and generate new knowledge to ensure best practice in the care of individuals with progressive dementia as well as their caregivers.

Resources

Alzheimer's Association www.alz.org
Alzheimer's Disease Education and Referral Center www.alzheimers.nia.nih.gov
The National Family Caregiver's Association (NFCA) www.nfcacares.org
American Association of Retired Persons (AARP) www.aarp.org/caregiving
ElderWeb www.elderweb.com
Nurse Competence in Aging http://www.ConsultGeriRN.org/
The Hartford Institute for Geriatric Nursing http://www.ConsultGeriRN.org/
National Conference of Gerontological Nurse Practitioners: Mental Health Toolkit http://www.ncgnp.org/

Box 6.1

Nursing Standard of Practice Protocol: Recognition and Management of Dementia

I. GOALS

  A. Early recognition of dementing illness.
  B. Appropriate management strategies in care of individuals with dementia.

II. OVERVIEW

The rapid growth of the aging population is associated with an increase in the prevalence of progressive dementias. It is imperative that a differential diagnosis be ascertained early in the course of cognitive impairment and that the patient is closely monitored for coexisting morbidities. Nurses have a central role in assessment and management of individuals with progressive dementia.

III. BACKGROUND

  A. Definitions/Distinctions
    1. Dementia is a clinical syndrome of cognitive deficits that involves both memory impairments and a disturbance in at least one other area of cognition (e.g., aphasia, apraxia, agnosia) and disturbance in executive functioning (American Psychiatric Association, 2000 [Level VI]).
    2. In addition to disruptions in cognition, dementias are commonly associated with changes in function and behavior.
    3. The most common forms of progressive dementia are Alzheimer's disease, vascular dementia, and dementia with Lewy bodies; the pathophysiology for each is poorly understood.
    4. Differential diagnosis of dementing conditions is complicated by the fact that concurrent disease states (i.e., co-morbidities) often coexist.
  B. Prevalence
    1. Dementia affects about 5% of individuals 65 and older (Richie & Lovestone, 2002 [Level VI]).
    2. Four to five million Americans have Alzheimer's disease (AD) (Hebert et al., 2003 [Level IV]).
    3. 13.2 million are projected to have AD by 2050 (Hebert et al., 2003 [Level IV]).
    4. Global prevalence of dementia is about 24.3 million, with 6 million new cases every year (Ferri et al., 2005 [Level IV]).
  C. Risk Factors
    1. Advanced age
    2. Mild cognitive impairment

3. Cardiovascular disease
4. Genetics: family history of dementia, Parkinson's disease, cardiovascular disease, stroke, presence of ApoE4 allele on chromosome 19
5. Environment: head injury, alcohol abuse

IV. PARAMETERS OF ASSESSMENT

No formal recommendations for cognitive screening are indicated in asymptomatic individuals. Clinicians are advised to be alert for cognitive and functional decline in older adults to detect dementia and dementia-like presentation in early stages. Assessment domains include cognitive, functional, behavioral, physical, caregiver, and environment.

A. Cognitive Parameters
1. Orientation: person, place, time
2. Memory: ability to register, retain, recall information
3. Attention: ability to attend and concentrate on stimuli
4. Thinking: ability to organize and communicate ideas
5. Language: ability to receive and express a message
6. Praxis: ability to direct and coordinate movements
7. Executive function: ability to abstract, plan, sequence, and use feedback to guide performance

B. Mental Status Screening Tools
1. Folstein Mini-Mental State Examination (Folstein et al., 1975 [Level IV]): the most commonly used test to assess serial cognitive change. On average, the MMSE declines 3 points per year in those with AD (Han et al., 2000 [Level I]). It is composed of items assessing orientation, attention, concentration, memory, language, and construction ability. Age, education, cultural background, and perceptual and physical abilities can affect performance. The MMSE might not detect mild cognitive loss and, as well, it is not diagnostic of decision-making capacity (Parker & Philp, 2004 [Level VI]).
2. Clock Drawing Test (CDT) (Royall et al., 1999 [Level IV]): a useful measure of cognitive function that correlates with executive-control functions (i.e., the cognitive process necessary to plan and carry out goal-directed behaviors). The patient is asked to draw a clock free-hand, put in all the numbers, and set a time asked for by the examiner. Physical ability and dexterity can influence performance.
3. Mini-Cognitive (Mini-Cog) (Borson et al., 2000 [Level IV]) combines the Clock Drawing Test with the three-word recall. The patient is asked to remember three unrelated words and later is asked to recall the three words. This clinically useful tool, rapidly administered, has a high level of sensitivity and

specificity and less bias than some other instruments (e.g., the MMSE) (Borson et al., 2003 [Level IV]).

When the diagnosis remains unclear, the patient may be referred for more extensive screening and neuropsychological testing, which might provide more direction and support for the patient and the caregivers.

C. Functional Assessment

1. Tests that assess functional limitations such as the Functional Activities Questionnaire (FAQ) (Pfeffer et al., 1982 [Level IV]) can detect dementia with sensitivity and specificity comparable to mental-status testing. They are also useful in monitoring the progression of functional decline.

2. The severity of disease progression in dementia can be demonstrated by performance decline in ADL and IADL tasks and is closely correlated with mental-status scores (Galasko et al., 1997 [Level IV]). See also chapter 3, *Assessment of Function,* for additional tools.

D. Behavioral Assessment

1. Assess and monitor for behavioral changes; in particular, the presence of agitation, aggression, anxiety, disinhibitions, delusions, and hallucinations.

2. Evaluate for depression because it commonly coexists in individuals with dementia (Zubenko et al., 2003 [Level IV]). Symptoms and signs may include the presence of neurovegetative signs (e.g., hypersomnia, insomnia, increased or decreased appetite, decreased energy, weight loss or gain, psychomotor agitation or slowing) or mood changes (e.g., depressed mood, feelings of worthlessness or helplessness, suicidal ideation). See also chapter 5, *Depression.* Determine if there is a diminished level of interest in life. Is there a lack of motivation, decreased initiation, or a poor ability to sustain effort?

E. Physical Assessment

1. A comprehensive physical examination with a focus on the neurological and cardiovascular system is indicated in individuals with dementia to identify the potential cause and/or the existence of a reversible form of cognitive impairment.

2. A thorough evaluation of all prescribed, over-the-counter, homeopathic, herbal, and nutritional products taken is done to determine the potential impact on cognitive status.

3. Laboratory tests are valuable in differentiating irreversible from reversible forms of dementia. Structural neuroimaging with noncontrast computed tomography (CT) or magnetic resonance imaging (MRI) scans are appropriate in the routine initial evaluation of patients with dementia.

F. Caregiver/Environment

The caregiver of the patient with dementia often has as many needs as the patient with dementia; therefore, a detailed assessment of the caregiver and the caregiving environment is essential.

1. Elicit the caregiver perspective of patient function and the level of support provided.
2. Evaluate the impact that the patient's cognitive impairment and problem behaviors have on the caregiver (mastery, satisfaction, and burden). Two useful tools include the Zarit Burden Interview (ZBI) (Bedard et al., 2001 [Level IV]) and the Caregiver Strain Index (CSI) Tool CSI–Caregiver strain Index (see www.ConsultGeriRN.org Topic: Caregiving).
3. Evaluate the caregiver experience and patient–caregiver relationship. The caregiving experience is a stressful one and the potential for elder mistreatment and caregiver illness exists.

V. NURSING CARE STRATEGIES

Based on evidence provided under the Interventions and Care Strategies in this chapter; specifically, use of the PLST that provides a framework for the nursing care of individuals with dementia (Smith et al., 2006 [Level V]).

A. Monitor the effectiveness and potential side effects of medications given to improve cognitive function or delay cognitive decline.
B. Provide appropriate cognitive-enhancement techniques and social engagement.
C. Ensure adequate rest, sleep, fluid, nutrition, elimination, pain control, and comfort measures.
D. Avoid the use of physical and pharmacologic restraints.
E. Maximize functional capacity: Maintain mobility and encourage independence as long as possible, provide graded assistance as needed with ADLs and IADLs, provide scheduled toileting and prompted voiding to reduce urinary incontinence, encourage an exercise routine that expends energy and promotes fatigue at bedtime, establish bedtime routine and rituals.
F. Address behavioral issues: Identify environmental triggers, medical conditions, caregiver–patient conflict that may be causing the behavior, define the target symptom (i.e., agitation, aggression, wandering) and pharmacological (psychotropics) and nonpharmacological (manage affect, limit stimuli, respect space, distract, redirect) approaches, provide reassurance, refer to appropriate mental health care professionals as indicated.
G. Ensure a therapeutic and safe environment: Provide an environment that is modestly stimulating, avoiding overstimulation that can cause agitation and increase confusion, and understimulation that can cause sensory deprivation and withdrawal. Utilize patient identifiers (name tags), medic alert systems and bracelets, locks, wander guard; eliminate any environmental hazards and modify the environment to enhance safety; provide environmental cues or sensory

aides that facilitate cognition; maintain consistency in caregivers and approaches.

H. Encourage and support advance-care planning: Explain trajectory of progressive dementia, treatment options, and advance directives.

I. Provide appropriate end-of-life care in terminal phase: Provide comfort measures including adequate pain management; weigh the benefits/risks of the use of aggressive treatment (tube feeding, antibiotic therapy).

J. Provide caregiver education and support: Respect family systems/dynamics and avoid making judgments, encourage open dialogue, emphasize the patient's residual strengths, provide access to experienced professionals, teach caregivers the skills of caregiving.

K. Integrate community resources into the plan of care to meet the needs for patient and caregiver information; identify and facilitate both formal (i.e., Alzheimer's Association, Respite Care, Specialized Long Term Care) and informal (i.e., churches, neighbors, extended family/friends) support systems.

VI. EVALUATION/EXPECTED OUTCOMES

A. Patient Outcomes: The patient remains as independent and functional in the environment of choice for as long as possible, the co-morbid conditions the patient may experience are well managed, and the distressing symptoms that may occur at end of life are minimized or controlled adequately.

B. Caregiver Outcomes (lay and professional): Caregivers demonstrate effective caregiving skills; verbalize satisfaction with caregiving; report minimal caregiver burden; are familiar with, have access to, and utilize available resources.

C. Institutional Outcomes: The institution reflects a safe and enabling environment for delivering care to individuals with progressive dementia; the quality improvement plan addresses high risk problem-prone areas for individuals with dementia, such as falls and the use of restraints.

VII. FOLLOW-UP TO MONITOR CONDITION

A. Follow-up appointments are regularly scheduled; frequency depends on the patient's physical, mental, and emotional status and caregiver needs.

B. Determine the continued efficacy of pharmacological/nonpharmacological approaches to the care plan and modify as appropriate.

C. Identify and treat any underlying or contributing conditions.

D. Community resources for education and support are accessed and utilized by the patient and/or caregivers.

VIII. RELEVANT PRACTICE GUIDELINES

  A. American Academy of Neurology: Detection of Dementia, Diagnosis of Dementia, Management of Dementia, and Encounter Kit for Dementia: http://www.aan.com/professionals/practice/guideline/index
  B. American Geriatrics Society: Clinical Recommendations for Feeding Tube Placement in Elderly Patients with Advanced Dementia: http://www.americangeriatrics.org/education/cp_index.shtml
  C. American Association of Geriatric Psychiatry: Position Statement: Principles of Care for Patients with Dementia Resulting from Alzheimer's Disease: http://www.aagponline.org/prof/position_caredmnalz.asp
  D. Alzheimer's Foundation of America (AFA): Excellence in Care: www.alzfdn.org

References

Abraham, I. L., MacDonald, K. M., & Nadzam, D. M. (2006). Measuring the quality of nursing care to Alzheimer's patients. *Nursing Clinics of North America*, *41*(1), 95–104. Evidence Level VI: Expert Opinion.

Acton, C. J., & Winter, M. A. (2002). Interventions for family members caring for an elder with dementia. *Annual Review of Nursing Research*, *20*, 149–179. Evidence Level I: Systematic Review.

Adelman, A. M., & Daly, M. P. (2005). Initial evaluation of the patient with suspected dementia. *American Family Physician*, *71*(9), 1745–1750. Evidence Level VI: Expert Opinion.

Allain, H., Schuck, S., Bentuee-Ferrer, D., Bourin, M., Vercelletto, M., Reymann, J., et al. (2000). Anxiolytics in the treatment of behavioral and psychological symptoms of dementia. *International Psychogeriatrics 12* (Suppl.), 281–289. Evidence Level VI: Expert Opinion.

American Psychiatric Association (2000). Diagnostic and statistical manual of mental disorders: *DSM-IV-TR* (4th ed.). Evidence Level VI: Expert Opinion.

Ballard, C., & Waite, J. (2006). The effectiveness of atypical antipsychotics for the treatment of aggression and psychosis in Alzheimer's disease. *Cochrane Database of Systematic Reviews*, (1), CD003476. Evidence Level I: Systematic Review.

Bates, J., Boote, J., & Beverley, C. (2004). Psychosocial interventions for people with milder dementing illness: A systematic review. *Journal of Advanced Nursing*, *45*(6), 644–658. Evidence Level I: Systematic Review.

Bedard, M., Molloy, D. W., Squire, I., Dubois, S., Lever, J. A., & O'Donnell, M. (2001). The Zarit Burden Interview: A new short version and screening version. *Gerontologist*, *41*(5), 652–657. Evidence Level IV: Nonexperimental Study.

Bennett, D. A., Wilson, R. S., Schneider, J. A., Evans, D. A., Beckett, L. A., Aggarwal, N. T., et al. (2002). Natural history of mild cognitive impairment in older persons. *Neurology, 59*, 198–205. Evidence Level IV: Nonexperimental Study.

Borson, S., Scanlan, J., Brush, M., Vitaliano, P., & Dokmak, A. (2000). The Mini-Cog: A cognitive "vital signs" measure for dementia screening in multilingual elderly. *International Journal of Geriatric Psychiatry, 15*(11), 1021–1027. Evidence Level IV: Nonexperimental Study.

Borson, S., Scanlan, J. M., Chen, P., & Ganguli, M. (2003). The Mini-Cog as a screen for dementia: Validation in a population-based sample. *Journal of the American Geriatrics Society, 51*, 1451–1454. Evidence Level IV: Nonexperimental Study.

Borson, S., Scanlan, J. M., Watanabe, J., Tu, S. P., & Lessig, M. (2005) Simplifying detection of cognitive impairment: Comparison of the Mini-Cog and MMSE in a multi-ethnic sample. *Journal of the American Geriatrics Society, 53*, 871–874. Evidence Level IV: Nonexperimental Study.

Borson, S. M., Scanlan, J. M., Watanabe, J., Tu, S. P., & Lessig, M. (2006). Improving identification of cognitive impairment in primary care. *International Journal of Geriatric Psychiatry, 21*, 349–355. Evidence Level IV: Nonexperimental Study.

Brookmeyer, R., Corrada, M. M., Curriero, F. C., & Kawas, C. (2002). Survival following a diagnosis of Alzheimer's disease. *Archives of Neurology, 59*, 1764. Evidence Level IV: Nonexperimental Study.

Bullock, R. (2004). The needs of the caregiver in the long-term treatment of Alzheimer's disease. *Alzheimer's Disease Associative Disorders, 18* (Suppl. 1), 817–823. Evidence Level VI: Expert Opinion.

Burgener, S. C., Bakas, T., Murray, C., Dunahee, J., & Tossey, S. (1998). Effective caregiving approaches for patients with Alzheimer's disease. *Geriatric Nursing, 19*, 121–126. Evidence Level II: Single Experimental Study.

Burgener, S. C., & Twigg, P. (2002). Interventions for persons with irreversible dementia. *Annual Review of Nursing Research, 20*, 89–124. Evidence Level I: Systematic Review.

Carson, S., McDonaugh, M. S., & Peterson, K. (2006). A systematic review of the efficacy and safety of atypical antipsychotics in patients with psychological and behavioral symptoms of dementia. *Journal of the American Geriatrics Society, 54*(2), 354–361. Evidence Level I: Systematic Review.

Cummings, J. L.(2004). Alzheimer's disease. *New England Journal of Medicine, 35*(1), 56–67. Evidence Level VI: Expert Opinion.

Cummings, J. L., Mega, M., Gray, K., Rosenberg-Thompson, S., Carusi, D. A., et al. (1994). The neuropsychiatric inventory: Comprehensive assessment of psychopathology in dementia. *Neurology, 44*(12), 2308–2314. Evidence Level IV: Nonexperimental Study.

Del Ser, T., McKeith, I., Anand, R., Cicin-San, A., Ferrara, R., & Spiegel, R. (2000). Dementia with Lewy bodies: Findings from an international multicenter study. *International Journal of Geriatric Psychiatry, 15*(11), 1034–1045. Evidence Level I: Systematic Review.

Desai, A. K., & Grossberg, G. T. (2005). Diagnosis and treatment of Alzheimer's disease. *Neurology, 64*(12) (Suppl. 3), S34–S39. Evidence Level VI: Expert Opinion.

Dubinsky, R. M., Stein, A. C., & Lyons, K. (2000). Practice parameter: Risk of driving and Alzheimer's disease (an evidence-based review). Report of the Quality Standards Subcommittee of the American Academy of Neurology. *Neurology, 54*(12), 2205–2211. Evidence Level VI: Expert Opinion.

Erkinjuntti, T., Kurz, A., Gautheir, S., Bullock, R., Lilienfield, S., & Damaraju, C. V. (2002). Efficacy of galantamine in probable vascular dementia and Alzheimer's disease combined with cerebrovascular disease: A randomized trial. *Lancet, 359,* 1283–1290. Evidence Level II: Single Experimental Study.

Evans, D. A., Funkenstein, H. H., Albert, M. S., Scheer, P. A., Cook, N. R., Chown, M. J., et al. (1989). The prevalence of Alzheimer's disease in a community population of older persons. Higher than previously reported. *Journal of the American Medical Association, 262,* 2551–2556. Evidence Level IV: Nonexperimental Study.

Evers, M. M., Purohit, D., Perl, D., Khan, K., & Martin, D. B. (2002). Palliative and aggressive end-of-life care for patients with dementia. *Psychiatric Services, 53*(5), 609–613. Evidence Level IV: Nonexperimental Study.

Ferri, C. P., Prince, M., Brayne, C., Brodaty, H., Fratiglioni, L., & Ganguli, M., et al. (2005). Global prevalence of dementia: A Delphi consensus study. *Lancet, 366*(9503), 2112–2117. Evidence Level IV: Nonexperimental Study.

Finucane, T. E., Christmas, C., & Travis, K. (1999). Tube feedings in patients with advanced dementia: A review of the evidence. *Journal of the American Medical Association, 282,* 1365–1370. Evidence Level VI: Expert Opinion.

Folstein, M. F., Folstein, S. E., & McHugh, P. R. (1975). Mini-mental state. *Journal of Psychiatric Research, 12,* 189–198. Evidence Level IV: Nonexperimental Study.

Forbes, D. (2004). Cognitive stimulation therapy improved cognition and quality of life in dementia. *Evidence-Based Nursing, 7*(2), 54. Level II: Single Experimental Study.

Freund, B., & Gravenstein, S. (2004). Recognizing and evaluating potential dementia in office settings. *Clinics in Geriatric Medicine, 20*(1), 1–14. Evidence Level VI: Expert Opinion.

Freund, B, Gravenstein, S., & Ferris, R (2002). Use of the Clock Drawing Test as a screen for driving competency in older adults. *Journal of the American Geriatrics Society, 50*(4), S3. Evidence Level IV: Nonexperimental Study.

Freund, B., Gravenstein, S., Ferris, R., Burke, B. L., & Shaheen, E. (2005). Drawing clocks and driving cars. *Journal of General Internal Medicine, 20*(3), 240–244. Evidence Level IV: Nonexperimental Study.

Galasko, D., Bennett, D. A., Sano, M., Ernesto, C., Thomas, R., Grundman, M., et al. (1997). An inventory to assess activities of daily living for clinical trials in Alzheimer's disease: The Alzheimer's Disease Cooperative Study. *Alzheimer's Disease and Associative Disorders, 11* (Suppl. 2), S33–S39. Evidence Level IV: Nonexperimental Study.

Gauthier, S., Reisberg, B., Zaudig, M., Peterson, R. C., Richie, K., Broich, K., et al. (2006). Mild cognitive impairment: A seminar. *Lancet, 367*(9518), 1262–1269. Evidence Level VI: Expert Opinion.

Geldmacher, D. S. (2003). Alzheimer's disease: Current pharmacotherapy in the context of patient and family need. *Journal of the American Geriatrics Society, 51,* S289–295. Evidence Level VI: Expert Opinion.

Geldmacher, D. S. (2004). Differential diagnosis of dementia syndromes. *Clinics in Geriatric Medicine, 20*(1), 27–43. Evidence Level VI: Expert Opinion.

Geldmacher, D. S., Provenzano, G., McRae, T., Mastey, V., & Lein, J. R. (2003). Donepezil is associated with delayed nursing home placement in patients with Alzheimer's disease. *Journal of the American Geriatrics Society, 51*, 937–944. Evidence Level II: Single Experimental Study.

Gerdner, L. A. (2000). Music, art, and recreational therapies in the treatment of behavioral and psychosocial symptoms of dementia. *International Psychogeriatrics, 12* (Suppl. 1), 359–366. Evidence Level VI: Expert Opinion.

Gray, K. F. (2004). Managing agitation and difficult behavior in dementia. *Clinics in Geriatric Medicine, 20*(1), 69–82. Evidence Level VI: Expert Opinion.

Han, L., Cole, M., Bellavance, F., McCusker, J., & Primeau, F. (2000). Tracking cognitive decline in Alzheimer's disease using the Mini-Mental State Examination: A meta-analysis. *International Psychogeriatrics, 12*(2), 231–247. Evidence Level I: Systematic Review.

Hardy, J., & Selkoe, D. J. (2002). The amyloid hypothesis of Alzheimer's disease: Progress and problems on the road to therapeutics. *Science, 297*, 353–356. Evidence Level I: Systematic Review.

Hebert, L. E., Scheer, P. A., Bienias, J. L., Bennett, D. A., & Evans, D. A. (2003). Alzheimer's disease in the U.S. population: Prevalence estimates using the 2000 census. *Archives of Neurology, 60*, 1119–1122. Evidence Level IV: Nonexperimental Study.

Holroyd, S. (2004). Managing dementia in long-term care settings. *Clinics in Geriatric Medicine, 20*(1), 83–92. Evidence Level VI: Expert Opinion.

Horgas, A. L., & Tsai, P. (1998). Analgesic drug prescription and use in cognitively impaired nursing home residents. *Nursing Research, 47*, 235–242. Evidence Level IV: Nonexperimental Study.

Kane, R. L., Ouslander, J. G., & Abrass, I. B. (2004). Chapter 6: Delirium and Dementia in Essentials of Clinical Geriatrics (5th ed.), New York: McGraw Hill. Evidence Level VI: Expert Opinion.

Kaufer, D. I., Cummings, J. L., Ketchel, P., Smith, V., MacMillan, A., Shelley, T., et al. (2000). Validation of the NPI-Q, a brief clinical form of the Neuropsychiatric Inventory. *Journal Neuropsychiatry Clinical Neurosciences, 12*(2), 233–239. Evidence Level IV: Nonexperimental Study.

Kim S., Song, H. H., & Yoo, S. J. (2003). The effects of bright light on sleep and behavior in dementia: An analytic review. *Geriatric Nursing, 24*(4), 239–243. Evidence Level I: Systematic Review.

Knopman, D. S., DeKosky, S. T., Cummings, J. L., Chai, H., Corey-Bloom, J., Relkin, N., et al. (2001). Practice parameter: Diagnosis of dementia (an evidence-based review). Report of the Quality Standards Subcommittee of the American Academy of Neurology. *Neurology, 56*(9), 1143–1153. Evidence Level VI: Expert Opinion.

Langa, K. M., Foster, N. L., & Larson, E. B. (2004). Mixed dementia: Emerging concepts and therapeutic implications. *Journal of the American Medical Association, 292*(23), 2901–2908. Evidence Level V: Literature Review.

Leifer, B. P. (2003). Early diagnosis of Alzheimer's disease: Clinical and economic benefits. *Journal of the American Geriatrics Society, 51*(5), S281–S288. Evidence Level VI: Expert Opinion.

Lonergan, E., Luxenberg, J., & Colford, J. (2002). Haloperidol for agitation in dementia. *Cochrane Database of Systemic Reviews, 2,* CD002852. Evidence Level I: Systematic Review.

Lopez, O. L., Becker, J. T., Wisniewski, S., Saxton, J., Kaufer, D. I., & Dekosky, S. T. (2002). Cholinesterase inhibitor treatment alters the natural history of Alzheimer's disease. *Journal of Neurology, Neurosurgery, and Psychiatry, 72*(3), 310–314. Evidence Level III: Quasi-experimental Study.

Lou, M. (2001). The use of music to decrease agitated behavior of the demented elderly: State of the science. *Scandinavian Journal of Caring Sciences, 15*(2), 165–173. Evidence Level I: Systematic Review.

Lyketsos, C. G., Colenda, C. C., Beck, C., Blank, K., Doraiswamy, M. P., Kalunian, D. A., et al. (2006). Position statement of the American Association for Geriatric Psychiatry regarding principles of care for patients with dementia resulting from Alzheimer's disease. *American Journal of Geriatric Psychiatry, 14*(7), 561–573. Evidence Level VI: Expert Opinion.

Lyketsos, C. G., Toone, L., Tchanz, J. T., Rabins, P. V., Steinberg, M., Onyike, C. U., et al. (2005). A population-based study of medical co-morbidity in early dementia and cognitive impairment no dementia (CIND): Association with functional and cognitive impairment. *The Cache County Study. American Journal of Geriatric Psychiatry, 13,* 656–664. Evidence Level IV: Nonexperimental Study.

Manley, J. J., & Espino, D. V. (2004). Cultural influences on dementia recognition and management. *Clinics in Geriatric Medicine, 20*(1), 93–119. Evidence Level IV: Nonexperimental Study.

Manning, C. (2004). Beyond memory: Neuropsychologic features in differential diagnosis of dementia. *Clinics in Geriatric Medicine, 20*(1), 45–58. Evidence Level VI: Expert Opinion.

Masterman, D. (2004). Cholinesterase inhibitors in the treatment of Alzheimer's disease and related dementias. *Clinics in Geriatric Medicine, 20*(1), 59–68. Evidence Level VI: Expert Opinion.

McKeith, I. G., Burn, D. J., Ballard, C. G., Collerton, D., Jaros, E., Morris, C. M., et al. (2003). Dementia with Lewy bodies. *Seminar in Clinical Neuropsychiatry, 8*(1), 46–57. Evidence Level V: Literature Review.

McKeith, I. G., Dickson, D. W., Lowe, J., Emre, M., O'Brien, D. M., & Feldman, H., et al. (2005). Diagnosis and management of dementia with Lewy bodies: Third report of the DLB consortium. *Neurology, 65,* 1863–1872. Evidence Level VI: Expert Opinion.

McShane, R., Areosa Sastre, A., & Minakaran, N. (2006). Memantine for dementia. *Cochrane Database of Systematic Reviews, Apr. 19* (2), 003154. Evidence Level I: Systematic Review.

Mezey, M. D., Mitty, E. L., Bottrell, M. M., Ramsey, G. C., & Fisher, T. (2000). Advance directives: Older adults with dementia. *Clinics in Geriatric Medicine, 16,* 255–268. Evidence Level VI: Expert Opinion.

Milisen, K., Braes, T., Flick, D. M., & Foreman, M. D. (2006). Cognitive assessment and differentiating the 3 Ds (dementia, depression, delirium). *Nursing Clinics of North America, 41*(1), 1–22. Evidence Level VI: Expert Opinion.

Mittelman, M. S., Ferris, S. H., Shulman, E., Steinberg, G., & Levin, B. (1996). A family intervention to delay nursing home placement of patients with

Alzheimer's disease. *Journal of the American Medical Association, 276*(21), 1725–1731. Evidence Level II: Single Experimental Study.

Neal, M., & Briggs, M. (2003). Validation therapy for dementia. *Cochrane Database of Systematic Reviews* (3), CD001394. Evidence Level I: Systematic Review.

Olsen, C. E., Poulsen, H. D., & Lublin, H. K. F. (2005). Drug therapy in dementia in elderly patients: A review. *Nordic Journal of Psychiatry, 59*(2), 71–77. Evidence Level I: Systematic Review.

Onega, L. L. (2006). Assessment of psychoemotional and behavioral status in patients with dementia. *Nursing Clinics of North America, 41*(1), 23–41. Evidence Level VI: Expert Opinion.

Ostbye, T., Hill, G., & Steenhuis, R. (1999). Mortality in elderly Canadians with and without dementia: A 5-year follow-up. *Neurology, 53,* 521–526. Evidence Level IV: Nonexperimental Study.

Parker, C., & Philp, I. (2004). Screening for cognitive impairment among older people in Black and minority ethnic groups. *Age and Aging, 33,* 447–452. Evidence Level VI: Expert Opinion.

Peatfield, J. G., Futrell, M., & Cox, C. L. (2002). Wandering: An integrative review. *Journal of Gerontological Nursing, 28*(4), 44–50. Evidence Level I: Systematic Review.

Pfeffer, R. I., Kurosaki, T. T., Harrah, C. H., Chance, J. M., & Filos, S. (1982). Measurement of functional activities of older adults in the community. *Journal of Gerontology, 37*(3), 323–329. Evidence Level IV: Nonexperimental Study.

Reimer, M.A., Slaughter, S., Donaldson, C., Currie, G., & Eliasziw, M. (2004). Special care facility compared with traditional environments for dementia care: A longitudinal study of quality of life. *Journal of the American Geriatrics Society, 52*(7), 1085–1092. Evidence Level IV: Nonexperimental Study.

Richie, K., & Lovestone, S. (2002). The dementias. *Lancet, 360*(9347), 1767–1769. Evidence Level VI: Expert Opinion.

Robinson, B. (1983). Validation of a Caregiver Strain Index. *Journal of Gerontology, 38,* 344–348. Evidence Level IV: Nonexperimental Study.

Roman, G. C. (2003a). Stroke, cognitive decline, and vascular dementia: The silent epidemic of the 21st century. *Neuroepidemiology, 22*(3), 161–164. Evidence Level VI: Expert Opinion.

Roman, G. C. (2003b). Vascular dementia: Distinguishing characteristics, treatment, and prevention. *Journal of the American Geriatrics Society, 51,* S296–S304. Evidence Level VI: Expert Opinion.

Ropacki, S. A., & Jeste, D. V. (2005). Epidemiology of and risk factors for psychosis of Alzheimer's disease: A review of 55 studies published from 1990 to 2003. *American Journal of Psychiatry, 162*(11), 2022–2030. Evidence Level I: Systematic Review.

Royall, D. R., Mulroy, A. R., Chiodo, L. K., & Polk, M. J. (1999). Clock drawing is sensitive to executive control: A comparison of six methods. *Journal of Gerontology & Psychological Science and Social Science, 54B*(5), 328–333. Evidence Level IV: Nonexperimental Study.

Sampson, E. L., Ritchie, C. W., Lai, R., Raven, P. W., & Blanchard, M. R. (2005). A systematic review of the scientific evidence for the efficacy of a palliative care approach in advanced dementia. *International Psychogeriatrics, 17,* 31–40. Evidence Level I: Systematic Review.

Scherder, E., Oosterman, J., Swabb, D., Herr, K., Ooms, M., Ribbe, M., et al. (2005). Recent developments in pain in dementia. *British Medical Journal, 330,* 461–464. Evidence Level V: Literature Review.

Schneider, L., Tariot, P., Dagerman, K., Davis, S., Hsiao, J., Ismail, M. S., et al. (2006). Effectiveness of atypical antipsychotic drugs in patient with Alzheimer's disease. *New England Journal of Medicine, 355,* 1525–1538. Evidence Level II: Single Experimental Study.

Schulz, R., & Beach, S. R. (1999). Caregiving as a risk factor for mortality: The Caregiver Health Effects Study. *Journal of the American Medical Association, 282*(23), 2215–2219. Evidence Level IV: Nonexperimental Study.

Smith, G. E., Kokmen, E., & O'Brien, P. C. (2000). Risk factors for nursing home placement in a population-based dementia cohort. *Journal of the American Geriatrics Society, 48,* 519–525. Evidence Level IV: Nonexperimental Study.

Smith, M., Hall, G. R., Gerdner, L., & Buckwalter, K. C. (2006). Application of the progressively lowered stress threshold model across the continuum of care. *Nursing Clinics of North America, 41*(1), 57–81. Evidence Level V: Case Study.

Sunderland, T., Hill, J. L., Mellow, A. M., Lawlor, B. A., Gundersheimer, J., Newhouse, P. A., et al. (1989). Clock drawing in Alzheimer's disease: A novel measure of dementia severity. *Journal of the American Geriatrics Society, 37*(8), 725–729. Evidence Level IV: Nonexperimental Study.

Takahashi, J., Yoshida, K., Sugita, T., Higuchi, H., & Shimiqu, T. (2003). Quetiapine treatment of psychotic symptoms and aggressive behavior in patients with dementia with Lewy bodies: A case series. *Progress in Neuro-Psychopharmacology and Biological Psychiatry, 27*(3), 549–553. Evidence Level IV: Nonexperimental Study.

Tariot, P. N., Farlow, M. R., Grossberg, G. T., Graham, S. M., McDonald, S., & Gergel, I., for the Memantine Study Group (2004). Memantine treatment in patients with moderate to severe Alzheimer's disease already receiving donepezil: A randomized controlled trial. *Journal of the American Medical Association, 291*(3), 317–324. Evidence Level II: Single Experimental Study.

Tariot, P. N., Profenno, L. A., & Ismail, M. S. (2004). Efficacy of atypical antipsychotics in elderly patients with dementia. *Journal of Clinical Psychiatry, 65* (Suppl. 11), 11–15. Evidence Level I: Systematic Review.

Thorgrimsen, L., Spector, A., Wiles, A., & Orrell, M. (2006). Aroma therapy for dementia. *The Cochrane Library.* Evidence Level I: Systematic Review.

Volicer, L., & Hurley, A. C. (2003). Management of behavioral symptoms in progressive dementias. *Journal of Gerontology: Series A, Biological Sciences, 58*(9), M837–M845. Evidence Level V: Literature Review.

Volicer, L., Hurley, A. C., & Blasi, Z. V. (2001). Scales for evaluation of end-of-life care in dementia. *Alzheimer's Disease and Associated Disorders, 15*(4), 194–200. Evidence Level IV: Nonexperimental Study.

Zubenko, G. S., Zubenko, W. N., McPherson, S., Spoor, E., Marin, D. B., Farlow, M. R., et al. (2003). A collaborative study of the emergence and clinical features of the major depressive syndrome of Alzheimer's disease. *American Journal of Psychiatry, 160*(5), 857–866. Evidence Level IV: Nonexperimental Study.

Delirium: Prevention, Early Recognition, and Treatment

7

Dorothy F. Tullmann
Lorraine C. Mion
Kathleen Fletcher
Marquis D. Foreman

Educational Objectives

On completion of this chapter, the reader should be able to:

1. describe hospitalized older adults at risk for delirium

2. discuss the importance of early recognition of delirium

3. identify four clinical characteristics of delirium

4. develop a plan to prevent or treat delirium

5. list five outcomes associated with delirium

Overview

Delirium is a common syndrome in hospitalized older adults. Sometimes reversible, delirium is one of the major contributors to poor outcomes of health care and institutionalization for older patients. A significant proportion of delirium cases has been shown to be preventable by identifying modifiable risk factors and utilizing a standardized nursing practice protocol. If delirium does develop, early recognition is of paramount importance to treat the underlying pathology and minimize delirium's sequelae. Nurses play a key role in both the prevention and early recognition of this potentially devastating condition.

For a description of Evidence Levels cited in this chapter, see chapter 1, Developing and Evaluating Clinical Practice Guidelines, page 4

Background and Statement of Problem

Delirium is a disturbance of consciousness with impaired attention and disorganized thinking that develops rapidly and with evidence of an underlying physiologic or medical condition (American Psychiatric Association, 2000). Delirium is characterized by a reduced ability to focus, sustain, or shift attention; memory impairment, disorientation, and/or illusions; visual or other hallucinations; and misperceptions of stimuli. Delusional thinking may also occur. Unlike other chronic cognitive impairments, delirium develops over a short period and tends to fluctuate during the course of the day. A patient may present with either hyperactive, hypoactive, or mixed subtypes of delirium (de Rooij, Schuurmans, van der Mast, & Levi, 2005 [Level I]). Nurses typically associate delirium with hyperactivity and distressing, time-consuming, harmful patient behaviors. However, the hypoactive subtype with its lack of overt psychomotor activity is also common (O'Keeffe & Lavan, 1999 [Level IV]).

Delirium is present on admission (prevalence) to the hospital in 10% to 15% of older patients; the in-hospital incidence (new onset) is 10% to 40% in older medical and surgical patients (Fann, 2000 [Level I]). Among hip-surgery patients alone, the incidence of delirium is 43% to 61% (Holmes & House, 2000 [Level I]). Older adults admitted to intensive care units (ICUs) have both a prevalent and an incident delirium of 31% (McNicoll et al., 2003 [Level IV]) and up to 83% of mechanically ventilated patients (all ages) experience delirium (Ely et al., 2001a [Level IV]). The incidence of delirium superimposed on dementia ranges from 22% to 89% (Fick, Agostini, & Inouye, 2002 [Level I]). The onset of delirium generally occurs shortly after admission, has a varied and unpredictable course, and may persist for several weeks after hospital discharge (Kiely et al., 2003 [Level IV]; Marcantonio et al., 2003 [Level IV]; Rudberg, Pompei, Foreman, Ross, & Cassel, 1997 [Level IV]).

The pathophysiology of delirium is not well understood (Trzepacz & van der Mast, 2002 [Level VI]) and a number of risk factors have been identified suggesting that the etiology of delirium is multifactorial (Inouye & Charpentier, 1996 [Level VI]). The most common risk factors for delirium include dementia, male gender, advanced age, and medical illness (Elie, Cole, Primeau, & Bellavance, 1998 [Level I]). Other predisposing risk factors identified are poor functional status, alcohol abuse, and depression (Fann, 2000 [Level I]), as well as dehydration and sensory impairment (Inouye, Viscoli, Horwitz, Hurst, & Tinetti, 1993 [Level IV]).

Precipitating risk factors occurring during hospitalization include polypharmacy, malnutrition, physical restraints, a bladder catheter, or any iatrogenic event (Inouye & Charpentier, 1996 [Level IV]). Multiple medications have been implicated as precipitating factors for delirium. These include but are not limited to anticholinergics, narcotics (meperidine), sedative hypnotics (benzodiazepines), histamine (H_2) receptor antagonists, corticosteroids, centrally acting antihypertensives, and antiparkinsonian drugs (Fann, 2000 [Level I]). Other precipitating factors include under-treated pain (Morrison et al., 2003 [Level IV]) and care-setting relocation (especially to ICU) (McCusker et al., 2001 [Level IV]).

Delirium results in significant distress for the patient, their family members, and nurses (Breitbart, Gibson, & Tremblay, 2002 [Level IV]). In addition, delirium is associated with increased mortality, increased postoperative complications, longer hospital stay, functional decline, and new nursing home placement (Fann, 2000 [Level I]). Long-term cognitive decline (Ely et al., 2004a [Level IV]; McCusker, Cole, Dendukuri, Belzile, & Primeau, 2001 [Level IV]) and increased health care costs (Inouye, 2006 [Level VI]; Milbrandt et al., 2004 [Level IV]) have also been associated with delirium. Clearly, delirium is a high-priority nursing challenge for all who care for older adults.

Parameters of Assessment

Identifying the risk factors for delirium (stated previously) is critically important. Eliminating or reducing these risk factors can prevent delirium in many cases (Milisen, Lemiengre, Braes, & Foreman, 2005 [Level I]).

Recognizing the first signs of delirium is also important to further identify, eliminate, or reduce the precipitating factor(s) such as pain, infection, or other acute illnesses. The criteria used to distinguish delirium or acute confusion from other changes in mental status include the following:

- Disturbance of consciousness (i.e., reduced clarity and awareness of the environment) with reduced ability to focus, sustain, and shift attention. Patients have trouble following instructions or making sense of their environment, even with cues. They may also get "stuck" on a particular concern or thought.
- A change in cognition: memory deficit, disorientation, language disturbance, and/or perceptual disturbance. Symptoms are often associated with disturbances in the sleep/wake cycle and rapidly shifting emotional disturbances, with escalation of the disturbed behavior at night (i.e., sundowning). Hallucinations and delusions are common. Patients can be hyperactive and agitated or lethargic and less active. The latter presentation is particularly of concern because it is often not recognized by health care providers as delirium. The presentation may also be mixed, with the patient fluctuating from one to the other.
- The cardinal sign of delirium is that these changes occur rapidly over several hours or days.

It is important to remember that delirium may occur concurrently with dementia or depression. In fact, those patients are at increased risk to develop delirium. Family and caregivers can be invaluable in helping to distinguish cognitive changes in those circumstances when the patient is not well known to the nurse or physician.

Despite its importance, delirium is under-recognized by nurses and physicians (Ely et al., 2004b [Level IV]; Fick & Foreman, 2000 [Level IV]; Inouye, Foreman, Mion, Katz, & Cooney, Jr., 2001 [Level IV]). Personal philosophies about aging are a factor in nurses' inability to distinguish delirium from dementia (McCarthy, 2003 [Level IV]). In addition, the hypoactive subtype of delirium, with no agitated behavior to alert physicians and nurses to its presence, is another reason why delirium is not identified. Failure to recognize delirium means that the underlying cause cannot be identified and treated in a timely manner, contributing to the sequelae associated with delirium.

Nurses are in the best position to recognize delirium. Screening tools have been developed to assist nurses in their assessment (Schuurmans, Deschamps, Markham, Shortridge-Baggett, & Duursma, 2003 [Level V]). Experienced clinicians can train nurses to use these instruments in their routine assessment of older adults (Pun et al., 2005 [Level IV]). In the absence of such training, however, nurses can identify the clinical features of delirium and alert the physician or nurse practitioner to continue the diagnostic process (see Section IV, *Parameters of Assessment,* in Box 7.1, Nursing Standard of Practice Protocol).

Intervention and Care Strategies

Multicomponent nursing interventions, guided by the multiple risk factors for delirium, are modestly successful in preventing delirium (Cole, Primeau, & McCusker, 1996 [Level I]; Milisen, Lemiengre, Braes, & Foreman, 2005 [Level I]). However, such multicomponent interventions are not effective for treating delirium once it has developed (Milisen et al., 2005 [Level I]; Pitkala, Laurila, Strandberg, & Tilvis, 2006 [Level II]) and are possibly less effective for older medical than surgical patients (Cole, Primeau, & Elie, 1998 [Level I]). None of the multicomponent intervention studies focused on patients with chronic cognitive impairment—patients at greatest risk for delirium (Britton & Russell, 2004 [Level I]). Medications are not effective in preventing delirium (Kalisvaart et al., 2005 [Level II]).

Once it has been determined that the patient is either at risk for or has already developed delirium, a standardized delirium protocol should be initiated immediately. Protocols tested in two multicomponent interventions effectively prevented delirium (Inouye et al., 1999 [Level II]; Marcantonio, Flacker, Wright, & Resnick, 2001 [Level II]). The protocols varied somewhat but two principles emerged from the research: (1) minimize the risk for delirium by preventing or eliminating the etiologic agent(s); and (2) provide a therapeutic environment and general supportive nursing care (see Section V, *Nursing Care Strategies,* in Box 7.1 Protocol for details).

Although nonpharmacologic interventions are preferred, medications are also used in the treatment of delirium (Meagher, 2001 [Level VI]). Antipsychotics (e.g., haloperidol) are frequently used although their efficacy and safety have not been established by double-blind, randomized, placebo-controlled trials (Seitz, Gill, & van Zyl, 2007 [Level I]). Medications such as diazepam to enhance post-laparotomy sleep in older patients (Aizawa et al., 2002 [Level II]), risperidone (Parellada, Baeza, de Pablo, & Martinez, 2004 [Level II]), and olanzapine (Skrobik, Bergeron, Dumont, & Gottfried, 2004 [Level II]) may prevent delirium but more robust studies are needed. Diazepam should not be used in older adults (Fick et al., 2003 [Level IV]) and, given the adverse affects in older adults with many medications (see chapter 12, *Reducing Adverse Drug Events*), any new medication approved for delirium should be used with extreme caution in these patients.

Case Study and Discussion

Mr. Z. is an 82-year-old patient admitted to your unit for prostate surgery. He is a retired accountant, lives with his wife, and is very active. He drives a car, plays golf, and regularly participates in activities at the senior center. His Type II diabetes is well controlled on Actoplus-met (i.e., pioglitazone hydrochloride and metformin hydrochloride). Mr. Z. reports that he has decreased his fluid intake so he can avoid waking several times during the night to urinate. He also has a history of hypertension, moderate hearing loss (hearing aids bilaterally), and previous surgery for inguinal hernia repair. He wears bifocal glasses for distance and reading. He is alert, oriented, and expresses a good understanding of his upcoming surgery. His preoperative laboratory values are within normal limits except for a hematocrit of 28% and a blood urea nitrogen/creatinine (BUN/Cr) ratio slightly elevated at 21:1. His medications include Actoplus-met for his diabetes and verapamil for hypertension.

Which factors present on admission to the hospital put Mr. Z at risk for developing delirium?

- *Age.* Older adults are at greater risk for delirium, particularly if they have underlying dementia or depression. Physiologic changes that occur with aging can affect the ability of older adults to respond to physical and physiologic stress and to maintain homeostasis.
- *Dehydration.* An elevated BUN/Cr ratio indicates dehydration (from decreased fluid intake), a frequent contributing factor (along with electrolyte imbalance) to delirium of hospitalized older adults.
- *Anemia.* Because of a low hematocrit, the body has diminished ability to deliver adequate oxygen to the brain, making delirium more likely.
- *Sensory deficits.* Those with vision and hearing loss are more likely to misinterpret sensory input, which places them at increased risk for delirium.
- It is important to understand that it might not be one particular factor but the interplay of patient vulnerability (i.e., predisposing factors) and precipitating factors—common during hospitalization—that place older adults at risk for delirium.

What can you do to help prevent delirium in Mr. Z.?

- If possible, consult with a geriatric specialist (physician or nurse) for a thorough geriatric assessment of Mr. Z.
- Make sure his glasses and hearing aids are on and functioning.
- Explore reasons for the low hematocrit.

Care is again provided for Mr. Z. 2 days after surgery. He is confused and picking at the air and oriented to self only. An indwelling urinary catheter and peripheral intravenous line are in place. In his report, the day-shift nurse mentioned considering a physical restraint because Mr. Z. was increasingly restless and might be delirious.

What are the clinical features of delirium?

- *Disturbance of consciousness* characterized by reduced clarity and awareness of the environment; reduced ability to focus, sustain, and shift attention. Patients have trouble following instructions or making sense of their environment, even with cues. They may also get "stuck" on a particular concern or thought.
- *Cognitive changes*: memory deficit, disorientation, language disturbance, and/or perceptual disturbance.
- *Perceptual disturbances*: Hallucinations and delusions are common. Patients can be hyperactive and agitated or lethargic (i.e., hypoactive) and less active. The latter presentation is of particular concern because it is often not recognized as delirium by health care providers. The presentation may also be mixed, with the patient fluctuating from one to the other behavioral state.
- Delirium can be *characterized by* disturbances in the sleep/wake cycle and rapidly shifting emotional disturbances, with escalation of the disturbed behavior at night (i.e., sundowning).
- The cardinal sign of delirium is that these *changes occur rapidly* over several hours or days.

It is also important to consider that delirium may occur concurrently with dementia or depression. In fact, these patients are at increased risk to develop delirium. Family and caregivers can be invaluable in helping to identify or distinguish cognitive changes in circumstances when the patient is not well known to the nurse or physician.

Which additional factors may now be contributing to Mr. Z.'s delirium?

- *Anesthesia and other medications.* It takes several hours for the body to clear the effects of anesthesia. Inasmuch as older adults have a larger percentage of body fat than younger persons and many drugs are fat-soluble, drug effects will last longer. Also, older adults tend to have less cellular water; therefore, water-soluble drugs will be more concentrated and have a more pronounced effect. Nurses need to ask the patient or family if any new drugs other than pain medication have been added. What is the dose and frequency of the pain medications? Is the dose appropriate?
- *Pain.* What is Mr. Z.'s pain-control regimen and status? Poor pain control contributes to restlessness and is associated with delirium. Is the current drug the best for good pain relief in this patient?

■ *Hypoxemia*. Mr. Z. is at risk because of limited mobility and possible at-electasis after surgery. What is his oxygen saturation (SpO2)? Does he have crackles or diminished breath sounds?

■ *Infection, inflammation, or other medical illness*. Postoperative infections, intra-operative myocardial infarctions (MIs), or strokes are possible causes of delirium in this case. Could Mr. Z. have a urinary tract infection (UTI) because he is post-prostate surgery and particularly because he has a Foley catheter? An inflammatory response to a new medical problem may be the cause of the delirium.

■ *Unfamiliar surroundings*. Particularly for those with sensory deficits, an unfamiliar environment can lead to misinterpretations of information, which may contribute to delirium.

What steps should be taken now?

■ *Avoid the use of restraints*, which could worsen Mr. Z.'s agitation.

■ *Call the physician or nurse practitioner (NP)* immediately and report your findings; request that he or she evaluate the patient to determine the underlying cause of the delirium. If Mr. Z.'s delirium worsens, he may also need medication (e.g., haloperidol) to control his symptoms.

■ *Frequent reality orientation*. Frequent orientation, reassurance, and helping Mr. Z. interpret his environment and what is happening to him should be helpful. (Monitor the patient's reaction. If the patient becomes upset or angry, modify your approach to that of more reassurance and validating the patient's experience rather than reorienting.)

■ Are Mr. Z.'s *hearing aids and glasses* in place and clean? Functioning? Impaired sensory input contributes significantly to delirium. Also, he may seem more confused than he really is if he is not able to hear what you are saying.

■ Invite *family/significant others* to stay as long as they are able to assist with his orientation, reassurance, and sense of well-being. Monitor the effect of family visitation. If the patient has increased agitation or anxiety, then limit the visitation of the individual who seems to be triggering Mr. Z.'s upset.

■ *Mobilize the patient*. Mobility assists with orientation and helps prevent problems associated with immobility, such as atelectasis and deep venous thrombosis.

■ *Judicious use of medications* for pain, sleep, or anxiety. Drugs used to address these issues can exacerbate the delirium. Try nonpharmacologic approaches for sleep and anxiety first. If Mr. Z. is having pain, are the drug and dose appropriate for him? A regular schedule of a smaller dose or nonnarcotic pain medication almost always is better than prn dosing.

■ Try to *provide for adequate sleep*: noise reduction at night; soft, relaxing music; warm milk or herbal tea; massage; and rescheduling care in order not to interrupt sleep.

■ Make sure the patient is well *hydrated*.

■ Talk to the doctor or NP about removing the *indwelling urinary catheter*. Because of his surgery, Mr. Z. may need it immediately post-op, but it should be removed as soon as possible. Additionally, recommend a urinalysis to rule out UTI.

■ *Address safety concerns* (e.g., increase surveillance). Mr. Z. is now also at risk for falls and/or pressure ulcers.

Summary

Delirium is a common occurrence in hospitalized older adults and contributes to poor outcomes. Thus, it is important to promptly identify those patients at risk for delirium and implement preventive measures, as well as to promptly recognize delirium when it appears. Nursing assessments using validated delirium screening instruments must become routine. A standard of practice protocol provides concise information to guide nursing care of individuals at risk of or experiencing delirium (see Box 7.1.).

Acknowledgments

Our thanks to Suzann Rosenthal-Williams, MSN, GNP, for her real-life experiences in helping to prevent and treat delirium in older adults, and to Naomi Gorton, Clinical Nurse Leader student, for her assistance in preparing the references.

Resources

Recommended Delirium-Screening Instruments

Confusion Assessment Method (CAM) (Inouye, 2003; Inouye et al., 1990 [Level IV]). Recommended for verbal patients by Laurila, Pitkala, Strandberg, & Tilvis (2002 [Level IV]).

Confusion Assessment Method for the Intensive Care Unit (CAM-ICU) (Ely et al., 2001a [Level IV]; Ely et al., 2001b [Level IV]). Recommended for nonverbal patients by Schuurmans et al. (2003 [Level V]).

Other Delirium-Screening Instruments

Delirium-O-Meter (deJonge, Kalisvarrt, Timmers, Kat, & Jackson, 2005 [Level VI]) may be used for monitoring the different characteristics and the severity of delirium in geriatric patients.

Delirium Rating Scale (DRS)-98 (Trzepacz et al., 2001 [Level IV]) may be used to assess delirium severity.

Mini-Mental State Examination (MMSE) (Folstein, Folstein, & McHugh, 1975 [Level IV]) may be used to monitor course of delirium in hospitalized patients according to O'Keeffe, Mulkerrin, Nayeem, Varughese, and Pillay (2005 [Level IV]).

Additional On-line Information About Delirium

http://www.icudelirium.org/delirium/

http://elderlife.med.yale.edu/public/pubs.php?pageid=01.03.07

Box 7.1

Nursing Standard of Practice Protocol: Delirium: Prevention, Early Recognition, and Treatment

I. GOAL: To reduce the incidence of delirium in hospitalized older adults.

II. OVERVIEW

A. Delirium is a common syndrome in hospitalized older adults.

B. Although sometimes reversible, delirium is associated with increased mortality, increased hospital costs, and long-term cognitive and functional impairment.

C. Delirium can be prevented with recognition of high risk patients and the implementation of a standardized protocol.

D. Delirium, when it develops, may be under-recognized by physicians and nurses.

E. Routine screening for delirium should be part of comprehensive nursing care of older adults.

III. BACKGROUND

A. Definition: Delirium is a disturbance of consciousness with impaired attention and disorganized thinking or perceptual disturbance that develops acutely, has a fluctuating course, and with evidence that there is an underlying physiologic or medical condition causing the disorder.

B. Epidemiology

1. Prevalence (present on admission): 10% to 15% in acute care (Fann, 2000 [Level I]); 31% in ICU (McNicoll et al., 2003 [Level IV]).

2. Incidence (new onset): 10% to 40% in acute care (Fann, 2000 [Level I]); 43% to 61% post–hip surgery (Holmes & House, 2000 [Level I]); 31% in ICU (McNicoll et al., 2003 [Level IV]); 83% of mechanically ventilated patients (Ely et al., 2001a [Level IV]).

3. Duration: May resolve in a few hours to days or persist for weeks to months (Fann, 2000 [Level I]).

C. Etiology

1. Pathophysiologic mechanisms unclear (Trzepacz & Van der Mast, 2002 [Level VI]).

2. Risk factors for delirium are multifactorial:

   a. Advanced age (Fann, 2000 [Level I])

   b. Dementia (Elie et al., 1998 [Level I])

   c. Medical illness (Elie et al., 1998 [Level I])

   d. Multiple medications (Elie et al., 1998 [Level I]; see chapter 12, *Reducing Adverse Drug Events*)

e. Alcohol abuse (Elie et al., 1998 [Level I])
f. Male gender (Elie et al., 1998 [Level I])
g. Poor functional status (Fann, 2000 [Level I])
h. Depression (Fann, 2000 [Level I])
i. Pain (Fann, 2000 [Level I])
j. Increased blood urea nitrogen/creatinine (BUN/Cr) ratio (Inouye & Charpentier, 1996 [Level IV])
k. Sensory impairment (Inouye & Charpentier, 1996 [Level IV])

3. Potential outcomes of delirium:
a. Increased mortality (Fann, 2000 [Level I])
b. Increased morbidity (Fann, 2000 [Level I])
   i. Long-term cognitive impairment (Ely et al., 2004a; McCusker et al., 2001 [Level IV])
   ii. Postoperative complications (Fann, 2000 [Level I])
   iii. Decreased functional ability (Fann, 2000 [Level I])
   iv. Increased hospital length of stay (Ely et al., 2004a; Pompei et al., 1994 [Level IV])
   v. Institutionalization (Fann, 2000 [Level I])
   vi. Increased health care costs (Inouye, 2006 [Level VI])

IV. PARAMETERS OF ASSESSMENT

A. Assess for risk factors
  1. Baseline or pre-morbid cognitive impairment (see chapter 4, *Assessing Cognitive Function*)
  2. Medications review (see chapter 12, *Reducing Adverse Drug Events*)
  3. Pain
  4. Metabolic disturbances (i.e., hypoglycemia, hypercalcemia, hyponatremia, hypokalemia)
  5. Dehydration (physical signs/symptoms, intake/output, Na$^+$, BUN/Cr)
  6. Infection (fever, WBCs with differential, cultures)
  7. Environment (sensory overload or deprivation)
  8. Impaired mobility
B. Features of delirium—assess every shift (see Resources for validated instruments)
  1. Acute onset; evidence of underlying medical condition
  2. Alertness: Fluctuates from stuporous to hypervigilant
  3. Attention: Inattentive, easily distractible, and may have difficulty shifting attention from one focus to another; has difficulty keeping track of what is being said
  4. Orientation: Disoriented to time and place; should not be disoriented to person
  5. Memory: Inability to recall events of hospitalization and current illness; unable to remember instructions; forgetful of names, events, activities, current news, and so on

6. Thinking: Disorganized thinking; rambling, irrelevant, incoherent conversation; unclear or illogical flow of ideas; or unpredictable switching from topic to topic; difficulty in expressing needs and concerns; speech may be garbled
7. Perception: Perceptual disturbances such as illusions and visual or auditory hallucinations; and misperceptions such as calling a stranger by a relative's name
8. Psychomotor activity: May fluctuate between hypoactive, hyperactive, and mixed subtypes

V. NURSING CARE STRATEGIES

Based on protocols in multicomponent delirium prevention studies (Inouye, et al., 1999; Marcantonio, et al., 2001 [Level II])
A. Collaborate with physician/nurse practitioner to treat the underlying pathology and contributing factors. If available, consult with geriatrician and/or Geriatric Nurse Practitioner or Clinical Nurse Specialist.
B. Eliminate or minimize risk factors
   1. Administer medications judiciously; avoid high risk medications (see chapter 12, *Reducing Adverse Drug Events*).
   2. Prevent/promptly and appropriately treat infections.
   3. Prevent/promptly treat dehydration and electrolyte disturbances.
   4. Provide adequate pain control (see chapter 10, *Pain Management*).
   5. Maximize oxygen delivery (supplemental oxygen, blood, and BP support as needed).
   6. Use sensory aids as appropriate.
   7. Regulate bowel/bladder function.
   8. Provide adequate nutrition.
C. Provide a therapeutic environment.
   1. Foster orientation: frequently reassure and reorient patient (unless patient becomes agitated); utilize easily visible calendars, clocks, caregiver identification; carefully explain all activities; communicate clearly.
   2. Provide appropriate sensory stimulation: quiet room; adequate light; one task at a time; noise-reduction strategies.
   3. Facilitate sleep: back massage, warm milk or herbal tea at bedtime; relaxation music/tapes; noise-reduction measures; avoid awakening patient.
   4. Foster familiarity: encourage family/friends to stay at bedside; bring familiar objects from home; maintain consistency of caregivers; minimize relocations.
   5. Maximize mobility: avoid restraints (see chapter 22, *Physical Restraints and Side Rails in Acute and Critical Care Settings*) and urinary catheters; ambulate or active range of motion three times daily.
   6. Communicate clearly, provide explanations.
   7. Reassure and educate family.

8. Minimize invasive interventions.
9. Consider psychotropic medication as a last resort.

VI. EVALUATION/EXPECTED OUTCOMES

A. Patient
   1. Absence of delirium or
   2. Cognitive status returned to baseline (prior to delirium)
   3. Functional status returned to baseline (prior to delirium)
   4. Discharged to same destination as prehospitalization
B. Health Care Provider
   1. Increased detection of delirium
   2. Implementation of appropriate interventions to prevent/treat delirium
   3. Use of standardized delirium-prevention protocol
   4. Decreased use of physical restraints
   5. Decreased use of antipsychotic medications
   6. Increased satisfaction in care of hospitalized elderly
C. Institution
   1. Decreased overall cost
   2. Decreased length of stays
   3. Decreased morbidity and mortality
   4. Increased referrals and consultation to the specified specialists
   5. Improved satisfaction of patients, families, nursing staff

VII. FOLLOW-UP MONITORING OF CONDITION

A. Decreased delirium to become a measure of quality care
B. Incidence of delirium to decrease
C. Patient days with delirium to decrease
D. Staff competence in recognition and treatment of acute confusion/delirium
E. Documentation of a variety of interventions for acute confusion/delirium

Na^+ = sodium; BUN/Cr = blood urea nitrogen/creatinine ratio; BP = blood pressure; Hgb/Hct = hemoglobin and hematocrit; SpO_2 = pulse oxygen saturation; WBCs = white blood cells; URI = upper respiratory infection; UTI = urinary tract infection

References

Agostini, J. V., Leo-Summers, L. S., & Inouye, S. K. (2001). Cognitive and other adverse effects of diphenhydramine use in hospitalized older patients. *Archives of Internal Medicine, 161,* 2091–2097. Evidence Level IV: Nonexperimental Study.

Aizawa, K., Kanai, T., Saikawa, Y., Takabayashi, T., Kawano, Y., Miyazawa, N., et al. (2002). A novel approach to the prevention of postoperative delirium in the elderly after gastrointestinal surgery. *Surgery Today, 32,* 310–314. Evidence Level II: Single Experimental Study.

American Psychiatric Association (2000). *Diagnostic and statistical manual of mental disorders* (4th ed., text revision). Washington, DC: Author.

Breitbart, W., Gibson, C., & Tremblay, A. (2002). The delirium experience: Delirium recall and delirium-related distress in hospitalized patients with cancer, their spouses/caregivers, and their nurses. *Psychosomatics, 43,* 183–194. Evidence Level IV: Nonexperimental Study.

Britton, A., & Russell, R. (2004). Multidisciplinary team interventions for delirium in patients with chronic cognitive impairment. *Cochrane Data Base Systematic Reviews, 2,* CD000395. Evidence Level I: Systematic Review.

Cole, M. G., McCusker, J., Bellavance, F., Primeau, F. J., Bailey, R. F., Bonycastle, J. J., et al. (2002). Systematic detection and multidisciplinary care of delirium in older medical inpatients: A randomized trial. *Canadian Medical Association Journal, 167*(7), 753–759. Evidence Level II: Single Experimental Study.

Cole, M. G., Primeau, F. J., & Elie, L. M. (1998). Delirium: Prevention, treatment, and outcome studies. *Journal of Geriatric Psychiatry and Neurology, 11,* 126–137. Evidence Level I: Systematic Review.

Cole, M. G., Primeau, F., & McCusker, J. (1996). Effectiveness of interventions to prevent delirium in hospitalized patients: A systematic review. *Canadian Medical Association Journal, 155,* 1263–1268. Evidence Level I: Systematic Review.

de Jonge, J. F. M., Kalisvarrt, K. J., Timmers, J. F. M., Kat, M.G., & Jackson, J. C. (2005). Delirium-O-Meter: A nurses' rating scale for monitoring delirium severity in geriatric patients. *International Journal of Geriatric Psychiatry 20,* 1158–1166. Evidence Level IV: Nonexperimental Study.

de Rooij, S. E., Schuurmans, M. J., van der Mast, R. C., & Levi, M. (2005). Clinical subtypes of delirium and their relevance for daily clinical practice: A systematic review. *International Journal of Geriatric Psychiatry 20,* 609–615. Evidence Level I: Systematic Review.

Elie, M., Cole, M. G., Primeau, F. J., & Bellavance, F. (1998). Delirium risk factors in elderly hospitalized patients. *Journal of General Internal Medicine, 13,* 204–212. Evidence Level I: Systematic Review.

Ely, E. W., Inouye, S. K., Bernard, G. R., Gordon, S., Francis, J., May, L., et al. (2001a). Delirium in mechanically ventilated patients: Validity and reliability of the confusion assessment method for the intensive care unit (CAM-ICU). *Journal of the American Medical Association, 286,* 2703–2710. Evidence Level IV: Nonexperimental Study.

Ely, E. W., Margolin, R., Francis, J., May, L., Truman, B., Dittus, R., et al. (2001b). Evaluation of delirium in critically ill patients: Validation of the Confusion Assessment Method for the Intensive Care Unit (CAM-ICU). *Critical Care Medicine, 29,* 2091–2097. Evidence Level IV: Nonexperimental Study.

Ely, E. W., Shintani, A., Truman, B., Speroff, T., Gordon, S. M., Harrell, F. E., Jr., et al. (2004a). Delirium as a predictor of mortality in mechanically ventilated patients in the intensive care unit. *Journal of the American Medical Association, 291,* 1753–1762. Evidence Level IV: Nonexperimental Study.

Ely, E. W., Stephens, R. K., Jackson, J. C., Thomason, J. W., Truman, B., Gordon, S., et al. (2004b). Current opinions regarding the importance, diagnosis, and management of delirium in the intensive care unit: A survey of 912 health care professionals. *Critical Care Medicine, 32,* 106–112. Evidence Level IV: Nonexperimental Study.

Fann, J. R. (2000). The epidemiology of delirium: A review of studies and methodological issues. *Seminars in Clinical Neuropsychiatry, 5,* 64–74. Evidence Level I: Systematic Review.

Fick, D. M., Agostini, J. V., & Inouye, S. K. (2002). Delirium superimposed on dementia: A systematic review. *Journal of the American Geriatric Society, 50,* 1723–1732. Evidence Level I: Systematic Review.

Fick, D. M., Cooper, J. W., Wade, W. E., Waller, J. L., Maclean, J. R., & Beers, M. H. (2003). Updating the Beers criteria for potentially inappropriate medication use in older adults: Results of a U.S. consensus panel of experts. *Archives of Internal Medicine 163,* 2716–2724. Evidence Level IV: Nonexperimental Study.

Fick, D., & Foreman, M. (2000). Consequences of not recognizing delirium superimposed on dementia in hospitalized elderly individuals. *Journal of Gerontological Nursing, 26,* 30–40. Evidence Level IV: Nonexperimental Study.

Folstein, M. F., Folstein, S. E., & McHugh, P. R. (1975). "Mini-Mental State": A practical method for grading the cognitive state of patients for the clinician. *Journal of Psychiatric Research, 12*, 189–198. Evidence IV: Nonexperimental Study.

Holmes, J. D., & House, A. O. (2000). Psychiatric illness in hip fracture. *Age & Ageing, 29*, 537–546. Evidence Level I: Systematic Review.

Inouye, S. K. (2003). The Confusion Assessment Method (CAM): Training manual and coding guide. Yale University School of Medicine. Retrieved September 15, 2006, from http://elderlife.med.yale.edu/pdf/The%20Confusion%20Assessment%20Method.pdf

Inouye, S. K. (2006). Delirium in older persons. *New England Journal of Medicine, 354*, 1157–1165. Evidence Level VI: Expert Opinion.

Inouye, S. K., Bogardus, S. T., Charpentier, P. A., Leo-Summers, Acampora, D., Holford, T. R., et al. (1999). A multicomponent intervention to prevent delirium in hospitalized older patients. *The New England Journal of Medicine, 340*, 669–676. Evidence Level II: Single Experimental Study.

Inouye, S. K., & Charpentier, P. A. (1996). Precipitating factors for delirium in hospitalized elderly persons: Predictive model and interrelationship with baseline vulnerability. *Journal of American Medical Association, 275*, 852–857. Evidence Level IV: Nonexperimental Study.

Inouye, S. K., Foreman, M. D., Mion, L. C., Katz, K. H., & Cooney, Jr., L. M. (2001). Nurses' recognition of delirium and its symptoms: Comparison of nurse and researcher ratings. *Archives of Internal Medicine, 161*, 2467–2473. Evidence Level IV: Nonexperimental Study.

Inouye, S. K., VanDyck, C. H., Alessi, C. A., Balkin, S., Siegel, A. P., et al. (1990). Clarifying confusion: The Confusion Assessment Method. A new method for detecting delirium. *Annals of Internal Medicine, 113*(12), 941–948. Evidence Level IV: Nonexperimental Study.

Inouye, S. K., Viscoli, C. M., Horwitz, R. I., Hurst, L. D., & Tinetti, M. E. (1993). A predictive model for delirium in hospitalized elderly medical patients based on admission characteristics. *Annals of Internal Medicine, 119*, 474–481. Evidence Level IV: Nonexperimental Study.

Kalisvaart, K. J., de Jonghe, J. F., Bogaards, M. J., Vreeswijk, R., Egberts, T. C., Burger, B. J., et al. (2005). Haloperidol prophylaxis for elderly hip-surgery patients at risk for delirium: A randomized placebo-controlled study. *Journal of the American Geriatrics Society, 53*, 1658–1666. Evidence Level II: Single Experimental Study.

Kiely, D. K., Bergmann, M. A., Murphy, K. M, Jones, R. N., Orav, E. J., & Marcantonio, E. R. (2003). Delirium among newly admitted post-acute facility patients: Prevalence, symptoms, and severity. *Journal of Gerontology Medical Sciences, 58A*(5), 441–445. Evidence Level IV: Nonexperimental Study.

Laurila, J. V., Pitkala, K. H, Strandberg, T. E., & Tilvis, R. S. (2002). Confusion assessment method in the diagnostics of delirium among aged hospital patients: Would it serve better in screening than as a diagnostic instrument? *International Journal of Geriatric Psychiatry, 18*(12), 1112–1119. Evidence Level IV: Nonexperimental Study.

Marcantonio, E. R., Flacker, J. M., Wright, R. J., & Resnick, N. M. (2001). Reducing delirium after hip fracture: A randomized trial. *Journal of the American Geriatrics Society, 49*(3) 516–679. Evidence Level II: Nonexperimental Study.

Marcantonio, E. R., Simon, S. E., Bergmann, M. A., Jones, R. N., Murphy, K. M., & Morris, J. N. (2003). Delirium symptoms in post-acute care: Prevalent, persistent, and associated with poor functional recovery. *Journal of the American Geriatrics Society, 51*, 4–9. Evidence Level IV: Nonexperimental Study.

McCarthy, M. C. (2003). Detecting acute confusion in older adults: Comparing clinical reasoning of nurses working in acute, long-term, and community health care environments. *Research in Nursing and Health, 26*, 203–212. Evidence Level II: Single Experimental Study.

McCusker, J., Cole, M., Abrahamowicz, M., Han, L., Podoba, J. E., & Ramman-Haddad, L. (2001). Environmental risk factors for delirium in hospitalized older people. *Journal of the American Geriatrics Society, 49*, 1327–1334. Evidence Level IV: Nonexperimental Study.

McCusker, J., Cole, M., Dendukuri, N., Belzile, E., & Primeau, F. (2001). Delirium in older medical inpatients and subsequent cognitive and functional status: A prospective study. *Canadian Medical Association Journal, 165*, 575–583. Evidence Level IV: Nonexperimental Study.

McNicoll, L., Pisani, M. A., Zhang, Y., Ely, E. W., Siegel, M. D., & Inouye, S. K. (2003). Delirium in the intensive care unit: Occurrence and clinical course in older patients. *Journal of the American Geriatrics Society, 51*, 591–598. Evidence Level IV: Nonexperimental Study.

Meagher, D. J. (2001). Delirium: Optimizing management. *British Medical Journal, 322*(7279), 144–149. Evidence Level VI: Expert Opinion.

Milbrandt, E. B., Deppen, S., Harrison, P. L., Shintani, A. K., Speroff, T., Stiles, R. A., et al. (2004). Costs associated with delirium in mechanically ventilated patients. *Critical Care Medicine, 32*, 955–962. Evidence Level IV: Nonexperimental Study.

Milisen, K., Lemiengre, J., Braes, T., & Foreman, M. D. (2005). Multicomponent intervention strategies for managing delirium in hospitalized older people: Systematic review. *Journal of Advanced Nursing, 52*, 79–90. Evidence Level I: Systematic Review.

Morrison, R. S., Magaziner, J., Gilbert, M., Koval, K. J., McLaughlin, M. A., Orosz, G., et al. (2003). Relationship between pain and opioid analgesics on the development of delirium following hip fracture. *Journals of Gerontology Series A—Biological Sciences & Medical Sciences, 58*(1), 76–81. Evidence Level IV: Nonexperimental Study.

O'Keeffe, S. T., & Lavan, J. N. (1999). Clinical significance of delirium subtypes in older people. *Age and Ageing, 28*, 115–119. Evidence Level IV: Nonexperimental Study.

O'Keeffe, S. T., Mulkerrin, E. C., Nayeem, K., Varughese, M., & Pillay, I. (2005). Use of serial Mini-Mental State Examinations to diagnose and monitor delirium in elderly hospital patients. *Journal of the American Geriatrics Society, 53*, 867–870. Evidence Level IV: Nonexperimental Study.

Parellada, E., Baeza, I., de Pablo, J., & Martinez, G. (2004). Risperidone in the treatment of patients with delirium. *Journal of Clinical Psychiatry, 65*(3), 348–353. Evidence Level II: Single Experimental Study.

Pitkala, K. H., Laurila, J. V., Strandberg, T. E., & Tilvis, R. S. (2006). Multicomponent geriatric intervention for elderly inpatients with delirium: A randomized controlled trial. *Journals of Gerontology A, Biologic Sciences & Medical Sciences 61*(2), 176–181. Evidence Level II: Single Experimental Study.

Pompei, P., Foreman, M., Rudberg, M. A., Inouye, S. K., Braund, V., & Cassel, C. K. (1994). Delirium in hospitalized older persons: Outcomes and predictors. *Journal of the America Geriatrics Society, 42*, 809–815. Evidence Level IV: Nonexperimental Study.

Pun, B. T., Gordon, S. M., Peterson, J. F., Shintani, A. K., Jackson, J. C., Foss, J., et al. (2005). Large-scale implementation of sedation and delirium monitoring in the intensive care unit: A report from two medical centers. *Critical Care Medicine, 33*, 1199–1205. Evidence Level IV: Nonexperimental Study.

Rudberg, M. A., Pompei, P., Foreman, M. D., Ross, R. E., & Cassel, C. K. (1997). The natural history of delirium in older hospitalized patients: A syndrome of heterogeneity. *Age and Ageing, 26*, 169–174. Evidence Level IV: Nonexperimental Study.

Schuurmans, M. J., Deschamps, P. I., Markham, S. W., Shortridge-Baggett, L. M., & Duursma, S. A. (2003). The measurement of delirium: Review of scales. *Research Theory in Nursing Practice, 17*, 207–224. Evidence Level V: Literature Review.

Seitz, D. P., Gill, S. S., & van Zyl, L. T. (2007). Antipsychotics in the treatment of delirium: A systematic review. *Journal of Clinical Psychiatry, 68*(1), 11–21. Evidence Level I: Systematic Review.

Skrobik, Y. K., Bergeron, N., Dumont, M., & Gottfried, S. B. (2004). Olanzapine vs. haloperidol: Treating delirium in a critical care setting. *Intensive Care Medicine, 30*, 444–449. Evidence Level II: Single Experimental Study.

Trzepacz, P. T., Mittal, D., Torres, R., et al. (2001). Validation of the Delirium Rating Scale-revised-98: Comparison with the delriium rating scale and the cognitive test for delirium. *Journal of Neuropsychiatry and Clinical Neuroscience 13*(3), 229–242. Evidence Level IV: Nonexperimental Study.

Trzepacz, P. T., & Van Der Mast, R. C. (2002). The neuropathophysiology of delirium. In J. Lindesay, K. Rockwood, & A. Macdonald (Eds.), *Delirium in old age* (pp. 51–100). New York: Oxford University Press. Evidence Level VI: Expert Opinion.

Family Caregiving

8

Deborah C. Messecar

Educational Objectives

After completing this chapter, the reader will be able to:

1. describe characteristics and factors that put family caregivers at risk for strain and/or depression

2. identify key aspects of a family caregiving assessment

3. list specific interventions to support family caregivers of older adults

4. identify family caregiver outcomes expected from the implementation of this protocol

Overview

Prevalence of Caregiving

Being a family caregiver is a widespread experience in the United States. Depending on how family caregiving is defined, national surveys estimate that anywhere from 22.4 million to 52 million people provide care for a chronically ill, disabled family member or friend during any given year (National Alliance for Caregiving [NAC] & American Association of Retired Persons [AARP], 2004 [Level IV]; Opinion Research Corporation [OPC], 2005 [Level IV]; U.S.

For a description of Evidence Levels cited in this chapter, see chapter 1, Developing and Evaluating Clinical Practice Guidelines, page 4

Department of Health and Human Services [USDHHS], 1998 [Level IV]). The lower estimate of 22.4 million, or 23%, of all U.S. households, applies when the definition of family care is restricted to care provided in the past 12 months to an older adult with substantial activities of daily living (ADL) and instrumental activities of daily living (IADL) needs (NAC & AARP, 2004 [Level IV]). When the definition of caregiving is expanded to include all ages older than 18 and past and present care, close to 60% of adult Americans are providing or have provided unpaid care to an adult family member or friend. Family caregiving is prevalent across all socioeconomic levels and among all ethnic groups. For example, 59% of non-Hispanic Whites, 53% of African Americans, and 51% of Hispanic adults in the United States report that they are or have been caregivers (OPC, 2005 [Level IV]).

Profile of Caregivers

Reflecting an increasing trend, 44% of all family caregivers of adults older than age 18 are men, 56% are women, and the majority is older than age 45 (OPC, 2005 [Level IV]). Among the primary family caregivers of older disabled or ill adults older than age 65, the proportion of male caregivers is lower (about 32%), but this number has increased from prior years (Wolf & Kasper, 2006 [Level I]). The most common caregiver arrangement is that of an adult female child providing care to an elderly female parent (USDHHS, 1998 [Level IV]). Primary family caregivers are children (41.3%), spouses (38.4%), and other family or friends (20.4%) (Wolf & Kasper, 2006 [Level I]). Many caregivers are older and are at risk for chronic illness themselves. Nearly 45% of all primary caregivers are older than age 65, with 47.4% of spousal primary caregivers being age 75 or older (Wolf & Kasper, 2006 [Level I]). Caregiving work can be hard and time-consuming and is often a long-term commitment. It is estimated that 17% of family caregivers are providing 40 hours of care a week or more (NAC & AARP, 2004 [Level IV]). The average duration of years spent caregiving is 4.3 (NAC & AARP, 2004 [Level IV]; USDHHS, 1998 [Level IV]).

Trends in Caregiving

National surveys indicate a trend in the United States of care recipients being older and more disabled, and more caregivers acting as the primary source of care (i.e., an increase from 34.9% in 1989 to 52.8% in 1999) without help from secondary caregivers (Wolf & Kasper, 2006 [Level I]). In the future, the need for family caregivers will increase. The number of people older than age 65 is expected to increase at a rapid rate; however, the number of family members available to care for them will not keep pace (NAC & AARP, 2004 [Level IV]). Family and friends now provide more than 80% of all long term care services in the country. The cost of the unpaid care they provide is enormous and is estimated to be $306 billion a year, more than twice as much as was actually spent on home care and nursing home services combined (Arno, 2006 [Level IV]). A typical working family caregiver can expect to lose $109 per day in wages and health benefits due to the need to provide full-time care at home (Altman, Cooper, & Cunningham, 1999 [Level IV]). The loss in income is the direct result of needing to make adjustments in work life such as reporting late to work or giving up work entirely (NAC & AARP, 2004 [Level IV]).

Impact of Caregiving on Caregiver

Caregiving has documented negative consequences for the caregiver's physical and emotional health. Caregiving-related stress in a chronically ill spouse results in a 63% higher mortality rate than in their noncaregiving peers (Schulz & Beach, 1999 [Level II]). Stress from caring for an older adult with dementia has been shown to impact the caregiver's immune system for up to 3 years after their caregiving ends (Kiecolt-Glaser & Glaser, 2003 [Level III]). Spouse caregivers who provide heavy care (i.e., 36 or more hours per week) are six times more likely than noncaregivers to experience symptoms of depression or anxiety; for adult-child caregivers, the rate is twice as high (Cannuscio et al., 2002 [Level IV]). In addition to mental health morbidity, family caregivers also experience physical health deterioration. Family caregivers have chronic conditions at more than twice the rate of noncaregivers (NAC & AARP, 2004 [Level IV]; USDHHS, 1998 [Level IV]). Family caregivers experiencing extreme stress have also been shown to age prematurely. It is estimated that this stress can take as many as 10 years off a family caregiver's life (Arno, 2006 [Level IV]).

Background and Statement of The Problem

Definitions

Family Caregiving

Family caregiving is broadly defined and refers to a broad range of unpaid care provided in response to illness or functional impairment to a chronically ill or functionally impaired older family member, partner, friend, or neighbor that exceeds the support usually provided in family relationships (Schumacher, Beck, & Marren, 2006 [Level VI]).

Informal Caregiving

Informal caregiving is a more inclusive term that refers to help provided by all nonprofessional providers of care, including family members, friends, neighbors, and/or members of a religious or other type of community. In addition to family members or significant others, friends, neighbors, or members of a faith community may provide informal caregiving (Schumacher et al., 2006 [Level VI]).

Family Caregiving Activities

Family caregiving activities include assistance with day-to-day activities, illness-related care, care management, and invisible aspects of care. Day-to-day activities include personal care activities (e.g., bathing, eating, dressing, mobility, transferring from bed to chair, and using the toilet) and IADLs (e.g., meal preparation, grocery shopping, making telephone calls, and money manage-ment) (NAC & AARP, 2004 [Level IV]; Walker, Pratt, & Eddy, 1995 [Level I]). Illness-related activities include managing symptoms, coping with illness be-haviors, carrying out treatments, and performing medical or nursing proce-dures that include an array of medical technologies (Smith, 1994 [Level IV]). Care-management activities include accessing resources, communicating with and navigating the health care and social services systems, and acting as an advocate (Schumacher, Stewart, Archbold, Dodd, & Dibble, 2000 [Level IV]). Invisible aspects of care are protective actions the caregiver takes to ensure the older adult's safety and well-being without their knowledge (Bowers, 1987 [Level IV]).

Caregiving Roles

Caregiving roles can be classified into a hierarchy according to who takes on the majority of responsibilities versus only intermittent supportive assistance. Pri-mary caregivers tend to provide most of the everyday aspects of care, whereas secondary caregivers help out as needed to fill the gaps (Cantor & Little, 1985 [Level V]; Penning, 1990 [Level IV]; Tennstedt, McKinlay, & Sullivan, 1989 [Level IV]). Among caregivers who live with their care recipients, spouses account for the majority of primary caregivers, whereas adult children are more likely to be secondary caregivers. The range of the family caregiving role includes pro-tective caregiving such as "keeping an eye on" an older adult who is currently independent but at risk to full-time, around-the-clock care for a severely im-paired family member. Health care providers may fail to assess the full scope of the family caregiving role if they associate family caregiving only with the performance of tasks.

Caregiver Assessment

This term refers to an ongoing iterative process of gathering information that de-scribes a family caregiving situation and identifies the particular issues, needs, resources, and strengths of the family caregiver.

Risk Factors for Negative Outcomes with Caregiving

Female caregivers are more likely to provide a higher level of care than men, which is defined as helping with at least two ADLs and providing more than 40 care hours per week. Male caregivers are more likely to provide care at the lowest level, which is defined as no ADLs and devoting very few hours of care per week (NAC & AARP, 2004 [Level IV]; Pinquart & Sorensen, 2006 [Level I]). A number of studies have found that female caregivers are more likely than male caregivers to suffer from anxiety, depression, and other symptoms associated with emotional stress due to caregiving (Mahoney, Regan, Katona, & Livingston, 2005 [Level IV]; Yee & Schulz, 2000 [Level I]); lower levels of physical health and subjective well-being than caregiving men (Pinquart & Sorensen, 2006 [Level I]); and are at higher risk for adverse outcomes (Schultz, Martire, & Klinger, 2005 [Level I]). In the pooled analysis from the Resources for Enhancing Alzheimer's

Caregiver Health (REACH) trials, females had higher initial levels of burden and depression (Gitlin et al., 2003 [Level I]).

Ethnicity

Rates of caregiving vary somewhat by ethnicity. Among the U.S. adult population older than age 18, 17% of White and 15% of African American families are providing informal care, whereas slightly lower percentages of Asian Americans (14%) and Hispanic Americans (13%) are engaged in caregiving for persons older than age 50 (NAC & AARP, 2004 [Level IV]). However, in another national survey that looked only at people 70+ years old, 44% of Latinos were found to receive informal home care compared to 34% of African Americans and 25% of non-Hispanic Whites (Weiss, Gonzalez, Kabeto, & Langa, 2005 [Level IV]). Ethnic differences are also found with regard to the care recipient. Among people aged 70+ who require care, Whites are the most likely to receive help from their spouses, Hispanics are the most likely to receive help from their adult children, and African Americans are the most likely to receive help from a nonfamily member (National Academy on an Aging Society, 2000 [Level V]).

Studies show that ethnic minority caregivers provide more care (McCann et al., 2000 [Level IV]; Pinquart & Sorenson, 2005 [Level I]) and report worse physical health than White caregivers (Dilworth-Anderson, Williams, & Gibson, 2002 [Level I]; Pinquart & Sorenson, 2005 [Level I]). African American caregivers experience less stress and depression and get more rewards related to caregiving when compared to White caregivers (Cuellar, 2002 [Level IV]; Dilworth-Anderson, et al., 2002 [Level I]; Gitlin et al., 2003 [Level I]; Haley et al., 2004 [Level II]; Pinquart & Sorenson, 2005 [Level I]). However, Hispanic and Asian American caregivers exhibit more depression than White caregivers (Gitlin et al., 2003; Pinquart, & Sorenson, 2005 [both Level I]). In addition, formal services are rarely used by ethnic minorities, which puts them at further risk for negative outcomes (Dilworth-Anderson et al., 2002; Pinquart & Sorenson, 2005 [both Level I]). A meta-analysis of three qualitative studies examined African American, Chinese, and Latino caregiver impressions of their clinical encounters around their care receiver's diagnosis of Alzheimer's disease (Mahoney, Cloutterbuck, Neary, & Zhan, 2005 [Level I]). The primary issues identified in the analysis by Mahoney et al. were disrespect for concerns as noted by African American caregivers, stigmatization of persons with dementia as noted by Chinese caregivers, and fears that home care would not be supported as noted by Latino caregivers. These findings indicate a need for greater culturally sensitive communications from health care providers.

Income and Educational Level

Low income is also related to being an ethnic minority and being "non-White"; these are risk factors for poorer health outcomes. Persons who become caregivers may be more likely to have incomes below the poverty level and be in poorer health, independent of caregiving (Vitaliano, Zhang, & Scanlan, 2003 [Level I]). Usually, educational level has been combined with income in most caregiving studies, so there is a lack of data on this variable. One study (Buckwalter et al., 1999 [Level II]) reported that caregivers who were less educated tended to report slightly more depression than those who were better educated. This is consistent with the findings from the REACH trial meta-analysis (Gitlin et al., 2003 [Level I]). In the meta-analysis completed by Schultz, Martire, & Klinger (2005 [Level I]), caregivers with low incomes and low levels of education were more at risk for adverse outcomes.

Relationship (Spouse, Non-Spouse)

Past research conducted primarily among non-Hispanic White samples has shown that caregiving outcomes differ between non-spouse (who are mostly adult children) and spouse caregivers (Pinquart & Sorensen, 2004 [Level I]). In some literature reviews, authors noted that spousal caregivers have reported higher levels of depression than non-spouses (Pruchno & Resch, 1989 [Level I]). However, Gitlin and colleagues' (Gitlin, Corcoran, Winter, Boyce, & Hauck, 2001 [Level II]) intervention study found spouses reported less "upset" with the care receiver's behavior than non-spouses, who showed no decrease in "upset." In a meta-analysis of caregiving studies, spousal caregivers benefited less from existing interventions than adult children (Sorensen, Pinquart, & Duberstein, 2002 [Level I]).

Quality of Caregiver–Care Receiver Relationship

Disruption in the caregiver and care receiver relationship (Croog, Burleson, Sudilovsky, & Baume, 2006 [Level IV]; Flannery, 2002 [Level VI]) and/or a poor quality of relationship (Archbold, Stewart, Greenlick, & Harvath, 1990, 1992 [both Level II]) can make caregiving seem more difficult even if the objective caregiving situation (e.g., hours devoted to caregiving, number of tasks performed) does not seem to be too demanding. Archbold et al. reported that the deleterious effects of lack of preparedness on caregiver strain faded after 9 months; however, a poor relationship with the care receiver remained strongly related to caregiver strain. Reporting a poorer quality of relationship with the care receiver was associated with a 23.5% prevalence of anxiety and 10% prevalence of depression in Mahoney and colleagues' descriptive study (Mahoney, Regan, Katona, & Livingston, 2005 [Level IV]).

Lack of Preparedness

Most caregivers are not prepared for the many responsibilities they face and do not receive formal instruction in caregiving activities (NAC & AARP, 2004 [Level IV]). According to a national opinion survey, "Attitudes and Beliefs About Caregiving in the U.S.," 58% of respondents say they are only somewhat or not at all prepared to handle health insurance matters for an adult family member or friend, and 56% say they feel unprepared to assist with medications. Moreover, 64% worry about selling the home of a loved one and moving that person to another location or setting up a will or trust for that person (OPC, 2005 [Level IV]). Stewart and colleagues reported that although health care professionals were a caregiver's main source of information on providing physical care, the caregiver received no preparation on how to care for the patient emotionally or deal with the stresses of caregiving (Stewart, Archbold, Harvath, & Nkongho, 1993

[Level IV]). Lack of preparedness can greatly increase the caregiver's perceptions of strain, especially during times of transition from hospital to home (Archbold et al., 1990, 1992 [both Level II]).

Baseline Levels of Burden and Depressive Scores

In a meta-analysis of 84 caregiving studies, Pinquart and Sorensen (2003 [Level I]) found that caregivers have higher levels of stress and depression as well as lower levels of subjective well-being, physical health, and self-efficacy than noncaregivers. The strongest negative effects of caregiving were observed for clinician-rated depression. Differences in perceived stress and depression between caregivers and noncaregivers were larger in spouses than in adult children (Pinquart & Sorensen, 2003 [Level I]). Caregivers of care receivers who have dementia (Pinquart & Sorensen, 2006 [Level I]) have more problems with symptom management (Butler et al., 2005; Grande, Farquhar, Barclay, & Todd, 2004 [both Level II]) and problematic communication (Tolson, Swan, & Knussen, 2002 [Level II]) and have also reported increased burden, strain, and depression across studies.

Physical Health Problems

Vitaliano and colleagues' (2003 [Level I]) quantitative review of 23 studies from North America, Europe, and Australia examined relationships of caregiving with several health outcomes. They found that caregivers are at greater risk for health problems than noncaregivers. These studies included 1,594 caregivers of persons with dementia and 1,478 noncaregivers who were similar in age (i.e., mean 65.6 years old) and sex ratio (i.e., 65% women, 35% men). In this review, six physiological and five self-reported categories that are indicators of illness risk and illness were examined. The physiological categories included level of stress hormones, antibodies, immune counts and functioning, and cardiovascular and metabolic variables. Caregivers had a 23% higher level of stress hormones (e.g., ACTH, catecholamines, cortisol) and a 15% lower level of antibodies (e.g., EBV, herpes simplex, IgG) than noncaregivers. Co-morbid medical illnesses are important because many caregivers are middle-aged to older adults, and they may be ill before they become caregivers. It is interesting that the relationship between caregiver status and physiological risk was stronger for men than women (Vitaliano et al., 2003 [Level I]).

Assessment and Assessment Tools

Although systematic assessment of the patient is a routine element of clinical practice, assessment of the family caregiver is rarely carried out to determine what help the caregiver may need. Effective intervention strategies for caregivers should be based on an accurate assessment of caregiver risk and strengths. According to a broad consensus of researchers and family caregiving organizations (Family Caregiver Alliance, 2006 [Level VI]), assessing the caregiver should involve addressing the following topics, which are applicable across settings (e.g., home, hospital) but may not need to be measured in every assessment. Specific topics may differ for:

- initial assessments compared to reassessments (the latter focus on what has changed over time)
- new versus continuing-care situations
- an acute episode prompting a change in caregiving versus an ongoing need
- type of setting and focus of services (Family Caregiver Alliance, 2006 [Level VI])

Caregiving Context

The caregiving context includes the background on the caregiver and the caregiving situation. The caregiver's relationship to the care recipient (i.e., spouse, non-spouse) is important because spouse and non-spouse caregivers have different risks and needs (Gitlin et al., 2003 [Level I]; Sorensen et al., 2002 [Level I]). The caregiver's various roles and responsibilities can either take away from or enhance their ability to provide care. For example, working caregivers may have to develop strategies to juggle family and work responsibilities, so it is necessary to know their employment status (i.e., work/home/volunteer) (Pinquart & Sorensen, 2006 [Level I]). The duration of caregiving (Sorensen et al., 2002 [Level I]) can give the clinician clues about how new caregiving is for the caregiver or alert the clinician to the possibility of caregiver exhaustion with the role. Questions about household status, such as how many people are in the home and the existence and involvement of extended family and social support (Pinquart & Sorensen, 2006 [Level I]), can give the clinician clues about how much support the caregiver has readily available. Depending on the type of impairment of the care receiver, the physical environment of the home or facility where care takes place can be significant (Vitaliano et al., 2003 [Level I]). It is important to determine what the caregiver's financial status is—for example, are they getting by or are they short of funds to provide for everyday necessities (Vitaliano et al., 2003 [Level I])? The clinician should ask about potential resources that the caregiver could choose to use and list them (Pinquart & Sorensen, 2006 [Level I]). In addition, the clinician should explore the family's cultural background (Dilworth-Andersen et al., 2002 [Level I]), looking for clues on how to use this information as a resource.

Caregiver's Perception of Recipient's Health and Functional Status

List activities the care receiver needs help with, including both ADLs and IADLs (Pinquart & Sorensen, 2003, 2006 [both Level I]). Determine if there is any cognitive impairment of the care recipient; if the answer is yes, ask if there are any behavioral problems (Gitlin et al., 2003 [Level I]; Sorensen et al., 2002 [Level I]). The presence of mobility problems can also make caregiving more difficult—the clinician can assess this by simply asking if the care recipient has problems getting around (Archbold et al., 1990 [Level II]) (see chapter 3, *Assessment of Function*).

Caregiver Preparedness for Caregiving

Does the caregiver have the skills, abilities, and knowledge to provide the care recipient with needed care? To assess preparedness, the clinician can use the Preparedness for Caregiving Scale (PCGS) (see www.ConsultGeriRN.org, Caregiving topic). The PCGS was developed by Archbold et al. (1990, 1992 [both Level II]). The concept of preparedness was derived from role theory, in which socialization to a role is assumed to be important for role enactment and performance. The PCGS is a self-report questionnaire that measures four perspectives of domain-specific preparedness: physical needs, emotional needs, resources, and stress. The PCGS was evaluated in a longitudinal correlational study of family caregivers (N=103) of older patients with chronic diseases (Archbold et al., 1990, 1992 [both Level II]). The scale has five Likert-type items with possible responses ranging from 1 = not at all prepared to 4 = very well prepared. Overall scores are computed by averaging responses to the five items. Scores range from 1.00 to 4.00, the lowest score correlating with least preparedness. Archbold and colleagues (1992) reported internal reliability (Cronbach's alpha) of 0.72 at 6 weeks and 0.71 at the 9-month interview.

Quality of Family Relationships

The caregiver's perception of the quality of the relationship with the care receiver is a key predictor of the presence or lack of strain from caregiving (Archbold et al., 1990 [Level II]). The quality of the relationship can be assessed using the Mutuality Scale (see Mutuality Scale at www.ConsultGeriRN.org, Caregiving topic), developed by Archbold et al. (1990, 1992 [both Level II]). *Mutuality* is defined as the caregiver's perceived quality of the relationship with the care receiver. It is a self-report instrument that asks caregivers to rate how they feel about the care recipient, with possible responses ranging from 0 = not at all to 4 = a great deal. The caregiver's mutuality score is computed by taking the average of the scores on the 15 items. Internal reliability and consistency (Cronbach's alpha) of the scale was 0.91 at both 6 weeks and 9 months from discharge from the hospital (Archbold et al., 1990 [Level II]).

Indicators of Problems with Quality of Care

Indicators of problems with the quality of care can include evidence of an unhealthy environment, inappropriate management of finances, and demonstration of a lack of respect for the older adult (see Resources section). The nurse's observations can be guided by the Elder Assessment Instrument (EAI) (Fulmer, 2002 [Level VI]), which helps the nurse identify elder abuse and neglect issues (see EAI at www.ConsultGeriRN.org). The EAI consists of seven sections that reviews signs, symptoms, and subjective complaints of elder abuse, neglect, exploitation, and abandonment (Fulmer, Paveza, Abraham, & Fairchild, 2000 [Level II]; Fulmer, Street, & Carr, 1984 [Level II]; Fulmer & Wetle, 1986 [Level II]). There is no "score," but the elder should be referred to social services if there is evidence of mistreatment; a complaint by the elder; or high risk of or probable abuse, neglect, exploitation, or abandonment of the older adult.

Caregiver's Physical and Mental Health Status

The caregiver's perception of their own health (Pinquart & Sorensen, 2006 [Level I]) is one of the most reliable indicators of a physical health problem. Depression or other emotional distress (e.g., anxiety) can be assessed using the Center for Epidemiological Studies–Depression Scale (CES–D) (see Resources section) (Pinquart & Sorensen, 2003, 2006; Sorensen et al., 2002 [all Level I]). The CES–D was initially designed as a screen for the community dwelling at risk of developing major depressive symptomatology. It has been used widely in intervention studies with family caregivers, where it has been self-administered. The Brown University Center for Gerontology and Healthcare Research created a set of End-of-Life Care Toolkit instruments, which are available for use on its Web site at no charge. For each of the 20 items, participants rate its frequency of occurrence during the past week on a 4-point scale from 0 (*rarely*) to 3 (*most of the time*). Scores range from 0 to 60, with a higher score indicating the presence of a greater number and frequency of depressive symptoms. A score of 16 or higher has been identified as discriminatory between groups with clinically relevant and nonrelevant depressive symptoms (Radloff, 1977 [Level II]; Radloff & Teri, 1986 [Level II]).

Burden or strain can be assessed using the Caregiver Strain Index (CSI) (see www.ConsultGeriRN.org, Family Caregiving topic) (Sullivan, 2002 [Level II]). Preexisting burden or strain places caregivers at greater risk and may prevent them from benefiting from interventions (Schultz & Beach, 1999 [Level II]; Vitaliano et al., 2003 [Level I]; Sullivan, 2002 [Level II]). The CSI is a tool that can be used to quickly identify families with potential caregiving concerns. It is a 13-question tool that measures strain related to care provision. There is at least one item for each of the following major domains: employment, financial, physical, social, and time. Positive responses to seven or more items on the CSI indicate a greater level of strain. Internal consistency reliability is high (alpha = 0.86) and construct validity is supported by correlations with the physical and emotional health of the caregiver and with subjective views of the caregiving situation. A positive screen (seven or more items positive) on the CSI indicates a need for more in-depth assessment to facilitate appropriate intervention.

Rewards of Caregiving

Although early family caregiving research focused almost exclusively on negative outcomes of caregiving, clearly there are many positive aspects of providing care. Spouses can be drawn closer together by caregiving, which can act as an expression of love. Adult child caregivers can feel a sense of accomplishment from helping their parents. Caregivers should be asked to enumerate their perceived benefits of caregiving (Archbold et al., 1995 [Level II]). These can include the satisfaction of helping a family member, developing new skills and competencies, and or improved family relationships.

Self-Care Activities for Caregivers

Self-care activities can include setting aside time to exercise, getting time for oneself, and obtaining respite. Even if caregivers do not use this strategy, the clinician should ask them to think about strategies that would work for them. Caregivers need to be reminded that self-care is not a luxury, it is a necessity. At a minimum, caregivers need to learn how to put themselves first, manage stress, socialize, and get help.

Interventions

Definitions

Psychoeducational Interventions

Psychoeducational interventions involve a structured program geared toward providing information about the care receiver's disease process, resources and services, and training caregivers to respond effectively to disease-related problems, such as memory and behavior problems in dementia patients or depression and anger in cancer patients. These interventions use lectures, group discussions, and written materials and are always led by a trained leader. Support may be part of a psychoeducational group, but it is secondary to the educational content.

Supportive Interventions

This category subsumes both professionally led and peer-led unstructured support groups focused on building rapport among participants and creating a space in which to discuss problems, successes, and feelings regarding caregiving.

Respite/Adult Day Care

Respite care is either in-home or site-specific supervision, assistance with ADLs, or skilled nursing care designed to give the caregiver time off.

Psychotherapy

This type of intervention involves a therapeutic relationship between the caregiver and a trained professional. Most psychotherapeutic interventions with caregivers follow a cognitive–behavioral approach.

Interventions to Improve Care-Receiver Competence

These interventions include memory clinics for patients with dementia and activity therapy programs designed to improve affect and everyday competence.

Multicomponent Interventions

Interventions in this group included various combinations of educational interventions, support, psychotherapy, and respite in Sorensen et al.'s meta-analysis.

Individual studies included after the 2002 meta-analysis include nursing management and interdisciplinary-care interventions.

Overview of Interventions

Past reviews of caregiver interventions, such as support groups, individual counseling, and education confirm that there is no single, easily implemented, and consistently effective method for eliminating the stresses and/or strain of being a caregiver (Knight, Lutzky, & Macofsky-Urban, 1993 [Level I]; Toseland & Rossiter, 1989 [Level I]). Sorensen and colleagues (2002 [Level I]) performed a more recent meta-analysis on the effects of a second generation of 78 caregiver intervention studies. The most consistent significant improvements in all outcome domains (i.e., burden, depression, well-being, ability and knowledge, care-receiver symptoms) assessed in the meta-analysis resulted from psychotherapy and caregiver psychoeducational interventions aimed at improving caregiver knowledge and abilities. Multicomponent interventions, which combined features of psychotherapy and knowledge/skill-building, had the largest effect on burden and, in addition, were effective for improving well-being and ability and knowledge. The effects of different types of interventions on selected caregiver outcomes from the meta-analysis and studies completed since 2002 are presented in Table 8.1.

More current studies of psychotherapy and psychoeducational interventions (Akkerman & Ostwald, 2004 [Level II]; Burns et al., 2005 [Level II]; Coon, Thompson, Steffen, Sorocco, & Gallagher-Thompson, 2003 [Level II]; Hebert et al., 2003 [Level II]; Hepburn et al., 2005 [Level II]) and multicomponent interventions (Mittelman, Roth, Coon, & Haley, 2004 [Level II]; Mittelman, Roth, Haley, & Zarit, 2004 [Level II]) fit the same pattern of results. All of these interventions address key negative aspects of caregiving: being overwhelmed with the physical demands of care, feeling isolated, not having time for oneself, having difficulties with the care recipient's behavior, and dealing with one's own negative responses.

There are several characteristics across interventions that seem to have a moderating effect on caregiving outcomes. Focusing the caregiver training exclusively on care receivers to alter their symptoms has almost no effect on caregivers (Sorensen et al., 2002 [Level I]). In the Sorensen meta-analysis, group interventions were less effective at improving caregiver burden than individual and mixed interventions, which is consistent with Knight et al. (1993 [Level I]) but inconsistent with the meta-analysis performed by Yin, Zhou, and Bashford (2002 [Level I]). Length of an intervention appears to be important in alleviating caregiver depression and care-receiver symptoms. Caregivers do less well with shorter interventions with regard to depression because they lose the supportive aspects of prolonged contact with a group or a professional before they can benefit.

Characteristics of the caregiver are also associated with intervention effectiveness. Some caregivers benefit less from interventions than others. For example, Sorensen found that spouse caregivers benefited less from interventions than adult children (2002 [Level I]). Table 8.2 presents caregiver characteristics associated with various intervention outcomes.

8.1 Effects of Different Types of Interventions on Caregiver Outcomes

Type of intervention	Burden or strain	Depression or distress	CG (Caregiver) well-being	CG ability, knowledge	CR (Care Receiver) symptoms	Health Service Utilization Institutionalization Costs
Psychoeducation Skill-building	Significant effect (Sorensen et al., 2002 [Level I]) Decreased burden – 6 studies (Acton & Winter, 2002 [Level II])	Significant effect (Sorensen et al., 2002 [Level I]) Decreased depression – 6 studies (Acton & Winter, 2002 [Level II]) Significant reduction in depressive symptoms (Gallagher-Thompson et al., 2003 [Level III]) Decreased bother, anxiety, depression (Mahoney, Tarlow, & Jones, 2003 [Level III]) Decreased depression (Coon et al., 2003 [Level III]) Decreased distress (Hepburn et al., 2005 [Level III])	Significant effect (Sorensen et al., 2002 [Level II])	Significant effect (Sorensen et al., 2002 [Level II]) Increased knowledge – 9 studies (Acton & Winter, 2002 [Level II]) 14% improved reaction to CR symptoms (Hebert et al., 2003 [Level III])	Significant effect (Sorensen et al., 2002 [Level II])	
Supportive Interventions	Significant effect (Sorensen et al., 2002 [Level II])			Significant effect (Sorensen et al., 2002 [Level II])		

8.1 Effects of Different Types of Interventions on Caregiver Outcomes

Type of intervention	Burden or strain	Depression or distress	CG (Caregiver) well-being	CG ability, knowledge	CR (Care Receiver) symptoms	Health Service Utilization Institutionalization Costs
Psychotherapy	Significant effect (Sorensen et al., 2002 [Level II]) Decreased objective burden	Significant effect (Sorensen et al., 2002 [Level II]) Decreased anxiety (Akkerman & Ostwald, 2004 [Level III])	Significant effect (Sorensen et al., 2002 [Level II])	Significant effect (Sorensen et al., 2002 [Level II]) Some improved reaction to CR symptoms (Burns et al., 2005 [Level III])	Significant effect (Sorensen et al., 2002 [Level II])	
Respite	Significant effect (Sorensen et al., 2002 [Level II])	Significant effect (Sorensen et al., 2002 [Level II]) Decreased depression – 3 studies (Acton & Winter, 2002 [Level II])	Significant effect (Sorensen et al., 2002 [Level II])			Institutionalization treatment less than control – 1 study (Acton & Winter, 2002 [Level II])
Focus on care receiver (CR)			Significant effect (Sorensen et al., 2002 [Level II])		Significant effect (Sorensen et al., 2002 [Level II]) Improved quality of life (Clark et al., 2006 [Level III])	Reduction in care-receiver anxiety (Smith, Forster, & Young, 2004 [Level III])
Multicomponent added to this category	Large significant effect (Sorensen et al., 2002 [Level II])	Improved distress and depression (Callahan et al., 2006 [Level III]) (Bass et al., 2003 [Level III])	Significant effect (Sorensen et al., 2002 [Level II])	Significant effect (Sorensen et al., 2002 [Level II])	Improved perceptions of health, decreased negative emotion and dependence (Burton & Gibbon, 2005 [Level III])	No differences (Callahan et al., 2006 [Level III])

Nursing and interdisciplinary care management – includes hospital or rehabilitation at home and primary care	Improved carer strain (Burton & Gibbon. 2005 [Level III]) Decreased burden/strain – 2 studies (Acton & Winter. 2002 [Level I]) REACH intervention overall decreased burden (Gitlin et al., 2003 [Level I]) Decreased burden (Kalra et al., 2004 [Level III]) Burden and strain were responsive to intervention (Schultz et al., 2005 [Level I])	Less burden (Crotty, Whitehead. Miller. & Gray. 2003 [Level III]) Less strain (Harris et al., 2005 [Level III]) More strain after intervention (Wade et al., 2003 [Level III]) Significant decrease in depressive symptoms (Eisdorfer et al., 2003 [Level III]) Decreased depression. distress, anxiety – 4 studies (Acton & Winter. 2002 [Level I]) Decreased anxiety and depression (Kalra et al., 2004 [Level III]) Decreased depression (Mittleman. Roth, Coon et al., 2003 [Level III]) Decreased reaction ratings (Mittleman. Roth. Haley. et al., 2004 [Level III]) Clinically significant decreases in depression and anxiety (Schultz et al., 2005 [Level I])	Higher role rewards (Li et al., 2003 [Level I]) Caregiver affect improved (Gitlin et al., 2005 [Level III]) Well-being worse in control group (Burns et al., 2003 [Level III])	Worse mental health (Wade et al., 2003 [Level III])	Some but not all service utilization outcomes (Bass et al., 2003 [Level III]) Cost twice as much as usual inpatient care (Harris et al., 2005 [Level III]) Lower hospitalization. reduced ER use (Shelton et al., 2001 [Level III]) Lower costs due to lower readmission (Teng et al., 2003 [Level III]) Delayed institutionalization (Schultz et al., 2005 [Level I])
Focus on physical or emotional health of CG		Decreased psychological distress (King et al., 2002 [Level III]) Decreased depression & anxiety (Waelde et al., 2004 [Level III])			

8.2 Effects of Different Types of Caregiver Characteristics on Caregiver Outcomes

Characteristics of caregiving situation	Burden	Depression	CG (Caregiver) Well-being	CG ability knowledge	CR (Care Receiver) Symptoms
CR has dementia	Less effective (Sorensen et al., 2002 [Level II)	Less effective (Sorensen et al., 2002 [Level II)	Less effective (Sorensen et al., 2002 [Level II])	Less effective (Sorensen et al., 2002 [Level II])	No effect (Sorensen et al., 2002 [Level II])
Adult-child CGs	Greater improvement (Sorensen et al., 2002 [Level II])	Greater improvement (Sorensen et al., 2002 [Level II]) Non-spouses did better (Gitlin et al., 2003 [Level II])	Greater improvement (Sorensen et al., 2002 [Level II])	Greater improvement (Sorensen et al., 2002 [Level II])	Smaller improvement (Sorensen et al., 2002 [Level II])
Spouse CGs	Smaller improvement (Sorensen et al., 2002 [Level II])	Smaller improvement (Sorensen et al., 2002 [Level II]) Wives with low mastery and high anxiety benefited the most (Mahoney et al., 2003 [Level II]) Cuban husbands improved more on depressive symptoms (Eisdorfer et al., 2003 [Level II])	Smaller improvement (Sorensen et al., 2002 [Level II])	Smaller improvement (Sorensen et al., 2002 [Level II])	Greater improvement (Sorensen et al., 2002 [Level II])
Older CGs	Greater improvement (Sorensen et al., 2002 [Level II]) Higher risk for (Schulz et al., 2005 [Level II])	No effects (Sorensen et al., 2002 [Level II]) Higher risk for (Schulz et al., 2005 [Level II])	Greater improvement (Sorensen et al., 2002 [Level II])	Greater improvement (Sorensen et al., 2002 [Level II])	Greater improvement (Sorensen et al., 2002 [Level II])

Female CGs	Greater improvement (Sorensen et al., 2002 [Level I]) Better improvement (Gitlin et al., 2003 [Level I]) Higher risk for (Schulz et al., 2005 [Level I])	Females benefit more (Gallagher-Thompson et al., 2003 [Level II]) Cuban daughters improved more on depressive symptoms (Eisdorfer et al., 2003 [Level II]) Higher risk for (Schulz et al., 2005 [Level I])	Greater improvement (Sorensen et al., 2002 [Level I])	Greater improvement (Sorensen et al., 2002 [Level I])
Ethnicity	(Sorensen et al., 2002 [Level I])	Latinos benefit as much (Gallagher-Thompson et al., 2003 [Level II]) Cuban husbands and daughters improved more on depressive symptoms (Eisdorfer et al., 2003 [Level II]) Hispanics did better (Gitlin et al., 2003 [Level II])	(Sorensen et al., 2002 [Level I])	
Lower education	Better improvement (Gitlin, et al., 2003 [Level I]) Higher risk for (Schulz et al., 2005 [Level I])	Better improvement (Gitlin et al., 2003 [Level I]) Higher risk for (Schulz et al., 2005 [Level I])		

Intervention Approaches with Disappointing Results

Some intervention approaches have been consistently disappointing, either showing no significant effects or limited responses. In Lee and Cameron's 2004 ([Level I]) update of the Cochrane database review, reanalysis of three trials of respite care found no significant effects of respite on any outcome variable. Interventions focused on medication management of the care receiver's dementing condition (Lingler, Martire, & Schulz, 2005 [Level I]) and/or targeted to managing problematic behavior (Livingston et al., 2005 [Level I]) were similarly disappointing. A meta-analysis of habit training for the management of urinary-incontinence interventions showed that not only were there no significant differences in incontinence between the intervention and control groups but that caregivers also found the intervention labor-intensive (Ostaszkiewicz, Johnston, & Roe, 2004 [Level I]).

Interventions with Little Effect Due to Study Flaws

In Acton and Winter's (2002 [Level I]) meta-analysis of dementia caregiving studies, small, diverse samples; lack of intervention specificity; diversity in the length, duration, and intensity of the intervention strategies; and problematic outcome measures led to nonsignificant results for many tested interventions. Cooke, McNally, Mulligan, Harrison, and Newman (2001 [Level I]) also reported that two-thirds of the interventions they examined did not show any improvement in any outcome measures. Their analysis was hampered by lack of detailed description of the interventions in the studies they examined. Study limitations have also been a factor leading to disappointing results for some innovative caregiving interventions for caregivers of care receivers with other long-term, debilitating illnesses. For example, interventions designed to teach arthritis management as a couple (Martire et al., 2003 [Level II]), to decrease the gap between caregivers' expectations and patients' actual functional abilities with skill-building, and nurse-coached pain management all had disappointing results due to either small sample sizes or the complexity of the problems they were designed to address (Martin-Cook, Davis, Hynan, & Weiner, 2005 [Level II]; Schumacher et al., 2002 [Level IV]). According to Price, Hermans, Grimley, and Evans (2006 [Level I]), modification interventions for wandering have never been adequately tested due to the many flaws identified in the existing published research; outcome measurement has also been problematic. More distal outcomes, such as depression, perceived stress, caregiver strain, and self-efficacy, that are less directly related to the actual intervention, are less likely to change significantly (Bourgeois, Schulz, Burgio, & Beach, 2002 [Level II]; Burgio, Stevens, Guy, Roth, & Haley, 2003 [Level II]) than outcomes that are more specific to the intervention (Hebert et al., 2003 [Level II]).

Interventions with Little Effect Due to Debilitating Nature of Care Receiver Illness

Caregivers caring for care receivers who have conditions that worsen substantially over time (e.g., dementia, Parkinson's disease, stroke) have reported either less improvement, no improvement, or increased strain after intervention (Forster et al., 2006 [Level I]; Sorensen et al., 2002 [Level I]; Wright, Litaker,

Laraia, & DeAndrade, 2001 [Level II]). Across many studies, Sorensen et al (2002 [Level I]) reported that interventions with caregivers of dementia patients are less successful than with other caregivers. They also noted that if levels of caregiving are relatively high and cannot be reduced, as is the case for dementia caregivers, then burden and depression are also less amenable to change. A multidisciplinary rehabilitation program for Parkinson's patients resulted in no improvement in depression for caregivers after treatment (Trend, Kaye, Gage, Owen, & Wade, 2002 [Level III]). A meta-analysis of hospital and home care for stroke patients reported no evidence from clinical trials to support a radical shift in the care of acute stroke patients from hospital-based (Langhorne et al., 2006 [Level I]). Individual studies that examined other psychoeducational and/or support and counseling interventions for stroke caregivers (albeit with relatively small samples) found no significant changes between the intervention and control groups (Clark, Rubenach, & Winsor, 2003 [Level II]; Grasel, Biehler, Schmidt, & Schupp, 2005 [Level III]; Larson et al., 2005 [Level II]). Only an intensive, multicomponent, skills-training intervention significantly decreased burden anxiety and depression for this category of caregivers (Kalra et al., 2004 [Level II]). A number of family-based and symptom-management interventions for cancer patients have also found no significant intervention effects (Hudson, Aranda, & Hayman-White, 2005 [Level II]; Kozachik et al., 2001 [Level II]; Kurtz, Kurtz, Given, & Given, 2005 [Level II]; Northouse, Kershaw, Mood, & Schafenacker, 2005 [Level II]; Wells, Hepworth, Murphy, Wujcik, & Johnson, 2003 [Level II]). In several of these studies, there was a large dropout rate among the intervention participants due to the rapidly deteriorating condition of the care receivers.

Novel Caregiver-Focused Intervention Approaches That Show Promise

A moderate-intensity exercise program was tested among older women family caregivers. Exercise participants showed significant improvements in total energy expenditure, stress-induced blood pressure reactivity, and sleep quality along with a decrease in psychological distress (King, Baumann, O'Sullivan, Wilcox, & Castro, 2002 [Level II]). In another pilot study, 12 older female dementia caregivers participated in a six-session manualized combined yoga and meditation program (Waelde, Thompson, & Gallagher-Thompson, 2004 [Level III]) in which participants experienced significant decreases in depression and anxiety. Secker and Brown (2005 [Level II]) had very good success with a pilot intervention that used cognitive behavioral therapy to treat caregiver psychological distress.

Resources for Enhancing Alzheimer's Caregiver Health (Reach)

The REACH project was designed to test promising interventions for enhancing family caregiving for persons with dementia and to overcome several of the limitations of prior research (Schultz et al., 2003 [Level V]). More than 1,200 caregivers participated at six sites nationwide. The sample was more diverse than most caregiving studies due to the multisite design: participants were 56% White, 24% African American, and 19% Latino (Wisniewski et al., 2003 [Level II]).

1. In the REACH study, Mahoney and colleagues (2003 [Level II]) examined the main outcome effects of a 12-month, computer-mediated automated interactive voice response (IVR) intervention designed to assist family caregivers managing care receivers with dementia. There was a significant intervention effect for bother, anxiety, and depression. Wives who exhibited low mastery and high anxiety benefited most from the automated telecare intervention.
2. Gallagher-Thompson et al. (2003 [Level II]) tested a psychoeducational (skill-building) approach modeled after community-based support groups. The intervention was tailored to be sensitive to ethnic groups. In this study, female caregivers benefited more from the skill-building approach than from support group alone, and the Latino caregivers benefited as much as the other caregivers.
3. Burgio et al. (2003 [Level II]) developed a manual-guided intervention tailored on cultural preferences of White and African American caregivers. The intervention combined both care recipient-focused behavior management skill training and caregiver-focused, problem-solving training. White caregivers showed more improvement in the control condition, and African American caregivers had the greatest improvements in the skill-training condition. Spouse and non-spouse caregivers responded differently to the intervention, with non-spouse caregivers benefiting more than spouses.
4. Eisdorfer et al. (2003 [Level II]) used a family-systems approach to develop a family-therapy intervention designed to enhance communication between caregivers and other family members by identifying existing problems in communication and facilitating changes in interaction patterns that encourage caregivers to gather and more effectively manage available family and community resources. In the second experimental condition, they added a computer-telephone integrated system of support. The combined family-therapy and technology-intervention caregivers experienced a significant decrease in depressive symptoms, which was particularly beneficial for Cuban American husband and daughter caregivers.
5. Burns and colleagues (2003 [Level II]) tested two primary-care interventions delivered during a 24-month period: patient-behavior management only and patient-behavior management plus caregiver stress and coping. Participants who received patient-behavior management only had significantly worse outcomes for well-being. When caregiving issues were not addressed, care was inadequate for reducing caregiver distress.
6. Gitlin et al. (2005 [Level II]) tested an intervention that consisted of in-home occupational therapy visits designed to help families modify the environment to reduce caregiver burden. At 12 months, caregiver affect improved significantly, but no other caregiver outcomes were significantly different from baseline.

When the results from the REACH interventions were pooled, overall interventions decreased burden significantly compared to the control conditions (Gitlin et al., 2003 [Level I]). Only the family therapy with computer technology intervention was effective for reducing depressive symptoms. Interventions were superior to control conditions on burden for women and caregivers with lower education; on depression, Hispanics, non-spouses, and caregivers with lower education had bigger responses.

Aspects of Interventions That Improve Effectiveness

A key conclusion of the REACH trial and several of the meta-analyses (Gitlin et al., 2003 [Level I]; Schulz et al., 2005 [Level I]; Sorensen et al., 2002 [Level I]) reviewed in this chapter was that family-caregiver interventions need to be multicomponent and tailored. Multicomponent interventions have the potential to include a repertoire of various strategies that target different aspects of the caregiving experience. In focus groups conducted during a caregiving clinical trial, Farran, Loukissa, Perraud, and Paun (2003 [Level II]) identified and catalogued the information and skills that caregivers reported they needed to respond to their own needs or the caregiving process, including care-receiver issues such as managing difficult behaviors, worrisome symptoms, personal-care problems, and caregiver concerns such as managing competing responsibilities and stressors, finding and using resources, and handling their emotional and physical responses to care. Tailored interventions are interventions that are crafted to match a specific target population (e.g., spouse caregivers of Alzheimer's patients) and their specific caregiving issues and concerns identified through thorough assessment (Archbold et al., 1995 [Level II]; Horton-Deutsch, Farran, Choi, & Fogg, 2002 [Level III]). Interventions that are individualized or tailored in combination with skill-building demonstrated the best evidence of effectiveness (Pusey & Richards, 2001 [Level I]). Among the psychoeducational interventions, some of the most effective were predicated on a skills-building approach (Gallagher-Thompson et al., 2003 [Level II]; Hepburn, Tornatore, Center, & Ostwald, 2001 [Level II]). Collaboration or a partnership model with the caregiver is also a key component of making the tailoring process more effective (Harvath et al., 1994 [Level V]). Programs that work collaboratively with care receivers and their families and are more intensive and modified to the caregivers' needs are also more successful (Brodaty, Green, & Koschera, 2003 [Level I]).

Nursing Care Strategies

1. **Identify content and skills needed to increase preparedness for caregiving.**

   Psychoeducational skill-building interventions include information about the care needed by the care receiver and how to provide it, as well as coaching on how to manage the caregiving role. Tasks associated with taking on the caregiving role include dealing with change, juggling competing responsibilities and stressors, providing and managing care, finding and using resources, and managing the physical and emotional responses to care (Acton & Winter, 2002 [Level I]; Farran et al., 2003 [Level IV]; Farran et al., 2004 [Level II]; Gitlin et al., 2003 [Level I]; Sorensen et al., 2002 [Level I]).

2. **Form a partnership with the caregiver prior to generating strategies to address issues and concerns.**

   The goal of this partnership is blending the nurse's knowledge and expertise in health care with the caregiver's knowledge of the family member and the caregiving situation. Each party brings essential knowledge to the process of mutual negotiation between the family and the nurse. Together they develop ideas to address the issues and concerns that are most salient for the caregiver and care receiver. Every family situation will be different, and interventions cannot be individualized without nurse–family collaboration (Brodaty et al., 2003 [Level I]; Gitlin et al., 2005 [Level II]; Harvath et al., 1994 [Level V]; Nolan, 2001 [Level V]).

3. **Identify the caregiving issues and concerns on which the caregiver wants to work and generate strategies.**

   Multiple strategies should be generated for each caregiving issue and concern. One of the most important findings from the review of literature on caregiving is that multicomponent interventions are superior to narrow, single-approach problem solving (Acton & Winter, 2002 [Level I]; Gitlin et al., 2003 [Level I]; Sorensen et al. 2002 [Level I]; several Level II individual studies [see Table 8.1]).

4. **Assist the caregiver in identifying strengths in the caregiving situation.**

   Not all outcomes from caregiving are negative, and caregiving can be rewarding for some caregivers who derive pride and satisfaction from the important role they are filling. Incorporating pleasurable activities into the daily routine or incorporating into some caregiving task something that is either fun or meaningful are ways of enhancing caregiving. Even in really difficult situations, there may be some positive benefit derived, such as satisfaction in meeting an important commitment and/or recognition of personal growth (Archbold et al., 1995 [Level II]).

5. **Assist the caregiver in finding and using resources.**

   Navigating the health care system is one of the most difficult skills caregivers have to master (Archbold et al., 1995 [Level II]; Farran et al., 2004 [Level II]; Schumacher et al., 2002 [Level IV]). Caregivers rarely know how to translate a need that they have into a request for help from the health care system. Learning how to speak to health care providers, negotiate billing, request help with transportation—all of these tasks can be overwhelming. For some caregivers, Internet and other on-line sources of support and information can be helpful.

6. **Help caregivers identify and manage their physical and emotional responses to caregiving.**

   We know that caregiving is sometimes associated with deterioration of the caregiver's health or significant depression (Schulz et al., 2003 [Level V]). Generating strategies to take care of the caregiver is just as important as the strategies for caring for the care recipient.

7. **Use an interdisciplinary approach when working with family caregivers.**

   Multicomponent interventions have the strongest record in terms of alleviating some of the global negative consequences of caregiving. Involving a team of other health professionals helps the nurse and family generate new ideas for strategies and brings a fresh perspective to the idea-generating process (Acton & Winter, 2002 [Level I]; Farran et al., 2003 [Level IV]; Farran et al., 2004 [Level II]; Gitlin et al., 2003 [Level I]; Sorensen et al., 2002 [Level I]; several Level II studies [see Table 8.1]).

Expected Outcomes

Outcomes Specific to the Caregiver

The goal of the guideline is to lower strain, depression, and poor physical health for caregivers. Indicators of problems include reports of depression and/or fatigue, increased use of over-the-counter and prescription medications, increased use of health services, neglect of own health, and substance abuse. Increased focus on the caregiver system as the unit of service should increase a nurse's confidence in working with family caregivers.

Outcomes Specific to the Patient

These include improvement (where possible) in patient functional status, nutrition, and hygiene. Improved symptom management for care recipients with significant chronic disease is also a desired outcome. This could include better pain management for care recipients with cancer, improved glycemic control for care recipients with diabetes, and/or diminished problematic behaviors for care recipients with dementia. The emotional well-being of the care recipient should also be an outcome of interventions to aid the caregiver. Decreased use of emergency services and increased use of formal care supports are system outcomes we might expect.

Resources

Preparedness Scale at www.ConsultGeriRN.org, Caregiving topic.
Mutuality Scale at www.ConsultGeriRN.org, Caregiving topic.
Elder Assessment Instrument at www.ConsultGeriRN.org, Elder Mistreatment
    and Abuse topic.
CES-D at http://www.chcr.brown.edu/pcoc/cesdscale.pdf.
Caregiver Strain Index at www.ConsultGeriRN.org, Caregiving topic.

Box 8.1

Nursing Standard of Practice Protocol: Family Caregiving

I. GOAL

Identify viable strategies to monitor and support family caregivers.

II. OVERVIEW

Family caregivers provide more than 80% of the long-term care for older adults in this country. Caregiving can be difficult, time-consuming work added on top of job and other family responsibilities. If caregivers suffer negative consequences from their caregiving role and these are not mitigated, increased morbidity and mortality may result for caregivers. Not all outcomes from caregiving are negative; there are many caregivers that report rewards from caregiving.

III. BACKGROUND AND STATEMENT OF PROBLEM

A. Definitions
1. Family caregiving: This is broadly defined and refers to a wide range of unpaid care provided in response to illness or functional impairment to a chronically ill or functionally impaired older family member, partner, friend, or neighbor that exceeds the support usually provided in family relationships (Schumacher, Beck, & Marren, 2006 [Level VI]).
2. Informal caregiving: This is a more inclusive term that refers to help provided by all nonprofessional providers of care, including family members, friends, neighbors, and/or members of a religious or other type of community. In addition to family members or significant others, friends, neighbors, or members of a faith community may provide informal caregiving (Schumacher et al., 2006 [Level VI]).
3. Family caregiving activities: These include assistance with day-to-day activities, illness-related care, care management, and invisible aspects of care. Day-to-day activities include personal-care activities (e.g., bathing, eating, dressing, mobility, transferring from bed to chair, and using the toilet) and IADLs (e.g., meal preparation, grocery shopping, making telephone calls, and money management) (NAC & AARP, 2004 [Level IV]; Walker et al., 1995 [Level I]). Illness-related activities include managing symptoms, coping with illness behaviors, carrying out treatments, and performing medical or nursing procedures that include an array of medical technologies (Smith, 1994 [Level IV]). Care-management activities include accessing resources, communicating with and navigating the health care and social services systems, and acting as an advocate (Schumacher et al., 2000 [Level IV]). Invisible aspects of care are protective actions caregivers take to ensure the older adults' safety and well-being without their knowledge (Bowers, 1987 [Level IV]).
4. Caregiving roles: These can be classified into a hierarchy according to who takes on the majority of responsibilities versus only intermittent supportive assistance. Primary caregivers tend to provide most of the everyday aspects of care, whereas secondary caregivers help out as needed to fill the gaps (Cantor & Little, 1985 [Level V]; Penning, 1990 [Level IV]; Tennstedt et al., 1989 [Level IV]). Among caregivers who live with their care recipients,

spouses account for the majority of primary caregivers, whereas adult children are more likely to be secondary caregivers. The range of the family caregiving role includes protective caregiving such as "keeping an eye on" an older adult who is currently independent but at risk, to full-time, around-the-clock care for a severely impaired family member. Health care providers may fail to assess the full scope of the family caregiving role if they associate family caregiving only with the performance of tasks.

5. Caregiver assessment: This refers to an ongoing iterative process of gathering information that describes a family caregiving situation and identifies the particular issues, needs, resources, and strengths of the family caregiver.

B. Risk factors associated with negative outcomes for caregiving

1. Just being a caregiver puts an individual at increased risk for higher levels of stress and depression and lower levels of subjective well-being and physical health (Pinquart & Sorenson, 2003; Vitaliano et al., 2003 [both Level I]).

2. Female caregivers, on average, provide more direct care and report higher levels of burden and depression (Gitlin et al., 2003 [Level I]).

3. Ethnic minority caregivers provide more care, use less formal services, and report worse physical health than White caregivers (Dilworth-Anderson, et al., 2002 [Level I]; McCann et al., 2000 [Level IV]; Pinquart & Sorenson, 2005 [Level I]).

4. African American caregivers experience less stress and depression and get more rewards from caregiving than White caregivers (Cuellar, 2002 [Level IV]; Dilworth-Anderson et al., 2002 [Level I]; Gitlin et al., 2003 [Level I]; Haley, et al., 2004 [Level II]; Pinquart & Sorenson, 2005 [Level I]).

5. Hispanic and Asian American caregivers exhibit more depression (Gitlin et al., 2003; Pinquart & Sorenson, 2005 [both Level I]).

6. Less-educated caregivers report more depression (Buckwalter et al., 1999 [Level II]; Gitlin et al., 2003 [Level I]).

7. Spouse caregivers report higher levels of depression than non-spouse caregivers (Pinquart & Sorenson, 2005; Pruchno & Resch, 1989 [both Level I]).

8. Caregivers who have a poor-quality relationship with the care recipient report more strain (Archbold, et al., 1990, 1992 [Level II]; Croog, Burleson, Sudilovsky, & Baume, 2006 [Level IV]; Flannery, 2002 [Level VI]).

9. Caregivers who lack preparedness for the caregiving role also increases strain (Archbold, et al., 1990, 1992 [both Level II]).

10. Caregivers of care recipients who have dementia suffer from increased strain (Pinquart & Sorenson, 2006 [Level I]).

IV. PARAMETERS OF ASSESSMENT

A. Caregiving Context:
   1. Caregiver relationship to care recipient (spouse, non-spouse) (Gitlin et al., 2003; Sorensen et al., 2002 [both Level I])
   2. Caregiver roles and responsibilities
      a. Duration of caregiving (Sorensen et al., 2002 [Level I])
      b. Employment status (i.e., work, home, volunteer) (Pinquart & Sorensen, 2006 [Level I])
      c. Household status (e.g., number in home) (Pinquart & Sorensen, 2006 [Level I])
      d. Existence and involvement of extended family and social support (Pinquart & Sorensen, 2006 [Level I])
   3. Physical environment (i.e., home, facility) (Vitaliano et al., 2003 [Level I])
   4. Financial status (Vitaliano et al., 2003 [Level I])
   5. Potential resources that caregiver could choose to use—list (Pinquart & Sorensen, 2006 [Level I])
   6. Family's cultural background (Dilworth-Andersen et al., 2002 [Level I])
B. Caregiver's perception of health and functional status of care recipient:
   1. List activities care receiver needs help with; include both ADLs and IADLs (Pinquart & Sorensen, 2003, 2006 [both Level I]).
   2. Presence of cognitive impairment—if yes, any behavioral problems? (Gitlin et al., 2003 [Level I]; Sorensen et al., 2002 [Level I]).
   3. Presence of mobility problems—assess with single question (Archbold et al., 1990 [Level II]).
C. Caregiver preparedness for caregiving:
   1. Does caregiver have the skills, abilities, knowledge to provide care recipient with needed care? (see Preparedness for Caregiving Scale at www.ConsultGeriRN.org, Family Caregiving topic).
D. Quality of family relationships:
   1. The caregiver's perception of the quality of the relationship with the care receiver (Archbold et al., 1990 [Level II]) (see Mutuality Scale at www.ConsultGeriRN.org, Family Caregiving topic).
E. Indicators of problems with quality of care:
   1. Unhealthy environment
   2. Inappropriate management of finances
   3. Lack of respect for older adult (see Elder Assessment Instrument [EAI]) at http://www.hartfordign.org/publications/trythis/issue15.pdf).
F. Caregiver's physical and mental health status:
   1. Self-rated health: single item—asks what is caregivers' perception of their health (Pinquart & Sorensen, 2006 [Level I]).
   2. Health conditions and symptoms

       a. Depression or other emotional distress (e.g., anxiety) (Pin-quart & Sorensen, 2006, 2003; Sorensen et al., 2002 [all Level I]). (See CES-D in Resources section).

       b. Reports of burden or strain (Schultz & Beach, 1999 [Level II]; Vitaliano et al., 2003 [Level I]). (See Caregiver Strain Index at www.ConsultGeriRN.org, Family Caregiving topic).

    3. Rewards of caregiving:

       a. List of perceived benefits of caregiving (Archbold et al., 1995 [Level II])

       b. Satisfaction of helping family member

       c. Developing new skills and competencies

       d. Improved family relationships

    4. Self-care activities for caregiver

V. NURSING CARE STRATEGIES

A. Identify content and skills needed to increase preparedness for caregiving (Acton & Winter, 2002 [Level I]; Gitlin et al., 2003 [Level I]; Sorensen et al., 2002 [Level I]; Farran et al., 2003 [Level IV]; Farran et al., 2004 [Level II]).

B. Form a partnership with the caregiver prior to generating strategies to address issues and concerns (Brodaty et al., 2003 [Level I]; Gitlin et al., 2003 [Level I]; Harvath et al., 1994 [Level V]).

C. Identify the caregiving issues and concerns on which the caregiver wants to work and generate strategies (Acton & Winter, 2002 [Level I]; Gitlin et al., 2003 [Level I]; Sorensen et al., 2002 [Level I]; several Level II studies [see Table 8.1]).

D. Assist the caregiver in identifying strengths in the caregiving situation (Archbold, et al., 1995 [Level II]).

E. Assist the caregiver in finding and using resources (Archbold et al., 1995 [Level II]; Farran et al., 2004 [Level II]; Schumacher et al., 2002 [Level IV]).

F. Help caregivers identify and manage their physical and emotional responses to caregiving (Schulz & Beach, 1999 [Level II]).

G. Use an interdisciplinary approach when working with family caregivers (Acton & Winter, 2002 [Level I]; Gitlin et al., 2003 [Level I]; Farran et al., 2003 [Level IV]; Farran et al., 2004 [Level II]; Sorensen et al., 2002 [Level I]; several Level II studies [see Table 8.1]).

VI. EVALUATION AND EXPECTED OUTCOMES

A. Outcomes specific to caregiving

    1. Lower caregiver strain

    2. Decreased depression

    3. Improved physical health

B. Outcomes specific to patient
   1. Quality of family caregiving
   2. Care-recipient functional status, nutrition, hygiene, and symptom management
   3. Care-recipient emotional well-being
   4. Decreased occurrence of adverse events such as increased frequency of emergent care

References

Acton, G. J., & Winter, M. A. (2002). Interventions for family members caring for an elder with dementia. *Annual Review of Nursing Research, 20*, 149–179. Evidence Level I: Systematic Review.

Akkerman, R. L., & Ostwald, S. K. (2004). Reducing anxiety in Alzheimer's disease family caregivers: The effectiveness of a nine-week cognitive-behavioral intervention. *American Journal of Alzheimer's Disease and Other Dementias, 19*(2), 117–123. Evidence Level II: Individual Experimental Study.

Altman, B. M., Cooper, P. F., & Cunningham, P. J. (1999). The case of disability in the family: Impact on health care utilization and expenditures for non-disabled members. *Milbank Quarterly, 77*(1), 39–75. Evidence Level IV: Nonexperimental Study.

Archbold, P. G., Stewart, B. J., Greenlick, M. R., & Harvath, T. A. (1990). Mutuality and preparedness as predictors of caregiver role strain. *Research in Nursing & Health, 13*(6), 375–384. Evidence Level II: Individual Experimental Study.

Archbold, P. G., Stewart, B. J., Greenlick, M. R., & Harvath, T. A. (1992). Clinical assessment of mutuality and preparedness in family caregivers to frail older people. In S. G. Funk, E. M. Tornquist, M. T. Champagne, & L. A. Copp (Eds.), *Key aspects of elder care* (pp. 332–337). New York: Springer Publishing Company, Inc. Evidence Level II: Individual Experimental Study.

Archbold, P. G., Stewart, B. J., Miller, L. L., Harvath, T. A., Greenlick, M. R., Van Buren, L., et al. (1995). The PREP system of nursing interventions: A pilot test with families caring for older members—preparedness (PR), enrichment (E), and predictability (P). *Research in Nursing & Health, 18*(1), 3–16. Evidence Level II: Individual Experimental Study.

Arno, P. S. (2006). *Economic value of informal caregiving.* Paper presented at the Care Coordination and the Caregiving Forum, Department of Veterans Affairs, NIH, Bethesda, MD, January 25–27, 2006. Evidence Level IV: Nonexperimental Study.

Bass, D. M., Clark, P. A., Looman, W. J., McCarthy, C. A., & Eckert, S. (2003). The Cleveland Alzheimer's managed-care demonstration: Outcomes after 12 months of implementation. *Gerontologist, 43*(1), 73–85. Evidence Level II: Individual Experimental Study.

Bourgeois, M. S., Schulz, R., Burgio, L. D., & Beach, S. (2002). Skills training for spouses of patients with Alzheimer's disease: Outcomes of an intervention study. *Journal of Clinical Geropsychology, 8*(1), 53–73. Evidence Level II: Individual Experimental Study.

Bowers, B. J. (1987). Intergenerational caregiving: Adult caregivers and their aging parents. *Advances in Nursing Science, 9*(2), 20–31. Evidence Level IV: Nonexperimental Study.

Brodaty, H., Green, A., & Koschera, A. (2003). Meta-analysis of psychosocial interventions for caregivers of people with dementia. *Journal of the American Geriatrics Society, 51*(5), 657–664. Evidence Level I: Systematic Review.

Buckwalter, K. C., Gerdner, L., Kohout, F., Hall, G. R., Kelly, A., Richards, B., et al. (1999). A nursing intervention to decrease depression in family caregivers of persons with dementia. *Archives of Psychiatric Nursing, 13*(2), 80–88. Evidence Level II: Individual Experimental Study.

Burgio, L., Stevens, A., Guy, D., Roth, D. L., & Haley, W. E. (2003). Impact of two psychosocial interventions on White and African American family caregivers of individuals with dementia. *Gerontologist, 43*(4), 568–579. Evidence Level II: Individual Experimental Study.

Burns, A., Guthrie, E., Marino-Francis, F., Busby, C., Morris, J., Russell, E., et al. (2005). Brief psychotherapy in Alzheimer's disease: Randomised controlled trial. *British Journal of Psychiatry, 187*(2), 143–147. Evidence Level II: Individual Experimental Study.

Burns, R., Nichols, L. O., Martindale-Adams, J., Graney, M. J., & Lummus, A. (2003). Primary care interventions for dementia caregivers: 2-year outcomes from the REACH study. *Gerontologist, 43*(4), 547–555. Evidence Level II: Individual Experimental Study.

Burton, C., & Gibbon, B. (2005). Expanding the role of the stroke nurse: A pragmatic clinical trial. *Journal of Advanced Nursing, 52*(6), 640–650. Evidence Level II: Individual Experimental Study.

Butler, L. D., Field, N. P., Busch, A. L., Seplaki, J. E., Hastings, T. A., & Spiegel, D. (2005). Anticipating loss and other temporal stressors predict traumatic stress symptoms among partners of metastatic/recurrent breast cancer patients. *Psycho-Oncology, 14*(6), 492–502. Evidence Level II: Individual Experimental Study.

Callahan, C. M., Boustani, M. A., Unverzagt, F. W., Austrom, M. G., Damush, T. M., Perkins, A. J., et al. (2006). Effectiveness of collaborative care for older adults with Alzheimer's disease in primary care: A randomized controlled trial. *Journal of the American Medical Association, 295*(18), 2148–2157. Evidence Level II: Individual Experimental Study.

Cannuscio, C. C., Jones, C., Kawachi, I., Colditz, G. A., Berkman, L., & Rimm, E. (2002). Reverberation of family illness: A longitudinal assessment of informal caregiver and mental health status in the nurses' health study. *American Journal of Public Health, 92*, 305–311. Evidence Level IV: Nonexperimental Study.

Cantor, M. H., & Little, V. (1985). Aging and social care. In R. H. Binstock & E. Shanas (Eds.), *Handbook of aging and the social sciences* (2nd ed., pp. 745–781). New York: Van Nostrand Reinhold. Evidence Level V: Narrative Literature Review.

Clark, M. M., Rummans, T. A., Sloan, J. A., Jensen, A., Atherton, P. J., & Frost, M. H., et al. (2006). Quality of life of caregivers of patients with advanced-stage cancer. *American Journal of Hospice & Palliative Medicine, 23*(3), 185–191. Evidence Level II: Individual Experimental Study.

Clark, M. S., Rubenach, S., & Winsor, A. (2003). A randomized controlled trial of an education and counseling intervention for families after stroke. *Clinical Rehabilitation, 17*(7), 703–712. Evidence Level II: Individual Experimental Study.

Cooke, D. D., McNally, L., Mulligan, K. T., Harrison, M. J., & Newman, S. P. (2001). Psychosocial interventions for caregivers of people with dementia: A systematic review. *Aging & Mental Health, 5*(2), 120–135. Evidence Level I: Systematic Review.

Coon, D. W., Thompson, L., Steffen, A., Sorocco, K., & Gallagher-Thompson, D. (2003). Anger and depression management: Psychoeducational skill training interventions for women caregivers of a relative with dementia. *Gerontologist, 43*(5), 678–689. Evidence Level II: Individual Experimental Study.

Croog, S. H., Burleson, J. A., Sudilovsky, A., & Baume, R. M. (2006). Spouse caregivers of Alzheimer's patients: Problem responses to caregiver burden. *Aging & Mental Health, 10*(2), 87–100. Evidence Level IV: Nonexperimental Study.

Crotty, M., Whitehead, C. H., Gray, S., & Finucane, P. M. (2002). Early discharge and home rehabilitation after hip fracture achieves functional improvements: A randomized controlled trial. *Clinical Rehabilitation, 16*(4), 406–413. Evidence Level II: Individual Experimental Study.

Crotty, M., Whitehead, C., Miller, M., & Gray, S. (2003). Patient and caregiver outcomes 12 months after home-based therapy for hip fracture: A randomized controlled trial. *Archives of Physical Medicine and Rehabilitation, 84*(8), 1237–1239. Evidence Level II: Individual Experimental Study.

Cuellar, N. G. (2002). Comparison of African American and Caucasian American female caregivers of rural, post-stroke, bedbound older adults. *Journal of Gerontological Nursing 28*, 36–45. Evidence Level IV: Nonexperimental Study.

Dilworth-Anderson, P., Williams, I. C., & Gibson, B. E. (2002). Issues of race, ethnicity, and culture in caregiving research: A 20-year review (1980–2000). *Gerontologist, 42*(2), 237–272. Evidence Level I: Systematic Review.

Eisdorfer, C., Czaja, S. J., Loewenstein, D. A., Rubert, M. P., Arguelles, S., & Mitrani, V. B., et al. (2003). The effect of a family-therapy and technology-based intervention on caregiver depression. *Gerontologist, 43*(4), 521–531. Evidence Level II: Individual Experimental Study.

Family Caregiver Alliance (2006). *Caregiver assessment: Principles, guidelines and strategies for change. Report from a national consensus development conference. Volume I*. San Francisco: Family Caregiver Alliance.. Evidence Level VI: Expert Opinion.

Farran, C. J., Gilley, D. W., McCann, J. J., Bienias, J. L., Lindeman, D. A., Evans, D. A. (2004). Psychosocial interventions to reduce depressive symptoms of dementia caregivers: A randomized clinical trial comparing two approaches. *Journal of Mental Health and Aging, 10*(4), 337–350. Evidence Level II: Individual Experimental Study.

Farran, C. J., Loukissa, D., Perraud, S., & Paun, O. (2003). Alzheimer's disease caregiving information and skills, Part I: Care recipient issues and concerns. *Research in Nursing & Health, 26*(5), 366–375. Evidence Level IV: Nonexperimental Study.

Flannery, R. B. J. (2002). Disrupted caring attachments: Implications for long-term care. *American Journal of Alzheimer's Disease and Other Dementias, 17*(4), 227–231. Evidence Level VI: Expert Opinion.

Forster, A., Smith, J., Young, J., Knapp, P., House, A., & Wright, J. (2006). Information provision for stroke patients and their caregivers. *The Cochrane Library, 1*. Evidence Level I: Systematic Review.

Fulmer, T. (May 2002). Elder abuse and neglect assessment. Try this: Best practices in nursing care to older adults, *15*(2). Retrieved February, 8, 2007, from The Hartford Institute for Geriatric Nursing, College of Nursing, New York University Web site: www.ConsultGeriRN. org/publications/trythis/issue15.pdf. Evidence Level VI: Expert Opinion.

Fulmer, T., Paveza, G., Abraham, I., & Fairchild, S. (2000). Elder neglect assessment in the emergency department. *Journal of Emergency Nursing, 26*(5), 436–443. Evidence Level II: Individual Experimental Study.

Fulmer, T., Street, S., & Carr, K. (1984). Abuse of the elderly: Screening and detection. *Journal of Emergency Nursing, 10*(3), 131–140. Evidence Level II: Individual Experimental Study.

Fulmer, T., & Wetle, T. (1986). Elder abuse screening and intervention. *Nurse Practitioner, 11*(5), 33–38. Evidence Level II: Individual Experimental Study.

Gallagher-Thompson, D., Coon, D. W., Solano, N., Ambler, C., Rabinowitz, Y., & Thompson, L. W. (2003). Changes in indices of distress among Latino and Anglo female caregivers of elderly relatives with dementia: Site-specific results from the REACH national collaborative study. *Gerontologist, 43*(4), 580–591. Evidence Level II: Individual Experimental Study.

Gitlin, L. N., Belle, S. H., Burgio, L. D., Czaja, S. J., Mahoney, D., Gallagher-Thompson, D., et al. (2003). Effect of multicomponent interventions on caregiver burden and depression: The REACH multisite initiative at 6-month follow-up. *Psychology & Aging, 18*(3), 361–374. Evidence Level I: Systematic Review.

Gitlin, L. N., Corcoran, M., Winter, L., Boyce, A., & Hauck, W. W. (2001). A randomized controlled trial of a home environmental intervention: Effect on efficacy and upset in caregivers and on daily function of persons with dementia. *Gerontologist, 41*(1), 4–14. Evidence Level II: Individual Experimental Study.

Gitlin, L. N., Hauck, W. W., Dennis, M. P., & Winter, L. (2005). Maintenance of effects of the home environmental skill-building program for family caregivers and individuals with Alzheimer's disease and related disorders. *Journals of Gerontology: Series A: Biological Sciences and Medical Sciences, 60A*(3), 368–374. Evidence Level II: Individual Experimental Study.

Grande, G. E., Farquhar, M. C., Barclay, S. I. G., & Todd, C. J. (2004). Caregiver bereavement outcome: Relationship with hospice at home, satisfaction with care, and home death. *Journal of Palliative Care, 20*(2), 69–77. Evidence Level II: Individual Experimental Study.

Grasel, E., Biehler, J., Schmidt, R., & Schupp, W. (2005). Intensification of the transition between inpatient neurological rehabilitation and home care of stroke patients: Controlled clinical trial with follow-up assessment six months after discharge. *Clinical Rehabilitation, 19*(7), 725–736. Evidence Level III: Quasi-experimental Study.

Haley, W. E., Gitlin, L. N., Wisniewski, S. R., Mahoney, D. F., Cood, D. W., Winter, L., et al. (2004). Well-being, appraisal, and coping in African American and Caucasian dementia caregivers: Findings from the REACH study. *Aging and Mental Health, 8*, 316–329. Evidence Level II: Individual Experimental Study.

Harris, R., Ashton, T., Broad, J., Connolly, G., & Richmond, D. (2005). The effectiveness, acceptability and costs of a hospital-at-home service compared with acute hospital care: A randomized controlled trial. *Journal of Health Services Research and Policy, 10*(3), 158–166. Evidence Level II: Individual Experimental Study.

Harvath, T. A., Archbold, P. G., Stewart, B. J., Gadow, S., Kirschling, J. M., Miller, L., et al. (1994). Establishing partnerships with family caregivers: Local and cosmopolitan knowledge. *Journal of Gerontological Nursing, 20*(2), 29–35, 42–43. Evidence Level V: Narrative Literature Review.

Hebert, R., Levesque, L., Vezina, J., Lavoie, J., Ducharme, F., & Gendron, C., et al. (2003). Efficacy of a psychoeducative group program for caregivers of demented persons living at home: A randomized controlled trial. *Journals of Gerontology Series B: Psychological Sciences and Social Sciences, 58B*(1), S58–S67. Evidence Level II: Individual Experimental Study.

Hepburn, K. W., Lewis, M., Narayan, S., Center, B., Tornatore, J., & Bremer, K. L., et al. (2005). Partners in caregiving: A psychoeducation program affecting dementia family caregivers' distress and caregiving outlook. *Clinical Gerontologist, 29*(1), 53–69. Evidence Level II: Individual Experimental Study.

Hepburn, K. W., Tornatore, J., Center, B., & Ostwald, S. W. (2001). Dementia family caregiver training: Affecting beliefs about caregiving and caregiver outcomes. *Journal of the American Geriatrics Society, 49*(4), 450–457. Evidence Level II: Individual Experimental Study.

Horton-Deutsch, S. L., Farran, C. J., Choi, E. E., & Fogg, L. (2002). The PLUS intervention: A pilot test with caregivers of depressed older adults. *Archives of Psychiatric Nursing, 16*(2), 61–71. Evidence Level III: Quasi-experimental Study.

Hudson, P. L., Aranda, S., & Hayman-White, K. (2005). A psychoeducational intervention for family caregivers of patients receiving palliative care: A randomized controlled trial. *Journal of Pain and Symptom Management, 30*(4), 329–341. Evidence Level II: Individual Experimental Study.

Kalra, L., Evans, A., Perez, I., Melbourn, A., Patel, A., & Knapp, M., et al. (2004). Training caregivers of stroke patients: Randomised controlled trial. *British Medical Journal, 328*(7448), 1099–1101. Evidence Level II: Individual Experimental Study.

Kiecolt-Glaser, J. K., & Glaser, R. (2003). *Chronic stress and age-related increases in the proinflammatory cytokine IL-6.* Proceedings of the National Academy of Sciences, June 30, 2003. Evidence Level III: Quasi-experimental Study.

King, A. C., Baumann, K., O'Sullivan, P., Wilcox, S., & Castro, C. (2002). Effects of moderate-intensity exercise on physiological, behavioral, and emotional responses to family caregiving: A randomized controlled trial. *Journals of Gerontology. Series A: Biological Sciences and Medical Sciences, 57A*(1), M26–M36. Evidence Level II: Individual Experimental Study.

Knight, B. G., Lutzky, S. M., & Macofsky-Urban, F. (1993). A meta-analytic review of interventions for caregiver distress: Recommendations for future research. *Gerontologist, 33*(2), 240–248. Evidence Level I: Systematic Review.

Kozachik, S. L., Given, C. W., Given, B. A., Pierce, S. J., Azzouz, F., & Rawl, S. M., et al. (2001). Improving depressive symptoms among caregivers of patients with cancer: Results of a randomized clinical trial. *Oncology Nursing Forum, 28*(7), 1149–1157. Evidence Level II: Individual Experimental Study.

Kurtz, M. E., Kurtz, J. C., Given, C. W., & Given, B. (2005). A randomized controlled trial of a patient/caregiver symptom control intervention: Effects on depressive symptomatology of caregivers of cancer patients. *Journal of Pain and Symptom Management, 30*(2), 112–122. Evidence Level II: Individual Experimental Study.

Langhorne, P., Dennis, M. S., Kalra, L., Shepperd, S., Wade, D. T., & Wolfe, C. D. A. (2006). Services for helping acute stroke patients avoid hospital admission. *The Cochrane Library, 1.* Evidence Level I: Systematic Review.

Larson, J., Franzen-Dahlin, A., Billing, E., von Arbin, M., Murray, V., & Wredling, R. (2005). The impact of a nurse-led support and education programme for spouses of stroke patients: A randomized controlled trial. *Journal of Clinical Nursing, 14*(8), 995–1003. Evidence Level II: Individual Experimental Study.

Lee, H., & Cameron, M. (2004). Respite care for people with dementia and their carers. *Cochrane Database of Systematic Reviews, 2,* 004396. Evidence Level I: Systematic Review.

Li, H., Melnyk, B. M., McCann, R., Chatcheydang, J., Koulouglioti, C., & Nichols, L. W., et al. (2003). Creating Avenues for Relative Empowerment (CARE): A pilot test of an intervention to improve outcomes of hospitalized elders and family caregivers. *Research in Nursing & Health, 26*(4), 284–299. Evidence Level I: Systematic Review.

Lingler, J. H., Martire, L. M., & Schulz, R. (2005). Caregiver-specific outcomes in anti-dementia clinical drug trials: A systematic review and meta-analysis. *Journal of the American Geriatrics Society, 53*(6), 983–990. Evidence Level I: Systematic Review.

Livingston, G., Johnston, K., Katona, C., Paton, J., Lyketsos, C. G., & World Federation of Biological Psychiatry; Old Age Task Force (2005). Systematic review of psychological approaches to the management of neuropsychiatric symptoms of dementia. *American Journal of Psychiatry, 162*(11), 1996–2021. Evidence Level I: Systematic Review.

Mahoney, D. F., Cloutterbuck, J., Neary, S., & Zhan, L. (2005). African American, Chinese, and Latino family caregivers' impressions of the onset and diagnosis of dementia: Cross-cultural similarities and differences. *Gerontologist, 45*(6), 783–792. Evidence Level I: Systematic Review.

Mahoney, D. F., Tarlow, B. J., & Jones, R. N. (2003). Effects of an automated telephone support system on caregiver burden and anxiety: Findings from the REACH for TLC intervention study. *Gerontologist, 43*(4), 556–567. Evidence Level II: Individual Experimental Study.

Mahoney, R., Regan, C., Katona, C., & Livingston, G. (2005). Anxiety and depression in family caregivers of people with Alzheimer's disease: The LASER-AD study. *American Journal of Geriatric Psychiatry, 13*(9), 795–801. Evidence Level IV: Nonexperimental Study.

Martin-Cook, K., Davis, B. A., Hynan, L. S., & Weiner, M. F. (2005). A randomized controlled study of an Alzheimer's caregiver skills training program. *American Journal of Alzheimer's Disease and Other Dementias, 20*(4), 204–210. Evidence Level II: Individual Experimental Study.

Martire, L. M., Schulz, R., Keefe, F. J., Starz, T. W., Osial, T. A., Dew, M. A., et al. (2003). Feasibility of a dyadic intervention for management of osteoarthritis: A pilot study with older patients and their spousal caregivers. *Aging & Mental Health, 7*(1), 53–60. Evidence Level II: Individual Experimental Study.

McCann, J. J., Hebert, L. E., Beckett, L. A., Morris, M. C., Scherr, P. A., & Evans, D. A. (2000). Comparison of informal caregiving by Black and White older adults in a community population. *Journal of the American Geriatrics Society, 48*, 1612–1617. Evidence Level IV: Nonexperimental Study.

Mittelman, M. S., Roth, D. L., Coon, D. W., & Haley, W. E. (2004). Sustained benefit of supportive intervention for depressive symptoms in caregivers of patients with Alzheimer's disease. *American Journal of Psychiatry, 161*(5), 850–856. Evidence Level II: Individual Experimental Study.

Mittelman, M. S., Roth, D. L., Haley, W. E., & Zarit, S. H. (2004). Effects of a caregiver intervention on negative caregiver appraisals of behavior problems in patients with Alzheimer's disease: Results of a randomized trial. *Journals of Gerontology, Series B: Psychological Sciences and Social Sciences, 59B*(1), P27–P34. Evidence Level II: Individual Experimental Study.

National Academy on an Aging Society (2000). *Caregiving: Helping the elderly with activity limitations—Challenges for the 21st century: Chronic and disabling conditions, No. 7.* Washington, DC. Evidence Level V: Narrative Literature Review.

National Alliance for Caregiving (NAC) and American Association for Retired Persons (AARP) (2004). *Caregiving in the U.S.* Bethesda and Washington, DC. Evidence Level IV: Nonexperimental Study.

Nolan, M. (2001). Working with family carers: Towards a partnership approach. *Reviews in Clinical Gerontology, 11*(1), 91–97. Evidence Level V: Narrative Literature Review.

Northouse, L., Kershaw, T., Mood, D., & Schafenacker, A. (2005). Effects of a family intervention on the quality of life of women with recurrent breast cancer and their family caregivers. *Psycho-Oncology, 14*(6), 478–491. Evidence Level II: Individual Experimental Study.

Opinion Research Corporation (OPC) (2005). *Attitudes and beliefs about caregiving in the U.S.: Findings of a national opinion survey.* Opinion Research Corporation. Evidence Level IV: Nonexperimental Study.

Ostaszkiewicz, J., Johnston, L., & Roe, B. (2004). Habit retraining for the management of urinary incontinence in adults. *Cochrane Database of Systematic Reviews*, Issue 2. Art. No.: CD002801. DOI: 10.1002/14651858.CD002801.pub2. Evidence Level I: Systematic Review.

Penning, M. J. (1990). Receipt of assistance by elderly people: Hierarchical selection and task specificity. *Gerontologist, 30*, 220–227. Evidence Level IV: Nonexperimental Study.

Pinquart, M., & Sorensen, S. (2003). Differences between caregivers and noncaregivers in psychological health and physical health: A meta-analysis. *Psychology & Aging, 18*(2), 250–267. Evidence Level I: Systematic Review.

Pinquart, M., & Sorensen, S. (2004). Associations of caregiver stressors and uplifts with subjective well-being and depressive mood: A meta-analytic comparison. *Aging & Mental Health, 8*(5), 438–449. Evidence Level I: Systematic Review.

Pinquart, M., & Sorenson, S. (2005). Ethnic differences in stressors, resources, and psychological outcomes of family caregiving: A meta-analysis. *Gerontologist, 45,* 90–106. Evidence Level I: Systematic Review.

Pinquart, M., & Sorensen, S. (2006). Gender differences in caregiver stressors, social resources, and health: An updated meta-analysis. *Journals of Gerontology, Series B: Psychological Sciences and Social Sciences, 61B*(1), P33–P45. Evidence Level I: Systematic Review.

Price, J. D., Hermans, D. G., Grimley, E, J. (2006). Subjective barriers to prevent wandering of cognitively impaired people. *Cochrane Database of Systematic Reviews,* Issue 1. Art. No.: CD001932. DOI: 10.1002/14651858.CD001932. Evidence Level I: Systematic Review.

Pruchno, R. A., & Resch, N. L. (1989). Mental health of caregiving spouses: Coping as mediator, moderator, or main effect? *Psychology & Aging, 4,* 454–463. Evidence Level I: Systematic Review.

Pusey, H., & Richards, D. (2001). A systematic review of the effectiveness of psychosocial interventions for carers of people with dementia. *Aging & Mental Health, 5*(2), 107–119. Evidence Level I: Systematic Review.

Radloff, L. (1977). The CES-D scale: A self-report depression scale for research in the general population. *Applied Psychological Measurement 1*(3), 385–401. Evidence Level II: Individual Experimental Study.

Radloff, L. S., & Teri, L. (1986). Use of the CES-D with older adults. Clinical *Gerontologist, 5,* 119–136. Evidence Level II: Individual Experimental Study.

Schulz, R., & Beach, S. R. (1999). Caregiving as a risk factor for mortality: The caregiver health effects study. *Journal of the American Medical Association, 282*(23), 2215–2219. Evidence Level II: Individual Experimental Study.

Schulz, R., Burgio, L., Burns, R., Eisdorfer, C., Gallagher-Thompson, D., Gitlin, L. N., et al. (2003). Resources for Enhancing Alzheimer's Caregiver Health (REACH): Overview, site-specific outcomes, and future directions. *Gerontologist, 43*(4), 514–520. Evidence Level V: Narrative Literature Review.

Schulz, R., Martire, L. M., & Klinger, J. N. (2005). Evidence-based caregiver interventions in geriatric psychiatry. *Psychiatric Clinics of North America, 28*(4), 1007–1038. Evidence Level I: Systematic Review.

Schumacher, K. L., Beck, C. A., & Marren, J. M. (2006). *American Journal of Nursing, 106*(8), 40–49. Evidence Level VI: Expert Opinion.

Schumacher, K. L., Koresawa, S., West, C., Hawkins, C., Johnson, C., & Wais, E., et al. (2002). Putting cancer pain management regimens into practice at home. *Journal of Pain and Symptom Management, 23*(5), 369–382. Evidence Level IV: Nonexperimental Study.

Schumacher, K. L., Stewart, B. J., Archbold, P. G., Dodd, M. J., & Dibble, S. L. (2000). Family caregiving skill: Development of the concept. *Research in Nursing & Health, 23*(3), 191–203. Evidence Level IV: Nonexperimental Study.

Secker, D. L., & Brown, R. G. (2005). Cognitive behavioural therapy (CBT) for carers of patients with Parkinson's disease: A preliminary randomised controlled trial. *Journal of Neurology, Neurosurgery and Psychiatry, 76*(4), 491–497. Evidence Level II: Individual Experimental Study.

Shelton, P., Schraeder, C., Dworak, D., Fraser, C., & Sager, M.A. (2001). Caregivers' utilization of health services: Results from the Medicare Alzheimer's disease demonstration, Illinois site. *Journal of the American Geriatrics Society, 49*(12), 1600–1605. Evidence Level II: Individual Experimental Study.

Smith, C. E. (1994). A model of caregiving effectiveness for technologically dependent adults residing at home. *Advances in Nursing Science, 17*(2), 27–40. Evidence Level IV: Nonexperimental Study.

Smith, J., Forster, A., & Young, J. (2004). A randomized trial to evaluate an education programme for patients and carers after stroke. *Clinical Rehabilitation, 18*(7), 726–736. Evidence Level II: Individual Experimental Study.

Sorensen, S., Pinquart, M., & Duberstein, P. (2002). How effective are interventions with caregivers? An updated meta-analysis. *Gerontologist, 42*(3), 356–372. Evidence Level I: Systematic Review.

Stewart, B. J., Archbold, P., Harvath, T., & Nkongho, N. (1993). Role acquisition in family care-givers of older people who have been discharged from the hospital. In S. G. Funk, et al. (Eds.), *Key aspects of caring for the chronically ill: Hospital and home* (pp. 219–230). New York: Springer Publishing Company. Evidence Level IV: Nonexperimental Study.

Sullivan, M. T. (2002). Caregiver Strain Index (CSI). Try this: Best practices in nursing care to older adults: Issue #14. Retrieved February 8, 2007, from The Hartford Institute for Geri-atric Nursing, College of Nursing, New York University Web site: http://www.hartfordign.org/publications/trythis/issue14.pdf. Evidence Level II: Individual Experimental Study.

Teng, J., Mayo, N. E., Latimer, E., Hanley, J., Wood-Dauphinee, S., Cote, R., et al. (2003). Costs and caregiver consequences of early supported discharge for stroke patients. *Stroke, 34*(2), 528–536. Evidence Level II: Individual Experimental Study.

Tennstedt, S. L., McKinlay, J. B., & Sullivan, L. M. (1989). Informal care for frail elders: The role of secondary caregivers. *Gerontologist, 29*(5), 677–683. Evidence Level IV: Nonexperimental Study.

Tolson, D., Swan, I., & Knussen, C. (2002). Hearing disability: A source of distress for older peo-ple and carers. *British Journal of Nursing, 11*(15), 1021–1025. Evidence Level II: Individual Experimental Study.

Toseland, R. W., & Rossiter, C. M. (1989). Group interventions to support family caregivers: A review and analysis. *Gerontologist, 29*(4), 438–448. Evidence Level I: Systematic Review.

Trend, P., Kaye, J., Gage, H., Owen, C., & Wade, D. (2002). Short-term effectiveness of inten-sive multidisciplinary rehabilitation for people with Parkinson's disease and their carers. *Clinical Rehabilitation, 16*(7), 717–725. Evidence Level III: Quasi-experimental Study.

U.S. Department of Health and Human Services (USDHHS). (1998). *Informal caregiving: Com-passion in action*. Washington, DC. Evidence Level IV: Nonexperimental Study.

Vitaliano, P. P., Zhang, J., & Scanlan, J. M. (2003). Is caregiving "hazardous to one's physical health"? A meta-analysis. *Psychological Bulletin, 129*, 946–997. Evidence Level I: System-atic Review.

Wade, D. T., Gage, H., Owen, C., Trend, P., Grossmith, C., & Kaye, J. (2003). Multidisciplinary rehabilitation for people with Parkinson's disease: A randomised controlled study. *Journal of Neurology, Neurosurgery and Psychiatry, 74*(2), 158–162. Evidence Level II: Individual Experimental Study.

Waelde, L. C., Thompson, L., & Gallagher-Thompson, D. (2004). A pilot study of a yoga and meditation intervention for dementia caregiver stress. *Journal of Clinical Psychology, 60*(6), 677–687. Evidence Level III: Quasi-experimental Study.

Walker, A., Pratt, C. C., & Eddy, L. (1995). Informal caregiving to aging family members: A critical review. *Family Relations, 44*, 404–411. Evidence Level I: Systematic Review.

Weiss, C. O., Gonzalez, H. M., Kabeto, M. U., & Langa, K. M. (2005). Differences in amount of informal care received by non-Hispanic Whites and Latinos in a nationally representative sample of older Americans. *Journal of the American Geriatric Society, 53*, 146–151. Evidence Level IV: Nonexperimental Study.

Wells, N., Hepworth, J. T., Murphy, B. A., Wujcik, D., & Johnson, R. (2003). Improving cancer pain management through patient and family education. *Journal of Pain and Symptom Management, 25*(4), 344–356. Evidence Level II: Individual Experimental Study.

Wisniewski, S. R., Belle, S. H., Coon, D. W., Marcus, S. M., Ory, M. G., Burgio, L. D., et al. (2003). The Resources for Enhancing Alzheimer's Caregiver Health (REACH): Project design and baseline characteristics. *Psychology and Aging, 18*(3), 375–384. Evidence Level II: Individ-ual Experimental Study.

Wolf, J. L., & Kasper, J. D. (2006). Caregivers of frail elders: Updating a national profile. *Geron-tologist, 46*, 344–356. Evidence Level I: Systematic Review.

Wright, L. K., Litaker, M., Laraia, M. T., & DeAndrade, S. (2001). Continuum of care for Alzheimer's disease: A nurse education and counseling program. *Issues in Mental Health Nursing, 22*(3), 231–252. Evidence Level II: Individual Experimental Study.

Yee, J. L., & Schulz, R. (2000). Gender differences in psychiatric morbidity among family care-givers: A review and analysis. *The Gerontologist, 40*, 147–164. Evidence Level I: Systematic Review.

Yin, T., Zhou, Q., & Bashford, C. (2002, May–June). Burden on family members: Caring for frail elderly–A meta-analysis of interventions. *Nursing Research, 51*(3), 199–208. Evidence Level I: Systematic Review.

Preventing Falls in Acute Care

9

Deanna Gray-Miceli

Educational Objectives

At the completion of this chapter, the reader should be able to:

1. gain knowledge about the consequences of falls among older adults

2. identify factors contributing to risk for falls and serious injury and utilize this knowledge to further direct nursing plans of care for the primary prevention of falls

3. understand the etiological basis for falls among older adults, particularly those who are hospitalized

4. utilize findings from a comprehensive post-fall assessment to develop an individualized plan of nursing care for the secondary prevention of recurrent falls

5. identify accepted "general safety measures" to prevent falls from occurring and to provide a safe environment for hospitalized older adult patients

Overview

Spurred by the rising incidence of patient falls in health care organizations across the United States (e.g., fall-related sentinel events rose from 3% in 2002 to more than 5% in 2006), the Joint Commission on Accreditation of Healthcare Organizations (JCAHO) has sanctioned National Patient Safety Goals (NPSG) for all JCAHO-approved institutions across the health care continuum. Two specific aims of this new health policy in acute care institutions are (1) to reduce risk of injury from falls including fatal falls, and (2) to provide a program to prevent patient falls. Both aims seek to promote improvements in patient safety

For a description of Evidence Levels cited in this chapter, see chapter 1, Developing and Evaluating Clinical Practice Guidelines, page 4

by reducing preventable falls through systemwide solutions whenever possible (JCAHO, 2006 [Level VI]).

Overall, across *all* patient settings, evidence exists that fall-prevention programs are effective. The RAND report cites, from a meta-analysis of 20 randomized clinical trials (among all patient settings), that fall-prevention programs reduced either the number of older adults who fell or the monthly rate of falling (U.S. Department of Health and Human Services, 2004 [Level I]). In hospital settings, however, studies are lacking and sorely needed to provide solid scientific evidence of the effect of fall-prevention programs on fall rates among older adult patients.

Current literature of hospital-based fall-prevention programs and their effect on fall prevention is predominantly descriptive, often void of evidence relating to intervention effectiveness. Conclusions drawn from two systematic reviews during a 7-year period of published hospital fall-prevention programs, showed no significant benefit from individual components of the interventions (i.e., the pooled effect of 25% reduction in fall rate), potentially attributable to methodological design issues (Oliver, Hopper, & Seed, 2000 [Level I]). In a few hospital-based studies, some evidence exists that multi-faceted interventions reduce the number of falls (Oliver, Daly, Martin, & McMurdo, 2004 [Level I]). For example, a multipronged approach of education, intervention, and exercise reduced falls by 30% and had less injury outcomes observed among patients (Haines, Bennell, Osborne, & Hill, 2004 [Level II]). Although relatively few studies focus on interventions to prevent falls in hospitalized-based older adult populations, the state of the science supports its use. Findings from a large meta-analysis support multifactorial interventions for fall prevention in the elderly (Chang et al., 2004 [Level I]).

The call for national improvements in patient safety and fall prevention warrant further development and testing of approaches actually used in practice. Despite fall-prevention program variability (according to available resources), organizational and staff commitment, and fall program/intervention type, two factors are consistent: (1) *nurses* are central to any mission of patient safety, fall prevention, and injury reduction; and (2) *nurses who* utilize evidenced-based interventions and sound clinical judgment to prevent patient falls in hospital settings are likely to be successful.

Nursing: A Quintessential Component to Preventing Patient Falls

Although promoting a culture of safety is everyone's shared responsibility in health care organizations, nurses are essential core members and team leaders for any salient commitment to reduce patient falls at the bedside, on the unit, or anywhere in the health care encounter (e.g., in the operating room or outpatient clinic).

Markers of quality fall-prevention and -management programs in hospital settings call for adherence to the same principles that guide the delivery of quality health care for older adult patients in any other setting: coordinated, communicated, and continuous patient-centered care (Resnick, 2003 [Level VI]). Nurses provide individualized patient assessment and reassessment, manage environmental-control issues on the unit, and develop and implement comprehensive plans of care for fall assessment and management that range from early detection of those at risk to continually monitoring for fall-related problems post-fall.

Although we typically think of fall prevention as exclusive to the patient, fall-prevention activities assumed by nurses also extend to family caregivers of older patients planning discharge to the home. When professional nurses are at the helm of decision-making, policy and practice benefit. In daily practice, the nurse's primary commitment is to the recipient of nursing and health care services whether the recipient is an individual, family, group, or community (American Nurses Association, 2002 [Level VI]).

Effective Fall-Prevention Programs

Models of Effective Programs Used by Nurses

Best practice exemplars of effective, successful fall-prevention programs exist within several models of care of hospitalized elderly and incorporate an interdisciplinary team with a strong geriatric nurse-centered approach. Models of care, serving as exemplars of the geriatric nurse-centered approach, realize improvements in hospital lengths of stay and health outcomes as well as fewer iatrogenic geriatric syndromes, such as inpatient falls. These models of care include Acute Care of the Elderly (ACE) Units, Nursing Improving Care for Health System Elders (NICHE) program, and the Geriatric Resource Nurse (GRN) model. ACE units provide geriatric interdisciplinary models of care and physically supportive environments that focus on the unique needs of older adults during hospitalization and report higher patient, family, and staff satisfaction compared to control units (Counsell et al., 2000 [Level II]). (See Resources for more information on ACE units.)

NICHE is a national geriatric nursing program currently implemented in more than 200 hospitals in more than 40 states as well as parts of Canada and The Netherlands. Since 1996, The Hartford Institute has administered NICHE, a national program aimed at improving systems to achieve positive outcomes for hospitalized older adults. The focus of NICHE is on programs and protocols that are predominantly under the control of nursing practice; in other words, areas where nursing interventions have a substantive and positive impact on patient care of older adults. Through NICHE, evidence-based geriatric best practices are facilitated into hospital care.

Evidenced-based research of three different types of models of care that incorporated a geriatric nurse practitioner found that when the geriatric nurse practitioner and nurse manager addressed the issue of falls risk with an educational program for the staff, the fall rate decreased by 5.8% (Smyth, Dubin, Restrepo, Nueva-Espana, & Capezuti, 2001 [Level IV]).

Essential Components of Effective Fall-Prevention Programs

Expert agreement concludes that an effective response by health care organizations and professionals to prevent and reduce falls and associated injuries include a structured program of three important components: (1) fall risk assessment along with individually designed action-based interventions, (2) post-fall assessment and appropriate data collection, and (3) use of fall-reduction tools (ECRI Institute, 2006 [Level VI]). All of these fundamental programmatic components are carried out by nurses and are included in nursing policy and practice. Fall prevention (both primary and secondary) implemented by nurses follows the nursing assessment process, which allows for multiple and continual types of assessment, reassessment, and evaluation following a fall or intervention to prevent a fall. It is a dynamic process with a continuous feedback loop. Throughout the nursing process, there are discrete points for nursing assessment to be performed including (1) health assessment of the older adult patient "at risk" (fall risk assessment); (2) nursing assessment of the patient following a fall (post-fall assessment); (3) assessment of the environment, equipment, and other situational fall circumstances upon admission and during hospitalization; and (4) assessment of the older adult's knowledge of falls and their prevention, including willingness to change behavior, if necessary, to prevent falls.

There are many assessment tools available for use by nurses who perform fall risk assessment. In the acute care setting, these tools have been summarized in an analytic review by Perell and colleagues (2001 [Level V]). The nursing assessment of the older adult patient who falls does not stop with administration of these assessment tools or other types of assessment. Rather, the nursing assessment is a process, which extends to formulate an analysis of the information and situational context of the patient so that corrective plans of action can unfold.

Inherent in any fundamental fall-prevention program is current knowledge of fall etiology, its assessment and prevention strategies. To prevent falls among older adult patients in acute care, professional nurses must have an informed awareness of (1) what constitutes a fall, (2) why falls are so important to prevent in the acute care setting, (3) which older adult patient is at greatest risk to fall and/or develop serious injury, (4) why older adult patients in an acute care setting fall, (5) what can be done to prevent the older adult patient from falling, and (6) what should be done once a patient has fallen. This chapter outlines an overview of the approach to fall assessment and prevention when each of these questions is asked and answered.

Background and Statement of the Problem

Defining Falls

There are several operational definitions of a fall, each utilized for either administrative, research, or clinical purposes. The first consensus opinion–definition of falling is an "unintentional coming to the ground or some lower level *and other than* as a consequence of sustaining a violent blow, loss of consciousness, sudden onset of paralysis as in stroke, or epileptic seizure" (Kellogg International Working Group on Fall Prevention in the Elderly, 1987 [Level VI]). This definition is more consistent to the epidemiological definitions used in public health tabulating falls as intentional or unintentional events (Centers for Disease Control and Prevention [CDC], National Center for Injury Prevention and Control [NCIPC], 2007 [Level VI]). The Kellogg definition stipulates outcome but does not acknowledge potential antecedents or mechanisms of occurrence—for example, not from the identified medical problems. This definition is contrasted to clinical observations and diagnostic coding in practice—for instance, "syncopal-type falls or falls due to syncope" (International Classification of Disease Manual ICD-10, 2006 [Level VI]).

The strongest level of research evidence shows that falls in older adults are due to multifactorial clinical causes (Chang et al., 2004 [Level I]), as reflected in the Prevention of Falls Network Europe (ProFaNE) consensus definition that falls occurring from all causes is "an unexpected event in which the participant comes to rest on the ground, floor or lower level" (ProFaNE, 2006 [Level VI]).

The regulatory definition for the hospital setting, proposed by the Centers for Medicare and Medicaid Services (CMS), considers whether or not falls are witnessed and whether the person was lowered to the ground with assistance. In all practice settings, falls can occur while walking or during a transition from bed, chair, stretcher, or toilet. They may be witnessed or unwitnessed (i.e., where the patient is found on the floor or self-reported by the patient, visitor, or family member). Specific to the acute care facility and to nursing, falls are tabulated according to the National Database of Nursing Quality Indicators (NDNQI), which provides reference points of comparison to measure program effectiveness. Using the NDNQI fall definitions, any unplanned descent to the floor with or without injury to the patient is a fall, and any staff assistance of the patient to the floor is considered an assisted fall (NDNQI, 2005 [Level VI]). Referral to the hospital policy and procedure manual for the facility-specific definition of a fall is recommended for comparison.

Why Falls Are Important in Acute Care

Many of the known negative health care outcomes from falls, such as injury and/or functional decline, typically strike those patients older than age 85 *and* are typically preventable. Overall, state departments of health, which analyze patient safety data, have reported to JCAHO that up to 30% of adverse medical events are due to avoidable patient falls.

The most serious outcome of a fall concerning the older adult, the health care provider, and the organizational system is a *fatality due to a fall*. Although the exact fatal-fall incidence in the in-patient setting is not known, the most approximate estimate is reported through the Patient Safety Reporting System, adopted in several states in the United States. Because true point incidences on in-patient fatal falls are not aggregated from individual states, we rely on global fatal-fall incidences from all settings in the CDC's NCIPC analysis. The CDC's most recent report of fatalities from falls among older adults in the United States during a 10-year period (1993–2003) shows a 55% increase in fatal falls (CDC, Morbidity and Mortality Weekly Report [MMWR], 2006 [Level VI]). Although the most current national incidences of fatal falls are under-represented (due to limitations in cause of death certificate-coding limitations) each year, falls result in more than 14,000 fatalities among seniors, ranking as the seventh leading cause of unintentional injury–fatality (CDC, NCIPC, 2007 [Level VI]). The fatal-fall incidence increases with age, those older than age 85 being the most vulnerable. In 2002, there were 1,208 deaths per 100,000 due to falls for all sexes and races among those 70 to 74 years, more than 2,000 deaths for those 75 to 79 years, and more than 5,999 deaths for those 85 and older. In 2001, more than 1.6 million older adults were treated in emergency departments for fall-related injuries and nearly 388,000 were hospitalized (Runyan et al., 2005 [Level V]). About 30% to 40% of emergency room visits resulted in hospitalization with an average length of stay of 8 to 15 days at an average cost of $10,000 to $12,000 per stay. Hospital in-patient falls are estimated to vary according to the unit, with one study reporting 3.1 falls per 1,000 patient-days (Fischer et al., 2005 [Level IV]). In this study, bleeding or laceration occurred in 53.6%, fracture or dislocation in 15.9%, and hematoma or contusion in 13%. Patients older than age 75 and those in geriatric psychiatric units were more likely to develop serious fall-related injury. Other serious injuries documented from falls included hip fracture and traumatic brain injury (TBI), among others.

The actual incidence of falls with serious injury, such as hip fracture, in the acute care hospital are nationally tabulated through external injury codes and then reported in the National Hospital Discharge Survey (NHDS) data bank and the Patient Safety Indicator at the Agency for Healthcare Research and Quality (AHRQ) (see Resources for further information). The CDC's analysis of the NHDS shows a decrease in the overall age-adjusted hospitalization rate of hip fracture from 917.6 per 100,000 to 775.7 per 100,000 (CDC, MMWR, 2006 [Level VI]). As 1 of 20 patient safety indicators [PSI] monitored in hospitals, postoperative hip fracture occurred among 5,200 in-patients in 2000, with risk for this PSI increasing with age (Romano et al., 2003 [Level V]). Hip fracture is a serious problem for older adults in terms of mortality and the excess morbidity incurred, especially for adults older than 70 years of age; thus, it is important for targeted proactive nursing interventions. Strong evidence reveals the high mortality rate at 6 months post–hip fracture (from 10% to 28%) (Kenne, Parker, & Pryor, 1993, [Level II]; Magaziner, et al., 1997 [Level V]) with more than 50% never regaining prefracture status (Marottolli, Berkman, & Cooney, 1992 [Level II]).

Evaluation of hospital-unit effectiveness in fall prevention depends on the operational fall definition, fall measurement, and how falls are monitored. Unit-based analysis of fall rates are regularly conducted by nursing care managers and risk analysts. When one considers the multifactorial causes of falls in older adults, it becomes clear as to why fall rates fluctuate individually within and between units. Typically, an average medical–surgical unit fall rate may be much lower than a neurological intensive care unit or rehabilitation unit. The patient demography of these two units is very different. There may be fewer patients on a specialized unit; however, aggregately, the patient may have many more risk factors and individualized reasons to fall.

Research has demonstrated that there are many predisposing risk factors that contribute to falls in older adults in any setting. Fall risk means that a factor or condition is present, significantly more often, in a person who falls than a person who does not fall. Risk factors are of two varieties: (1) those occurring in the person's environment (called extrinsic risks); which include environmental and situational context that patients encounter; and (2) those occurring within the person, or intra-individually (called intrinsic risks) (Table 9.1). Intrinsic risks include the person's underlying medical problem or presence of chronic disease, physical status such as presence of weakness, and use of certain medications.

Hospital settings possess many environmental hazards, which for an acutely ill older adult signal risk. Hazards exist on the floor surface itself in terms of its glossiness (i.e., from bright lights glaring against shiny linoleum tile), wetness from spills (e.g., overfilled water pitchers that may drip onto the floor), and slippery surface areas. In health care settings, environmental falls are commonly

9.1 Examples of Extrinsic and Intrinsic Risks for Falls

Extrinsic Risks

Floor surfaces that are slippery, wet, extra-shiny, or uneven or cracked

Equipment that is faulty, nonsupportive, or collapsing when used, laden with debris

IV poles, stretchers, or beds that are not sturdy or move away from the patient when used for support

Poor lighting or extra-glaring "blinding" bright lights

Bathrooms lacking grabrails, bars, or nonskid appliqués or mats

Physical restraints

Inappropriate footwear

Intrinsic Risks

Lower extremity weakness

History of falls

Gait deficit

Balance deficit

Use of an assistive device

Visual deficit

Arthritis

Impaired ADLs

   Dependency in transferring/mobility

Depression

Cognitive impairment

   Agitated confusion

Older than age 80

Urinary incontinence/frequency

Culprit medications: benzodiazepines, sedatives/hypnotics, alcohol, antidepressants, neuroleptics, anti-arrhythmics, digoxin, and diuretics

Source: Adapted from ECRI Institute (2006). Falls prevention strategies in healthcare settings guide. Plymouth Meeting, PA: ECRI [Level VI].

Oliver, D., Daly, F., Martin, F. C., & McMurdo, M. E. (2004). Risk factors and risk assessment tools for falls in hospital in-patients: A systematic review. *Age and Ageing, 33*(2), 122–130 [Level I].

Papaioannou, A., Parkinson, W., Cook, R., Ferko, N., Corker, E., & Adachi, J. D. (2004). Prediction of falls using a risk assessment tool in the acute care setting. *BioMed Central, 1*, 1 [Level III].

Rubenstein, L. Z., & Josephson, K. R. (2002). The epidemiology of falls and syncope. *Clinics of Geriatric Medicine, 18*, 141–158 [Level II].

found where a slip may occur from a spill or wet surface (Connell, 1996 [Level VI]). Slippery surface areas pose threats if adequate precaution is not taken. For instance, if an older adult does not wear anti-skid slippers while walking, a slip and fall can occur. Built-up debris on bed wheels, stretchers wheels, bedside tables, or intravenous poles can lead to poor contact between two surfaces and a slippage or sliding of the equipment can occur when used for support.

When brakes are not used on wheelchairs or a bed, slides can occur when a patient attempts to stand up (the wheelchair can slide away from the person) or sit down on a bed (the bed slides away from the person). Uneven floor surfaces are problematic in doorways when a ledge or raised tile is present. An older patient with lack of steppage height (e.g., from Parkinson's disease, loss of lower extremity sensation, or Type II diabetes) can trip over the uneven edge. Improper footwear constitutes a hazard; a few studies have found evidence for risk of falls in older adults related to footwear. In one study, greater heel height was associated with increased risk of a fall, whereas greater sole contact area was associated with reduced fall risk (Tencer et al., 2004 [Level IV]). Shoes such as those worn by athletes appear to be beneficial for older adults with lower risks of falling (Koepsell et al., 2004 [Level IV]).

Assistive devices and other types of equipment need to be routinely assessed for function and structural support. If they are defective, bedrails or assistive devices may collapse when weight is applied. Grabrails in the bathroom, around the toilet, and in the shower stall are essential to help maintain upright postural stability for older adult patients. Bedside commodes should be placed against a wall or another source of support and used only with assistance of nursing staff. A bedside commode (and the patient) can easily topple over when a patient exiting from a bed or chair leans on one handrail of the bedside commode when it is not secured against a supportive structure such as a wall or piece of furniture.

Physical Restraint Use

Capezuti and colleagues (2002 [Level III]) cite physical restraint use as a contributor to risk for falling, not a solution for fall prevention. Also noted by Capezuti et al., neither physical restraints nor side rails have ever been shown to reduce falls or associated injury. In fact, in the last 20 years, there have been numerous reports of restraint-related injuries reported in the professional literature, by the U.S. Food and Drug Administration (FDA), and the Joint Commission on Accreditation of Healthcare Organizations (JCAHO). Many of these injuries are due to a patient's attempts to remove restraints or to ambulate while restrained (Agostini, Baker, & Bogardus, 2001 [Level VI]). The injuries include neurological injuries (DiMaio, Dana, & Bux, 1986 [Level V]), stress-induced complications (related to agitation secondary to restraint), and strangulation (Dube & Mitchell, 1986 [Level VI]; Miles, 2002 [Level VI]). The most common mechanism of restraint-related death is by asphyxiation—that is, the person is suspended by a restraint from a bed or chair and the ability to inhale is inhibited by gravitational chest compression (DiNunno, Vacca, Costantinedes, & DiNunno, 2003 [Level V]). Clearly, the risk of serious injury or fatality due to physical restraint is substantial and must be considered when deciding about using restraints.

Intrinsic Risks to Fall

A summary of 16 studies defined the most common intrinsic risk factors for falling among older adults in any setting (Rubenstein & Josephson, 2002 [Level II]) (see Table 9.1). When their relative risk was determined, lower extremity weakness ranked as the most potent risk factor, with a four times greater risk to fall than if the restraint were not present. History of falls ranked second,

9.2 Examples of Co-morbidity Impact on Aging Changes	
Changes	**Impact**
Visual changes	
Presbyopia (reduced accommodation)	Difficulty may be encountered with descending steps, particularly the last step may be missed, or surface edges
Senile miosis (smaller pupils)	Dimly lit rooms or hallways difficult to visualize Surface edges without bold, contrast colors may visually "blend" together
Cardiovascular changes	
Orthostatic hypotension (OH)	Positional changes (e.g., lying to sitting up in bed or standing from sitting) may cause sudden drop in blood pressure precipitating a fall
Neuromuscular changes	
Reduced steppage height	Stumbles, trips with ascending steps or walking on uneven surfaces
Impaired reaction time	Trips, stumbles, or pushes causing a sudden loss of balance can result in impaired ability to maintain upright stance

Source: Adapted from Maki, B. E., & McIllroy, W. E. (2003). Effects of aging on control of stability. In L. Luxon et al. (Eds.), *A textbook of audiological medicine: Clinical aspects of hearing and balance* (pp. 671–690). London: Marin Dunitz Publishers.

increasing the risk of falling threefold; gait or balance deficit ranked third and fourth, respectively, increasing fall risk about threefold. Other factors increasing risk of falling at least twofold were use of an assistive device, visual deficit, arthritis, impaired activities of daily livings (ADLs), and depression. Cognitive impairment and being older than age 80 increased fall risk 1.8 and 1.7 times, respectively. Evidence-based research of fall risks seen among older adults in hospital in-patient settings have confirmed similar findings (see Table 9.1) and include gait instability, agitated confusion, urinary incontinence/frequency, history of falls, and use of "culprit" medications (Oliver, Daly, Martin, & McMurdo, 2004 [Level I]). Positive predictive validity of falls has also been evidenced by intrinsic risk of a history of falls, visually impaired, toileting assistance, dependency in transfer and mobility, and mental impairment (Papaioannou et al., 2004 [Level III]). Of all these associated risks for falling, Papaioannou et al. found that cognitive impairment was the most significant predictor. Some intrinsic risks are also implicated as underlying causative agents (Rubenstein & Josephson, 2006 [Level I]), such as diseases causing cognitive impairment or gait and balance instability. The contribution of chronic disease to increased fall risk is notable (Tinetti, Williams, & Mayewski, 1986 [Level II]) as well as the co-morbidity of changes related to aging (Table 9.2).

Age-Related Changes Contributing to Fall Risk

There may be subtle changes in older persons' organ systems; coupled with the effects of co-morbidities and acute or chronic illness, the risk for falls increases significantly. Experts agree that it is the co-morbidity of the aging changes, and not age per se, that increases the risk of falls (Public Health Agency of Canada, 2007 [Level VI]). Some of the visual changes experienced by older adults include presbyopia—a reduction in accommodation. The effects of presbyopia are most obvious when descending steps. Because of this condition, older adults may miss the last step (an important reason why handrails must end on the landing surface and why the use of handrails is essential). A reduction in the diameter of the pupil, a condition called *senile miosis*, results in smaller pupils. Dimly lit rooms and hallways or surface edges that do not have bold contrasting colors can lead to trips and falls. The presence of a cataract, more prevalent in older age groups and with certain conditions, obstructs central vision and can contribute to falls when steps or obstacles are not visualized. In a study of older adults with cataracts, removal of the cataracts was associated with a reduced risk for recurrent falling (Brennan et al., 2003 [Level III]). Neuromuscular aging changes include reduced steppage height. If reduced steppage height is evident, stumbles, trips, and falls can occur when ascending a step or walking on an uneven surface. Also, transitioning from a flat floor surface to a thicker carpeted surface can reproduce similar fall occurrences. Other changes include impaired ability to react to sudden loss of balance (from a push or trip) or impaired ability to maintain upright stance (Maki & McIllroy, 2003 [Level VI]). In addition to disease and co-morbidities of aging, other sources of intrinsic risk to falls includes medications.

Medications Contributing to Fall Risk

Medications implicated in increasing fall risk are those causing potentially dangerous side effects, including drowsiness, mental confusion, problems with balance, loss of urinary control, and sudden drops in blood pressure with standing (i.e., postural hypotension). All of these effects may lead to a slip and fall (Ensrud et al., 2002 [Level II]; Neutel, Perry, & Maxwell, 2002 [Level VI]; Smith, 2003 [Level VI]). Classifications of medications implicated in falls for older adults include psychotropic agents (e.g., benzodiazepines, sedatives and hypnotics, antidepressants, and neuroleptics), anti-arrhythmics, digoxin, and diuretics (Leipzig, Cumming, & Tinetti, 1999 [Level I]).

Factors Increasing the Risk to Develop Serious Injury

Risk factors for the development of serious injury such as hip fracture have been isolated to include advancing age, lack of physical activity, presence of osteoporosis, low body mass index, and a previous hip fracture (Stevens, 2000 [Level V]). Almost all older individuals with hip fractures have osteoporosis, yet from findings from a retrospective analysis of records of patients receiving hip-fracture surgery, it appears that the frequency of treating these high risk older patients for osteoporosis is less than optimal (Kamel, 2004 [Level IV]). Kamel further points out that inadequate treatment for osteoporosis increases risk for osteoporotic fractures, including recurrent hip fractures. Advancing age is a significant risk for those older than age 85 who experience nearly an eightfold increase in hospitalization due to hip facture. TBI is another serious injury that can occur from a fall and is caused by a "blow to the head or jolt to the head or penetrating head injury that disrupts function of the brain; however, not all blows result in TBI (CDC, NCIPC, 2007 [Level VI]). Of all causes, falls are the leading cause of TBI (CDC, NCIPC, 2007 [Level VI]), with adults age 75 and older having the highest rate of TBI-related hospitalization and death (Langlois, Rutland-Brown, & Thomas, 2006 [Level V]). Groups at risk for the development of TBI include men, who are twice as likely to sustain a TBI; adults age 75 or older; and African Americans, who have the highest death rate from TBI (CDC, NCIPC, 2007 [Level VI]). There is strong clinical reason to suspect that anticoagulated older adults are at higher risk for TBI, should they sustain a fall with head injury, but empiric research in this age group is lacking. Still, best practice approaches to care of older adults must include a risk-benefit evaluation of medications, such as Coumadin, Plavix, and/or aspirin, among others, that place the older adult at increased risk of bleeding following a fall (Resnick, 2003 [Level VI]).

The quality and quantity of life for older adults at risk for falling in the acute care setting depends on the reduction of risk factors so as to prevent a fall, especially one resulting in serious injury. In licensed medical-care settings, the onus of responsibility rests on the licensed practitioner to follow appropriate standards of care to ensure that patients are safe and free from injury during periods of illness and treatment recovery. Nurses share in this enormous responsibility to provide both safe care and safe environments. Just how this is accomplished occurs when knowledge is integrated in the nursing assessment so that fall-prevention interventions are individualized. Answers to the question: "Why do older adult patients in an acute care setting fall?" begin with a focused patient assessment.

Assessment of Older Adults Post-Fall

The assessment of an older adult who has fallen in any setting is complex because falls in this age group are due to multifactorial and interacting predisposing intrinsic and extrinsic risks (see Tables 9.1 and 9.2) and precipitating causes (Rubenstein & Josephson, 2006 [Level I]), as illustrated in Table 9.3 (Gray-Miceli, Johnson, & Strumpf, 2005 [Level VI]). Through many interactive mechanisms, we are learning much more about why patients in hospital settings fall. This knowledge has been mostly realized through improved reporting systems, such as the electronic medical record and greater attention to the types of information gathered from assessment tools. When this information is coupled with results from a root-causes analysis performed following a sentinel event and funneled to patient safety databanks, a clearer understanding of patient falls is evident.

The most up-to-date knowledge of root causes of *all* patient falls in the inpatient setting in 2005 is derived from tabulated reported incidences to JCAHO (2006 [Level V]) and includes inadequate:

- patient assessment—accounting for 70% of patient falls
- communication—accounting for more than 60% of patient falls
- environmental safety and security—accounting for 50% of patient falls

9.3 Medical Events and Diseases Associated With Falls in Older Adults

Age-Related

Dizziness with standing from physiological age-related changes
Dizziness with head rotation from physiological age-related changes

Accidental/Environmental

Slipping or tripping on a wet/slippery surface
Trip/slip
Lack of support from equipment or assistive device

Acute (Treatable) Sudden Symptoms

Mental confusion/delirium
Heart racing or skipping beats (arrhythmia)
Dizziness with standing up (orthostatic hypotension)
Dizziness with room spinning (vertigo)
Generalized weakness (infection, sepsis)
Involuntary movement of limbs accompanied by confusion, unresponsiveness, or
    absent facial features (seizure)
Lower extremity weakness (electrolyte imbalance)
Gait ataxia associated with acute alcohol ingestion
Feeling faint or dizzy or unable to sustain consciousness (hypoglycemia)
Blacking out or loss of recall of fall event (syncope)
Unilateral weakness, sudden speech change, and/or facial droop (TIA/CVA)

Chronic (Manageable) Gradual or Recurrent Symptoms

Lower extremity numbness (neuropathy, diabetes, PVD, B_{12} deficiency)
Lower extremity weakness (arthritis, CVA, thyroid disease)
Fatigue (anemia, CHF)
Dyspnea on exertion (emphysema, pneumonia)
Weakness (frailty, disuse, anemia)
Lightheadedness (carotid stenosis, cerebrovascular disease, emphysema)
Dizziness with standing (OH secondary to diabetes)
Dizziness with head rotation (carotid stenosis, hypersensitivity)
Dizziness with movement (labyrinthitis)
Forgetting the fall (dementia)
"I don't know" responses (depression)
Lower extremity joint pain (arthritis)
Unsteadiness with walking (dementia, CVA/MID)
Poor balance (Parkinson's disease)

Reprinted with permission from Gray-Miceli, D., Johnson, J. C., & Strumpf, N. E. (2005). A step-wise approach to a comprehensive post-fall assessment. *Annals of Long Term Care, 13*(12), 16–24, Table II, p. 20.

9.4	Some Examples of Fall Causes

Accident/environment (31%)

Gait and balance disorders or weakness (17%)

Dizziness and vertigo (13%)

Drop attack (9%)

Confusion (5%)

Postural hypotension (OH; 3%)

Visual disorder (2%)

Syncope (0.03%)

Source: Adapted from Rubenstein, L. Z., & Josephson, K. R. (2006). Falls and their prevention in elderly people: What does the evidence show? *Medical Clinics of North America, 90*(5), 807–824 [Level I].

Multifactorial Causes of Falls

Falls among older adults are a multifactorial phenomenon, attributable to medications (Ensrud et al., 2002 [Level II]; Leipzig et al., 1999 [Level I]; Neutel et al., 2002 [Level VI]; Smith, 2003 [Level VI]), chronic diseases (Shaw, 2002; Stolze et al., 2004 [both Level VI]), the co-morbidity of aging and age-related changes, environmental causes, prodromal causes (Gray-Miceli, Waxman, Cavalieri, & Lage, 1991 [Level IV]); Rubenstein et al., 2000 [Level II]), or other acute illness.

Falls related to acute cardiovascular events include heart blocks, arrhythmia causing rate disturbances, and disorders causing orthostatic hypotension [OH] (Heitterachi, Lord, Meyerkorf, McCloskey, & Fitzpatrick, 2002 [Level III]; Ooi, Hossain, & Lipsitz, 2000 [Level IV]). OH can occur from acute illnesses such as volume depletion or blood loss, chronic illness such as Type II diabetes with autonomic neuropathy, or from adverse medication effects (e.g., from diuretics or vasodilators). Hospitalized adults older than age 85 frequently possess many of these acute and chronic conditions (see Table 9.3) and when coupled with frailty, associated functional decline can lead to lower extremity weakness and subsequent falling.

Evidence-based research by Rubenstein and Josephson (2006 [Level I]) on fall etiology in older persons is summarized from 12 large studies (with a sample size of 3,628 reported falls) in Table 9.4. The data are drawn from six studies conducted in community-dwelling populations and six studies conducted among institutionalized populations and is limited by factors such as patient recall, reporting, and classification methods of falls.

Fall Assessment

There are several interrelated components of the fall assessment of an older adult recommended by geriatric experts and national guidelines for fall prevention in older adults (American Geriatrics Society [AGS], 2001 [Level VI];

American Medical Directors Association [AMDA], 1998 [Level VI]). One component outlined in the guidelines is primary prevention, or screening for "risk to fall" among all older adults admitted to a medical facility. For those at high risk to fall or who have recently experienced a fall, a more comprehensive multidimensional assessment (inclusive of a review of fall risk) is appropriate (AGS, 2001 [Level VI]) and is often provided by an interdisciplinary team in the medical-care setting.

Assessment Tools Used for Fall-Risk Determination

The purpose of fall-risk assessment is to identify risk for falling in advance and to correct problems so as to prevent patient falls. Fall-risk determination is also performed following a patient fall to help direct interventions. Many published tools are available to assist clinicians in fall-risk determination. Tools selected for use in practice should ideally have been empirically tested for determinations of reliability, validity, and predictability of future falls; sensitivity scores are reported for some tools (Table 9.5). Because of wide availability of fall-risk screening tools for use with older adults, home-grown tools developed by the facility that are not empirically tested should be avoided because they lack validity, reliability, and often sensitivity testing. Fall-risk status is likely to fluctuate over time, especially among hospitalized older adults experiencing acute illness. For this reason, the standard of care calls for fall-risk assessment to be done on admission, when transferred to a new unit or when level of care changes, if a change in condition occurs, and after a fall. Fall-risk assessment tools used for patient assessment tend to focus on intrinsic and, to a lesser degree, extrinsic risks. They tend to be brief in length, some taking only a few minutes to administer. Used in isolation, they provide limited information and often lack sufficient detail about the fall history and situational context, patient symptoms, or important examination findings (as can be obtained through a comprehensive post-fall assessment [PFA]). Intrinsic items assessed range from a yes or no response to presence or absence of visual impairment, confusion, high risk medications, OH, and gait or balance impairment. Summed scores help to identify risk profiles and specific areas of impairment and to monitor patient status over time.

Assessment tools are always used along with sound nursing judgment. In the case of PFA, fall-risk tools do not replace it, rather, the complement it. It is important to recognize nursing judgment in the process of fall-risk assessment. Although the relative odds of falling are statistically much higher for older persons with one, two, or multiple risk factors, falls can still occur if no risk factors are present; therefore, the scores with certain patients are sometimes misleading. Some tools, particularly homegrown ones, may fail to detect known risk factors because their presence is lacking on the tool itself. For this reason, sole reliance on tools becomes problematic in practice.

This clinical concern is supported by evidenced-based research of the Timed Get Up and Go Test (TUG), a tool used in practice to predict falls. Among a sample of elderly patients admitted to a hospital who were followed prospectively, the TUG test, used in isolation, failed to identify those patients likely to fall. In short, it did not possess predictive validity for acutely ill older adults when used alone (Lindsay, James, & Kippen, 2004 [Level III]).

9.5 Listing of Some Empirically Tested Fall Assessment Tools

Name of Tool	Author	Setting	Training	Time to Administer	Sensitivity
Assessment of High Risk to Fall	Spellbring	IP	Y	17 minutes	UK
Berg Balance Test	Berg	OP	Y	15 minutes	77
Patient Fall Questionnaire	Rainville	IP	Y	UK	UK
STRATIFY	Oliver	IP	N	UK	93
Fall Prediction Index	Nyberg	IP-CVA	UK	UK	100
Resident Assessment Instrument	Morris	NH	Y	80 minutes	UK
Post-Fall Index	Gray-Miceli	NH	Y	22 minutes	UK
Morse Fall Scale	Morse	IP	Y	<1 minute	78
Fall Risk Assessment Tool	MacAvoy	IP	N	UK	93
Hendrich Fall Risk Model	Hendrich	IP	N	<1 minute	77
Timed Get Up and Go	Shumway-Cook	OP	Y	<1 minute	87
Tinetti Performance Oriented Mobility	Tinetti	IP	Y	20 minutes	80

Key: IP: in-patient; IP-CVA: cerebrovascular accident; OP: outpatient; NH: nursing home; Y: yes; N: no; UK: unknown

Source: Adapted from ECRI: *Fall Prevention Strategies in Healthcare Settings* (2006): In ECRI and Perell, et al. (2001), Fall risk assessment measures: An analytic review. *Journal of Gerontology. 56A*(12), 761–766.

Extrinsic risk assessment is another vital component, particularly in an in-patient setting where environmental slips and falls are commonplace. Checklists are available to guide health care providers in conducting environmental and equipment assessment for risks. Fall-risk assessment results in identification of individualized risks for falling, which are communicated to other members of the team so that plans of care can be targeted to the older adult's needs.

Post-Fall Assessment

Another component of patient assessment after a fall is referred to as "post-fall assessment" (PFA) and is designated for the secondary prevention of falls. PFAs are recommended in clinical guidelines and are multifactorial in nature, focusing on identifying intrinsic and extrinsic risks and other causative etiology. The purpose of PFA is to identify the underlying causes of the fall and to respond to it appropriately. Components of the PFA are typically routinely performed by professional nurses in all patient settings, although this evaluation may be skeletal or limited according to the completeness of questions and examination included on the tool used. Few empirically published tools for PFA exist, and previous research has shown that fall-risk determination, using short forms, asking five to eight questions about risk, often replace (inappropriately) PFA in institutionalized settings (Gray-Miceli, Strumpf, Reinhard, Zanna, & Fritz, 2004 [Level IV]). There is evidence that comprehensive PFA tools are useful and available to assist professional registered nurses in performing a PFA, especially in institutionalized settings (Gray-Miceli, Strumpf, Johnson, Dragascu, & Ratcliffe, 2006 [Level III]). In settings where teams are unavailable, comprehensive PFA may be carried out through consultation with a specially trained geriatrician, neurologist, or advanced practice nurses.

The PFA is a comprehensive yet fall-focused history and physical examination of the present problem (i.e., falling), often coupled with a functional assessment and review of past medical problems and medications. Clinical guidelines are clear about all of the necessary components for inclusion for patients who have fallen, including fall history, fall circumstance, medical problems, medication review, mobility assessment, vision assessment, and neurological examination including mental status and cardiovascular assessment. In addition to this information, data are collected about the patient's physical status through administration of selected tools to assess gait and balance (see Table 9.5 for additional information on tools; TUG test [see chap. 3, *Assessment of Function*]; Tinetti Performance Oriented Mobility; The Berg Balance Test). Performing a comprehensive PFA allows the clinician to identify intrinsic risks such as balance impairment or OH determination, as well as historical or physical examination findings consistent with a range of underlying fall causes such as brady- or tachy-arrhythmia associated with dizziness. Until recently, there have been no comprehensive, empirically tested PFA tools that allow registered nurses to determine potential underlying fall causes (Gray-Miceli, et al. 2006 [Level III]).

In the hospital setting, certain components of a PFA can be elicited immediately following a patient's fall, whereas other questions will follow later during an intermediate period. The decision to ask certain questions immediately depends on the medical stability of the patient and nursing judgment. A PFA can help determine the underlying cause of the fall, whenever possible, if the right set of questions is asked. Furthermore, this information can be communicated to senior-level providers, staff, and family.

The PFA begins with eliciting a clear history of the fall event by asking the older adult patient to describe the details and what he or she recalls occurring. In cases of aphasia or poor recall from delirium or dementia, a piece of the history can be obtained by using alterative communication methods such as nods of the head, eliciting details from observers such as other health care providers

9.6 Sample of Key Symptoms Associated With Falls

Symptoms to Elicit	Possible Etiology
Cardiovascular	
Lightheadedness	Carotid stenosis, medications, CAD; arrhythmia
Dizziness with standing	OH (Orthostatic hypotension)
Dizziness with head rotation	Carotid stenosis/hypersensitivity
Shortness of breath	Arrhythmia
Syncope	Vaso vagal, neurological, carotid hypersensitivity
Neurological/musculoskeletal	
Gait unsteadiness	Dementia, PD, CVA, foot problems
Lower extremity weakness (bilateral)	Disuse, thyroid disease, and electrolyte disorders
Lower extremity weakness (unilateral)	CVA, arthritis
Lower extremity numbness	Neuropathy, DM, B_{12} deficiency, PD
General	
Sudden weakness	Disuse, anemia
Fatigue	Infection, CHF
Focal bone pain	Bone fracture
Genito urinary	
Urinary frequency/urgency	UTI
Urinary incontinence	UTI
Behavioral	
Thirst, hunger	Unmet physical needs
Continuous wandering/motor restlessness	Dementia

Reprinted with permission from Gray-Miceli, D., Johnson, J. C., & Strumpf, N. E. (2005). A step-wise approach to a comprehensive post-fall assessment. *Annals of long term care: clinical care and aging*, *13*(12), 16–24. Table I, p. 19.

who may have witnessed the fall, from visitors, or from roommates. Much of the historical information seeks to determine the presence of symptoms, which might further explain the fall, and to recreate a visual image of the fall event. Lists of key symptoms, which often herald an acute or chronic medical cause, are listed in Table 9.6. In the hospital setting, key symptoms such as OH, syncope, or dizziness can be further evaluated, monitored, and/or treated as directed by the medical plan of care.

9.7   Immediate Post-Fall Assessment

Actions Taken by Professional Nurses and Nursing Staff

If an older adult patient is found on the floor, remain with the patient, summon additional help, and proceed to:

- Ask the older adult to explain what happened, if possible
- Ask the how he or she is feeling and if there is pain
- Control any bleeding (follow unit protocol) from injured site
- Assess level of consciousness and perform neurological assessment, including pupillary checks (according to unit protocol)
- Gather and document vital signs: note the apical pulse rate and the supine blood pressure
- Examine for signs of external injury to the head, spine, neck, and extremities
- Determine oxygenation status
- Determine finger-stick glucose if hypoglycemia is suspected
- If stable, sit the patient up with support and assess sitting blood pressure
- Gather and review pertinent symptoms at the time of the fall
- Immobilize an extremity if fracture is suspected
- Reassure the older patient
- If the patient is stable, assist with transfer to bed or appropriate area for further evaluation
- Diagnosis and treatment

Reprinted with permission from ECRI. Gray-Miceli, D. (2006). *Fall Prevention Strategies in Healthcare Settings*, chap. 5, Patient Post-Fall Assessment: ECRI. Level VI.

The Immediate Post-Fall Assessment

As soon as possible after a patient has fallen or a resident is discovered, an assessment is made by the RN to determine the extent of any sustained injuries. Before any intervention is taken, any staff member should remain with the patient and call for help. During this time, the older adult patient is verbally reassured and kept warm (but not moved) until help arrives. There are many key observations to be noted about the fallen individual's medical and psychological condition, as well as the condition of the environment. The medical stability of the patient determines the sequence of information gathered either immediately or in the interim period, according to current standards of practice followed by licensed professionals. For instance, if the patient is unconscious from a head injury sustained during the fall, neurological checks, vital signs with apical pulse rate, and pulse oxygenation are assessed first. Other assessments of gait or functional status are conducted after the patient has stabilized. While this is being performed, other staff members can assess environmental spills or if shoes or slippers are worn. The nursing staff can use the intercom system to call for help, reassure the other residents in a calm manner, and keep the fallen resident comfortable. Information about the lighting and use of assistive devices can be gathered. Any verbalizations made by the patient should be noted about his or her condition. There are certain key actions that

9.8 Critical Observations Made During the Immediate Post-Fall Assessment

Expressions or verbalizations of pain (facial grimacing, crying, screaming, agitation)

Changes in behavior or function, which may indicate pain

Swelling of an extremity (wrist, arm, leg) or head (hematoma, skull pain)

Unstable vital signs

Discolored cyanotic skin

Skin temperature (cold, clammy, diaphoretic)

Skin lacerations, contusions

Loss of consciousness, no response to stimuli or significant change in level of consciousness

Changed range of motion of extremities

Evidence of neck, head, or spinal-cord injury

Abnormal or erratic neurological responses, such as absent pupil response, fixed or dilated pupils, seizures, or abnormal changes in posture

Reprinted with permission from ECRI (2006). *Fall prevention strategies in healthcare settings*, chapter 5, Patient Post-Fall Assessment: ECRI Institute [Level VI].

should be taken by licensed professional nursing staff when evaluating a fallen patient (Table 9.7); some of these areas can be expanded on later when obtaining more detailed information about the fall. Critical observations made during the immediate PFA that should be communicated to the primary-care provider (Table 9.8) include observation or verbalizations of pain, extremity swelling, unstable vital signs, discolored skin, temperature, laceration or contusions of the skin, loss of consciousness, decreased range of motion, evidence of head or neck injury and abnormal or erratic neurological responses, uncontrollable bleeding, and incontinence of bowel or bladder at the time of the fall.

Interim Post-Fall Assessment

During the interim period of PFA and monitoring (from several days to weeks), professional nurses continue to review, determine, and communicate pertinent findings from this assessment and its progression or resolution. Once the patient is medically stable, fall-risk assessment can be reassessed by the interdisciplinary team revaluating intrinsic and extrinsic risks so that a plan of care can be determined. The interim PFA period often requires a different set of assessments, and this may be an ideal time to administer a cognitive, functional, and/or emotional assessment, such as use of the Geriatric Depression Scale, or a problem-focused mobility assessment. Develop a plan of care and request a change in physician orders for level of supervision required by nursing staff of the older patient or specific activity restrictions, depending on the fall assessment findings.

Longitudinal Post-Fall Assessment

Following a patient fall, the presence of injury may not be apparent until days or even weeks later. When cognitive impairment exists, the accuracy of the historical accounts of pain obtained immediately after the fall may be questioned. Observations of functional status with attention to any subtle or blatant changes in mobility can signal an underlying fracture or a looming unstable joint that was not previously reported. Likewise, during a patient fall in which the older adult is cognitively intact and then later develops an acute delirium or post-fall confusional state should signal to the professional nurse the possibility of injury. In these two instances, the standard of care is warranted as part of the ongoing PFA to monitor vital signs and neurological status for a period of several days or more, as clinically indicated. Fall policy and procedures should reflect this provision because any change in patient condition warrants follow-through, documentation, and communication to senior-level providers, other nursing staff, and family.

Interventions for Fall Prevention and Management

Influencing the nursing plan of care are decisions made at discrete points in time about which nursing interventions should be selected. Decisions about intervention choice are formed by clinical judgment, which always factors in the medical stability of the older adult patient (including whether his or her judgment or cognition is impaired) and the range of possible measures to promote safety and minimize risks of injury. Often, a panorama of interventions is chosen, which may or may not be effective in fall prevention. The most important determining factor hinges on findings obtained during an individualized assessment—for example, standard of care calls for stuporous or delirious patients with impaired level of consciousness, cognition, and judgment to receive more intense observation and clinical care. Likewise, although research evidence is lacking, the standard of care calls for a patient at risk for serious injury (e.g., hip fracture, subdural hematoma, or other type of TBI), secondary to bleeding disorders or use of anticoagulants, to be carefully assessed and more intensely monitored in an acute care setting.

Evidenced-based interventions and their clinical effectiveness are evolving. Action-based interventions range from imminent threats to patient safety requiring "emergency treatment" to interventions requiring routine monitoring and surveillance. Because available resources vary among facilities, a central component of any fall prevention program is for health care organizations to ensure that available toolkits exist to help staff manage patient falls (ECRI, 2006 [Level VI]).

Nursing judgment and team discussion about risks versus benefits of an intervention is central to the nurse's mission to protect older adults from harm. Some best practice exemplars for fall prevention are presented, which can help determine what is in the best nursing intervention for a particular patient at a particular moment in time. As the status of the patient changes, so too do interventions, which range from various types and degrees of surveillance and supervision to actual physical assistance. Also keep in mind, many nursing practices and interventions once thought to prevent falls, now outdated, are found to either cause harm or are ineffectual in preventing falls, as in the case of physical-restraint use. See chapter 22, *Physical Restraints*.

The most current evidenced-based research from systematic review and meta-analysis of randomized controlled trials (until 2002) concludes that individualized multifactorial risk assessment combined with risk-reducing interventions are the most effective fall-prevention strategies (Chang et al., 2004 [Level I]). Further research on effective interventions applicable to in-patient hospital settings support use of tailored exercise to improve gait and balance or muscular strength (Close et al., 1999 [Level II]), geriatric consultation with medication review and management (Ray et al., 1997 [Level II]), visual correction, and patient education.

Instituting General Safety Measures

Hospitals have a legal responsibility to ensure that the facility is free from environmental hazards and safe for patients as well as staff and visitors. Routine environmental assessment includes the unit, corridors, entrances, and exits, as well as patient holding areas, patient rooms, and areas to which patient are transported (e.g., radiology, nuclear imaging, operating room). In each area, an environmental assessment is performed focusing on floor surfaces, furniture, hallways, steps, safety devices (e.g., stretchers, wheelchairs, and other types of chairs), clutter, bathrooms with appropriate grabrails, and routine assessment of equipment. Use of a checklist signed by the designated employee allows for audit review of compliance.

As part of general safety, some facilities designate any adult older than age 65 admitted to be on "safety precautions," which can include various other safety measures (discussed herein). Clinically, it is important to recognize—in advance, whenever possible—that if instructions are given to patients for general safety precautions, they are actually able to hear, understand, and demonstrate that they can follow instructions. Simply "telling the older adult" to be careful or to not get up without assistance is insufficient and negligent in the face of an ongoing or new onset of delirium or cognitive impairment. Rather, other safety measures need to be immediately instituted, discussed with the team and the family caregiver, and incorporated as part of the plan of care. Immediate options always include (1) increasing surveillance by either continuously staying with the patient; (2) moving the patient to a closer location (provided there is a staff member constantly observing the patient); (3) providing a one-on-one type of sitter service for continual surveillance; or (4) engaging the older patient in activities or other forms of recreation and therapeutic or diversional activity. Sitter-type services can be provided by hospital staff, volunteers, or through private-duty services. Discussion with family caregivers and the interdisciplinary team are essential in these cases.

Exercise for Older Adults Who Fall

More than a decade of research evidence supports use of exercise in improving muscular weakness, balance, and gait and in reducing the risk and incidence of falls compared to control groups among older adults (Carter, Kannus, & Khan,

2001 [Level I]). Specific use of exercise in older adults who are impaired has also been found to be beneficial (Rubenstein et al., 2000 [Level II]). In the community, exercise also has beneficial outcomes for older adults at risk. In a study using a community-based exercise intervention, consisting of weekly group exercises and ancillary home exercises, the rate of falls in the intervention group was reduced by 40% compared to the control group (Barnett, Smith, Lord, Williams, & Baumand, 2003 [Level II]). A narrative review of the epidemiological evidence of prospective and case-control studies showed that higher levels of leisure-time physical activity is associated with a 20% to 40% reduced risk of hip fracture (Gregg, Pereira, & Caspersen, 2000 [Level V]).

Many opportunities exist for older adult patients in a hospital setting to benefit from focal lower extremity strengthening exercises, offered through physical therapy, and/or more global types of exercise, such as walking and mobility programs or group exercises and the use of a pool in rehabilitation hospitals. Once a prescription is written, medical clearance may often be needed or a pre-screening performed by the physical therapist. In the case initiating focal lower extremity exercise for an identified "intrinsic fall risk factor," referrals should be made by the primary care provider because symptoms of lower extremity weakness may be due to other coexisting but treatable illnesses. Two classic examples of treatable illness manifesting as "lower extremity weakness" (which is considered an intrinsic risk factor) in an older adult are thyroid disease and giant cell arteritis (i.e., polymyalgia rheumatica).

Hospitalized older adults carry an increased risk for co-morbidities, such as coronary artery disease, vertigo, and dizziness, which are likely to require a medical clearance prior to engaging in strenuous, aerobic types of exercise. Falls among this population can also occur during exercise due to peripheral neuropathy, particularly in diabetics who may be unable to sense their feet on the floor.

A thorough assessment of co-morbidities in frail older adults can help to minimize potential safety concerns or risks that may exist on the part of the clinician. This is an important aspect of the overall decision to institute strenuous exercise in frail older adults but is beyond the scope of this chapter. Research evidence supports use of strengthening, functional motor activities, and balance exercises during rehabilitation in an outpatient hospital setting in high risk geriatric patients with a history of injurious falls (Hauer et al., 2001 [Level II]).

Early Mobility for Older Patients Who Fall

Early mobility, whenever the older patient is medically stable, is a fundamental and basic aspect of care for all older adult patients to receive during their hospitalization. It is a step toward the prevention of deconditioning, reduced mobility, and immobility and other cascading problems that can result when less sedentary (e.g., statis pneumonia or atelectasis). Early mobility as an intervention begins with the simple and conscious decision by nursing to assist the patient out of bed to walk to the bathroom whenever possible rather than to use a bedpan or even a bedside commode that offers little opportunity for mobility. Wearing proper footwear, corrective lenses, and clearing a path that is clutter- and spill-free are essential. Use of a walking aid such as a standard cane or walker may also be required; appropriate assistive devices can be ascertained through an occupational or physical therapist (OT, PT) consultation.

Another essential aspect for older adults with co-morbidities is for nurses to preemptively ask the older patients "Who is assisting you, from sitting to standing?" and then, while walking, "How are you feeling"? Of concern is the detection of symptoms such as lightheadedness, vertigo with rotational movement, or muscular stiffness. If significant enough to prohibit mobility, these symptoms can be managed and monitored once they are detected. Another concern exists for older adult patients with OH. In this instance, gradual upright incline with assistance while monitoring for symptoms of lightheadedness are important. If an older adult experiences symptoms or develops acute physiological evidence of a problem (e.g., near syncope, syncope, or changes in heart rate or blood pressure), slowly easing the older adult back to a recumbent position and notifying the physician for further evaluation is warranted.

Mobility programs build on the positive feedback that the patient is feeling and objectively gaining strength each day that mobility is instituted. A checklist can monitor progress and serve to validate clinical progression to the patient. Care must be taken, however, to remind persons who are restricted from independent mobility to always wait for assistance. Recommendations are set to a similar time each day and to use consistent staff.

Fall-Prevention Program

Fall prevention begins with an integrated and coordinated approach including fall-risk determination and PFA to identify risk factors. Accurate documentation should be provided in the plan of care, nursing and interdisciplinary notes, and other aspects of the medical record such as the problem-list to help to ensure communication and ongoing monitoring. Review of fall-related information collected about a fall event, or a person deemed at risk to fall by the interdisciplinary team adds an important dimension to fall care. The team offers input from their unique perspective of the fall circumstance and how to best manage a fall or a patient at high risk for falls. The interdisciplinary team consists of the medical provider (physician or advance practice nurse), nurse, PT or OT, risk manager, pharmacist, and other direct health care providers.

Hospital-based fall-prevention programs have been described in the literature but few clinical trails have been conducted demonstrating their effectiveness. One study examined the effect of a program of fall prevention that includes multifactorail components of fall-risk assessment, a choice of interventions, patient and staff education, as well as labels or "graphics alerting others to at risk patients." Use of this model and its outcomes were examined prospectively for 5 years by Dempsey (2004 [Level IV]), who reported a significant reduction in fall rates. However, over time, compliance deteriorated, warranting further nursing inquiry considering use of a process approach to increase nurse autonomy in fall prevention.

Some Best Practice Exemplars Used by Acute Care Hospitals

The difference between environmental safety assessment and safety rounds is that the latter are a regular, systematic observation by one or two key personnel of the hospital unit; when assumed by the same personnel, hazards may be more quickly appreciated. Further, they occur at regular points in time, such as every 2 or 4 hours around the clock and also detect patients in need of assistance. This level of frequency is likely to detect problems early so that intervention can ensure the prevention of environmental type of falls. Use of a checklist can help ensure compliance and monitor for patterns and types of hazards that need correction.

Many hospital-based fall-prevention programs include toileting rounds. Toileting rounds utilize nurses' aides to regularly assess older adult patients for the need to urinate and to provide the patient with assistance. The purpose of toileting rounds is to prevent patients from incurring urinary accidents (and potential falls) by encouraging regular voiding. In many circumstances, urinary accidents can lead to falls. Scenarios include the older adult sensing a need to urinate, getting up out of bed unassisted, and incurring a fall by an unrecognized physiologic mechanism (e.g., OH). Another scenario is en route to the bathroom: the older adult has a urinary accident on the floor and slips and falls on the wet floor. By offering toileting rounds on a regular basis, the potential for these occurrences are minimized, reducing fall rates as well as the iatrogenic complications (e.g., hip fracture). Toileting is a fundamental element of basic care that has an important place in the prevention of patient falls but its importance is under-recognized. In a study by Brown, Vittinghoff, & Wyman (2000 [Level III]), urge incontinence (and not stress), especially if occurring weekly or more often, increased the risk of falls and nonspinal, nontraumatic fractures in older White women living in the community.

Specific Nursing Interventions

Personal alarms are routinely used to alert nursing staff to impending falls or changes in patient mobility status. Care should be taken when deciding to use these devices because they do no prevent a fall from occurring; rather, they heighten staff's awareness by sounding an alarm, indicating that a change in position has occurred. There are many commercial products available, but generally they are of two types: personal alarms clipped to a patient's gown or chair and bed-chair pressure sensors. Despite their widespread use, there is little evidence as to their effectiveness in reducing falls in an acute care hospital setting. Use of a bed-sensor alarm was studied in a geriatric rehabilitation unit with older adult patients who were deemed by nurses to be at increased risk for falling (Kwok, Mok, Chien, & Tam, 2006 [Level II]). In this study, the availability of bed-sensor devices neither reduced physical-restraint use nor improved the clinical outcomes of older adults with perceived fall risk. In a nursing home–based study, however, use of the "NOC WATCH," a nonintrusive monitor used with older adults at high risk for falling (Kelly, Phillips, Cain, Polissar, & Kelly, 2002 [Level IV]), reduced the fall rate by 91%, thereby supporting other clinical trails using a randomized design.

The use of both floor mats and low-rise beds has an important place in the armamentarium of clinical interventions to prevent the occurrence of serious injury when a bed fall occurs. Floor mats are simply placed surrounding the bed and serve to cushion the impact of the fall. They vary in thickness and, if portions of an area are uncovered, substantial injury could still occur if a patient attempts to get out of bed and a bed fall ensues. Little if any empirical research evidence exists as to their effectiveness in preventing bed falls causing fractures to the hip or TBI. Other common interventions used in hospitals also potentially relevant in reducing serious injury in the aftermath from a bed fall are low-rise beds. In principle, they shorten the height of the fall and thus potentially minimize any serious injury. Theoretically, however, use of either floor mats or low-rise beds could still result in serious injury in an older adult with co-morbidities such as osteoporosis. More research is needed to explore this relationship.

The minimization of physical-restraint use has been the subject of case reports and descriptive research in residential- and acute care facilities, with few randomized controlled trials evaluating its effectiveness, especially in acute care. See chapter 22, *Physical Restraints and Side Rails in Acute and Critical Care Settings*, for an evidence-based review of restraints and side-rail use.

The standard of care recommends that older adults at risk for falling or who have fallen be offered a hip protector, which is especially important in the acute care setting, where limited scientific evidence exists to the contrary. Older adults compliance for use of a hip protector is limited by issues related to the feasibility of applying them and then getting them off quickly enough for toileting. Esthetically, they may appear too bulky and cumbersome and thus be a deterrent to the potential user. Facilities may not even stock hip protectors, which are not covered by Medicare and average an out-of-pocket expense of up to $100 each. A recent meta-analysis of their effectiveness from studies conducted in institutionalized settings or the community indicates that hip protectors are an ineffective intervention for those living at home and that their effectiveness in the institutional setting is uncertain (Parker, Gillespie, & Gillespie, 2006 [Level I]).

Technological advances have offered staff and patients a greater variety of solutions to the problem of falling. Improvements have occurred with walking aides such as canes that "talk" and provide feedback to the user, balance retraining that helps patients learn about where their body is in space and how to compensate for muscular impairments, and other types of equipment used at the bedside when transitioning patients. Although these devices are available, research is evolving and limited in terms of their effectiveness in fall prevention (Nelson et al., 2004 [Level VI]).

An integral component of any fall-prevention educational intervention for hospitalized older adults or preparing for discharge home concerns their working knowledge of what caused their fall and what can be done about it. Exploring the older adults' beliefs and attitudes is important and can lead to dispelling myths they may hold about falling (e.g., it is a normal part of aging or that nothing can be done about it). An older person's view and conceptualization about falling is a starting point for a tailored educational intervention. A systematic review of the literature of many studies examining older adults' preferences, views, and experiences relative to fall-prevention strategies reported several important findings (McInnes & Askie, 2004 [Level I]): (1) in clinical practice, it is important to consult with individuals to find out what they are willing to modify; and (2) what changes they are prepared to make to reduce their risk of falling. Otherwise, they may not attend fall-prevention educational programs.

Case Study and Discussion

Mrs. S. is an 80-year-old White female admitted to the step-down rehabilitation unit at the hospital following a 3-week admission for treatment of a community-acquired pneumonia. Mrs. S. received IV antibiotics and fluids for management of the infiltrate and associated dehydration. Mrs. S.'s hospitalization was complicated by development of acute confusion, which escalated following use of IV theophylline and Atrovent and Proventil nebulizers. Mrs. S. also developed a deep-vein thrombosis of the leg, which was treated with IV heparin, and she now receives Coumadin. Mrs. S.'s fall-risk score was significant for visual impairment due to a cataract, delirium, focal lower extremity weakness due to osteoarthritis, chronic obstructive lung disease, osteoporosis, and forgetfulness with short-term memory loss.

Prior to this hospitalization, Mrs. S. was functioning independently in her home until her son and daughter found her on the floor, mildly confused and disoriented, complaining of dizziness. Mrs. S. was transported to the emergency room for further evaluation. She was diagnosed with a right-lung infiltrate via chest x-ray and moderate to severe dehydration. An IV line was started, and she was treated with antibiotics and admitted for observation. A 12-lead EKG showed a sinus bradycardia at 54 beats per minute. A CT scan of the head was not performed; instead, Mrs. S. was placed on observation and admitted to a medical–surgical unit.

After the 3-week-long hospitalization, Mrs. S. is transferred via wheelchair to the rehabilitation unit. During the admission assessment, you note Mrs. S.'s total fall-risk score increased by 4 points due to increased confusion and disorientation, periods of restlessness, and reduced mobility. Mrs. S.'s vital signs are stable. You learn from the nursing report that Mrs. S. needs constant supervision or she wanders off the unit. During the physical examination, you are paged overhead and respond by going to the nursing station. When you return to examine Mrs. S., she is gone. A second overhead page is called "stat" for assistance on your unit. Apparently, Mrs. S. was found sitting on the floor outside of the elevator, complaining of pain in her right hip and right ankle.

The immediate post-fall assessment shows possible loss of consciousness because Mrs. S. was observed unresponsive for a few seconds. There is evidence of a head injury with a laceration and hematoma to the scalp, as well as right lower leg pain and swelling. Mrs. S.'s sitting BP is 80/50 and her pulse is 60, regular but weak. Ice is applied to her scalp and her leg is immobilized. The physician is notified immediately and a STAT CT scan of the head is ordered, which later confirmed an acute intracranial bleed. Mrs. S. is prepared for cranial surgery and then hip-fracture repair the following day.

1. **What nursing actions should have been taken to prevent the fall and serious injury?**

   Mrs. S. is at high risk for serious injury due to her fall-risk screen score and use of an anticoagulation medication, Coumadin. The standard of practice for caring for an older adult hospitalized with increased risk for falls with serious injury requires the nurse to recognize that this patient is likely to have impaired judgment and inability to follow directions due to her disorientation, relocation to a new unit, and evidence of restlessness. Because she is ambulatory but forgetful, this creates a situation in which the patient needs constant supervision. Mrs. S. should be allowed to ambulate but only with 1:1 supervision and/or physical assistance whenever possible. The nurse failed to recognize the importance of providing constant supervision to the patient. Actions that should have been undertaken include constant supervision by support staff, such as volunteers and/or a special assignment of a nurse's aide to stay with the patient. Family would need to be notified of this decision and to enlist their support for considering a private-duty nursing assistant. Acute confusion or delirium renders Mrs. S. unsafe to make the necessary decisions or judgments about her care.

In terms of preventing serious injury, Mrs. S. should be offered a hip protector, which are indicated in the standard of practice, especially for older adults who are deemed of high risk for fracture. Osteoporotic older adults who fall are likely to fracture an extremity or incur serious injury. Thus, the standard of practice also calls for the use of a low-rise bed and floor mats in the event of a potential bed fall. Anticipating the patient's needs by regular rounds and toileting can help prevent urinary accidents and/or falls en route to the bathroom.

It is imperative for Mrs. S.'s mobility that she be allowed to continue to move freely and ambulate, provided she is supervised and/or assisted because of her disorientation. Daily walking on the unit, in the patient's room, and whenever possible to increase mobility is essential.

2. **How should the nursing assessment be focused?**
Further assessment for reversible causes of delirium is warranted. Because the Theophylline and Atrovent may have exacerbated the confusion, thus they may need to be discontinued. A pharmacy consultation as part of the interdisciplinary assessment would be appropriate. Alternative respiratory interventions for increased pulmonary secretions such as clapping, postural drainage deep breathing, and use of an inspirometery could be instituted.

Further assessment of Mrs. S.'s falls (i.e., a fall evaluation) is clinically indicated. She has had two falls recently, one at home and one at the hospital. The etiology of these falls is not clear. The history of "being dazed" occurring in both falls warrants additional workup. In the emergency room, the patient did not receive a CT scan of her head. The fall evaluation includes, among other tests, a 24-hour Holter monitor. A consultation with a geriatrician and /or neurologist is clinically warranted.

Summary

Fall prevention is a shared responsibility by all health care providers and professionals caring for older adult patients. National recommendations exist to guide practice and should be routinely incorporated into any fall-prevention program and practice policy. Some of the evidence-based research presented in this chapter can help clinicians make choices about the most efficacious or effective interventions, remembering that this choice changes with changes in the patient's condition. Therefore, selecting the most appropriate intervention will always depend on what the nursing and medical assessment determine the likely cause of the fall to be and the medical stability of the patient at that time. Among older adults with advanced years of age with complex illness and multiple co-morbidites and geriatric syndromes, this determination becomes increasingly more challenging but not impossible to determine. The safety of older adults in the hospital and continuing on discharge to home depends on continual assessment and reevaluation of their condition coupled with education, use of the most effective and safest technology, and the older adult's knowledge and willingness to participate in evidenced-based care.

Resources

ACE Units

www.NICHE.org

Patient Safety Goals for Fall Prevention

http://www.jointcommission.org/PatientSafety/NationalPateintsSafetyGoals

Evidenced-Based Clinical Practice Guidelines for Falls Prevention

http://www.ngc.gov/search/searchresults.aspx?Type=3&txtSearch=falls+
    prevention&num=20

Clinical Practice Guidelines for Falls Prevention

http://www.amda.com/clinical/falls
http://www.americangeriatrics.org/products/postionpapers/Falls.pdf

Fall Prevention Strategies in Healthcare Settings

http://www.ecri.org

Best Practice Examples Related to Falls Prevention

Institute for Healthcare Improvement http://www.ihi.org National Center for
    Injury Prevention and Control What You Can Do to Prevent Falls: Senior
    Falls, A Toolkit to Prevent Falls http://www.cdc.gov/ncipc/pub-res/toolkit/
    WhatYouCanDoToPreventFalls.htm Accessed May 9, 2007.

Medical Standards and Guidelines

Clinical Guidelines for the Assessment and Implementation of Bedrails in Hos-
    pitals, Long Term Care Facilities http://www.medmalrx.com Accessed May
    9, 2007

Box 9.1

Nursing Standard of Practice Protocol: Fall Prevention

I. GOALS

A. Prevent falls and serious injury outcomes in hospitalized older adults.

B. Recognize multifactorial risks and causes of falls in older adults.

C. Institute recommendations for falls prevention and management consistent with clinical practice guidelines and standards of care.

II. OVERVIEW

Falls among older adults are not a normal consequence of aging; rather, they are considered a geriatric syndrome most often due to discrete multifactorial and interacting, predisposing (intrinsic and extrinsic risks), and precipitating (dizziness, syncope) causes (Rubenstein & Josephson, 2006 [Level I]; Gray-Miceli et al., 2005 [Level VI]). Fall epidemiology varies according to clinical setting. In acute care, fall incidence ranges from 2.3 to 7 falls per 1,000 patient days depending on the unit (Fletcher, 2005). Nearly one-third of older adults living in the community fall each year in their home. The highest fall incidence occurs in the institutional long term care setting (i.e., nursing home), where 50% to 75% of the 1.63 million nursing home residents experience a fall yearly. Falls rank as the eighth leading cause of unintentional injury for older Americans and were responsible for more than 16,000 deaths in 2006 (CDC, NCIPC, 2007 [Level VI]).

III. BACKGROUND AND STATEMENT OF THE PROBLEM

A. Definition

1. Fall: A fall is an unexpected event in which the participant comes to rest on the ground, floor, or lower level (ProFaNE, 2006 [Level VI]).

B. Fall Etiology

1. Fall risk factors include intrinsic risks of cognitive, vision, gait or balance impairment, high risk/contraindicated medications, and/or the extrinsic risks of assistive devices, inappropriate footwear, restraint, use of nonsturdy furniture or equipment, poor lighting, uneven or slippery surfaces (Chang et al., 2004 [Level I]).

2. Fall causes include, among others, orthostatic hypotension, arrhythmia, infection, generalized or focal muscular weakness, syncope, seizure, hypoglycemia, neuropathy, and medication.

IV. PARAMETERS OF ASSESSMENT

A. Assess and document all older adult patients for intrinsic risk factors to fall:
   1. Advancing age, especially if older than 75
   2. History of a recent fall
   3. Specific co-morbidities: dementia, hip fracture, Type II diabetes, Parkinson's disease, arthritis, and depression
   4. Functional disability: use of assistive device
   5. Alteration in level of consciousness or cognitive impairment
   6. Gait, balance, or visual impairment
   7. Use of high risk medications (Chang et al., 2004 [Level I])
   8. Urge urinary incontinence (Brown, Vittinghoff, & Wyman, 2000 [Level III])
   9. Physical restraint use (Capezuti, Maislin, Strumpf, & Evans, 2002 [Level III])
   10. Bare feet or inappropriate footwear
   11. Identify risks for significant injury due to current use of anticoagulants such as Coumadin, Plavix, or aspirin and/or those with osteoporosis or risks for osteoporosis (Resnick, 2003 [Level VI])
B. Assess and document patient-care environment routinely for extrinsic risk factors to fall and institute corrective action:
   1. Floor surfaces for spills, wet areas, unevenness
   2. Proper level of illumination and functioning of lights (night light works)
   3. Table tops, furniture, beds are sturdy and are in good repair
   4. Grabrails and grabbars are in place in the bathroom
   5. Use of adaptive aides work properly and are in good repair
   6. Bedrails do not collapse when used for transitioning or support
   7. Patient gowns/clothing do not cause tripping
   8. IV poles are sturdy if used during ambulation and tubing does not cause tripping
C. Perform a PFA following a patient fall to identify possible fall causes (if possible, begin the identification of possible causes within 24 hours of a fall) as determined during the immediate, interim, and longitudinal post-fall intervals. Because of known incidences of delayed complication of falls, including fractures, observe all patients for about 48 hours after an observed or suspected fall (AGS, 2001 [Level VI]; ECRI, 2006 [Level VI]; Gray-Miceli et al., 2006 [Level III]):
   1. Perform a physical assessment of the patient at the time of the fall, including vital signs (which may include orthostatic blood pressure readings), neurological assessment, and evaluation for head, neck, spine, and/or extremity injuries.
   2. Once the assessment rules out any significant injury:
      a. obtain a history of the fall by the patient or witness description and document

        b. note the circumstances of the fall: location, activity, time of day, and any significant symptoms

        c. review of underlying illness and problems

        d. review medications

        e. assess functional, sensory, and psychological status

        f. evaluate environmental conditions

        g. review risk factors for falling (AGS, 2001; AMDA, 1998; ECRI, 2006; UIGN, 2004; Resnick, 2003 [all Level VI])

D. In the acute care setting, an integrated multidisciplinary team (consisting of the physician, nurse, health care provider, risk manager, physical therapist, and other designated staff) plans care for the older adult, at risk for falls or who has fallen, hinged on findings from an individualized assessment (ECRI, 2006; JCAHO, 2006 [both Level VI]).

E. The process approach to an individualized PFA includes use of standardized measurement tools of patient risk in combination with a fall-focused history and physical examination, functional assessment, and review of medications (AGS, 2001; AMDA, 1998; Resnick, 2003; UIGN, 2004 [all Level VI]). When plans of care are targeted to likely causes, individualized interventions are likely to be identified. If falling continues despite attempts at individualized interventions, the standard of care warrants a reexamination of the older adult and their falls

V. NURSING CARE STRATEGIES

A. General safety precaution and fall prevention measures that apply to all patients, especially older adults:

    1. Assess the patient care environment routinely for extrinsic risk factors and institute appropriate corrective action.

        a. Use standardized environmental checklists to screen; document findings.

        b. Communicate findings to risk managers, housekeeping, maintenance department, all staff and hospital administration, if needed.

        c. Reevaluate environment for safety (ECRI, 2006 [Level VI]).

    2. On admission, assess/screen older adult patient for multifactorial risk factors to fall, following a change in condition, on transfer to a new unit, and following a fall (ECRI, 2006 [Level VI]):

        a. Use standardized or empirically tested fall-risk tools in conjunction with other assessment tools to evaluate risk for falling (e.g., Tinetti Performance Oriented Mobility, The Timed Get Up and Go Test; AGS, 2001 [Level VI]).

        b. Document findings in nursing notes, interdisciplinary progress notes, and the problem list.

        c. Communicate and discuss findings with interdisciplinary team members.

d. In the interdisciplinary discussion, include review and reduction or elimination of high risk medications associated with falling.

e. As part of falls protocol in the facility, flag the chart or use graphic or color display of the patient's risk potential to fall.

f. Communicate to the patient and the family caregiver identified risk to fall and specific interventions chosen to minimize the patient's risk.

g. Include patient and family members in the interdisciplinary plan of care and discussion about fall-prevention measures.

h. Promote early mobility and incorporate measures to increase mobility, such as daily walking, if medically stable and not otherwise contraindicated.

i. Upon transfer to another unit, communicate the risk assessment and interventions chosen and their effectiveness in fall prevention.

j. Upon discharge, review with the older patient and or family caregiver the fall risk factors and measures to prevent falls in the home. Provide patient literature/brochures if available. If not readily available, refer to the Internet for appropriate Web sites and resources.

k. Explore with the older patient and/or family caregiver avenues to maintain mobility and functional status; consider referral to home-based exercise or group exercises at community senior centers. If discharge is planned to a subacute or rehabilitation unit, label the older adult's mobility status, functional status, and other forms of activity in the home to increase gait or balance on the transfer form.

3. Institute general safety precautions according to facility protocol, which may include:

a. Referral to a falls-prevention program

b. Use of a low-rise bed that measures 14 inches from floor

c. Use of floor mats if patient is at risk for serious injury, such as osteoporosis

d. Easy access to call light

e. Minimization and/or avoidance of physical restraints

f. Use of personal or pressure sensors alarms

g. Increased observation and surveillance

h. Use of rubber-soled healed shoes or nonskid slippers

i. Regular toileting at set intervals and/or continence program; provide easy access to urinals and bedpans

j. Observation during walking rounds or safety rounds

k. Use of corrective glasses for walking

l. Reduction of clutter in traffic areas

m. Early mobility program (ECRI, 2006 [Level VI])

4. Provide staff with clear, written procedures describing what to do when a patient fall occurs.

B. Identify specific patients requiring additional safety precautions and/or evaluation by a specialist, or:
   1. those with impaired judgment or thinking due to acute or chronic illness (delirium, mental illness)
   2. those with osteoporosis, at risk for fracture
   3. those with current hip fracture
   4. those with current head or brain injury (standard of care)

C. Review and discuss with interdisciplinary team findings from the individualized assessment and develop a multidisciplinary plan of care to prevent falls (Chang et al., 2004 [Level I]).
   1. Communicate to the physician or advance practice nurse important PFA findings (ECRI, 2006 [Level VI]).
   2. Monitor the effectiveness of the falls prevention interventions instituted.
   3. Following a patient's fall, observe for serious injury due to a fall and follow facility protocols for management (standard of care).
   4. Following a patient's fall, monitor vital signs, level of consciousness, neurological checks, and functional status per facility protocol. If significant changes in patient's condition occurs, consider further diagnostic tests such as plain film x-rays, CT scan of the head/spine/extremity, neurological consultation, and /or transfer to a specialty unit for further evaluation (standard of care).

VI. EVALUATION/EXPECTED OUTCOMES

A. Patient:
   1. Safety will be maintained.
   2. Falls will be avoided.
   3. Will not develop serious injury outcomes from a fall if it occurs.
   4. Will know their risks for falling.
   5. Will be prepared on discharge to prevent falls in their homes.
   6. Prehospitalization level of mobility will continue.
   7. Who develops fall-related complications such as injury or change in cognitive function will be promptly assessed and treated to prevent adverse outcomes.

B. Nursing Staff:
   1. Will be able to accurately detect, refer, and manage older adults at risk for falling or who have experienced a fall.
   2. Will integrate into their practice comprehensive assessment and management approaches for falls prevention in the institution.
   3. Will gain appreciation for older adults' unique experience of falling and how it influences their daily living, functional, physical, and emotional status.

4. Will educate older adult patients anticipating discharge about falls prevention strategies.

VII. FOLLOW-UP MONITORING OF CONDITION

A. Monitor fall incidence and incidences of patient injury due to a fall, comparing rates on the same unit over time.
B. Compare falls per patient month against national benchmarks available in the National Database of Nursing Quality Indicators.
C. Incorporate continuous quality improvement criteria into falls prevention program.
D. Identify falls team members and roles of clinical and nonclinical staff (ECRI, 2006 [Level VI]).
E. Educate patient and family caregivers about falls prevention strategies so they are prepared for discharge (JHF, 2003 [Level VI]; UIGN, 2004 [Level VI]).

VIII. RELEVANT PRACTICE GUIDELINES

A. American Geriatrics Society, British Geriatrics Society, American Academy of Orthopedic Surgeons (AGS/BGS/AAOS) Guidelines for the Prevention of Falls in Older Persons (2001). *Journal of American Geriatrics Society, 49*, 664–672. Evidence Level VI: Expert Opinion.
B. American Medical Directors Association (AMDA). Falls and fall risk. Columbia, MD: American Medical Directors Association. Evidence Level VI: Expert Opinion.
C. University of Iowa Gerontological Nursing Interventions Research Center (UIGN). (2004). Falls prevention for older adults. Iowa City, IA: University of Iowa Gerontological Nursing Interventions Research Center, Research Dissemination Core. Evidence Level VI: Expert Opinion.
D. ECRI Institute: Falls Prevention Strategies in Healthcare Settings (2006). Plymouth Meeting, PA. Evidence Level VI: Expert Opinion.
E. Resnick, B. (2003). Preventing falls in acute care. In: M. Mezey, T. Fulmer, I. Abraham (Managing Ed.) & D. Zwicker (Eds.). *Geriatric nursing protocols for best practice* (2nd ed., pp. 141–164). New York: Springer Publishing Company, Inc. Evidence Level VI: Expert Opinion.

References

Agostini, J. V., Baker, D. I., & Bogardus, S. T. (2001). Making health care safer: A critical analysis of patient safety practices. Agency for Healthcare Research and Quality (AHRQ). File Inventory, Evidence Report/Technology Assessment Number 43. AHRQ Publication No. 01-E058, Rockville, MD. Chapter 26: Prevention of Falls in Hospitalized and Institutionalized Older People. Retrieved May 15, 2004, from http://www.ahrq.gov/clinic/ptsftinv.htm. Evidence Level VI: Expert Opinion.

American Geriatrics Society, British Geriatrics Society, American Academy of Orthopedic Surgeons Panel on Falls Prevention (AGS, BGS, AAOS) (2001). Guidelines for the prevention of falls in older persons. *Journal of the American Geriatrics Society, 49*(5), 664–681. Evidence Level VI: Expert Opinion.

American Medical Directors Association (AMDA) (1998). *Falls and fall risk*. Columbia, MD: AMDA. Evidence Level VI: Expert Opinion.

American Nurses Association (ANA) (2002). *Code of ethics*. Evidence Level VI: Expert Opinion.

Barnett, A., Smith, B., Lord, S. R., Williams, M., & Baumand, A. (2003). Community-based group exercise improves balance and reduces falls in at-risk older people: A randomized controlled trial. *Age & Ageing, 32*(4), 407–414. Evidence Level II: Randomized Controlled Trial.

Brennan, S., Dewar, C., Sen, J., Clarke, D., Marshall, T., & Murray, P. I. (2003). A prospective study of the rate of falls before and after cataract surgery. *British Journal of Ophthalmology, 87,* 560–562. Evidence Level III: Quasi-experimental Study.

Brown, J. S., Vittinghoff, E., & Wyman, J. F. (2000). The study of osteoporotic fractures research group. Urinary incontinence: Does it increase risk for falls and fractures? *Journal of the American Geriatric Society, 48,* 721–725. Evidence Level III: Quasi-experimental Study.

Capezuti, E., Maislin, G., Strumpf, N., & Evans, L. K. (2002). Side-rail use and bed-related fall outcomes among nursing home residents. *Journal of the American Geriatrics Society, 50*(1), 90–96. Evidence Level III: Quasi-experimental Study.

Carter, N. D., Kannus, P., & Khan, K. M. (2001). Exercise in the prevention of falls in older people: A systematic literature review examining the rationale and the evidence. *Sports Medicine, 31*(6), 427–438. Evidence Level I: Systematic Integrative Review.

Centers for Disease Control and Prevention (CDC), National Center for Injury Prevention and Control (NCIPC) (2007). Preventing falls among older adults. Retrieved May 29, 2007, from cdc.gov/ncipc/duip/preventadultfalls.htm. Evidence Level VI: Expert Opinion.

Centers for Disease Control (CDC) (2006). Fatalities and injuries from falls among older adults: United States, 1993–2003 and 2001–2005. November 17, 2006, *Morbidity and Mortality Weekly Report, 55,* 45. Evidence Level VI: Expert Opinion.

Chang, J. T., Morton, S. C., Rubenstein, L. Z., Mojica, W. A., Maglione, M., Suttorp, M. J., et al. (2004). Interventions for the prevention of falls in older adults: Systematic review and meta-analysis of randomized controlled trials. *British Medical Journal, 328*(7441), 680. Evidence Level I: Systematic Meta-analysis Review.

Close, J., Ellis, M., Hooper, R., Glucksman, E., Jackson, S., & Swift, C. (1999). Prevention of falls in the elderly trial (PROFET): A randomized controlled trial. *Lancet, 353,* 93–97. Evidence Level II: Randomized Controlled Trial.

Connell, B. R. (1996). Role of the environment in falls prevention. *Clinics in Geriatric Medicine, 12*(4), 859–880. Evidence Level VI: Expert Opinion.

Counsell, S. R., Holder, C. M., Liebenauer, L. L., Palmer, R. M., Fortinsky, R. H., Kresevic, D. M., et al. (2000). Effects of a multicomponent intervention on functional outcomes and process of care in hospitalized older patients: A randomized controlled trial of Acute Care for Elders (ACE) in a community hospital. *Journal of the American Geriatrics Society, 48*(12), 1572–1581. Evidence Level II: Randomized Controlled Trial.

Dempsey, J. (2004). Fall prevention revisited: A call for a new approach. *Journal of Clinical Nursing, 13*(4), 479–485. Evidence Level IV: Quasi-experimental Study.

DiMaio, V. J. M., Dana, S. E., & Bux, R. C. (1986). Deaths caused by vest restraint. *Journal of the American Medical Association, 255,* 905. Evidence Level V: Case Report.

DiNunno, N., Vacca, M., Costantinedes, F., & DiNunno, C. (2003). Death following atypical compression of the neck. *American Journal of Forensic Medicine and Pathology, 24,* 364–368. Evidence Level V: Case Report.

Dube, A. H., & Mitchell, E. K. (1986). Accidental strangulation from vest restraints. *Journal of the American Medical Association, 256,* 2725–2726. Evidence Level VI: Expert Opinion.

ECRI Institute (2006). *Falls prevention strategies in healthcare settings guide*. Plymouth Meeting, PA: ECRI Publishers. Evidence Level VI: Expert Opinion.

Ensrud, K. E., Blackwell, T. L., Mangione, C. M., Bowman, P. J., Whooley, M. A., Bauer, D. C., et al. (2002). Study of Osteoporotic Fractures Research Group. Central nervous system–active medications and risk for falls in older women. *Journal of the American Geriatrics Society, 50*(10), 1629–1637. Evidence Level II: Randomized Controlled Trial.

Fischer, I. D., Krauss, M. J., Dunagan, W. C., Birge, S., Hitcho, E., Johnson, S., et al. (2005). Patterns and predictors of in-patient falls and fall-related injuries in a large academic hospital. *Infection Control Hospital Epidemiology*, *26*(10), 822–827. Evidence Level IV: Nonexperimental Study.

Gray-Miceli, D., Johnson, J. C., & Strumpf, N. E. (2005). A step-wise approach to a comprehensive post-fall assessment. *Annals of Long Term Care: Clinical Care and Aging*, *13*(12), 16–24. Evidence Level VI: Expert Opinion.

Gray-Miceli, D., Strumpf, N. E., Johnson, J. C., Dragascu, M., & Ratcliffe, S. (2006). Psychometric properties of the post-fall index. *Clinical Nursing Research*, *15*(3), 157–176. Evidence Level III: Quasi-experimental Study.

Gray-Miceli, D., Strumpf, N. E., Reinhard, S. C., Zanna, M. T., & Fritz, E. (2004). Current approaches to post-fall assessment. *Journal of the American Medical Directors Association*, *5*(6), 387–394. Evidence Level IV: Nonexperimental Study.

Gray-Miceli, D. G., Waxman, H., Cavalieri, T., & Lage, S. (1991). Prodromal falls among older nursing home residents. *Applied Nursing Research*, *7*(1), 18–27. Evidence Level IV: Nonexperimental Study.

Gregg, E. W., Pereira, M. A., & Caspersen, C. J. (2000). Physical activity, falls, and fractures among older adults: A review of epidemiological evidence. *Journal of the American Geriatrics Society*, *48*(8), 883–893. Evidence Level V: Systematic Integrative Review.

Haines, T. P., Bennell, K. L., Osborne, R. H., & Hill, K. D. (2004). Effectiveness of targeted falls prevention program in subacute hospital setting: Randomized controlled trial. *British Medical Journal*, *328*, 676. Evidence Level II: Randomized Controlled Trial.

Hauer, K., Roos, B., Rutschle, K., Opitz, H., Specht, N., & Bartsch, P., et al. (2001). Exercise training for rehabilitation and secondary prevention of falls in geriatric patients with a history of injurious falls. *Journal of the American Geriatric Society*, *49*(1), 10–20. Evidence Level II: Randomized Controlled Trial.

Heitterachi, E., Lord, S. R., Meyerkorf, P., McCloskey, I., & Fitzpatrick, R. (2002). Blood pressure changes on upright tilting predict falls in older people. *Age & Ageing*, *31*(3), 181–186. Evidence Level III: Quasi-experimental Study.

International Classification of Disease Manual ICD-10 (2006). World Health Organization, Geneva: Switzerland. Evidence Level VI: Expert Opinion.

Joint Commission on Accreditation of Healthcare Organizations (JCAHO). (2006). Root causes of patient falls. Joint Commission on Accreditation of Healthcare Organizations. Retrieved on March 31, 2007, from http://www.jointcommission.org/NR/rdonlyres/FA5A080F-C259-47CC-AAC8-BAC3F5C. Evidence Level V: Case Report.

Joint Commission on Accreditation of Healthcare Organizations (JCAHO). (2006). Joint Commission on National Patient Safety Goals (NPSG). Joint Commission on Accreditation of Healthcare Organizations. Retrieved on May 2, 2007, from http://www.jcaho.org. Evidence Level VI: Expert Opinion.

Kamel, H. K. (2004). Secondary prevention of hip fractures among hospitalized elderly: Are we doing enough? *The Internet Journal of Geriatrics and Gerontology*, *1*(1), 1–5. Available on the Internet at http://www.ispub.com/ostia/index.php?xmlFilePath=journals/ijgg/vol1n1/hip.xml. Evidence Level IV: Nonexperimental Study.

Kellogg International Working Group on Fall Prevention in the Elderly (1987). The prevention of falls in later life. *Danish Medical Bulletin* (Suppl. 4), 1–24. Evidence Level VI: Expert Opinion.

Kelly, K. E., Phillips, C. L., Cain, K. C., Polissar, N. L., & Kelly, P. B. (2002). Evaluation of a nonintrusive monitor to reduce falls in nursing home patients. *Journal of the American Medical Directors Association*, *3*(6), 377–382. Evidence Level IV: Nonexperimental Study.

Kenne, G. S., Parker, M. J., & Pryor, G. A. (1993). Mortality and morbidity of hip fracture. *British Medical Journal*, *307*, 1248–1250. Evidence Level II: Single Experimental Study.

Koepsell, T. D., Wolf, M. E., Buchner, D. M., Kukull, W. A., LaCroix, A. Z., Tencer, A. F., et al. (2004). Footwear style and risk of falls in older adults. *Journal of the American Geriatrics Society*, *52*(9), 1495–1501. Evidence Level IV: Nonexperimental Study.

Kwok, T., Mok, F., Chien, W. T., & Tam, E. (2006). Does access to bed-chair pressure sensors reduce physical restraint use in the rehabilitation setting? *Journal of Clinical Nursing*, *15*(5), 581–587. Evidence Level II: Randomized Controlled Trial.

Langlois, J. A., Rutland-Brown, W., & Thomas, K. E. (2006). *Traumatic brain injury in the United States: Emergency department visits, hospitalization and deaths*. Atlanta, GA: CDC and the National Center for Injury Prevention and Control. Evidence Level V: Narrative Review.

Leipzig, R. M., Cumming, R. G., & Tinetti, M. E. (1999). Drugs and falls in older people: A systematic review and meta-analysis: Cardiac and analgesic drugs. *Journal of the American Geriatrics Society, 47*(1), 40–50. Evidence Level I: Systematic Meta-analysis.

Lindsay, R., James, E. L., & Kippen, S. (2004). The timed Get Up and Go Test: Unable to predict falls on the acute medical ward. *Australian Journal of Physiotherapy, 50*(4), 249–251. Evidence Level III: Quasi-experimental Study.

Magaziner, J., Lydick, E., Hawkes, W., Fox, K. M., Zimmerman, S. I., & Epstein, R. S. (1997). Excess mortality attributable to hip fracture in White women aged 70 years and older. *American Journal of Public Health, 87*(10), 1630–1636. Evidence Level V: Narrative Literature Review.

Maki, B. E., & McIllroy, W. E. (2003). Effects of aging on control of stability. In L. Luxon et al. (Eds.), *A textbook of audiological medicine: Clinical aspects of hearing and balance* (pp. 671–690). London: Marin Dunitz Publishers. Evidence Level VI: Expert Opinion.

Marottolli, R. A., Berkman, L. F., & Cooney, L. M. (1992). Decline in physical function following hip fracture. *Journal of the American Geriatrics Society, 40*(9), 861–866. Evidence Level II: Randomized Controlled Trial.

McInnes, E., & Askie, L. (2004). Evidence review on older people's views and experiences of falls-prevention strategies. *Worldviews on Evidenced-Based Nursing, 1*(1), 20–37. Evidence Level I: Systematic Integrative Review.

Miles, S. H. (2002). Deaths between bedrails and air-pressure mattresses. *Journal of the American Geriatrics Society, 50*, 1124–1125. Evidence Level VI: Expert Opinion.

National Database of Nursing Quality Indicators (NDNQI) (2005). Retrieved April 20, 2007, from www.nursingworld.org/quality/database.htm. Evidence Level VI: Expert Opinion.

Nelson, A., Powell-Cope, G., Gavin-Dreschnack, D., Quigley, P., Bulat, T., & Baptiste, A.S., et al. (2004). Technology to promote safe mobility in the elderly. *Nursing Clinics of North America, 39*(3), 649–671. Evidence Level VI: Expert Opinion.

Neutel, C. I., Perry, S., & Maxwell, C. (2002). Medication use and risk of falls. *Pharmacoepidemiological Drug Safety, 11*(2), 97–104. Evidence Level VI: Expert Opinion.

Oliver, D., Daly, F., Martin, F. C., & McMurdo, M. E. (2004). Risk factors and risk assessment tools for falls in hospital in patients: A systematic review. *Age & Ageing, 33*(2), 122–130. Evidence Level I: Systematic Integrative Review.

Oliver, D., Hopper, A., & Seed, P. (2000). Do hospital fall-prevention programs work? A systematic review. *Journal of the American Geriatrics Society, 48*(12), 1679–1689. Evidence Level I: Systematic Integrative Review.

Ooi, W. L., Hossain, M., & Lipsitz, L. A. (2000). The association between orthostatic hypotension and recurrent falls in nursing home residents. *American Journal of Medicine, 108*(2), 106–111. Evidence Level IV: Nonexperimental Study.

Papaioannou, A., Parkinson, W., Cook, R., Ferko, N., Corker, E., & Adachi, J. D. (2004). Prediction of falls using a risk assessment tool in the acute care setting. *BioMed Central, 21*, 21. Evidence Level III: Quasi-experimental Study.

Parker, M. J., Gillespie, W. J., & Gillespie, L. D. (2006). Effectiveness of hip protectors for preventing hip fractures in elderly people. *BMJ, 332*(7541), 571–574. Evidence Level I: Systematic Integrative Review.

Perell, K. L., Nelson, A., Goldman, R., Luther, S. L., Prieto-Lewis, N., Rubenstein, L. Z. (2001). Fall-risk assessment measures: An analytic review. *Journal of Gerontology, 56*(A) (12), 761–766. Evidence Level V: Narrative Review.

Prevention of Falls Network Europe (ProFaNE) (2006). Retrieved April 19, 2007, from http://www.profane.eu.org. Evidence Level VI: Expert Opinion.

Public Health Agency of Canada (2007). Aging and seniors. Retrieved March 21, 2007, from http://www.phac-aspc.gc.ca/seniors-aines/pubs/seniorsfalls/chapter3e.htm. Evidence Level VI: Expert Opinion.

Ray, W. A., Taylor, J. A., Meador, K. G., Thapa, P. B., Brown, A. K., Kajihara, H. K., et al. (1997). A randomized trial of a consultation service to reduce falls in nursing homes. *Journal of the American Medical Association, 278*, 557–562. Evidence Level II: Randomized Controlled Trial.

Resnick, B. (2003). Preventing falls in acute care. In M. Mezey, T. Fulmer, I. Abraham, & D. Zwicker (Eds.), (Managing Ed.) *Geriatric nursing protocols for best practice* (2nd ed., pp. 141–164). New York: Springer Publishing Company, Inc. Evidence Level VI: Expert Opinion.

Romano, P. S., Geppert, J. J., Davies, S., Miller, M. R., Elixhauser, A., & McDonald, K. (2003). A national profile of patient safety in U.S. hospitals. *Health Affairs, 22*(2), 154–166. Evidence Level V: Case Report.

Rubenstein, L. Z., & Josephson, K. R. (2002). The epidemiology of falls and syncope. *Clinic Geriatrics Medicine 18*, 141–158. Evidence Level II: Randomized Control Trial.

Rubenstein, L. Z., & Josephson, K. R. (2006). Falls and their prevention in the elderly: What does the evidence show? *Medical Clinics of North American, 90* (5), 807–824. Evidence Level I: Systematic Integrative.

Rubenstein, L. Z., Josephson, K. R., & Trueblood, P. R., et al. (2000). Effects of group exercise on strength, mobility, and falls among fall-prone elderly men. *Journal of Gerontology A: Biological Science Med Sci, 55*(6), M317–M321. Evidence Level II: Randomized Controlled Trial.

Runyan, C. W., Perkis, D., Marshall, S. W., Johnson, R. M., Coyne-Beasley, T., Waller, A. E., et al. (2005). Unintentional injuries in the home in the United States, Part II: Morbidity. *American Journal of Preventive Medicine, 28*(1), 80–87. Evidence Level V: Case Report.

Shaw, F. E. (2002). Falls in cognitive impairment and dementia. *Clinical Geriatric Medicine, 18*(2), 159–173. Evidence Level VI: Expert Opinion.

Smith, R. G. (2003). Fall-contributing adverse effects of the most frequently prescribed drugs. *Journal of the American Podiatric Medical Association, 93*(1), 42–50. Evidence Level VI: Expert Opinion.

Smyth, C., Dubin, S., Restrepo, A., Nueva-Espana, H., & Capezuti, E. (2001). Creating order out of chaos: Models of GNP practice with hospitalized older adults. *Clinical Excellence for Nurse Practitioners, 5*(2), 88–95. Evidence Level IV: Nonexperimental Study.

Stevens, J.A. (2000). Reducing falls and resulting hip fractures among older women. In Centers for Disease Control, Morbidity and Mortality Weekly Report, March 31, 2000/49(RRO2); 1–12. Retreived May 23, 2007, from http:cdc.gov/mmwr/preview/mmwrhtml/rr4902a2.htm. Evidence Level V: Review.

Stolze, H., Klebe, S., Zechlin, C., Baecker, C., Friege, L., & Deuschl, G. (2004). Falls in frequent neurological diseases: Prevalence, risk factors, and etiology. *Journal of Neurology, 251*(1), 79–84. Evidence Level VI: Expert Opinion.

Tencer, A. F., Koepsell, T. D., Wolf, M. E., Frankenfeld, C. L., Buchner, D. M., Kukull, W. A., et al. (2004). Biomechanical properties of shoes and risk of falls in older adults. *Journal of the American Geriatrics Society, 52*(11), 1840–1846. Evidence Level IV: Nonexperimental Study.

Tinetti, M. E., Williams, T. S., & Mayewski, R. (1986). Fall risk index for elderly patients based on number of chronic disabilities. *American Journal of Medicine, 80*(3), 429–434. Evidence Level II: Randomized Controlled Trial.

University of Iowa Gerontological Nursing Interventions Research Center (UIGN). (2004). Fall prevention for older adults. Iowa City, Iowa: University of Iowa Gerontological Nursing Interventions Research Center, Research Dissemination Core. http://www.nursing.uiowa.edu/consumers_patients/evidence_based.htm. Evidence Level VI: Expert Opinion.

U. S. Department of Health and Human Services (USDHHS) (2004). Centers for Medicare and Medicaid Services. Evidence report and evidence-based recommendations: Fall prevention interventions in the Medicare population. RAND; Contract No. 500-98-0281; Period September 30, 1998, to September 29, 2003. Evidence Level I: Systematic Review.

Pain Management

10

Ann L. Horgas
Saunjoo L. Yoon

Educational Objectives

At the completion of this chapter, the reader will be able to:

1. discuss the importance of effective pain management for older adults

2. describe best methods of assessing pain

3. discuss pharmacological and nonpharmacological strategies for managing pain

4. state at least two key points to include in education for patients and families

Background and Significance

Physical pain is a significant problem for many older adults. It has been estimated that at least 50% of community-dwelling older adults suffer from pain (Herr, 2002a; Sha et al., 2005), and among nursing home residents, as many as 85% reportedly experience pain (American Geriatrics Society [AGS], 2002 [Level VI]; Thomas, Flaherty, & Morley, 2001).

The high prevalence of pain is primarily related to the high rate of chronic health disorders among older adults, particularly painful musculoskeletal

---

For a description of Evidence Levels cited in this chapter, see chapter 1, Developing and Evaluating Clinical Practice Guidelines, page 4

conditions such as arthritis, gout, and peripheral vascular disease (Helme & Gibson, 1999). In addition, there is a high prevalence of more acute conditions, such as cardiovascular disease or infection, and other painful medical diseases and syndromes in this age group (Feldt, Warne, & Ryden, 1998). Cancer, in particular, is associated with significant pain for one-third of patients with active disease and for two-thirds of those with advanced disease (Reiner & Lacasse, 2006 [Level I]). Thus, pain among older adults is quite common and also often complicated by the concomitant presence of different types, locations, and causes of pain.

Why is knowledge about pain in older adults so important? There are several key reasons. First, pain has major implications for older adults' health, functioning, and quality of life (AGS, 2002 [Level VI]) and is associated with depression, withdrawal, sleep disturbances, impaired mobility, decreased activity engagement, and increased health care use (Gordon et al., 2002 [Level I]; Herr, 2002a). Other geriatric conditions that can be exacerbated by pain include falls, deconditioning, malnutrition, gait disturbances, and slowed rehabilitation (AGS, 2002 [Level VI]; Gordon et al., 2002 [Level I]). Thus, pain has major implications for physical, functional, and mental health among older adults.

Second, nurses have a key role in assessing and managing pain. The promotion of comfort and relief of pain is fundamental to nursing practice and, as integral members of interdisciplinary health care teams, nurses must work effectively to both assess and treat pain. Given that the prevalence of pain in older adults is substantially higher than among younger adults, this nursing role becomes increasingly important in the older population. In addition, nurses have the primary responsibility to teach the patient and family about pain and how to manage it, both pharmacologically and nonpharmacologically. As such, nurses must be knowledgeable about pain management in general and about managing pain in older adults in particular.

Third, the Joint Commission on Accreditation of Healthcare Organizations (JCAHO), the accrediting body for health care organizations that provide direct care, mandates pain assessment and management as part of the survey and accreditation process (JCAHO, 2001). The Joint Commission declared that "patients have the right to appropriate assessment and management of pain" and considers pain as the fifth vital sign (JCAHO, 2001). Thus, provider compliance with regulatory guidelines about pain management helps guarantee patients' rights, but this does not address pain management needs of older adults experiencing significant pain unless they are hospitalized.

Definitions of Pain

Pain is a multidimensional, subjective experience with sensory, cognitive, and emotional dimensions (AGS, 2002 [Level VI]); Melzack & Casey, 1968). For clinical practice, McCaffery's classic definition of pain is perhaps the most relevant. She states, "Pain is whatever the experiencing person says it is, existing whenever he says it does" (McCaffery, 1968; McCaffery & Pasero, 1999). This definition serves as a reminder that pain is highly subjective and that patients' self-report and description of pain is paramount in the pain assessment process.

Types of Pain

There are several different types and classifications of pain. The most basic distinction is whether the pain is acute or persistent (e.g., chronic pain). Although *persistent pain* and *chronic pain* have been used interchangeably, the term *persistent pain* has recently been adopted because it is believed to have fewer negative connotations (AGS, 2002 [Level VI]; Weiner, Herr, & Rudy, 2002).

Acute pain results from an injury, surgery, or disease-related tissue damage (Panda & Desbiens, 2001). Usually associated with autonomic activity, such as tachycardia and diaphoresis, acute pain is usually relatively brief and subsides with healing. In contrast, *persistent pain* is defined as a painful experience that continues for a prolonged period of time (usually more than 3 to 6 months) (AGS, 2002 [Level VI]; Harkins, 2002). Persistent pain may or may not be associated with a diagnosable disease process and autonomic activity is usually absent (AGS, 2002 [Level VI]; Panda & Desbiens, 2001). Persistent pain can lead to functional loss, reduced quality of life, and mood and behavior changes, especially when it is untreated (Gordon et al., 2002 [Level I]). Persistent and acute pain often coexist among older adults due to high rates of co-morbidity.

Pain is further classified as either *nociceptive* or *neuropathic*, depending on the cause. Nociceptive pain results from disease processes (e.g., osteoarthritis), soft-tissue injuries (e.g., falls), and medical treatment (e.g., surgery, venipuncture, and other procedures) and is associated with stimulation of specific peripheral or visceral receptors. Nociceptive pain is usually localized and responsive to treatment. Neuropathic pain, caused by pathology in the peripheral or central nervous system, is often associated with diabetic neuropathies, phantom-limb pain, post-herpetic and trigeminal neuralgias, stroke, and chemotherapy treatment for cancer. Neuropathic pain is more diffuse and less responsive to analgesics. However, these pain types often overlap and are not always clearly differentiated.

Pain Assessment Strategies

Despite the prevalence and consequences of pain, evidence suggests that pain is under-detected and poorly managed among older adults (Horgas & Tsai, 1998 [Level IV]; Miller, Nelson, & Mezey, 2000; Smith, 2005 [Level I]). There are several factors that contribute to this situation, including individual- and caregiver-based factors. Individual factors that may impair pain assessment include (1) belief that pain is a normal part of aging, (2) concern of being labeled a hypochondriac or complainer, (3) fear of the meaning of pain relative to disease progression or prognosis, (4) fear of narcotic addiction and analgesics, (5) worry about health care costs, and (6) a belief that pain is not important to health care providers (AGS, 2002 [Level VI]; Gordon et al., 2002 [Level I]). Other factors, such as hearing and speech difficulties, may prevent older adults from effectively communicating pain to health care providers (Feldt et al., 1998). In addition, cognitive impairment is an important factor in reducing older adults' ability to report pain (Smith, 2005 [Level I]).

Pain detection and management are also influenced by provider-based factors. Health care providers have been found to share the mistaken belief that pain is a part of the normal aging process and to avoid using opioids due to fear about potential addiction and adverse side effects (Wells, Kaas, & Feldt, 1997). Similarly, cognitive status influences providers' assessment and treatment of pain. For instance, it has been found that cognitively impaired nursing home residents were prescribed and administered significantly less analgesic medication than were cognitively intact older adults (Horgas & Tsai, 1998 [Level IV]). This finding may reflect cognitively impaired adults' inability to recall and report the presence of pain to their health care providers. It may also reflect caregivers' inability to detect pain, especially among frail older adults. In one nursing home study, it was found that patients' and caregivers' reports of pain were congruent in only about one-third of cases (Horgas & Dunn, 2001 [Level IV]). Furthermore, it was noted that depression was highest in residents for whom pain was not perceived by their caregivers. Pain assessment and management can be a complicated clinical issue. Health care providers should face the challenge of pain assessment by first systematically examining their own biases and beliefs about pain and eliciting and understanding the challenges and beliefs their patients bring to the situation as well.

Self-Reported Pain

There is no objective biological marker or laboratory test for the presence of pain. Thus, the most accurate and reliable measure of pain is the patient's self-report. This is also consistent with the definition provided earlier in this chapter—that pain is defined as "whatever the experiencing person says it is, existing whenever he [or she] says it does" (McCaffery, 1968; McCaffery & Pasero, 1999). Evidence suggests that patients with mild to moderate cognitive impairment can report their pain when asked clear questions and given sufficient time to respond (Ferrell, Ferell, & Rivera, 1995 [Level IV]).

The first principle of pain assessment is to *ask* about the presence of pain in regular and frequent intervals (AGS, 2002 [Level VI]). It is mandatory to allow patients sufficient time to consider questions and formulate answers, especially when working with cognitively impaired older adults. It is also important to explore different words that patients may use synonymously with pain, such as *discomfort* or *aching*.

Pain intensity can be measured in various ways. Some commonly used tools include the visual analog scale (VAS), the verbal descriptor scale, and the faces scale (Herr, 2002a). In the VAS, widely used in hospital settings, patients are asked to rate the intensity of their pain on a 0 to 10 scale. The VAS requires the ability to discriminate subtle differences in pain intensity and may be difficult for some older adults to complete. The verbal descriptor scale, however, has been specifically recommended for use with older adults (Herr, 2002a). This tool measures pain intensity by asking participants to select a word that best describes their present pain (e.g., no pain to worst pain imaginable). This measure has been found to be a reliable and valid measure of pain intensity and is reported to be the easiest to complete and the most preferred by older adults (Taylor, Harris, Epps, & Herr, 2005 [Level V]). Pictures of faces (i.e., the faces scales) are also used to measure pain intensity, especially among cognitively impaired older adults. The Faces Pain Scale (FPS), initially developed to assess pain intensity in children, consists of seven cartoon facial depictions, ranging from the least pain to the most pain possible (Bieri, Reeve, Champion, Addicoat, & Ziegler, 1990). Among adults, the FPS is considered more appropriate than other pictorial scales because the cartoon faces are not age-, gender-, or race-specific. However, the FPS has relatively low reliability and validity when used among older adults with cognitive impairment and is not recommended for use in this population (Taylor et al., 2005 [Level V]). See the Resources section for information on accessing these measurement tools.

Observed Pain Indicators

Because some older adults cannot adequately report pain due to dementia and deficits such as compromised cognitive and verbal skills (i.e., memory loss, loss of judgment, confusion, and attention and language deficits), observational assessment of pain behaviors is often necessary. Several researchers have developed methods to directly observe pain behaviors (Feldt, 2000; Hurley, Volicer, Hanrahan, House, & Volicer, 1992; Keefe & Block, 1982; Snow et al., 2004). These methods include recognizing behaviors such as guarded movement, bracing, rubbing the affected area, grimacing, painful noises or words, and restlessness. For instance, Hurley and colleagues (1992) developed the Discomfort Scale-DAT to assess discomfort in persons with advanced Alzheimer's disease. They identified nine indicators of discomfort associated with fever: noisy breathing, absence of a look of contentment, looking sad, looking frightened, frowning, absence of a relaxed body posture, looking tense, negative vocalizations, and fidgeting. This measure, however, has been reported to require significant training and to be too complex for routine nursing care (Miller, Moore, Schofield, & Ng'andu, 1996). Feldt and colleagues developed the Checklist for Nonverbal Pain Behaviors to assess the presence of six pain behaviors during rest and movement (Feldt et al., 1998). This tool is based on naturalistic observations of hospitalized older adults, has shown high inter rater reliability (93% agreement; Kappa = 0.63 – 0.82), and is positively associated with self-reports of pain (Feldt, 2000). More recently, Snow and colleagues developed the NOPPAIN scale for assessing pain in noncommunicative nursing home residents (Snow et al., 2004). The NOPPAIN is used by certified nursing assistants to rate the presence and intensity of pain among residents following usual care activities. The results of preliminary studies testing the NOPPAIN indicate that it is reliable and valid but that further testing is needed in different clinical settings (Taylor et al., 2005 [Level VI]). Taken together, several tools are available to measure behavioral indicators of pain, but all of them need further development and testing before they can be adopted for widespread use in clinical practice (Herr, Bjoro, & Decker, 2006 [Level I]).

In summary, pain assessment is a clinical procedure that can be hampered by many factors. Systematic and thorough assessment, however, is a critical first step in appropriately managing pain in older adults. Assessment issues are summarized in the recommended pain management protocol. The use of a standardized pain assessment tool is important in measuring pain: it enables health care providers to document their assessment; measure change in pain; evaluate treatment effectiveness; and communicate to other health care providers, the patient, and the family. Comprehensive pain assessment includes measures of self-reported pain and pain behaviors and includes information from patients and families as well.

Pain Management Strategies

Managing pain in older adults can be a challenging process. The main goal is to maximize function and quality of life (Herr, 2002b) by minimizing pain whenever possible (Wisconsin Medical Society Task Force on Pain Management, 2004 [Level VI]). Pain treatments that use a multidimensional approach and are tailored to the patient, however, are often effective (Gibson, Farrell, Katz, & Helme, 1996). Thus, a combination of pharmacological and nonpharmacological strategies should be used to ease the pain.

Several excellent pain assessment protocols have been developed for use with older adults. For instance, the American Geriatrics Society (AGS) published clinical practice guidelines for managing persistent pain in older adults (AGS, 2002 [Level VI]) and evidence-based exercise practice recommendations for older adults with osteoarthritis pain (AGS, 2001 [Level VI]). These guidelines provide comprehensive information specific to the needs of geriatric patients. In addition, there are other published guidelines for the management of pain in osteoarthritis, rheumatoid arthritis, and juvenile chronic arthritis (American Pain Society, 2002) and for the relief of cancer pain (American Pain Society, 2005; World Health Organization, 1996). These guidelines are disease-specific, rather than age-group specific but provide comprehensive information for managing these chronic pain conditions. See the Treatment Guidelines section of Box 10.1 for information on how to access this information.

Pharmacological Pain Treatment

Pain treatment with medications involves a complex decision-making process based on multiple considerations. Ideally, it is a mutual process among health care providers, patients, and caregivers. It includes a careful discussion of risks versus benefits, frequent reviews of drug regimens used by older adults, and the establishment of clear goals of therapy. Often it is a process of trial and error that aims to balance medication effectiveness with management of side effects. Other considerations included in the process are frequency of use, type of pain, severity of pain, duration of treatment, and cost.

The World Health Organization (WHO, 1996) provides a three-step analgesic ladder that has been widely used as a guide for treating cancer pain. Choices are made from three drug categories based on three levels of pain severity: nonopioids, opioids, and adjuvant agents. Combinations of drugs are used because two or more drugs can treat different underlying pain mechanisms and different types of pain and allow for smaller doses of each analgesic to be used, thus minimizing side effects. The WHO (1996) recommends choosing analgesics based on the principles of by mouth, by the clock, by the ladder, for the individual, and attention to detail. These principles can be applied to effectively manage persistent noncancer pain. Adjuvant drugs are those with a primary purpose other than pain relief but that can be used for analgesic effects in certain painful conditions (AGS, 2002 [Level VI]).

Special Considerations for Administering Analgesics

Older adults are at higher risk for side effects with drug therapies due to age-related physiologic decline in drug metabolism and elimination. Specific age-related changes influence the pharmacodynamics (i.e., mechanisms of drug action in the body) and pharmacokinetics (i.e., processes of drug absorption, distribution, metabolism, and elimination in the body) of medications (Buxton, 2006). Some pharmacokinetic changes with advanced age include altered body composition (e.g., decreased lean body mass and total body water, increased percentages of body fat) and changes in function of drug-eliminating organs (e.g., declined renal function, reduced hepatic blood flow with reduction of serum albumin and certain drug-metabolizing enzymes). Some pharmacodynamic changes in older adults are due in part to physiological changes and decreased homeostatic resilience. These changes can result in increased drug side effects (Nies, 2001).

Recommendations for beginning medication treatment include starting at low doses and gradually titrating upward, while monitoring and managing side effects. The adage "start low and go slow" is often used. Titrate doses upward to desired effect using short-acting medications first, and consider using longer duration medications for long-lasting pain. Choose a drug with a short half-life and the fewest side effects if possible (Pasero, Reed, & McCaffery, 1999).

Multiple drug routes are available for administration of pain medications. As long as patients are able swallow safely, the oral route is the first choice because it is the least invasive and very effective. The onset of action is within 30 minutes to 2 hours. For more immediate pain relief, intravenous administration is recommended, although topical and rectal routes may also be used. However, relief from pain with intravenous medication has a shorter duration; therefore, it may be particularly useful for relieving breakthrough pain. Intramuscular injections should be avoided in the elderly, however, because of tissue injury and because they typically produce pain. Overall, adopting a preventive approach to pain management, whenever possible, is recommended. By treating pain before it occurs, less medication is required than to relieve it (American Pain Society, 2002 [Level VI]). Examples of pain prevention are around-the-clock dosing, dosing prior to a painful treatment or event, and giving the next dose before the previous dose wears off.

Pain Management in Dementia

People with dementia are often under-treated and poorly assessed for pain, although they have diagnoses (e.g., osteoarthritis) known to cause pain (Horgas & Tsai, 1998 [Level IV]). In situations in which clinicians suspect a patient may be experiencing pain (e.g., direct observation, patient has a condition known to cause pain, or patient has agitation), a clinical trial of pain medication and nonpharmacologic strategies should be initiated. The Assessment of Discomfort in Dementia (ADD) protocol has been designed to assess and treat physical pain and affective discomfort in persons with late-stage dementia. See Treatment

10.1 Common Pain Medications for Use with Older Adults

Indication and Effects	Type	Medication	Starting Dose (Maximum Daily Dose)	Half-Life	Special Considerations (Adverse Reactions)
Mild Pain	Nonopioids	Acetaminophen (Tylenol)	325–650 mg po q4–6h [4000 mg/day]	1–3h	Decreased maximum dose in patients (50%–75%) with hepatic disease, excessive alcohol use (if ≥3 alcoholic drinks/day), impaired renal dysfunction (Renal insufficiency with chronic use)
		NSAIDs: Ibuprofen (Advil, Motrin)	200–400 mg po q6–8h (3200 mg)	1.8–2.5h	Caution with hepatic and renal disease, may cause central nervous system symptoms (gastrointestinal bleeding)
		COX–2 Inhibitor: Celecoxib (Celebrex)	100–200 mg po q12–24h [400 mg/day]	11h	Higher doses may cause higher risk of GI side effects Contraindicated in patients with sulfa sensitivity (GI bleeding, nausea, diarrhea, headache)
Mild to Moderate Pain	Opioids	Tramadol (Ultram) for mild to moderate pain	25–50 mg po q 4–6 hr (300 mg/day)	5–9h	Caution in patients with renal or liver impairment, avoid in patients with risk for seizures (Nausea, constipation, sedation, fatigue)
		Codeine	15–30 mg po q 4–6 h No maximum	2–4h	Usually not recommended for older adults due to greater risk of having nausea and constipation (Central nervous system depression, nausea, constipation, respiratory depression, hypotension, dizziness)
		Hydrocodone: (Vicodin, Lorcet, Lortab)*	2.5–5 mg po q 4–6 h See comments	3–4h	*Dose limitation by fixed-dose combinations with acetaminophen and/or NSAIDs (CNS depression, nausea, constipation, respiratory depression)

	Oxycodone: (OxyContin) (Percocet, Tylox) *	10 mg po q 12 2.5–5 mg po q 4–6 h (oxycodone) (Variable)	2–3h 4.5h	Decrease dose in patients with severe hepatic impairment *Dose limitation by fixed-dose combinations with acetaminophen and/or NSAIDs (CNS depression, nausea, constipation, respiratory depression)
Moderate to Severe Pain	Morphine immediate release (Roxanol)	10–30 mg po q 4 h (Variable)	2–4h	Recommended for breakthrough pain (CNS depression, nausea, constipation, respiratory depression)
	Morphine sustained release (MS Contin)	15 mg po q 12h (Variable)		Limited usefulness in patients with renal insufficiency (CNS depression, nausea, constipation, respiratory depression)
	Transdermal Fentanyl (Duragesic)	25 μg/hr patch q 72h (Variable)	13–24h	The lowest patch (25 μg/hr) recommended for patients requiring oral morphine 60 mg per day. peak effects of first dose between 18–24 hours (CNS depression, nausea, constipation, respiratory depression)
	Hydromorphone (Dilaudid)	2–4 mg po q 3–4h (Variable)	2–3h	Can be used for breakthrough pain or for around-the-clock dosing (CNS depression, nausea, constipation, respiratory depression)

Source. Adapted from: American Geriatrics Society Panel on Persistent Pain in Older Adults (2002). The management of persistent pain in older persons. Journal of the American Geriatrics Society, 50, S205–S224 [Level VI].
Glen, V. L., & St. Marie, B. (2002). Overview of pharmacology. In B. St. Marie (Ed.), American Society of Pain Management Nurses: Core curriculum for pain management nursing (pp. 181–237). Philadelphia: W. B. Saunders Company [Level VI].
McCaffery, M., & Portenoy, R. (1999). Nonopioids. In M. McCaffery & C. Pasero (Eds.), Pain clinical manual (2nd ed.). St. Louis, MO: Mosby [Level VI].

Guidelines (access to ADD tool) in Box 10.1. Use of the protocol has shown significant decrease in discomfort in dementia patients (Herr et al., 2006 [Level VI]; Kovach, Weissman, Griffie, Matson, & Muchka, 1999) and may be employed to improve pain control in this population.

Analgesic Drug Tolerance, Dependency, and Addiction

The use of opioids in treating severe, long-lasting pain or in terminal conditions may lead to drug tolerance or dependency. Fear of developing dependency, however, does not justify withholding these medications, especially in terminally ill patients or for any condition known to cause pain. Understanding tolerance, dependency, and addiction is important in effectively managing pain in older adults. *Drug tolerance* is defined as a decline in drug effectiveness over time due to continual use (Panda & Desbiens, 2001). Increasing the dose can overcome this effect. *Drug dependence* is identified by uncomfortable symptoms that occur with abrupt withdrawal of the drug (Panda & Desbiens, 2001). Opioid tapering is recommended when discontinuing use to alleviate this effect. The American Pain Society (2003) defines *drug addiction* as a psychological condition characterized by compulsive drug use and an uncontrollable craving to obtain effects other than relief of pain. It occurs rarely when opioids are used as medications for pain control and occurs even more rarely in older adults (American Pain Society, 2003 [Level VI]; Pasero, Portenoy, & McCaffery, 1999).

Types of Analgesic Medication

Medications commonly used to treat pain in older adults are summarized in Table 10.1, which also includes recommended dosages and special considerations. Specific information about these types of medications is discussed herein.

Nonopioids are the first line in pharmacologic pain treatment. This group includes acetaminophen, nonsteroidal anti-inflammatory drugs (NSAIDs), and cyclooxygenase-2 (COX-2) inhibitors (AGS, 2002 [Level VI]). They are generally used for a wide variety of painful conditions, both acute and chronic, from mild to moderate severity. Acetaminophen (e.g., Tylenol) is considered the drug of choice for relief of musculoskeletal pain (AGS, 2002 [Level VI]) because it has few side effects and is probably the safest nonopioid for most people. However, it should be used with caution in people with underlying hepatic or renal disease. The NSAIDs (e.g., ibuprofen and naproxen sodium) are also effective for treating mild to moderate pain and, along with acetaminophen, are often used in combination with opioids for moderate to severe pain.

The most common side effect of the NSAIDs is gastric damage. This occurs locally (as gastric irritant) and systemically (through inhibition of prostaglandin synthesis), resulting in increased gastrointestinal(GI) tract susceptibility to injury. Older adults are more likely to develop ulcer disease and renal insufficiency and have a greater incidence of death from the GI effects of NSAIDs. Other side effects include increased bleeding time, central nervous system effects, hepatic disease, and worsening asthma. When NSAIDs are used as single doses, in low doses, and for short periods, side effects are usually less common than with long-term use.

The COX-2 inhibitor, celecoxib (e.g., Celebrex), has been shown to be as effective as NSAIDs for pain relief and is indicated for mild to moderate pain but should not be used in persons with sulfa sensitivities (Wiholm, 2001 [Level IV]). Although this COX-2 inhibitor is often prescribed instead of nonselective NSAIDs to reduce risk of GI bleeding, one study showed no significant reduction of GI risk (Stockl, Cyprien, & Change, 2005 [Level IV]) and a similar risk of other side effects such as cardiovascular events (e.g., myocardiac infarction, stroke), hypertension, acute renal failure, and nephritic syndrome (Mukherjee, Nissen, & Topol, 2001 [Level I]; Whelton, 2006 [Level V]). Celecoxib loses its GI benefit, if there is any, over traditional NSAIDs when it is combined with low-dose aspirin (Lanas, 2005 [Level V]). Because proton-pump inhibitor (PPI) therapy reduces the incidence of gastroduodenal ulcers and reduces the risk and incidence of GI complications in patients taking NSAIDs, it may be helpful to recommend or to prescribe this form of gastro-protection for older patients who must combine NSAIDs and aspirin (Kimmey & Lanas, 2004 [Level V]).

Tramadol (e.g., Ultram, Ultracet) has characteristics of both nonopioids and opioids in analgesic properties. It is effective for moderate to severe pain, and its mechanism of action is not completely understood. Nausea and vomiting are common side effects associated with the use of tramadol, along with dizziness, sedation, restlessness, diarrhea or constipation, dyspepsia, weakness, diaphoresis, seizures, and respiratory depression (Glen & St. Marie, 2002 [Level VI]). It should not be used in people with a history of codeine allergy, and it should be used cautiously in persons with hepatic or renal impairment.

Opioid drugs (e.g., codeine and morphine) are effective at treating moderate to severe pain from multiple causes. They provide effective pain relief for elderly people, although many older adults and health care providers are reluctant to use them due to fears of overdose, side effects, and intolerance. Potential side effects include nausea, constipation, drowsiness, cognitive effects, and respiratory depression. The Agency for Healthcare Research and Quality (AHRQ) recommends achieving safe administration of opioids to older adults by reducing the dose to 25% to 50% of the usual adult dose (U.S. Department of Health and Human Services, 1992). Tolerance to the side effects develops with use over time, but it is strongly recommended that stool softeners or routine laxatives are co-administered with opioids from the outset (AGS, 2002 [Level VI]).

Adjuvant drugs, drugs administered in conjunction with analgesics, are often administered with nonopioids and opioids to achieve optimal pain control through additive analgesic effects or to enhance response to analgesics, especially for neuropathic pain (AGS, 2002 [Level VI]). Although tricyclic antidepressants (e.g., nortriptyline, desipramine) have shown dual effects on both pain and depression, they are inappropriate for pain management in older adults due to high rates of serious side effects (AGS, 2002 [Level VI]; Fick et al., 2003 [Level VI]). Anticonvulsants (e.g., gabapentin), often used for trigeminal neuralgia, may be used as adjuvant drugs with fewer side effects than tricyclic antidepressants (AGS [Level VI], 2002). Local anesthetics, such as lidocaine as a patch, gel, or cream, can be used as an additional treatment for the pain of post-herpetic neuralgia.

Equianalgesia refers to equivalent analgesia effects. Understanding of equianalgesic dosing (e.g., dose conversion chart, conversion ratio) improves prescribing practices for managing pain in older adults. Equianalgesic dosing charts provide lists of drugs and doses of commonly prescribed pain medications that are approximately equal in providing pain relief. They can provide practical information for selecting appropriate starting doses or when changing from one drug to another (Pasero et al.). In addition, utilizing equianalgesic dosing practices (Pasero et al.) and the WHO analgesic ladder (WHO, 1996) may provide more optimal pain relief with fewer side effects in older adults as opposed to trying to alleviate pain with maximum daily doses of mild analgesics alone.

Drugs to Avoid in Older Adults

Some medications should be generally avoided in older adults because they are either ineffective for them or cause higher risk of having side effects. Inappropriate analgesic medications for older adults are meperidine (e.g., Demerol), propoxyphene and its combination products (e.g., Darvon, Darvocet, Darvon-N, and Davocet-N), ketorolac (e.g., Toradol), and pentazocine (e.g., Talwin). These medications cause central nervous system side effects including confusion or hallucinations, may not be effective enough when administered at the commonly prescribed dose, or may produce more side effects than positive analgesic effect (Fick et al., 2003 [Level VI]). Additionally, sedatives, antihistamines, and antiemetics should be avoided, if possible, or used with caution due to long duration of action, risk of falls, hypotension, anticholinergic effects, and sedating effects (Fick et al., 2003; Pasero et al., 1999a [both Level VI]).

Nonpharmacological Pain Treatment

Older adults are at higher risk of having side effects from pharmacological treatment due to age-related physiological changes (Buxton, 2006) and increased use of multiple medications (i.e., polypharmacy) for managing multiple chronic health conditions (Helme & Gibson, 1999). Therefore, nonpharmacological treatments should be implemented, whenever possible, to accomplish maximum pain relief with the fewest side effects (Nikolaus & Zeyfang, 2004). It is recommended that nonpharmacological pain treatments be used as complementary therapy rather than as a substitute for pharmacological pain treatments (Herr, 2002b).

Many older adults are willing to use nonpharmacological modalities to manage pain (Herr, 2002b). In fact, one study indicated that more than 50% of older adults reported using three or more strategies for pain (Barry, Gill, Kerns, & Reid, 2005 [Level IV]). The most commonly reported nonpharmacological strategies reported were activity restriction, heat/cold application, and exercise. Another study reported that 96% of older adults reported using at least one complementary/alternative therapy modality and that prayer was the most commonly reported strategy (Dunn & Horgas, 2000 [Level IV]).

Types of Nonpharmacological Treatment Strategies

Nonpharmacological pain treatment strategies generally fall into two categories: physical pain relief approaches and cognitive-behavioral approaches (Herr, 2002b). Physical strategies include but are not limited to transcutaneous electrical nerve stimulation (TENS), physical therapies, use of heat and cold, massage, exercise, and various complementary/alternative therapies (e.g., acupuncture, chiropractic services). Cognitive-behavioral strategies are designed to change the person's perception of the pain and improve coping strategies (Rudy, Hanlon, & Markham, 2002). These include strategies such as relaxation, distraction guided imagery, hypnosis, and biofeedback. Other nonpharmacological pain treatment includes self-management and low-level laser therapy (LLLT). To date, few of these nonpharmaceutical strategies have been empirically evaluated for their effectiveness in pain management.

Several physical strategies to relieve pain—exercise, electrical stimulation (ES) including TENS, and LLLT—have been evaluated and revealed conflicting results (Furlan et al., 2001 [Level I]). However, exercise prescriptions for older adults recommended by the American Geriatrics Society Panel on Exercise and Osteoarthritis (AGS, 2001 [Level VI]) should be considered for those with osteoarthritis pain. ES has shown significant benefits for passive humeral lateral rotation of shoulder pain after stroke but no improvement in the quality of life (Price, 2001 [Level I]). Although only limited data are available, ES seems to be a low-risk intervention with no negative effects for managing post-stroke shoulder pain (Price, 2001 [Level I]). LLLT can be considered for short-term relief of pain with few side effects for adults with rheumatoid arthritis. The therapeutic effect of LLLT for persons with osteoarthritis, however, is supported by some empirical findings and needs further investigation (Brosseau et al., 2000 [Level I]). Laser therapy for chronic low-back pain, however, showed no effect (Furlan et al., 2001 [Level I]).

Cognitive-behavioral strategies include, among others, self-management, cognitive behavioral therapy, biofeedback, and attentional pain control strategy (i.e., distraction). Biofeedback may be beneficial for selected older adults with persistent pain (Middaugh & Pawlick, 2002 [Level V]). Attentional pain control strategies, those that manipulate attention to alter perception of pain, for cancer pain seem to be beneficial but need further study (Buck & Morley, 2006 [Level III]). Self management programs have not indicated clinical benefit in pain management or improved function for older adults with osteoarthritis (Chodosh et al., 2005 [Level I]), and self-management in a group format appears to have limited benefit (Ersek, Turner, McCurry, Gibbons, & Kraybill, 2003 [Level II]). For example, older adults with chronic pain showed improvement in their physical role function and pain intensity after group self-management interventions but not in their pain-related activity, depression, or beliefs about pain relief (Ersek et al., 2003 [Level II]). These psychoeducational therapies, however, appear to be effective as adjuvant therapy for treating pain in older adults with cancer (Devine, 2003 [Level I]).

Special Considerations of Using Nonpharmacological Treatment for Older Adults

It is essential for nurses to understand an individual's barriers to and preferences for using nonpharmacological treatments, his or her cognitive status, and the availability and effectiveness of such treatments when they are recommended to older adults with pain. Personal barriers may include limited access to the treatment modality, individual preferences for the type of program (e.g., group versus individual) or treatment (e.g., physical versus cognitive), and personal beliefs and attributions (Austrian, Kerns, & Reid, 2005 [Level IV]). For example, some older adults may lack financial resources or transportation to attend group interventions, whereas others may fear adverse effects of the treatment (e.g., more pain/injury). Some may have low energy or simply lack interest in a specific program being offered to them (Austrian et al., 2005 [Level IV]). Other personal barriers include reluctance to add more pain management strategies to existing medication regimens, belief that pain is a normal part of aging, knowledge deficits about pain management methods, and poor communication with health care providers (Davis, Hiemenz, & White, 2002 [Level IV]).

Thus, individuals differ widely in their preferences for and ability to use nonpharmacologic interventions to manage pain. Spiritual and/or religious coping strategies, for instance, must be consistent with individual values and beliefs. Other strategies, such as imagery, biofeedback, or relaxation techniques, may not be feasible for cognitively impaired older adults. Psychoeducational interventions may be burdensome for some patients (Devine, 2003 [Level I]); therefore, it is important for health care providers to consider a broad array of nonpharmacological pain management strategies and to tailor selections to the individual. It is also important to gain individual and family input about the use of home and folk remedies because use of herbals or home remedies is often not disclosed to health care providers and may result in negative drug–herb interactions (Yoon & Horne, 2001 [Level IV]; Yoon, Horne, & Adams, 2004 [Level IV]; Yoon & Schaffer, 2006 [Level IV]).

Summary

Pain is a significant problem for older adults, which has the potential to negatively impact independence, functioning, and quality of life. For pain to be effectively managed, it must first be carefully and systematically assessed. Pain assessment in older adults should start with self-reported pain. It should also incorporate assessment of nonverbal pain behaviors and family input about usual pain responses and patterns, particularly in patients unable to communicate their pain. The use of established pain assessment/measurement tools is recommended. Pain treatment in older adults should be tailored to the type and severity of pain, with medications that can be safely used in older adults (or combined with nonpharmacological treatment for heightened effectiveness). Older adults, their families, and their care providers should be knowledgeable about pain and how to manage it. Thus, education is an important part of the process and should not be overlooked. Empowering individuals and their caregivers to effectively manage pain is a critical nursing role that can improve quality of life for older adults.

Case Study and Discussion

Mr. J. is an 87-year-old man living in a skilled nursing facility. He has been diagnosed with Alzheimer's disease and has an MMSE score of 17. He has a history of osteoarthritis, diabetes, and hypertension. He has been residing in the residential facility for 1 year and his memory has been slowly declining during that time. Recently, Mr. J. has exhibited a change in behavior. He usually walks around the facility frequently throughout the day but now sits in his chair. The nursing assistants note that he has been frequently rubbing his knees. He denies pain when asked.

The nursing assistants informed the nurse of their observations and the change in Mr. J.'s usual behavior. The nurse initiated a more thorough

pain assessment, starting with self-report questions and also asking Mr. J.'s wife for her observations about his behavior. The nurse also conducted a thorough nursing assessment to rule out physical causes such as infection or sensory changes (e.g., lost glasses, which would impair walking). Then the nurse completed the NOPPAIN to assess behavioral indicators of pain. Although Mr. J. verbally denied pain, he demonstrated facial grimacing, non-verbal vocalization, and rigidity/guarding while transferring from the chair to bed. The nurse consulted the medication orders and then initiated a trial of Tylenol ES 1 tab q 6 hours. Mr. J. demonstrated a reduction in his pain behaviors and began to resume his walking routine.

Among older adults, it is important to routinely ask about the presence of pain and when there is a change in behavior. Older adults are often reluctant to complain about pain, and persons with dementia are often unable to recall the presence of pain due to memory changes. Thus, it is important to use an observational tool to assess the presence of pain behaviors in older adults. It is also important to investigate the causes of pain when behavioral pain indicators are present. For instance, onset of abdominal pain would be considered a more emergent condition than knee pain. Thus, thorough patient assessment is necessary, particularly in older adults who are likely to experience persistent and acute pain conditions simultaneously.

Box 10.1

Nursing Standard of Practice Protocol: Pain Management in Older Adults

STANDARD: All older adults will either be pain free or their pain will be controlled to a level that is acceptable to the patient and allows the person to maintain the highest level of functioning possible.

OVERVIEW: Pain, a common, subjective experience for many older adults, is associated with a number of chronic (e.g., osteoarthritis) and acute (e.g., cancer, surgery) conditions. Despite its prevalence, evidence suggests that pain is often poorly assessed and poorly managed, especially in older adults. Cognitive impairment due to dementia and/or delirium represents a particular challenge to pain management because older adults with these conditions may be unable to verbalize their pain. Nurses, an integral part of the interdisciplinary care team, need to understand myths associated with pain management, including addiction and belief that pain is a normal result of aging, to provide optimal care and to educate patients and families about managing pain.

I. BACKGROUND

A. Definitions
   1. *Pain*: Pain is defined as "an unpleasant sensory and emotional experience" (AGS, 2002; Melzack & Casey, 1968) and also as "whatever the experiencing person says it is, existing whenever he says it does" (McCaffery, 1968; McCaffery & Pasero, 1999). These definitions highlight the multidimensional and highly subjective nature of pain. Pain is usually characterized according to the duration of pain (e.g., acute versus persistent) and the cause of pain (e.g., nociceptive versus neuropathic). These definitions have implications for pain management strategies.
   2. *Acute Pain*: Defines pain that results from injury, surgery, or tissue damage. It is usually associated with autonomic activity, such as tachycardia and diaphoresis. Acute pain is usually time-limited and subsides with healing.
   3. *Persistent Pain*: Defines pain that *persists* for a prolonged period (usually more than 3 to 6 months) (AGS, 2002; Harkins, 2002). Persistent pain may or may not be associated with a diagnosable disease process and autonomic activity is usually absent. Persistent pain is often associated with functional loss, mood and behavior changes, and reduced quality of life.
   4. *Nociceptive Pain*: The term refers to pain caused by stimulation of specific peripheral or visceral pain receptors. This type of pain results from disease processes (e.g., osteoarthritis), soft-tissue injuries (e.g., falls), and medical treatment (e.g., surgery, venipuncture, and other procedures). It is usually localized and responsive to treatment.
   5. *Neuropathic Pain*: Refers to pain caused by damage to the peripheral or central nervous system. This type of pain is associated with diabetic neuropathies, post-herpetic and trigeminal neuralgias, stroke, and chemotherapy treatment for cancer. It is usually more diffuse and less responsive to analgesic medications.
B. Epidemiology
   1. Approximately 50% of community-dwelling older adults have pain.
   2. Approximately 85% of nursing home residents experience pain.
C. Etiology
   1. More than 80% of older adults have chronic medical conditions that are typically associated with pain, such as osteoarthritis and peripheral vascular disease.
   2. Older adults often have multiple medical conditions, both chronic and/or acute, and may suffer from multiple types and sources of pain.

D. Significance
   1. Pain has major implications for older adults' health, functioning, and quality of life. If unrelieved, pain is associated with the following:
      a. depression
      b. sleep disturbances
      c. withdrawal and decreased socialization
      d. functional loss and increased dependency
      e. exacerbation of cognitive impairment
      f. increased health care utilization and costs
   2. Nurses have a key role in pain management. The promotion of comfort and relief of pain is fundamental to nursing practice. Nurses need to be knowledgeable about pain in late life to provide optimal care, to educate patients and families, and to work effectively in interdisciplinary health care teams.
   3. The Joint Commission on Accreditation of Healthcare Organizations (JCAHO) now requires regular and systematic assessment of pain in all hospitalized patients. Because older adults constitute a significant portion of the patient population in many acute care settings, nurses need to have the knowledge and skill to address specific pain needs of older adults.

II. ASSESSMENT PARAMETERS

A. Assumptions
   1. The majority of hospitalized older patients suffer from both acute and persistent pain.
   2. Older adults with cognitive impairment experience pain but are often unable to verbalize it (Smith, 2005 [Level I]).
   3. Both patients and health care providers have personal beliefs, prior experiences, insufficient knowledge, and mistaken beliefs about pain and pain management that (a) influence the pain management process, and (b) must be acknowledged before optimal pain relief can be achieved [AGS, 2002 [Level VI]).
   4. Pain assessment must be regular, systematic, and documented to accurately evaluate treatment effectiveness (AGS, 2002 [Level VI]).
   5. Self-report is the gold standard for pain assessment (AGS, 2002 [Level IV]).
B. Strategies for Pain Assessment
   1. Review medical history, physical exam, and laboratory and diagnostic tests to understand sequence of events contributing to pain (AGS, 2002 [Level VI]).
   2. Assess present pain, including intensity, character, frequency, pattern, location, duration, and precipitating and relieving factors (AGS, 2002 [Level VI]).

3. Review medications, including current and previously used prescription drugs, over-the-counter drugs, and home remedies. Determine which pain control methods have previously been effective for the patient. Assess patient's attitudes and beliefs about use of analgesics, adjuvant drugs, and nonpharmacological treatments (AGS, 2002 [Level VI]).

4. Use a standardized tool to assess self-reported pain. Choose from published measurement tools and recall that older adults may have difficulty using 10-point visual analog scales. Vertical verbal descriptor scales or faces scales may be more useful with older adults (Taylor et al., 2005 [Level V]).

5. Assess pain regularly and frequently but at least every 4 hours. Monitor pain intensity after giving medications to evaluate effectiveness.

6. Observe for nonverbal and behavioral signs of pain, such as facial grimacing, withdrawal, guarding, rubbing, limping, shifting of position, aggression, agitation, depression, vocalizations, and crying. Also watch for changes in behavior from the patient's usual patterns (Taylor et al., 2005 [Level V]).

7. Gather information from family members about the patient's pain experiences. Ask about the patient's verbal and nonverbal/behavioral expressions of pain, particularly in older adults with dementia.

8. When pain is suspected but assessment instruments or observation is ambiguous, institute a clinical trial of pain treatment (i.e., in persons with dementia). If symptoms persist, assume pain is unrelieved and treat accordingly (Herr, et al., 2006 [Level VI]).

III. NURSING CARE STRATEGIES

A. Prevention of Pain

1. Assess pain regularly and frequently to facilitate appropriate treatment (AGS, 2002 [Level VI]).

2. Anticipate and aggressively treat for pain before, during, and after painful diagnostic and/or therapeutic treatments (AGS, 2002 [Level VI]).

3. Educate patients, families, and other clinicians to use analgesic medications prophylactically prior to and after painful procedures (AGS, 2002 [Level VI]).

4. Educate patients and families about pain medications and their side effects; adverse effects; and issues of addiction, dependence, and tolerance (AGS, 2002 [Level VI]).

5. Educate patients to take medications for pain on a regular basis and to avoid allowing pain to escalate (AGS, 2002 [Level VI]).

6. Educate patients, families, and other clinicians to use nonpharmacological strategies to manage pain, such as relaxation, massage, and heat/cold (AGS, 2002 [Level VI]).

B. Treatment Guidelines
   1. Pharmacologic (AGS, 2002 [Level VI])
      a. Older adults are at increased risk for adverse drug reactions.
      b. Monitor medications closely to avoid over- or under-medication.
      c. Administer pain drugs on a regular basis to maintain therapeutic levels; avoid PRN drugs.
      d. Document treatment plan to maintain consistency across shifts and with other care providers.
      e. Use equianalgesic dosing and the WHO three-step ladder to obtain optimal pain relief with fewer side effects.
   2. Nonpharmacologic (AGS, 2002 [Level VI])
      a. Investigate older patients' attitudes and beliefs about, preference for, and experience with nonpharmacological pain-treatment strategies.
      b. Tailor nonpharmacologic techniques to the individual.
      c. Cognitive-behavioral strategies focus on changing the person's perception of pain (e.g., relaxation therapy, education, and distraction) and may not be appropriate for cognitively impaired persons.
      d. Physical pain relief strategies focus on promoting comfort and altering physiologic responses to pain (e.g., heat, cold, TENS units) and are generally safe and effective.
   3. Combination approaches that include both pharmacological and nonpharmacological pain treatments are often the most effective.
C. Follow-up Assessment
   1. Monitor treatment effects within 1 hour of administration and at least every 4 hours.
   2. Evaluate patient for pain relief and side effects of treatment.
   3. Document patient's response to treatment effects.
   4. Document treatment regimen in patient care plan to facilitate consistent implementation.

IV. EXPECTED OUTCOMES

A. Patient:
   1. Will be either pain free or pain will be at a level that the patient judges as acceptable.
   2. Maintains highest level of self-care, functional ability, and activity level possible.
   3. Experiences no iatrogenic complications, such as falls, GI upset/bleeding, or altered cognitive status.
B. Nurse:
   1. Will demonstrate evidence of ongoing and comprehensive pain assessment.
   2. Will document evidence of prompt and effective pain management interventions.

3. Will document systematic evaluation of treatment effectiveness.
4. Will demonstrate knowledge of pain management in older patients, including assessment strategies, pain medications, non-pharmacological interventions, and patient and family education.

C. Institution
   1. Facilities and institutions will provide evidence of documentation of pain assessment, intervention, and evaluation of treatment effectiveness.
   2. Facilities and institutions will provide evidence of referral to specialists for specific therapies (e.g., psychiatry, psychology, biofeedback, physical therapy, or pain treatment centers).
   3. Facilities and institutions will provide evidence of pain management resources for staff (e.g., care-planning and pain management references, pain management consultants).

V. TREATMENT GUIDELINES

A. Pain
   1. The Hartford Institute for Geriatric Nursing: Try This Series: Assessing Pain in Older Adults http://www.ConsultGeriRN.org/resources/zeducation/tryThis.html
   2. American Geriatric Society Guideline on the Management of Persistent Pain http://www.americangeriatrics.org/education/manage_pers_pain.shtml
   3. Herr, K., Steffensmeier, J., Rakel, B. (2006). University of Iowa Gerontological Nursing Interventions Research Center, Research Translation and Dissemination Core, Iowa City, IA.
   4. American Association of Pain Management Nurses (ASPMN): Geriatric Pain Assessment: Self-Directed Learning https://www.commercecorner.com/aspmn/productlist1.aspx
   5. American Pain Society: Pain Guidelines and Online Resource Centers http://www.ampainsoc.org/links/clinician1.htm
   6. International Association for the Study of Pain: Curriculum on Pain for Schools of Nursing; Pain in Older Persons Book http://www.iasp-pain.org/

B. Pain in Persons with Dementia and Long Term Care
   1. American Medical Directors Association (AMDA): Clinical Practice Guideline: Pain Management in the Long Term Care Setting http://www.amda.com/tools/cpg/chronicpain.cfm
   2. City of Hope: State-of-the-Art Review of Tools for Assessing Pain in Nonverbal Older Adults http://www.cityofhope.org/prc/elderly.asp
   3. American Association of Pain Management Nurses (ASPMN): Pain Assessment in the Nonverbal Patient: Position Statement with Clinical Practice Recommendations. http://www.aacn.org/AACN/practice.nsf/vwdoc/PainAssmt

C. Measurement Tools
   1. See City of Hope Web site listed previously for comprehensive review of tools for persons with dementia

References

American Geriatrics Society Panel on Exercise and Osteoarthritis. (2001). Exercise prescription for older adults with osteoarthritis pain: Consensus practice recommendations. *Journal of American Geriatrics Society, 49,* 808–823. Evidence Level VI: Expert Opinion.

American Geriatrics Society Panel on Persistent Pain in Older Persons. (2002). The management of persistent pain in older persons. *Journal of the American Geriatrics Society, 50,* S205–S224. Evidence Level VI: Expert Opinion.

American Pain Society (APS) (2002). *Guideline for the management of pain in osteoarthritis, rheumatoid arthritis, and juvenile chronic arthritis* (2nd ed.). Glenview, IL: APS. Evidence Level VI: Expert Opinion.

American Pain Society. (2003). *Principles of analgesic use in the treatment of acute and cancer pain* (5th ed.). Glenview, IL: APS. Evidence Level VI: Expert Opinion.

American Pain Society. (2005). *Guidelines for the management of cancer pain in adults and children.* Glenview, IL: APS. Evidence Level VI: Expert Opinion.

Austrian, J. S., Kerns, R. D., & Reid, M. C. (2005). Perceived barriers to trying self-management approaches for chronic pain in older persons. *Journal of American Geriatrics Society, 53,* 856–861. Evidence Level IV: Nonexperimental Study.

Barry, L. C., Gill, T. M., Kerns, R. D., & Reid, M. C. (2005). Identification of pain-reduction strategies used by community-dwelling older persons. *Journal of Gerontology: Medical Sciences, 60A,* 1569–1575. Evidence Level IV: Nonexperimental Study.

Bieri, D., Reeve, R. A., Champion G. D., Addicoat L., & Ziegler, J. B. (1990). The Faces Pain Scale for the self-assessment of the severity of pain experienced by children: Development, initial validation, and preliminary investigation for ratio scale properties. *Pain, 41,* 139–150.

Brosseau, L., Welch, V., Wells, G., Tugwell, P., de Bie, R., Gam, A., et al. (2000). Low- level laser therapy for osteoarthritis and rheumatoid arthritis: A meta-analysis. *Journal of Rheumatology, 27,* 1961–1969. Evidence Level IV: Nonexperimental Study.

Buck, R., & Morley, S. (2006). A daily process design study of attentional pain-control strategies in the self-management of cancer pain. *European Journal of Pain, 10,* 385–398. Evidence Level III: Quasi-experimental Study.

Buxton, I. L. O. (2006). Pharmacokinetics and pharmacodynamics: The dynamics of drug absorption, distribution, action, and elimination: Introduction. In L. L. Brunton (Ed.), *Goodman & Gilman's the pharmacological basis of therapeutics* (11th ed., pp. 1–39). New York: McGraw-Hill.

Chodosh, J., Morton, S. C., Mojica, W., Maglione, M., Suttorp, M. J., Hilton, L., et al. (2005). Meta-analysis: Chronic disease self-management programs for older adults. *Annals of Internal Medicine, 143,* 427–438. Evidence Level I: Systematic Review.

Davis, G. C., Hiemenz, M. L., & White, T. L. (2002). Barriers to managing chronic pain of older adults with arthritis. *Journal of Nursing Scholarship, 34,* 121–126. Evidence Level IV: Nonexperimental Study.

Devine, E. C. (2003). Meta-analysis of the effect of psychoeducational interventions on pain in adults with cancer. *Oncology Nursing Forum, 30,* 75–89. Evidence Level I: Systematic Review.

Dunn, K., & Horgas, A. L. (2000). The prevalence of prayer as a spiritual self-care modality in elders. *Journal of Holistic Nursing, 18,* 337–351. Evidence Level IV: Nonexperimental Study.

Ersek, M., Turner, J. A., McCurry, S. M., Gibbons, L., & Kraybill, B. M. (2003). Efficacy of a self-management group intervention for elderly persons with chronic pain. *The Clinical Journal of Pain, 19,* 156–167. Evidence Level I: Systematic Review.

Feldt, K. S. (2000). The checklist of nonverbal pain indicators (CNPI). *Pain Management Nursing, 1*(1): 13–21.

Feldt, K. S., Warne, M. A., & Ryden, M. B. (1998). Examining pain in aggressive cognitively impaired older adults. *Journal of Gerontological Nursing, 24,* 14–22.

Ferrell, B. A., Ferrell, B. R., & Rivera, L. (1995). Pain in cognitively impaired nursing home patients. *Journal of Pain and Symptom Management, 10,* 591–598. Evidence Level IV: Nonexperimental Study.

Fick, D. M., Cooper, J. W., Wade, W. E., Waller, J. L., Maclean, R., & Beers, M. H. (2003). Updating the Beers criteria for potentially inappropriate medication use in older adults: Results of a U.S. consensus panel of experts. *Archives of Internal Medicine, 163*, 2716–2724. Evidence Level VI: Expert Opinion.

Furlan, A. D., Clarke, J., Esmail, R., Sinclair, S., Irvin, E., & Bombardier, C. (2001). A critical review of reviews on the treatment of chronic low-back pain. *Spine, 26*, E155–E162. Evidence Level I: Systematic Review.

Gibson, S., Farrell, M., Katz, B., & Helme, R. (1996). Multidisciplinary management of chronic nonmalignant pain in older adults. In B. R. Ferrell & B. A. Ferrell (Eds.), *Pain in the elderly* (pp. 91–99). Seattle: IASP Press.

Glen, V. L., & St. Marie, B. (2002). Overview of pharmacology. In B. St. Marie (Ed.), *American Society of Pain Management Nurses: Core curriculum for pain management nursing* (pp. 181–237). Philadelphia: W. B. Saunders Company. Evidence Level VI: Expert Opinion.

Gordon, D. B., Pellino, T. A., Miaskowski, C., McNeill, J. A., Paice, J. A., Laferriere, D., et al. (2002). A 10-year review of quality improvement monitoring in pain management: Recommendations for standardized outcome measures. *Pain Management Nursing, 3*, 116–230. Evidence Level I: Systematic Review.

Harkins, S. W. (2002). What is unique about the older adult's pain experience? In D. K. Weiner, K. Herr, & T. E. Rudy (Eds.), *Persistent pain in older adults: An interdisciplinary guide for treatment* (pp. 4–17). New York: Springer Publishing Company.

Helme, R. D., & Gibson, S. J. (1999). Pain in older people. In I. K. Crombie, P. R. Croft, S. J. Linton, et al. (Eds.), *Epidemiology of pain* (pp. 103–112). Seattle: IASP Press.

Herr, K. (2002a). Chronic pain: Challenges and assessment strategies. *Journal of Gerontological Nursing, 28*(1), 20–27.

Herr, K. (2002b). Chronic pain in the older patient: Management strategies. *Journal of Gerontological Nursing, 28*(2), 28–34.

Herr, K., Bjoro, K., & Decker, S. (2006). Tools for assessment of pain in nonverbal older adults with dementia: A state-of-the-science review. *Journal of Pain and Symptom Management, 31*(2), 170–192. Evidence Level I: Systematic Review.

Herr, K., Coyne, P. J., Key, T., Manworren, R., McCaffery, M., Merkel, S., et al. (2006). Pain assessment in the nonverbal patient: Position statement with clinical practice recommendations. *Pain Management Nursing, 7*(2), 44–52. Evidence Level VI: Expert Opinion.

Horgas, A. L., & Dunn, K. (2001). Pain in nursing home residents: Comparison of residents' self-report and nursing assistants' perceptions. *Journal of Gerontological Nursing, 27*, 44–53. Evidence Level IV: Nonexperimental Study.

Horgas, A. L., & Tsai, P. F. (1998). Analgesic drug prescription and use in cognitively impaired nursing home residents. *Nursing Research, 47*, 235–242. Evidence Level IV: Nonexperimental Study.

Hurley, A. C., Volicer, B. J., Hanrahan, P. A., House, S., & Volicer, L. (1992). Assessment of discomfort in advanced Alzheimer patients. *Research in Nursing and Health, 15*(5), 367–377.

Joint Commission on the Accreditation of Healthcare Organization (2001). *Accreditation manual for hospitals*. Oakbrook Terrace, IL: JCAHO.

Keefe, F. J., & Block, A. R. (1982). Development of an observation method for assessing pain behavior in chronic low-back pain patients. *Behavior Therapy, 13*, 363–375.

Kimmey, M. B., & Lanas, A. (2004). Review article: Appropriate use of proton pump inhibitors with traditional nonsteroidal anti-inflammatory drugs and COX-2 selective inhibitors. *Alimentary Pharmacology and Therapeutics, 19* (Suppl. 1), 60–65. Evidence Level V: Literature Review.

Kovach, C., Weissman, D., Griffie, J., Matson, S., & Muchka, S. (1999). Assessment and treatment of discomfort for people with late-stage dementia. *Journal of Pain and Symptom Management, 18*, 412–419.

Lanas, A. (2005). Gastrointestinal injury from NSAID therapy: How to reduce the risk of complications. *Postgraduate Medicine, 117*(6), 23–31. Evidence Level V: Narrative Literature Review.

McCaffery, M. (1968). *Nursing practice theories related to cognition, bodily pain, and man-environment interaction*. Los Angeles: UCLA Students Store.

McCaffery, M., & Pasero, C. (1999). *Pain: Clinical manual* (2nd ed.). St. Louis, MO: Mosby.

McCaffery, M., & Portenoy, R. (1999). Nonopiods. In M. McCaffery & C. Pasero (Eds.), *Pain clinical manual* (2nd ed.). St. Louis, MO: Mosby. Evidence Level VI: Expert Opinion.

Melzack, R., & Casey, K. L. (1968). Sensory, motivational, and central control determinants of pain: A new conceptual model. In D. R. Kenshalo (Ed.), *The skin senses* (pp. 423–443). Springfield, IL: Charles C. Thomas Press.

Middaugh, S. J., & Pawlick, K. (2002). Biofeedback and behavioral treatment of persistent pain in the older adult: A review and a study. *Applied Psychophysiology and Biofeedback, 27*, 185–202. Evidence Level V: Care Report/Narrative Literature Review.

Miller, J., Moore, K., Schofield, A., & Ng'andu, N. (1996). A study of discomfort and confusion among elderly surgical patients. *Orthopedic Nursing, 16*(5), 12–13.

Miller, L. L., Nelson, L. L., & Mezey, M. (2000). Comfort and pain relief in dementia: Awakening a new beneficence. *Journal of Gerontological Nursing, 26*, 32–40.

Mukherjee, B., Nissen, S. E., & Topol, E. (2001). Risk of cardiovascular events associated with selective COX-2 inhibitors. *Journal of American Medical Association, 286*, 954–959. Evidence Level I: Systematic Review.

Nies, A. S. (2001). Principles of therapeutics. In J. G. Hardman & L. M. Limbird (Eds.), *Goodman & Gilman's the pharmacological basis of therapeutics* (10th ed,.pp. 45–66). New York: McGraw-Hill.

Nikolaus, T., & Zeyfang, A. (2004). Pharmacological treatments for persistent nonmalignant pain in older persons. *Drugs & Aging, 21*(1), 19–41.

Panda, M., & Desbiens, N. A. (2001). Pain in elderly patients: How to achieve control. *Consultant, 41*, 1597–1604.

Pasero, C., Portenoy, R. K., & McCaffery, M. (1999a). Opioid analgesics. In M. McCaffery and C. Pasero (Eds.), *Pain: Clinical manual* (2nd ed., pp. 161–299). St. Louis, MO: Mosby. Evidence Level VI: Expert Opinion.

Pasero, C., Reed, B., & McCaffery, M. (1999). Pain in the elderly. In M. McCaffery and C. Pasero (Eds.), *Pain: Clinical manual* (2nd ed., pp. 674–710). St. Louis, MO: Mosby.

Price, C. I. M. (2001). Electrical stimulation for preventing and treating post-stroke shoulder pain: A systematic Cochrane review. *Clinical Rehabilitation, 15*, 5–19. Evidence Level I: Systematic Review.

Reiner, A., & Lacasse, C. (2006). Symptom correlates in the gero-oncology population. *Seminars in Oncology Nursing, 22*, 20–30. Evidence Level I: Systematic Review.

Rudy, T. E., Hanlon, R. B., & Markham, J. R. (2002). Psychosocial issues and cognitive-behavioral therapy: From theory to practice. In D. K. Weiner, K. Herr, & T. E. Rudy (Eds.), *Persistent pain in older adults: An interdisciplinary guide for treatment*. New York: Springer Publishing Company.

Sha, M. C., Callahan, C. M., Counsel, S. R., Westmoreland, G. R., Stump, T. E., & Kroenke, K. (2005). Physical symptoms as a predictor of health care use and mortality among older adults. *The American Journal of Medicine, 118*, 301–306.

Smith, M. (2005). Pain assessment in nonverbal older adults with advanced dementia. *Perspectives in psychiatric care, 41*, 99–113. Evidence Level I: Systematic Review.

Snow, A. L., Weber, J. B., O'Malley, K. J. Cody, M., Beck, C., Bruera, E., et al. (2004). NOPPAIN: A nursing assistant–administered pain assessment instrument for use in dementia. *Dementia and Geriatric Cognitive Disorders, 17*, 240–246.

Stockl, K., Cyprien, L., & Chang, E. Y. (2005). Gastrointestinal bleeding rates among managed-care patients newly started on COX-2 inhibitors or nonselective NSAIDs. *Journal of Managed Care Pharmacy, 11*, 550–558. Evidence Level IV: Nonexperimental Study.

Taylor, L., J., Harris, J., Epps, C. D., & Herr, K. (2005). Psychometric evaluation of selected pain-intensity scales for use with cognitively impaired and cognitively intact older adults. *Rehabilitation Nursing, 30*, 55–61. Evidence Level V: Care Report/Narrative Literature Review.

Thomas, D. R., Flaherty, J. H., & Morley, J. E. (2001). The management of chronic pain in long term care settings. *Annals of Long Term Care, 11* (Suppl.), 3–20.

U.S. Department of Health and Human Services (1992). *Acute pain management: operative or medical procedures and trauma* (AHCPR Publication No. 92-0032). Rockville, MD: Author.

Weiner, D. K., Herr, K., & Rudy, T. E. (Eds.) (2002). *Persistent pain in older adults*. New York: Springer Publishing Company.

Wells, N., Kaas, M., & Feldt, K. (1997). Managing pain in the institutionalized elderly: The nursing role. In D. I. Mostofsky & J. Lomranz (Eds.), *Handbook of pain and aging* (pp. 129–151). New York: Plenum Press.

Whelton, A. (2006). Clinical implications of nonopioid analgesia for relief of mild to moderate pain in patients with or at risk for cardiovascular disease. *American Journal of Cardiology, 97* (Suppl. 1), 3–9. Evidence Level V: Narrative Literature Review.

Wiholm, B. E. (2001). Identification of sulfonamide-like adverse drug reactions to celecoxib in the World Health Organization database. *Current Medical Research and Opinion, 17,* 210–216. Evidence Level IV: Nonexperimental Study.

Wisconsin Medical Society Task Force on Pain Management. (2004). Guidelines for the assessment and management of chronic pain. *Wisconsin Medical Journal, 103*(3), 19–42. Evidence Level VI: Expert Opinion.

World Health Organization (WHO). (1996). *Cancer pain relief and palliative care (technical report series)* (2nd ed). World Health Organization: Geneva, Switzerland.

Yoon, S. L., & Horne, C. H. (2001). Herbal products and conventional medicines used by community-residing older women. *Journal of Advanced Nursing, 33,* 51–59. Evidence Level IV: Nonexperimental Study.

Yoon, S. L., Horne, C. H., & Adams, C. (2004). Herbal product use by African American older women. *Clinical Nursing Research, 13,* 271–288. Evidence Level IV: Nonexperimental Study.

Yoon, S. L., & Schaffer, S. D. (2006). Herbal, prescribed, and over–the–counter drug use in older women: Prevalence of drug interactions. *Geriatric Nursing, 27,* 118–129. Evidence Level IV: Nonexperimental Study.

Iatrogenesis: The Nurse's Role in Preventing Patient Harm

11

Deborah C. Francis

Educational Objectives

At the completion of this chapter, the reader will be able to:

1. define *iatrogenesis* and the most common types of iatrogenic events affecting older adults

2. understand the scope of the problem of iatrogenic events

3. describe the nurse's role in preventing iatrogenic harm in hospitalized patients

4. recognize the increasing incidence of hospital-acquired infections and the nurse's role in prevention

5. identify the nursing and organizational priorities needed to promote geriatric patient safety

Overview

Iatrogenesis is a common and serious hazard of hospitalization and health care interventions that is associated with significant adverse patient outcomes. Iatrogenic illness and injury is known to prolong hospital stays and increase patient morbidity and mortality at significant cost to health care organizations, third-party payers, and patients alike. From the Greek word *iatros*, meaning healer, iatrogenesis means "brought forth by a healer." It has also been referred to as *nursigenic* when the harm is caused by nurses. A more appropriate term might be *comiogenic illness*, which comes from the Greek *komein*, meaning to

For a description of Evidence Levels cited in this chapter, see chapter 1,
Developing and Evaluating Clinical Practice Guidelines, page 4

223

care, and referring to any adverse event associated with the "care" of patients (Sharpe & Faden, 1998 [Level VI]). Iatrogenic harm refers to an unintended adverse patient outcome due to any therapeutic, diagnostic, and prophylactic intervention that is not considered the natural course of the disease. Common iatrogenic illnesses include adverse drug events (ADEs), complications of diagnostic and therapeutic procedures, and nosocomial complications that occur in the course of medical and health care. The latter includes hospital-acquired infections (HAIs), geriatric syndromes, and falls or other injuries related to the environment or equipment defects. Less well recognized are the harmful effects to patients' values, beliefs, prejudices, fears, and attitudes of well-intentioned health care providers.

Background and Significance of The Problem

Steele, Gertman, Crescenzi, & Anderson (1981, 2004 [both Level IV]) were some of the first to recognize iatrogenesis as a problem in older adults when they found that 38% of geriatric patients suffered an iatrogenic illness during a hospital stay. Citing the lack of progress made since a similar report was published 15 years earlier, they raised the alarm about the extent of adverse events in hospitalized patients. Iatrogenesis came to the forefront when medical errors causing patient harm made headlines with the release of the Institute of Medicine (IOM) landmark report entitled "To Err Is Human: Building a Safer Health System" (Kohn, Corrigan, & Donaldson, 1999 [Level I]). It demonstrated that errors made by medical practitioners cause between 44,000 and 98,000 deaths per year at a cost of up to $29 billion in unnecessary health care costs, disability, and lost income. The report strongly urged immediate, vast, and comprehensive systemwide changes, including both voluntary and mandatory reporting programs by health care organizations, and jump-started the patient safety movement of today. Starfield (2000 [Level VI]) estimates that 1 million persons are injured and up to 250,000 persons die every year as a direct result of iatrogenic complications, making it the third most common cause of death after cancer and heart disease. A national study of 37 million Medicare patients found that an average of 195,000 people die every year due to potentially preventable patient safety incidents (Health Grades, Inc., 2004 [Level IV]). Particularly concerning is the fact that despite dramatic improvements made in recent years, especially in the reduction of infections and anesthesia-associated mortality, an alarming increase in adverse events among Medicare beneficiaries has been noted (Villanueva & Anderson, 2001 [Level IV]). Most recently, a 2005 survey conducted by the Kaiser Family Foundation, AHRQ, and the Harvard School of Public Health revealed that one-third of respondents reported that they or a family member had been harmed by a medical error during their lifetime, while one in five noted that it caused serious health consequences (Kaiser Family Foundation, 2004 [Level IV]). The literature available on medical-error–related iatrogenesis is vast and will not be covered in this chapter. Readers are referred to the Resources section of this chapter for more information on medical errors.

The true extent of the problem of iatrogenesis is not well understood and is complicated by various factors. The majority of the research has occurred in acute care and, to a lesser degree, nursing home settings, with the incidence of iatrogenic events in the community not well understood yet. Lack of standardization in the literature as to what constitutes an iatrogenic event and different methods of data collection and analysis make it difficult to understand the true extent of the problem. In addition, there is both a lack of recognition and standardized reporting procedures by hospitals and providers. As such, what we know of the problem of iatrogenesis may be but the tip of the iceberg.

Retrospective chart reviews of patients in the United States, Canada, England, New Zealand, Australia, and Denmark have demonstrated that between 3% and 16.6% of patients experience one or more adverse events during the course of hospitalization (Baker et al., 2004 [Level IV]; Brennan et al., 1991 [Level IV]; Brennan et al., 2004 [Level IV]; Davis et al., 2002 [Level IV]; Forster et al., 2004 [Level IV]; Schioler et al., 2001 [Level IV]; Thomas et al., 2000 [Level IV]; Vincent, Neale, & Woloshynowych, 2001 [Level IV]; Wilson et al., 1995 [Level IV]). Evidence suggests that admissions to U.S. emergency rooms for iatrogenic complications are on the rise, accounting for 3.1 visits per 1,000 patients in 1992 and 5.2 visits per 1,000 in 1999, with substantially higher rates noted for older adults (Burt, 2001). More than 50% of adverse events occur prior to hospitalization, up to 70% of which are considered preventable (Sharpe & Faden, 1998 [Level VI]), whereas close to 25% occur after hospital discharge (Forster et al., 2004 [Level IV]). Of those adverse events that occur during hospitalization, 20% to 51% were considered preventable and 2% to 26% life-threatening or fatal (Brennan et al., 1991, 2004; Forster et al., 2004; Giraud et al., 1993; Lefevre et al., 1992; Steele et al., 2004 [all Level IV]). Up to 75% of iatrogenic disease in the hospital is thought to be due to medications or adverse events after medical or surgical procedures. It is difficult to estimate the human and financial cost of this problem and it is thought to be underestimated.

The risk of an iatrogenic event is highest among patients 65 years and older, with evidence suggesting it affects between 36% and 58% of hospitalized older adults (Steele et al., 1981, 2004 [both Level IV]; Lefevre, 1992 [Level IV]; Rothschild, Bates, & Leape, 2000 [Level V]). Other high risk groups include patients in the emergency room and interventional radiology and those admitted to intensive care units (ICUs) and thoracic, cardiac surgery, and vascular units. Studies of patients admitted to an ICU have found that between 1.2% and 31% suffer an adverse event, with 45% considered preventable and 13% life-threatening or fatal (Darchy, LeMiere, Figueredo, Bavoux, & Domart, 1999 [Level IV]; Giraud et al., 1993 [Level IV]; Lehmann, Puopolo, Shaykevich, & Brennan 2005 [Level IV]; Rothschild et al., 2005 [Level IV]).

Iatrogenesis in Older Adults

The landmark Harvard Medical Practice Study (1991) found that patients 65 years and older suffered twice as many diagnostic complications, two and a half times as many medication reactions, four times as many therapeutic mishaps, and nine times as many falls as compared to younger patients. A more recent review corroborated these data, finding that older adults experience 2.2% more adverse events due to perioperative complications and 10% more falls than those patients younger than 65 years (Rothschild et al., 2000 [Level V]). The reasons include normal age-related physiological changes and concomitant chronic medical conditions that place older adults at much greater risk of harm. The increase in medical or psychiatric conditions with age requires more medications and diagnostic or therapeutic procedures, making older adults far more prone to be harmed by medical care. Age-related diminished physiologic reserve (especially in hepatic, renal, and cognitive function) and impaired homeostatic and compensatory mechanisms impede the ability of older adults to respond to physiological and psychological stressors. Age-associated physiologic changes tend to exaggerate the effects of medications, leading to more adverse side effects and iatrogenic harm. This risk is potentiated by the increased number of co-morbid conditions that occur with age and drug–drug and drug–disease interactions from subsequent polypharmacy.

In addition to the increased potential for adverse effects of medications, aging is associated with an increased risk of infection. An age-related blunted febrile response can mask the early signs of infection, which may be missed by the clinician who relies on a spike in temperature or increased white blood cell count to recognize an infection. A blunted thirst sensation dramatically increases the risk of dehydration in older patients who may, for functional or cognitive reasons, be unable to independently drink adequate amounts of fluids. An older adult with age-associated decline in cardiac reserve who is receiving continuous intravenous fluids is at increased risk of iatrogenic congestive heart failure (CHF).

Another important consideration is the atypical presentation of disease in the elderly. Early symptoms of acute medical conditions tend to be more vague, insidious, and atypical and therefore are often missed or misinterpreted by clinicians, family/caregivers, and patients alike. This complicates accurate diagnosis and timely treatment and, consequently, results in a high number of emergent, high risk interventions. For example, an acute appendicitis in an older adult may present as nonlocalized abdominal discomfort or may not manifest symptoms until perforation occurs; or a person with a myocardial infarction may have no pain at all. More common in older adults is a urinary tract infection (UTI) or pneumonia presenting with confusion, falls, or functional impairment, rather than the typical symptoms of infection in younger persons.

Older adults are at a particularly high risk for cascade iatrogenesis, which is a phenomenon that occurs when an initial medical intervention triggers a series of complicating events, initiating a cascade of decline, which is often irreversible. For example, a patient who is medicated for agitated behaviors associated with delirium becomes lethargic from over-sedation, aspirates, and develops aspiration pneumonia. Subsequent functional decline due to prolonged bedrest results in a fractured hip when a patient falls while trying to get to the bathroom. This then increases the length of stay and further increases the potential for complications. Iatrogenic cascades have been found to occur most frequently among the oldest, most functionally impaired patients and those with a higher severity of illness on admission (Potts et al., 1993 [Level IV]).

To further complicate matters, most physicians and nurses are inadequately trained in geriatric care and therefore are not prepared to manage the complex, chronic care needed by frail older patients. Without a solid understanding of the geriatric approach, providers can inadvertently cause more harm during the course of treatment. The purpose of this chapter is to describe the role of the nurse in preventing iatrogenic harm, as well as to briefly summarize the organizational priorities needed to minimize adverse events in hospitalized older adults.

Assessment and Proactive Intervention for Iatrogenesis

Adverse Drug Events (ADEs)

Adverse effects of medications are the most common type of iatrogenesis in older adults. It is estimated that 35% of older persons experience ADEs, almost half of which are preventable (Safran et al., 2005 [Level IV]). The majority of cases in which patients are admitted to the hospital with an iatrogenic illness or injury can be attributed to ADEs (Darchy et al., 1999 [Level IV]). A study of four ambulatory care clinics in Boston found that 25% of patients in primary care reported an ADE, with 13% considered serious and 11% preventable (Gandhi et al., 2003 [Level IV]). McDonnell (2002 [Level IV]) found that not only were 62% of ADEs resulting in hospital admission during an 11-month period potentially preventable but also that 25% were deemed life-threatening. Most resulted from inadequate drug-monitoring therapy or inappropriate dosing. Despite widespread recognition of the adverse effects of medications, the incidence of ADE-related hospital admissions has not decreased during the past 20 years. Perhaps most concerning is the fact that the absolute numbers may have increased (Green, Mottram, Rowe, & Pirmohamed, 2000 [Level IV]).

Once admitted, ADEs tend to be the most common type of treatment-caused injury in the hospitalized patient, with at least one-third related to errors and thus considered preventable. Baune et al. (2003 [Level IV]) noted a 9.9% prevalence rate of ADEs in a Paris hospital, concluding that 73% were serious and 25% preventable. Lazarou, Pomeranz, & Corey (1998 [Level I]) demonstrated that there were approximately 106,000 fatal ADEs in hospitalized patients in the United States in 1994.

The potential for ADEs is highest among older adults, who are the greatest consumers of medications. It is well known that the risk increases exponentially with the increase in number of drugs (Gandhi et al., 2003 [Level IV]). Polypharmacy, which is prevalent among older patients, increases the risk of drug–drug interactions, whose effect on this population is more dramatic. It has been shown to be a significant predictor of hospitalization, nursing home placement, death, hypoglycemia, fractures, impaired mobility, pneumonia, and malnutrition (Frazier, 2005 [Level I]). Any and all medications can cause ADEs, although certain classes, such as antibiotics and cardiovascular drugs, have been identified in studies of hospitalized patients to be particularly problematic. (See chapter 12, *Reducing Adverse Drug Events,* for assessment and interventions to prevent ADEs).

Nosocomial or Health Care-Acquired Complications

Nosocomial or health care–acquired injuries that are not directly related to the illness or specific treatment of the acute problem occur in hospitalized older patients with far greater frequency (Rothschild et al., 2000 [Level V]. The most common preventable and potentially life-threatening iatrogenic complications in hospitalized older adults include nosocomial infection and certain geriatric syndromes. The latter include but are not limited to delirium, functional decline/deconditioning, falls, malnutrition, pressure ulcers, depression, and incontinence that occur in the course of receiving medical and nursing care. The reader is referred to the appropriate book chapters (chapters 3, 5, 7, 9, 13, 15, and 18, respectively) in this text for protocols to identify, prevent, and manage these common iatrogenic geriatric syndromes.

HAI, first defined in 1970 by the Centers for Disease Control (CDC) as one that develops in a patient after hospital admission, is a serious risk for any patient and, like other iatrogenic harm, the risk rises dramatically with age (Beaujean et al., 1997 [Level IV]). HAI is one of the leading causes of death and morbidity in hospitalized patients (WHO, 2002 [Level I]). It is estimated that HAIs affect more than 2 million patients in the United States every year and cause at least 90,000 deaths (Leape, 2005a [Level V]), at a cost exceeding $4.5 billion (Hollenbeak et al., 2006 [Level IV]). Although the true incidence is difficult to determine, evidence suggests that 5% to 10% of patients develop an HAI, which increases morbidity, mortality, length of stay, and cost of care (Hugonnet, Chevrolet, & Pittet, 2007 [Level IV]; Hussain et al., 1996 [Level IV]). In addition, a disturbing increase in risk has been noted in recent decades (Burke, 2003 [Level V]). The state of Pennsylvania, which recently mandated hospitals to report catheter-associated bloodstream infections (CABSIs), UTIs from catheters, and HAIs from specified surgeries, found that 19,154 patients acquired an infection in 2005. The mortality rate was 12.9% compared to 2.3% for all patients, whereas the length of stay for those patients who acquired an infection was 20.6 days compared to 4.5 days for all patients. Of note, the average cost was six times higher for a patient who acquired an infection and, in some cases, the charges exceeded the reimbursement (Hollenbeak et al., 2006 [Level IV]).

The rate of HAI is highest among older and critically ill patients, who tend to be the sickest and most immune-compromised, undergo more invasive procedures, and receive more intravascular devices, which significantly increases the risk of secondary infection. Studies of older adults in geriatric and rehabilitation units of acute care facilities suggest an even higher rate of HAI, noting a prevalence rate of 2.7% to 32.7% and an incidence rate of between 10.7% and 32.7% (Beaujean et al., 1997; Eveillard et al., 1998; Hussain et al., 1996 [all Level IV]). Once infected with an HAI, an older patient is much more likely to experience subsequent adverse complications and a prolonged hospital stay (Rothschild et al., 2000). It has been suggested that 25% of HAIs occur in patients in critical care units (CCUs) and up to 70% are due to resistant microorganisms. A 4-year prospective study of patients admitted to a medical–surgical ICU found that 34% of patients developed an HAI after a median of 9 days. The infection not only prolonged the length of hospital stay by 8 to 9 days but also doubled the risk of death (Appelgren et al., 2001 [Level IV]). Analysis of the National Nosocomial Surveillance Index found that the most common infections in an ICU are urinary tract (31%), pneumonia (27%), and bloodstream infections (19%) and are related to invasive devices in the vast majority of cases (Richards, Edwards, Culver, & Gaynes, 1999 [Level IV]).

UTIs are the most common HAIs, accounting for 30% to 40% of all nosocomial infections and increasing patient morbidity, length of stay, and costs of care (Brosnahan & Kent, 2004 [Level I]). The risk is directly related to the use and duration of indwelling bladder catheters, accounting for approximately

80% of hospital-acquired UTIs. The risk for developing a catheter-associated UTI (CAUTI) increases by approximately 5% for every hospital day (Nicolle, 2005 [Level V]). In one series, 9% of older patients who received an indwelling catheter developed a nosocomial UTI during the acute hospital stay; 50% of catheters used were determined to be inappropriate (Hazelett, Tsai, Gareri, & Allen, 2006 [Level IV]). A systematic review of the effects of duration of indwelling catheters on patient outcomes during a 37-year period revealed both a significant increase in UTIs when the catheter was removed after 48 hours and a reduction in hospital length of stay when removed within 24 to 48 hours (Fernandez & Griffiths, 2006 [Level I]). Coates, Hu, Bax, & Page (2002 [Level V]) found that catheter duration over 6 days was the highest risk factor for CAUTI and that by day 30, 100% of patients with catheters developed a UTI. Older patients are at particular risk for a UTI due to functional abnormalities (e.g., obstruction, prostate enlargement), certain medications, and chronic diseases (e.g., diabetes and cardiovascular and neurological diseases).

Hospital-acquired bloodstream infections are common, serious, and costly infections that appear to be the eighth leading cause of death in the United States (Wenzel & Edmond, 2001 [Level V]). These infections are most often related to the use of an invasive device and occur more than 50% of the time in ICU patients. CABSIs are serious and costly infections in ICU patients, occurring in 3% to 7% of all patients with central venous catheters (Warren, Zack, Cox, Cohen, & Fraser, 2003 [Level III]). A recent 3-year study of patients in the ICU and CCUs found a disturbingly high mortality and disability rate in 54 patients with CABSIs: 20 of the 54 patients died and only 9 were discharged home. Of note is the significant cost of care imposed by these infections, with the hospital losing money in 50 of 54 cases (Shannon et al., 2006 [Level IV]). The rising proportion of infections due to antibiotic-resistant organisms, as demonstrated in the largest multisite prospective surveillance study to date of nosocomial bloodstream infections in the United States, is of great concern (Wisplinghoff et al., 2004 [Level IV]).

Hospital-acquired pneumonia (HAP) is the second most common type of nosocomial infection after UTI, with an estimated mortality rate of 20% to 46% (Arozullah, Khuri, Henderson, & Daley, 2001 [Level IV]) and is the third most common postoperative complication after urinary tract and wound infections. Patients receiving continuous mechanical ventilation have a 6- to 21-fold increased risk of developing bacterial HAP (CDC, 2003 [Level I]). Pulmonary aspiration of secretions from the orophargeal or gastrointestinal tract is the most common cause of HAP and is considered preventable in the majority of cases (Brooks-Brunn, 1995 [Level V]). Although there is good evidence that the rate of aspiration pneumonia can be reduced by routine oral care (Hockenbury & Litwiller, 2004 [Level V]; Schleder, Stott, & Lloyd, 2002 [Level III]; Simmons-Trau, Cenek, Counterman, 2004 [Level V]), oral hygiene continues to be a nursing function of "low priority" in most health care settings (Weitzel, Robinson, & Holmie, 2006 [Level III]).

Surgical-site infections (SSIs) are the most common type of nosocomial infection in patients undergoing surgery, with incidence rates ranging from 5.6% to 24.5% of patients (de Oliveira, Ciosak, Ferraz, & Grinbaum, 2006 [Level IV]; Segers, de Jong, Kloek, Spanjaard, & de Mol, 2006 [Level IV]). Patients who develop an SSI have prolonged and more costly hospitalizations. They are also twice as likely to die, 60% more likely to be admitted to an ICU, and five times more likely to be rehospitalized than patients who do not develop an SSI (Kirkland, Briggs, Trivette, Wilkinson, & Sexton, 1999 [Level III]). Although the risk of an SSI varies according to type of surgery and patient-specific factors, Hollenbeak et al. (2006 [Level IV]) clearly demonstrated that factors related to the hospital itself, such as practice patterns and the environment of care, significantly increase the risk of patient harm.

Other infections that commonly affect hospitalized older patients include those affecting the skin (e.g., methicillin-resistant streptococcal aureus [MRSA]), the gastrointestinal tract (e.g., clostridium difficile [c. difficile] colitis), and candida infections of the oropharyngeal cavity. Clostridium difficile infections are affecting significant numbers of hospitalized older patients. It is estimated that 20% to 40% of hospitalized patients are colonized with the c. difficile toxin as compared to 2% to 3% of healthy adults (Bartlett, 2006 [Level V]). Of patients with antibiotic-associated diarrhea, 15% to 25% and more than 95% of patients with pseudomembranous colitis carry the c. difficile toxin. Since 2003, there has been an increase in frequency and severity of c. difficile infections, which are also becoming more refractory to treatment and more apt to relapse (Bartlett, 2006 [Level V]).

The alarming increase in antimicrobial-resistant organisms, such as MRSA and vancomycin resistant enterococcus (VRE), is of great concern to all health care providers and organizations. MRSA has increased in prevalence from 2% of staph aureus infections in 1974 to 63% in 2004, whereas VRE has steadily increased from <1% in 1990 to 28.5% of enterococcol isolates in 2003 (CDC, 2006 [Level I]). Vancomycin resistance has been shown to be an independent risk factor for death and is associated with poor patient outcomes, including longer length of stay, increased mortality, and higher costs of care (Salgado & Farr, 2003 [Level I]). More recently, the increase in multi drug resistant organisms has been associated with significantly longer hospital stays, increased cost, and mortality. The CDC has responded with the management of *Multi-Drug Resistant Organisms in Health Care Settings Guideline,* which outlines administrative priorities, education and training, judicious use of antibiotics, surveillance procedures, infection-control precautions, and environmental measures that must be implemented to prevent transmission of these potentially deadly organisms (CDC, 2006 [Level I]).

Nursing Strategies for HAI

Reducing the rate of HAI of is one of the Joint Commission's National Patient Safety Goals and comprises three of the six goals of the Institute for Healthcare Improvement's (IHI) 100,000 Lives Campaign. To that end, it is imperative that evidence-based medical and nursing care be implemented and that a system be in place to effectively and efficiently translate this into practice. The WHO and the CDC have published numerous guidelines for the prevention of health care infections with recommendations based on levels of evidence from the literature (see the Resources section). The CDC Guideline for Hand Hygiene in Health Care Settings (2002) includes the ban on artificial and long nails, mandated surveillance programs, and use of waterless-based antiseptic hand rubs before and after contact with a patient (CDC, 2002 [Level I]). Additional CDC guidelines include prevention of intravascular site-related infections (2002), infection control (2003), health care–associated pneumonia (2003), and MRSA (2006).

Hand washing and disinfection remains the most effective strategy to eliminate HAI (Rotter, 1998 [Level V]), and strict hand hygiene as outlined by the CDC guideline needs to be maintained at all times (Boyce & Pittet, 2002 [Level I]). Yet, despite widespread knowledge of the problem, health care providers continue to remain a major source of nosocomial infection. Studies of hand-hygiene practices have demonstrated low compliance rates, although coordinated efforts to address this problem have demonstrated significant improvements in adherence to hand hygiene (Eldridge et al., 2006 [Level V]), and subsequent reduction in nosocomial infection rates (Aragon, Sole, & Brown, 2005 [Level V]); Halwani, Solaymani-Dodaran, Grundmann, Coupland, & Slack (2006 [Level IV]) demonstrated a clear link between cross transmission of nosocomial infection in the ICU and understaffing, and factors that result in multiple staff–patient contacts, emphasizing the importance of good hand hygiene. Basic nursing interventions consisting of strict adherence to hand hygiene and gloves, elevating the head of the bed (HOB) for patients at risk for aspiration, and routine oral care can effectively reduce the rate of HAP in ICU patients (Weitzel, Robinson, & Holmie, 2006 [Level III]).

Encouraging deep breathing and coughing and incentive spirometry for high risk patients, as well as early mobilization, are critical nursing interventions to prevent pneumonia. Patients on mechanical ventilation are at substantially greater risk of ventilator-associated pneumonia (VAP), one of the infections targeted for reduction by the use of the IHI bundles. Elevating the HOB between 30 and 45 degrees has been shown to decrease the incidence of VAP from 34% to 8% in mechanically ventilated patients (Drakulovic et al., 1999 [Level II]). Nursing-specific strategies to reduce the risk of VAP are critical and include hand hygiene; HOB elevation; oral care with an antiseptic rinse for cardiac-surgery patients; noninvasive positive pressure ventilation; early extubation; subglottic secretion drainage; and avoiding gastric over-distension, condensate collection, and unplanned extubation (Hsieh & Tuite, 2006 [Level V]). A reduction in the rates of VAP and length of stay in the ICU was demonstrated through development of an evidence-based guideline that included five nursing interventions (i.e., HOB elevation, oral care, ventilator tubing condensate removal, hand hygiene, and glove use) (Abbott, Dremsa, Stewart, Mark, & Swift, 2006 [Level V]). Tolentino-DelosReyes, Ruppert, & Shiao (2007 [Level III]) demonstrated a significant improvement in critical care nurses' knowledge and adherence to evidence-based practice after an educational program on the ventilator "bundle," or set of interventions, to decrease VAP.

Nurses must be alert to and proactively collaborate with the physician to ensure the necessity of all invasive devices. Nurse-generated daily reminders to remove indwelling catheters within 5 days significantly reduced the duration of catheter use, rate of CAUTI, and the associated costs of care (Huang et al., 2004 [Level III]). Decision support tools, such as computerized physician order entry (CPOE) prompts, or standardized orders, have demonstrated the potential to decrease variation in care and improve patient care (Morris, 2004 [Level V]; Quinn & Mannion, 2005 [Level III]). A collaborative physician–nurse practice model utilizing computerized prompts and evidence-based guidelines for catheter use effectively decreased the use of indwelling bladder catheters and the subsequent nosocomial infection rate (Conklin, 2006 [Level III]). A 3-year prospective cohort study of all patients admitted to four general medical units at Yale–New Haven Hospital demonstrated that a multidisciplinary approach using technology (i.e., computerized prompts and bladder scans), staff education, and nurse empowerment to encourage timely removal resulted in an 81% reduction in catheter use and a 73% decrease in nosocomial UTIs (Topal et al., 2005 [Level III]). When clinically indicated, the use of antimicrobial bladder catheters (i.e., nitrofurazone-coated silicone or silver-coated latex) can prevent bacteriuria in hospitalized patients in need of short-term catheterization (Johnson, Kuskowski & Wilt, 2006 [Level I]). Gentry & Cope (2005 [Level III]) found that silver-alloy hydrogel-coated catheters reduced the risk of nosocomial UTIs by at least 33.5%. The authors reported that had an assessment for the appropriate indication for the catheter been performed in the first place, the increased the risk of infection may have been avoided; therefore, every effort must be made to address clinical necessity. In addition, the cost of these specialty catheters may offset the benefits if the use of inappropriate catheterization is not addressed (Gentry & Cope, 2005). A prospective study to determine risk factors for CAUTI found not only fecal incontinence to be a major risk but also that the hospital that used the silver-alloy catheters had a higher rate of CAUTIs, suggesting that overdependence on this technology may lead to laxity in care (Tsuchida et al., 2006 [Level IV]). As such, nurses need to be aware of the evidence-based criteria for an indwelling catheter (Griffiths & Fernandez, 2005 [Level I]) and collaborate with the primary provider to ensure that the device is clinically justified and not used for convenience or prevention of iatrogenic skin breakdown and pressure ulcers rather than good nursing care. When needed, select and maintain a closed catheter system with a small-size catheter, and insert using aseptic technique. Properly securing the catheter to avoid any movement that can introduce bacteria, ensuring unobstructed flow of urine, and properly positioning the drainage bag are additional interventions that can decrease the risk of UTI. Routine catheter irrigation should also be avoided (Smith, 2003 [Level IV]).

Risk-screening tools used to identify and stratify a patient's risk for nosocomial infections such as the National Nosocomial Infections Surveillance (NNIS) should be used not only for ongoing surveillance and reporting but also considered to target evidence-based interventions. Golliot et al. (2001 [Level IV]) suggest that all geriatric patients need to be considered as high risk for infection and closely monitored, and a risk index for nosocomial infection in geriatric rehabilitation and long term care facilities should be implemented. Segers et al. (2006 [Level IV]) demonstrated a steady decline in incidence of SSIs during a 2-year period with the implementation of risk assessment, novel treatment strategies, and a good surveillance program. A postoperative risk index, which was developed to identify patients at highest risk of nosocomial pneumonia and better guide perioperative respiratory care, successfully decreased the rate of pneumonia in patients undergoing major noncardiac surgery (Arozullah et al., 2001 [Level IV]). The risk factors included older than 60 years, functional impairment, and weight loss, suggesting that optimizing nutritional status preoperatively and promoting timely perioperative physical therapy and nursing mobilization of a surgical patient can reduce the risk of infection. Central venous catheter infections can be reduced significantly using nontechnologic strategies such as strict hand washing, maximal sterile barrier precautions, use of antiseptic solutions, insertion and management by trained personnel, and continuing quality improvement programs (Gnass et al., 2004 [Level IV]). Caparros, Lopez, & Grau (2001 [Level II]) decreased the incidence of catheter-related sepsis by enriching high-protein formula in critically ill patients receiving enteral feeding with arganine, fiber, and antioxidants. It is well known that SSIs are reduced with antibiotic prophylaxis within 2 hours of incision, and the incidence of nosocomial infection can be safely and effectively reduced by tightening glycemic control in the critically ill patient population (Grey & Perdrizet, 2004 [Level II]). To reduce the incidence of SSI, the timing of antibiotic administration must be a nursing priority and attention given to processes of care (Vazquez-Aragon, Lizan-Garcia, Cascales-Sanchez, Villar-Canovas, & Garcia-Olmo, 2003 [Level IV]).

Approximately one-third of nosocomial infections can be prevented by effective evidence-based infection control programs (Haley et al., 1985 [Level I]). Active, continuous infection control surveillance (rather than passive, voluntary-reporting programs) must be implemented to decrease hospital infection rates. infection control staff must be actively involved in implementing the guidelines, training staff, and performing ongoing surveillance and reporting processes with strong support from hospital leadership. In addition, because of increasing problems with bacterial resistance, antibiotic therapy needs to be prescribed judiciously and the use of vancomycin restricted. infection control efforts need to address strict adherence to appropriate cleansing of equipment and the environment, isolation of colonized patients, and appropriate surveillance programs.

Processes of care need to be reviewed and interdisciplinary quality improvement efforts initiated to minimize infection. A 5-year nurse-led interdisciplinary patient safety initiative that addressed systems problems, human factors, staff education, and reporting systems effectively reduced VAP (from 47.8 to 10.9 per 1,000 ventilator days) and CABSI (from 90th to 50th percentile). In addition, the rate of serious ADEs decreased by 45%, length of hospital stay was reduced from 8.1 to 4.5 days, RN vacancy rate decreased, and the use of contracted nurses was reduced by more than half (50% ICU, 65% medical–surgical) (Luther et al., 2002 [Level III]. In a study by Coopersmith et al. (2002 [Level III]), monthly feedback of infection rates was provided to staff along with an educational program; this intervention resulted in a 66% reduction in the occurrence of CABSI in the ICU. Performance feedback to individual surgeons has also been shown to decrease surgical-wound infection rates (Garcia-Rodriguez et al., 2006 [Level IV]). Education and performance feedback to staff and physicians on compliance with catheter care and hand hygiene led to a significant reduction in the CAUTI rate (Rosenthal, Guzman, & Safdar, 2004 [Level III]). Providing nursing staff with quarterly unit-specific data on CAUTI rates reduced the overall rate of CAUTI from 32 to 17.4 per 1,000 catheter-patient days at a cost savings of $403,000 during an 18-month period (Goetz, Kedzuf, Wagener, & Muder, 1999 [Level III]). Gastmeier et al. (2002 [Level II]) demonstrated that nosocomial infection rates can be reduced by introducing quality-improvement efforts such a quality circles and continuous surveillance.

Geriatric Syndromes

Geriatric syndromes are increasingly being recognized as serious and pre-ventable iatrogenic complications. Those that occur as a direct result of medical and nursing care (iatrogenesis) cause serious adverse outcomes in older pa-tients. The reader is referred to chapters 3, 7, 9, 12, 13, 15, and 18, which discuss geriatric syndromes that may be iatrogenic in origin. Geriatric syndromes are generally defined as highly prevalent, atypical, single-symptom states with var-ious causes; they need to be recognized as a valuable theoretical framework and used to train medical students (Olde-Rikkert, Rigaud, van Hoeyweghen, & de Graaf, 2003 [Level V]) and nurses (Stierle et al., 2006 [Level V]). Geriatric syndromes are also considered indicative of the quality of care of older adults in the nursing home setting (Sloss et al., 2000 [Level III]).

Tsilimingras, Rosen, and Berlowitz (2003 [Level V]) contend that the pati-ent-safety initiatives sparked by the "To Err Is Human" publications do not go far enough to address the unique needs of older patients who are at greatest risk of iatrogenic harm. They suggest that geriatric syndromes need to be recognized as distinct iatrogenic events—going so far as to call them medical errors—and urge major system reform to address these preventable and costly problems. Strategies include the need to routinely identify and report all geriatric syn-dromes and, when they occur, proactively identify and address system failures, reduce ADEs, improve the continuity of care, improve geriatric training pro-grams, and establish dedicated geriatric units (Tsilimingras et al., 2003 [Level V]). Covinsky et al. (1998 [Level III]) demonstrated that functional outcomes can be improved at no additional cost with the use of a dedicated acute care for the elderly (ACE) unit, which utilized patient-centered care (i.e., routine nursing assessment of patient functional status and use of nursing protocols, rounds by a multidisciplinary team), a specially designed environment, regu-lar review of medical care, and emphasis on discharge planning. Recognizing that older patients are at greatest risk of costly adverse outcomes, many health care organizations are utilizing geriatric specialists, dedicated acute care units for older patients, interdisciplinary teams, and other innovative models of care delivery that have dramatically improved geriatric patient care and outcomes. Berntsen (2006 [Level V]) calls for the implementation of patient centeredness as a way of minimizing patient harm. One of the original six aims to maintain patient safety outlined in a major IOM report (2001 [Level I]), patient centered-ness expects that the needs, wants, and preferences of the patient should drive health care interventions. Nurses providing patient-centered care compassion-ately and empathetically respond to the needs of the patient and offer ample opportunities for patients and families to direct their care through involved and informed decision making (Berntsen, 2006 [Level V]). Kane (2002 [Level V]) provides a compelling argument that major system reform for chronic disease is needed if quality geriatric patient care is to be achieved. He suggests reevalu-ating the roles of not only patients and their families but also hospital personnel at all levels and utilizing information technology to more closely monitor and quickly intervene with higher risk patients.

Hospital staff needs to understand the increased vulnerability of older and critically ill patients, to readily identify those at higher risk, and to proactively intervene to prevent patient harm. Evidence-based medical care and nursing standards of practice for falls, delirium, pressure ulcers, and other geriatric syndromes as outlined in this book need to be adopted. Screening tools, such as the High Risk Diagnoses for the Elderly Scale, designed to predict 1-year mortality in hospitalized elders (Desai, Bogardus, Williams, Vitagliano, & Inouye, 2002 [Level IV]), can be used to target patients for interventions to minimize patient harm and suffering and cost of care. Screening hospitalized older adults for malnutrition and dehydration early is effective in decreasing protein-calorie malnutrition (Rypkema et al., 2003 [Level III]). It is widely accepted that hospitalized patients with dementia are at greatest risk of developing delirium (Fick, Agnostini, & Inouye, 2002 [Level I]). Seminal work by Inouye and others in the area of delirium demonstrated that this serious and costly complication can be prevented with early preventive strategies, as outlined in chapter 7, *Delirium: Prevention, Early Recognition, and Treatment* (Inouye et al., 1999 [Level II]; Inouye, 2004 [Level VI]; Milisen, Lemiengre, Braes, & Foreman, 2005 [Level I]).

Adverse Effects of Diagnostic, Medical, and Surgical Procedures

Patients in CCUs and the elderly are at increased risk of iatrogenic harm due to the need for more medical procedures and therapies. Iatrogenic pneumothorax due to either barotraumas or invasive procedures is a life-threatening complication in 3% of ICU patients (de Lassence et al., 2006 [Level IV]), whereas ICU-acquired paresis (generalized weakness) appears to affect 25.3% of patients (de Jonghe et al., 2002 [Level IV]). Patients requiring prolonged mechanical ventilation in the ICU are well known to be at significantly greater risk of developing VAP and suffering poorer outcomes. A 2-year retrospective study of 11,119 patients who underwent cardiac catheterization and/or percutaneous interventions with femoral artery access found that patients older than 70 were at higher risk of vascular complications (Dumont, Keeling, Bourguignon, Sarembock, & Turner, 2006 [Level IV]).

Diagnostic tests and procedures involve some degree of risk based on whether they are invasive or administer a pharmacologically inert agent such as contrast dye or radiation therapy. Contrast dye, commonly used in CT scans and myelography, can produce both allergic and nonallergic reactions ranging from urticaria and angioedema to anaphylaxis. Radiocontrast infusion in patients with renal impairment can cause acute renal failure or an exacerbation of CHF. Intrathecal use of contrast media in myelography is known to produce various adverse effects including vasovagal syncope, nausea, postural headache, hearing loss, aseptic meningitis, and encephalopathy.

Medical procedures, such as thoracentesis and cardiac catheterization, have also been linked to significantly more preventable adverse effects, such as cardiac arrhythmias, bleeding, infection, and pneumothorax, in older adults (Thomas & Brennan, 2000 [Level IV]). The literature is full of case reports of iatrogenic injuries and deaths due to procedures such as venous embolism caused by the injection of CT contrast (Imai, Tamada, Gyoten, Yamashita, & Kajihara, 2004 [Level V]), aspiration deaths due to barium (Blackmore,

Cranshaw, & Soar, 2005 [Level V]), emollient laxatives and contrast medium (Hunsaker & Hunsaker, 2002 [Level V]), and colonic perforations due to endoscopy or enema (Bobba & Arsura, 2004 [Level V]). As mentioned previously, device-related infections, particularly central venous catheter bloodstream infection, VAP, and CAUTIs, pose an enormous threat to geriatric and critically ill patients and are of even greater concern in developing countries (Rosenthal et al., 2006 [Level IV]).

Even relatively risk-free medical and nursing procedures such as the administration of intravenous fluids can be dangerous in an older patient with age-related reduced cardiac reserve, leading to preventable CHF or hypokalemia. Sherman (2005 [Level V]) identifies three new forms of geriatric iatrogenesis, referred to as the "hypos" of hospitalization, that can delay discharge, increase costs, and lead to adverse patient outcomes. Iatrogenic-induced hypokalemia occurs when intravenous fluids are given without potassium, whereas hypotension can be induced when an as-needed antihypertensive is administered for a high blood pressure taken while the patient is in the supine position. Transient decreases in oral intake in patients receiving oral hypoglycemic agents or standing insulin orders can cause preventable hypoglycemia, if the lower limit at which the insulin is administered is not at least a blood glucose of 200 or 250g/dl. Hospital-acquired acute renal failure is common, with iatrogenic causes implicated in half of all patients (Finn, 2003 [Level V]). Unnecessary bedrest, in and of itself, can have serious negative effects on older patients, including functional decline, venous thrombotic embolism (VTE), pressure ulcers, falls, delirium, orthostatic hypotension, anorexia, and constipation and fecal impaction, among others adverse outcomes.

Surgical and perioperative complications are also common, although great strides have been made, especially in the areas of perioperative management, anesthesia, surgical technique, and intensive care. A 5-year study examining iatrogenic ureter injuries found that incidence of injuries declined from 31.7% to 11.8%, attributing the decline to the use of prophylactic J stent or ureteric catheter placement (Al-Awadi, Kehinde, Al-Hunayan, & Al-Khayat, 2005 [Level IV]). Although age per se is not an independent risk factor for perioperative complications, pathologic changes associated with age especially in the cardiovascular and pulmonary systems tend to place an older patient at greater risk. Age-associated changes and atypical presentation of disease further complicate the picture, making diagnosis more difficult. As such, geriatric patients account for half of all surgical emergencies and three-fourths of all operative deaths; therefore, timely diagnosis and optimal perioperative care is critical for survival.

Assessment and Interventions to Reduce Adverse Effects of Diagnostic, Medical, and Surgical Procedures

Nurses have a responsibility to recognize the increased risk to older patients of any diagnostic, prophylactic, and medical procedures. Collaboration with the physician is important to ensure that the patient is giving informed consent and that the patient is appropriately screened, assessed, and managed to prevent unnecessary harm. Nurses must also ensure the patient clearly understands the inherent risks and benefits. Given the significantly greater risk of harm in older adults, a geriatric patient requires a careful and comprehensive assessment of the appropriateness of all invasive procedures and devices. Although health care professionals are trained to always weigh the risk and benefits, it is critical to heighten one's assessment of the situation and to err on the side of caution with older patients. Potentially harmful diagnostic and therapeutic procedures may well be contraindicated if the potential benefit does not clearly increase the potential for improving patient outcomes. This is particularly important, given the strong evidence that the older population tends to have lower rates of informed consent (Sugarman, McCrory, & Hubal, 1998 [Level I]). Ensuring that an older patient clearly understands the risks and benefits of any and all invasive procedures and is truly making an "informed" decision is critical and may warrant several discussions to evaluate the patient's understanding of the situation. Given the age-associated increase in sensory deficits (see chapter 21, *Sensory Changes*), it is critical to identify visual or hearing loss that may impair patient understanding and provide the patient with appropriate sensory aides (e.g., glasses, hearing amplifier).

Nurses must take a more active role in identifying patients at higher risk of surgical complications, given the evidence that only a small percentage of surgeons and anesthetists recognized the higher risk patients or ordered improved postoperative monitoring (Pirret, 2003 [Level III]). A simple nursing preoperative assessment tool identified the higher risk patients in need of improved postoperative monitoring and reduced acute admissions to the ICU from 40% to 19%. Barbosa-Silva and Barros (2005 [Level IV]) determined that a new method of nutritional screening is an important nutritional prognostic variable that can be used to identify the risk of postoperative complications. Collaborating with nutrition services to identify the higher risk patient, nursing can intervene to increase postoperative monitoring and management.

Contrast dye needs to be avoided in patients with renal insufficiency, and nursing staff needs to closely monitor the patient's hydration status before and after the use of contrast dye in diagnostic studies. Careful monitoring and stabilization of all active medical problems and attention to age-adjusted approaches during the perioperative phase is equally important. Administering age-adjusted appropriate medications to premedicate prior to procedures is critical, as is the ability of the nurse to question what may be a high risk dose or drug. A geriatric patient's oral intake needs to be carefully monitored and reported, and insulin needs to be adjusted to prevent hypoglycemia (Sherman, 2005 [Level V]). Nursing staff needs to routinely take orthostatic vital signs or to at least measure the blood pressure of older patients in at least the sitting position to ensure that standing systolic and diastolic hypotension is not induced by treating supine systolic hypertension (Sherman, 2005 [Level V]).

Evidence-based guidelines need to be adopted, with fastidious attention to the implementation process. Nursing care focused on preventing infection, reducing tension at the surgical site, and optimizing nutritional status has been shown to effectively prevent surgical-wound dehiscence, a serious complication with up to 50% mortality (Hahler, 2006 [Level V]). Given the plethora of evidence that communication and other systems problems cause iatrogenic patient harm, the Joint Commission recently mandated timeouts and other verification procedures at high risk times to prevent wrong-site surgeries and other errors (Edmonds, Liguori, & Stanton, 2005 [Level V]).

Provider Beliefs and Attitudes

Although the majority of the literature focuses on iatrogenic illness and injuries that result from either the commission or omission of a physical act, arguments can be made that equally detrimental effects to patients can occur as a direct result of a health care practitioner's values, beliefs, fears, prejudices, and attitudes. For example, the early belief that ulcers were due to psychological problems and that leprosy was a contagious disease that warranted lifetime quarantine resulted in undue suffering by large numbers of people. A nurse's perception of older adults as chronically ill and frail may foster increasing dependence and functional decline when the patient is not provided the opportunity or assistance to routinely ambulate or engage in self-care skills. A diagnosis of dementia may lead a prejudiced or uneducated health care practitioner to expect less of a patient and to subsequently offer fewer treatment options.

Providers who fail to place the patient's values ahead of their own can cause undue suffering and harm when these values are in conflict. It is well known that a significant number of nursing home patients suffer needlessly in pain, sometimes due to a clinician's fear of narcotic dependence that takes precedence over comfort. Older adults, more than any other age group, tend to be under-treated for pain (Robinson, 2007 [Level V]; Lovheim, Sandman, Kallin, Karlsson, & Gustafson, 2006 [Level IV]) and other conditions, including osteoporosis (Davis, Ashe, Guy, & Khan, 2006 [Level IV]) and depression (Harman et al., 2002 [Level IV]). In a study examining the attitudes of family physicians toward late-life depression, the authors attributed its under-treatment to overconfidence by providers with no recent training in the condition, 41% of whom identified depression as the most common geriatric problem (Harman et al., 2002 [Level IV]). The assumption that the quality of life of the demented person is "poor" may contribute to the assumption by the nurse or physician that palliation or institutionalization is the most appropriate goal of care, regardless of the values of the older adult. Kenny (1990 [Level V]) asserts that the present system of hospital care not only perpetuates dependency and iatrogenesis among geriatric patients but also tends to "erode their self-esteem, identity and individuality." In addition, prolonged hospital stays are known to increase social isolation and foster dependence (Mayo, Wood-Dauphinee, Gayton, & Scott, 1997 [Level IV]). One is left to wonder how much this may contribute to the high rates of depression in hospitalized older patients. To make matters worse, older patients are known to under-report or deny symptoms, in part because they have grown accustomed to living with chronic aches and pains and may interpret new symptoms as yet another symptom of a long-standing health problem. They may believe the symptom is a normal part of aging or fear a loss of independence or, worse, institutionalization if they admit to a physical or cognitive deficit. Older adults today are also from a generation who respect and more readily accept the word of the physician and are less inclined to be assertive with the provider or aggressive in seeking a second opinion. These factors can have disastrous results when it is considered that most physicians are poorly trained in geriatric health care and may be unaware of core concepts of geriatric medicine, such as the importance of a functional approach to care and the atypical presentation of disease that makes diagnosis more difficult. As such, it is important that health care practitioners examine their belief systems and educate themselves and not unwittingly contribute to the patient's suffering and despair because of biases toward older patients that can compromise clinical objectivity and patient care.

Medical and Nursing Error and Other Care-Related Factors

The plethora of literature and research sparked by the patient-safety movement has documented that the provision of medical and nursing care itself places older patients at increased risk of health care–related harm. It is now well recognized that a significant proportion of iatrogenic complications are directly related to the complex interplay of organizational and human factors that create opportunities for patient harm. A prospective study of patients admitted for CHF found that 7% of admissions were the result of improper treatment, including fluid overload, and inappropriate medications and procedures. In addition, hospital mortality for this group was three times greater than older patients admitted without iatrogenic CHF (Rich et al., 1996 [Level IV]). The Harvard Medical Practice Study found that a disturbing 20.7% of adverse events was due to negligence, with a significantly greater proportion occurring among older patients (Brennan et al., 1991, 2004 [both Level IV]).

Lack of provider and organizational awareness of the risk and lack of attention to patient and environmental safety further increase the risk of iatrogenic harm. As such, maintaining patient safety depends on understanding and proactively addressing measures to ensure systems and processes of care that foster safe, evidence-based patient care. An in-depth discussion of medical and nursing error and the organizational interventions needed to maintain patient safety is beyond the scope of this chapter. However, nurses need to be at the forefront and engaged in interdisciplinary efforts to prevent unnecessary patient harm. Nurses play a pivotal role in preventing patient harm. They are not only the largest workforce of health care providers, they also provide the final "barrier a patient has to being a victim of error" (Hughes & Clancy, 2005 [Level V]). Significant strides in improving patient care have been made with nurses actively involved in identifying care-related problems. For example, the Institute for Healthcare Improvement (IHI) and The Robert Wood Johnson Foundation–sponsored national initiative, *Transforming Care at the Bedside* (TCAB), creates, tests, and implements nurse-generated practice changes (Viney, Batcheller, Houston, & Belcik, 2006 [Level V]) to improve patient care and safety. A 6-week nationwide study of the effect of nursing rounds at least every 2 hours demonstrated a significant decrease in call-light use and a subsequent reduction in patient falls and increase in patient satisfaction (Meade, Bursell & Ketelsen, 2006 [Level III]. Connor (2002 [Level IV]) reports on effective multidisciplinary approaches that include patient safety rounds and problem-specific teams that created and implemented evidence-based opiate guidelines, improved pain management through a multidisciplinary educational program, and routinely reviewed and addressed medication events. Of import, a recent survey of 1,200 critical care nurses demonstrated that nurses in hospitals who had adopted an oral care protocol were more apt to implement evidence-based care than those who did not use the protocol, and that there is inconsistent adoption and adherence to the CDC guidelines for VAP in the United States (Cason, Tyner, Saunders, Broome, & Centers for Disease Control and Prevention, 2007 [Level IV]). The critical need for optimal implementation of and adherence to evidence-based guidelines, including adoption of nursing protocols, cannot be underemphasized.

National and Organizational Priorities

Despite early recognition of the problem, better care, and prophylaxis for iatrogenic events, progress has been slow and the rate of preventable adverse events remains alarmingly high; several appear to be increasing. The IOM *To Err Is Human* report increased provider awareness to the dangers of diagnostic and therapeutic interventions and led to a significant increase in patient-safety research, literature, and initiatives (Stelfox, Palmisani, Scurlock, Orav, & Bates, 2006 [Level V]). Continued funding for patient-safety research and major patient-safety initiatives by organizations such as Agency for Healthcare Research and Quality (AHRQ), the IHI, Leapfrog Group, IOM, and others must be a priority (Leape, 2005a [Level V]). IHI's "5 Million Lives Campaign" aims to protect that many patients from incidents of medical error in the 2 years preceding. Affonso, Jeffs, Doran, & Ferguson-Pare (2003 [Level V]) and Johnstone and Kanitsaki (2006 [Level V]) contend that health professional groups and organizations are morally obligated to make patient-safety research a priority and that nursing organizations need to provide active leadership and commitment to this endeavor.

Developing, implementing, and regularly updating evidence-based interventions at the national and local levels are critical. National evidence-based guidelines and standards of practice, especially in the areas of infection control by the CDC and WHO, and geriatric best practice by geriatric nursing experts working with The John A. Hartford Foundation, have been and continue to be developed and regularly updated. Health care organizations have not only a responsibility to ensure that these standards are implemented and adhered to but also an economic imperative, due to the unnecessary costs associated with iatrogenesis (Hwang & Herndon, 2007 [Level V]). Inouye and colleagues (2003 [Level III]) demonstrated that effective delirium prevention in acutely ill patients was dependent on nurse's adherence to nonpharmacologic protocols. The Joint Commission has taken the lead in hospitals by mandating adherence to annual patient safety goals, such as improving the accuracy of patient identification and communication between caregivers, improving medication safety, reducing the risk of infection, and preventing falls and pressure ulcers.

Efforts must continue to increase education and training to all medical, nursing, and ancillary health care professionals (HCPs) in the areas of iatrogenesis, gerontological nursing, geriatric syndromes, patient safety, and teamwork. Wakefield et al. (2005 [Level V]) argue that nursing and medical schools must integrate patient-safety principles into their curricula in order to teach HCPs to more effectively prevent and manage errors and to ease the burden on an already overstretched health care system. More emphasis needs to be placed on teaching the aviation model, which emphasizes teamwork and communication, and for nurses to understand human factors as a cause of and means to prevent error and patient harm (Sherwood, Thomas, Bennett, & Lewis, 2002 [Level V]). Of concern is the disturbing lack of geriatric education in health care professions schools that is only beginning to be addressed. Research in the area of delirium, restraints, and CHF has demonstrated that nurses with training in geriatrics provide significantly better care to older patients (Foreman, Wakefield, Culp, & Milisen, 2001 [Level V]; Lacko et al., 2000 [Level III], Naylor, 2004 [Level V]; Neufeld et al., 1999 [Level IV]). Initiatives to promote more geriatric education in nursing schools and geriatric competence for all nurses need to continue and to be supported (Stierle et al., 2006 [Level V]). Medical trainees need additional training in malnutrition (Singh, Watt, Veitch, Cantor, & Duerksen, 2006 [Level III]), geriatric syndromes (Olde-Rikkert et al., 2003 [Level V]), and functional and diagnostic assessment of frail older patients in order to prevent iatrogenic harm, including cascade iatrogenesis (Potts et al., 1993 [Level IV]). Every effort must be taken to ensure that nursing and other health-professional students receive similar training. Although improvements have been made in the past decade integrating more gerontological nursing education into nursing-school curricula, Berman et al. (2005 [Level IV]) demonstrated a critical need to address the shortage of nursing faculty qualified in gerontology.

Nurse staffing and competence is imperative, given strong evidence that both staffing levels and educational preparation inversely affect patient care. The groundbreaking AHRQ report entitled "Keeping Patients Safe: Transforming the Work Environment of Nurses" demonstrated that staffing and workflow design clearly impact errors and patient-safety outcomes (Page, 2004 [Level I]). A study of HAIs in the ICU confirmed previous data that nurse staffing is directly related to infection rate. The authors noted an increase in infection several days after heavy workload, and they advocate maintaining staffing at higher levels to minimize the risk of infection (Hugonnet, Chevrolet, & Pittet, 2007 [Level IV]). Yet, despite increased attention and major research done in this area, lack of standardized data and other problems continue to hinder attempts to find a clear solution to the optimal staffing needed to minimize error (Blegen, 2006 [Level I]). Research must continue in this area so that improvements in nurse staffing, work areas, and transfer of knowledge both within the organization and between providers is optimized to maintain patient safety.

Health care organizations need to ensure that coordinated and effective training in both patient safety and geriatric patient care is well integrated into staff orientation and ongoing in-service and annual mandatory and competency training programs. Collaboration between education and risk management, quality and infection control is important to effectively identify educational priorities and the most effective training strategies. Lee, Fletcher, Westley, & Fankhauser (2004 [Level V]) successfully enhanced the competence of nursing staff in geriatric nursing using a series of self-paced learning modules in conjunction with the implementation of the geriatric resource nurse (GRN) model of care and staff development. Parke, Ross, & Moss (2003 [Level V]) created and implemented the gerontological enrichment program in which knowledge, skills, and abilities were successfully integrated into existing acute care nursing competencies.

Hospital and nursing leadership need to embrace patient safety as an explicit organizational goal and actively promote a culture of safety in which everyone is aware of the significance of iatrogenesis and accepts that human beings make mistakes even in perfect systems (Dennison, 2005 [Level V]). Leadership must foster a safety-oriented environment in which all staff and physicians are encouraged to identify, report, and actively work in a positive manner to eliminate potentially harmful situations (Leape, 2000 [Level VI]). A national survey of nurses in 25 U.S. hospitals found a large percentage of iatrogenic harm is not reported by nurses, a mere 36% of whom felt near misses should be reported (Blegen et al. (2004 [Level IV]). Leape, a leading and respected authority on patient safety, considers it an ethical imperative to "first, do no harm," and encourages physicians to do everything practical to keep patients safe, including being open and honest with patients and ensuring the competence of colleagues (Leape, 2005b [Level VI]).

Safe patient care cannot be ensured without the appropriate organizational structure and processes that promote efficient communication of pertinent information. It is imperative that hospitals address systems problems, including staffing and workflow design, processes of care such as communication and teamwork, and human factors such as fatigue, all of which are known to jeopardize patient safety. Communication and collaboration is vital "to ensure appropriate exchange of information and coordination of care" (IOM, 2001 [Level I]), whereas lack of communication is considered a major contributor to iatrogenic complications. The Joint Commission recognized that communication breakdown is the cause of close to 70% of all sentinel events, although a study to elicit stories of preventable physical or psychological harm due to medical error found breakdown in communication was a far greater problem than technical error (Kuzel et al., 2004 [Level IV]).

Hospitals need to examine information processes to ensure that pertinent data are routinely and consistently shared with the health care team, including the patient. It is critical to evaluate and optimize which patient information is communicated during any handoff report, especially at high risk times, and create evidence-based guidelines regarding what needs to be included during this process (Alvarado et al., 2006 [Level IV]). Inaccurate or absent information can dramatically increase the risk of harmful effects on older patients. The "kardex" and care plan for an older patient that lacks critical baseline functional and cognitive data can hamper recognition of subtle changes in condition and may contribute to functional decline and other adverse outcomes, including cascade iatrogenesis. Nursing staff needs to include daily functional priorities and goals that have been developed with the patient and/or family into every shift or handoff report.

Evidence suggests that patient transfer from either another unit or hospital may be independently associated with the development of nosocomial infections (Eveillard, Quenon, Rufat, Mangeol, & Fauvelle, 2001 [Level IV]). Boockvar et al. (2004 [Level IV]) demonstrated that patient transfer from hospital to a skilled nursing facility was a significant risk factor for ADEs. Every effort must be made to also address the communication of appropriate data during these high risk times. It is widely recognized that hospital discharge is a potentially high risk opportunity for ADEs; therefore, posthospital medication-management strategies using interdisciplinary teams, information technology, and transitional-care models need to be considered (Foust, Naylor, Boling, & Cappuzzo, 2005 [Level V]). Telephone calls to recently discharged patients can be an effective measure to minimize adverse events and prevent unnecessary readmissions (Forster et al., 2004 [Level IV]). Because so many hospital admissions are related to ADEs, hospitals should consider screening for them in the emergency department to better understand and address the problem in the outpatient setting (Hafner, Belknap, Squillante, & Bucheit, 2002 [Level IV]).

Information technology has the potential to significantly improve our ability to provide safe patient care by enhancing communication and providing decision support. The electronic medical record (EMR) needs to be a considered a priority by organizations as a means to ensure that evidence-based patient care is implemented and monitored (IOM, 2001 [Level I]). A well-designed EMR with CPOE has been shown to reduce the number of medication errors by 81% (Koppel et al., 2005 [Level IV]). Not only are prescription errors due to illegible handwriting prevented, but the EMR can also ensure best-practice prescribing using standardized order sets and preprogrammed medication alerts to prevent adverse drug–drug interactions. The EMR also has the capability to provide decision support, promote continuity of care, and decrease adverse events with more efficient communication between care providers, especially at high risk times such as during cross-coverage (Petersen, Orav, Teich, O'Neil, & Brennan, 1998 [Level III]) and during handoff. However, after identifying 22 types of error risks with the CPOE system, Koppel et al. (2005 [Level IV]) warn that attention needs to be given to the role of the EMR in facilitating medication errors and every measure taken to reduce this risk,. It is also important that health care professionals with geriatric background be involved from the onset with the building of the EMR to ensure that best-practice geriatric assessment and management protocols are included. Nurses need to be aware of the limitations of CPOE and remain vigilant partners in care to ensure patient safety.

Health care organizations need to recognize both what constitutes high risk situations and those populations most at risk for adverse outcomes and implement effective patient-safety strategies designed to minimize harm. Other evidence-based priorities needed by health care organizations to address all the factors required to promote patient safety are critical; however, they are beyond of scope of this chapter. The IHI has developed an eight-step process for leaders to follow to improve patient safety (http://www.ihi.org/IHI/Results/WhitePapers/LeadershipGuidetoPatientSafetyWhitePaper.htm), whereas Dennison (2005 [Level V]) suggests hospital leadership use the "PATIENT SAFE" mneumonic to ensure that the numerous, necessary steps are taken to ensure patient safety.

Nurses are in a unique role to prevent the cascade of iatrogenesis (Jacelon, 1999 [Level V]) and must use their knowledge of aging to proactively intervene to promote and advocate safe, quality geriatric patient care to members of the health care team, including physicians. For example, knowledge of the concept of diminishing physiologic reserve capacity with aging should prompt the nurse to understand the need to balance diagnostic and therapeutic interventions with the need for rest and sleep (Hart, Birkas, Lachmann, & Saunders, 2002 [Level V]). Closely monitoring sleep patterns in order to prevent sleep deprivation and scheduling tests and therapy only after the patient has adequate rest are critical to prevent delirium and promote healing. Computerized prompts to use a nonpharmacological sleep protocol, which is as effective and less harmful than sedative-hypnotic medications and promotes higher quality sleep (McDowell,

Mion, Lydon, & Inouye, 1998 [Level III]), have decreased the use of higher risk sleeping medications (Agostini et al., 2007 [Level III]).

Promoting a more collaborative relationship between the nurse and the patient to attain mutually agreed-upon goals is an important but often overlooked process of care that can foster more patient control, self-care, and autonomy. Faulkner (2001 [Level III]) developed a tool that measures the extent to which a nursing unit empowers or disempowers patients, implying that the latter will increase their risk of becoming dependent, and suggests that the tool can positively augment quality-improvement efforts. Nurses must effectively encourage patients to be vigilant and proactive partners in care in order to prevent unnecessary harm (Hibbard, Peters, Slovic, & Tusler, 2005 [Level IV]). Providing patient education about medical errors and what they could do about them has been shown to increase actual protective behaviors in patients (Hibbard et al., 2005 [Level IV]). Given the evidence, the Joint Commission is following suit with its 2007 patient-safety goal mandating more active involvement of patients in their plan of care. Hospitals are encouraged to provide patients with fall prevention and restraint-reduction patient-safety information upon admission in order to encourage more active involvement of the patient and significant others in maintaining safety.

Conclusion

Significant progress has been made in better understanding and addressing the problem of iatrogenesis with the work of agencies such as the AHRQ, IHI, Joint Commission, National Patient Safety Foundation, IOM, Leapfrog Group, and others. Major strides have been made in the Veterans Administration health system, which implemented systemwide patient-safety and training initiatives and created four patient-safety research centers, emerging as a leader in patient safety. Yet, there remains much work to be done, especially in the area of preventing harm to vulnerable geriatric patients.

Nurses must recognize their critical role in preventing these iatrogenic complications, which far too often can and do trigger a cascade of inevitable decline that could have been prevented if the initial iatrogenic event had not occurred. Nurses have a responsibility to advocate for their patients, and this duty is critical for patients who cannot do so for themselves, such as cognitively impaired elders and those without family support. They depend on the nurse's knowledge of their baseline functional and cognitive status and risk factors to appreciate the goals of and barriers to care. They rely on the nursing staff's ability to recognize subtle changes and to proactively intervene to keep older patients safe while hospitalized. Involving family and caregivers as much as possible and providing predischarge training and referral to community resources can help discharge at-risk patients in a timelier manner and minimize recidivism. No longer should iatrogenic harm be the unfortunate price that patient's pay for medical progress, nor should we accept the fact that random, unlucky events happen in a chaotic environment. Rather, nurses need to take a stand to educate themselves and others to the problem of iatrogenesis and to take every precaution necessary to ensure a culture and practice of patient safety that will one day result in a decline in this major public health problem.

Resources

Patient Safety

Agency for Health Care Research and Quality (AHRQ): Patient Safety Network http://www.psnet.ahrq.gov/

Institute for Healthcare Improvement http://www.ihi.org/IHI/

Institute of Medicine http://www.iom.edu/

IOM Crossing the Quality Chasm http://www.iom.edu/CMS/8089.aspx

Joint Commission www.jointcommission.org/PatientSafety

National Patient Safety Foundation http://www.npsf.org/

U.S. Department of Veterans Affairs National Center for Patient Safety http://www.patientsafety.gov/

World Health Organization World Alliance on Patient Safety http://www.who.int/patientsafety/en/

Infection Control Centers for Disease Control and Prevention (CDC) http://www.cdc.gov

Association for Professionals in Infection Control and Epidemiology (APIC), Society of Healthcare Epidemiology of America (SHEA) http://www.apic.org/Content/NavigationMenu/GovernmentAdvocacy/MandatoryReporting/PositionPapers/mrpositionpapers.htm

National Nosocomial Infection Surveillance System http://www.cdc.gov/ncidod/dhqp/nnis.html

Handwashing Guidelines http://www.mrw.interscience.wiley.com/cochrane/clsysrev/articles/CD005186/frame.html

World Health Organization's World Alliance for Patient Safety

Guidelines on Hand Hygiene in Health Care (Advanced Draft, 2005) http://www.who.int/patientsafety/events/05/HH_en.pdf

Clinical Practice

AHRQ (Agency for Healthcare Research and Quality) Clinical Practice Guidelines http://www.ahrq.gov/clinic/cpgsix.htm

EPIQ (Effective Practice, Informatics and Quality Improvement) Supports effective, evidence-based practice, health informatics, and quality improvement initiatives http://www.health.auckland.ac.nz/population-health/epidemiology-biostats/epiq/

National Guideline Clearinghouse
A public resource for evidence-based clinical practice guidelines http://www.guideline.gov/

Joanna Briggs Institute (Promote and Support Best Practice) International, interdisciplinary evidence-based resources http://www.joannabriggs.edu.au/about/home.php

References

Abbott, C. A., Dremsa, T., Stewart, D. W., Mark, D. D., & Swift, C. C. (2006). Adoption of a ventilator-associated pneumonia clinical practice guideline. *Worldviews on Evidence-Based Nursing*, 3(4), 139–152. Evidence Level V: Review.

Affonso, D. D., Jeffs, L., Doran, D., & Ferguson-Pare, M. (2003). Patient safety to frame and reconcile nursing issues. *Canadian Journal of Nursing Leadership, 16*(4), 69–81. Evidence Level V: Review.

Agostini, J. V., Zhang, Y., & Inouye, S. K. (2007). Use of computer-based reminder to improve sedative-hypnotic prescribing in older hospitalized patients. *American Geriatrics Society, 55*(1), 43–48. Evidence Level III: Quasi-experimental Study.

Al-Awadi, K., Kehinde, E. O., Al-Hunayan, A., & Al-Khayat, A. (2005). Iatrogenic ureteric injuries: Incidence, aetiological factors and the effect of early management on subsequent outcome. *International Urology & Nephrology, 37*(2), 235–241. Evidence Level IV: Nonexperimental Study.

Alvarado, K., Lee, R., Christoffersen, E., Fram, N., Boblin, S., Poole, N., et al. (2006). Transfer of accountability: Transforming shift handover to enhance patient safety. *Healthcare Quarterly, 9*, 75–79. Evidence Level IV: Nonexperimental Study.

Appelgren, P., Hellstrom, I., Weitzberg, E., Soderlund, V., Bindslev, L., & Ransjo, U. (2001). Risk factors for nosocomial intensive care infection: A long-term prospective analysis. *Acta Anaesthesiologica Scandinavica, 45*(6), 710–719. Evidence Level IV: Nonexperimental Study.

Aragon, D., Sole, M. L., & Brown, S. (2005). Outcomes of an infection prevention project focusing on hand hygiene and isolation practices. *AACN Clinical Issues, 16*(2), 121–132. Evidence Level V: Program Evaluation.

Arozullah, A. M., Khuri, S. F., Henderson, W. G., & Daley, J. (2001). Development and validation of a multifactorial risk index for predicting postoperative pneumonia after major noncardiac surgery. *Annals of Internal Medicine, 135*(10), 647–657. Evidence Level IV: Nonexperimental Study.

Baker, G. R., Norton, P. G., Flintoft, V., Blais, R., Brown, A., Cox, J., et al. (2004). The Canadian Adverse Events Study: The incidence of adverse events among hospital patients in Canada. *Canadian Medical Association Journal, 170*(11), 1678–1686. Evidence Level IV: Nonexperimental Study.

Barbosa-Silva, M. C., & Barros, A. J. (2005). Bioelectric impedance and individual characteristics as prognostic factors for postoperative complications. *Clinical Nutrition, 24*(5), 830–838. Evidence Level IV: Nonexperimental Study.

Bartlett, J. G. (2006). Narrative review: The new epidemic of *Clostridium difficile. Annals of Internal Medicine, 145*(10), 758–764. Evidence Level V: Review.

Baune, B., Kessler, V., Patris, S., Descamps, V., Casalino, E., Quenon, J. L., et al. (2003). Medicinal iatrogenics in hospitals: A survey on a given day. *Presse Med, 32*(15), 683–688. Evidence Level IV: Nonexperimental Study.

Beaujean, D. J., Blok, H. E., Vandenbroucke-Grauls, C. M., Weersink, A. J., Raymakers, J. A., & Verhoef, J. (1997). Surveillance of nosocomial infections in geriatric patients. *Journal of Hospital Infection, 36*(4), 275–284. Evidence Level IV: Nonexperimental Study.

Berman, A., Mezey, M., Kobayashi, M., Fulmer, T., Stanley, J., Thornlow, D., et al. (2005). Gerontological nursing content in baccalaureate nursing programs: Comparison of findings from 1997 and 2003. *Journal of Professional Nursing, 21*(5), 268–275. Evidence Level IV: Nonexperimental Study.

Berntsen, K. J. (2006). Implementation of patient centeredness to enhance patient safety. *Journal of Nursing Care Quality, 21*(1), 15–19. Evidence Level V: Review.

Blackmore, S. J., Cranshaw, J., & Soar, J. (2005). Barium sulphate aspiration and lung injury. *Care of the Critically Ill, 21*(1), 26–28. Evidence Level V: Case Report.

Blegen, M. A. (2006). Patient safety in hospital acute care units. *Annual Review of Nursing Research, 24*, 103–125. Evidence Level I: Systematic Review.

Blegen, M. A., Vaughn, T., Pepper, G., Vojir, C., Stratton, K., Boyd, M., et al. (2004). Patient and staff safety: Voluntary reporting. *American Journal of Medical Quality, 19*(2), 67–74. Evidence Level IV: Nonexperimental Study.

Bobba, R. K., & Arsura, E. L. (2004). Septic shock in an elderly patient on dialysis: Enema-induced rectal injury confusing the clinical picture. *Journal of the American Geriatrics Society, 52*(12), 2144. Evidence Level V: Case Report.

Boockvar, K., Fishman, E., Kyriacou, C. K., Monias, A., Gavi, S., & Cortes, T. (2004). Adverse events due to discontinuations in drug use and dose changes in patients transferred between acute- and long-term care facilities. *Archives of Internal Medicine, 164*(5), 545–550. Evidence Level IV: Nonexperimental Study.

Boyce, J. M., & Pittet, D. (2002). Guideline for Hand Hygiene in Health-Care Settings. Recommendations of the Healthcare Infection Control Practices Advisory Committee and the HIPAC/SHEA/APIC/IDSA Hand Hygiene Task Force. *American Journal of Infection Control, 30*(8), S1–S46. Evidence Level I: Systematic Review.

Brennan, T. A., Leape, L. L., Laird, N. M., Hebert, L., Localio, A. R., Lawthers, A. G., et al. (2004). Incidence of adverse events and negligence in hospitalized patients: Results of the Harvard Medical Practice Study. *Quality and Safety in Health Care, 13*(2), 145–151. Evidence Level IV: Nonexperimental Study.

Brennan, T. A., Leape, L. L., Laird, N. M., Hebert, L., Localio, A. R., Lawthers, A. G., et al. (1991). Incidence of adverse events and negligence in hospitalized patients: Results of the Harvard Medical Practice Study. *New England Journal of Medicine, 324*, 370–376. Evidence Level IV: Nonexperimental Study.

Brooks-Brunn, J. A. (1995). Postoperative atelectasis and pneumonia: Risk factors. *American Journal of Critical Care, 4*(5), 340–349. Evidence Level V: Review.

Brosnahan, J. E., & Kent, B. (2004). Short-term indwelling catheters (a systematic review): Evidence for a primarily nursing decision. *Worldviews Evidence-Based Nursing, 1*(4), 228. Evidence Level I: Systematic Review.

Burke, J. P. (2003). Infection control: A problem for patient safety. *New England Journal of Medicine, 348*(7), 651–656. Evidence Level V: Review.

Burt, C. W. (2001). Emergency health care encounters for adverse effects of medical treatment. *Managed Care Interface, 14*(12), 39–42.

Caparros, T., Lopez, J., & Grau, T. (2001). Early enteral nutrition in critically ill patients with a high-protein diet enriched with arginine, fiber, and antioxidants compared with a standard high-protein diet: The effect on nosocomial infections and outcome. *Journal of Parenteral & Enteral Nutrition, 25*(6), 299–308. Evidence Level II: Individual Experimental Study.

Cason, C. L., Tyner, T., Saunders, S., Broome, L., & Centers for Disease Control and Prevention. (2007). Nurses' implementation of guidelines for ventilator-associated pneumonia from the Centers for Disease Control and Prevention. *American Journal of Critical Care, 16*(1), 28–36. Evidence Level IV: Nonexperimental Study.

Centers for Disease Control (CDC). (2002). Guideline for hand hygiene in healthcare settings. Atlanta, GA: U.S. Department of Health and Human Services, CDC. Retrieved May 4, 2007, from http://www.cdc.gov/handhygiene/. Evidence Level I: Systematic Review.

Centers for Disease Control (CDC). (2003). Guideline for preventing health-care–associated pneumonia. Atlanta, GA: U.S. Department of Health and Human Services, CDC. Retrieved May 4, 2007, from http://www.cdc.gov/ncidod/dhqp/gl_hcpneumonia.html. Evidence Level I: Systematic Review.

Centers for Disease Control (CDC). (2006). Management of multidrug-resistant organisms in healthcare settings. Atlanta, GA: U.S. Department of Health and Human Services, CDC. Retrieved May 4, 2007, from http://www.cdc.gov/ncidod/dhqp/pdf/ar/mdroGuideline2006.pdf.

Coates, A., Hu, Y., Bax, R., & Page, C. (2002). The future challenges facing the development of new antimicrobial drugs. *National Reviews Drug Discovery, 1*(11), 895–910. Evidence Level V: Review.

Conklin, S. M. (2006). A collaborative practice model reduces indwelling catheter use and risk for nosocomial urinary tract infections. *Worldviews on Evidence-Based Nursing, 1*(4), 232. Evidence Level III: Prospective Cohort with Intervention Study.

Connor, M., Ponte, P. R., & Conway, J. (2002). Multidisciplinary approaches to reducing error and risk in a patient care setting. *Critical Care Nursing Clinics of North America, 14*(4) 359–367. Evidence Level IV: Nonexperimental Study.

Coopersmith, C. M., Rebmann, T. L., Zack, J. E., Ward, M. R., Corcoran, R. M., Schallom, M. E., et al. (2002). The effect of education programs on decreasing catheter-related bloodstream infection in the surgical intensive care unit. *Critical Care Medicine, 30*, 59–64. Evidence Level III: Pre- and Post-Intervention Observational Study.

Covinsky, K. E., Palmer, R. M., Kresevic, D. M., Kahana, E., Counsell, S. R., Fortinsky R. H., et al. (1998). Improving functional outcomes in older patients: Lessons from an acute care for elders unit. *Joint Commission Journal on Quality Improvement, 24*(2), 63–76. Evidence Level III: Quasi-experimental Study.

Darchy, B., LeMiere, E., Figueredo, B., Bavoux, E., & Domart, Y. (1999). Iatrogenic diseases as a reason for admission to the intensive care unit: Incidence, causes and consequences.

Archives of Internal Medicine, 159(1), 71–78. Evidence Level IV: Nonexperimental Study.

Davis, J. C., Ashe, M. C., Guy, P., & Khan, K. M. (2006). Under-treatment after hip fracture: A retrospective study of osteoporosis overlooked. *Journal of the American Geriatrics Society, 54*(6), 1019–1020. Evidence Level IV: Nonexperimental Study.

Davis, P., Lay-Yee, R., Briant, R., Ali, W., Scott, A., & Schug, S. (2002). Adverse events in New Zealand public hospitals I: Occurrence and impact. *New Zealand Medical Journal, 115*, 1167: U271 Evidence Level IV: Nonexperimental Study.

de Jonghe, B., Sharshar, T., Lefaucheur, J., Authier, F., Durand-Zaleski, I., Boussarsar, M., et al. (2002). Caring for the critically ill patient. Paresis acquired in the intensive care unit: A prospective multicenter study. *Journal of the American Medical Association, 288*(22), 2859–2867. Evidence Level IV: Nonexperimental Study.

de Lassence, A., Timsit, J. F., Tafflet, M., Azoulay, E., Jamali, S., Vincent, F., et al. (2006). Pneumothorax in the intensive care unit: Incidence, risk factors, and outcome. *Anesthesiology, 104*(1), 5–13. Evidence Level IV: Nonexperimental Study.

de Oliveira, A. C., Ciosak, S. I., Ferraz, E. M., & Grinbaum, R. S. (2006). Surgical site infection in patients submitted to digestive surgery: Risk prediction and the NNIS risk index. *American Journal of Infection Control, 34*(4), 201–207. Evidence Level IV: Nonexperimental Study.

Dennison, R. D. (2005). Creating an organizational culture for medication safety. *Nursing Clinics of North America, 40*(1), 1–23. Evidence Level V: Review.

Desai, M. M., Bogardus, S. T., Jr., Williams, C. S., Vitagliano, G., & Inouye, S. K. (2002). Development and validation of a risk-adjustment index for older patients: The high risk diagnoses for the elderly scale. *Journal of the American Geriatrics Society, 50*(3), 474–481. Evidence Level IV: Nonexperimental Study.

Drakulovic, M. B., Torres, A., Bauer, T. T., Nicolas, J. M., Nogue, S., & Ferrer, M. (1999). Supine body position as a risk factor for nosocomial pneumonia in mechanically ventilated patients: A randomized trial. *Lancet, 354*(9193), 1851–1858 Evidence Level II: Single Experimental Study.

Dumont, C. J. P., Keeling, A. W., Bourguignon, C., Sarembock, I. J., & Turner, M. (2006). Predictors of vascular complications post-diagnostic cardiac catheterization and percutaneous coronary interventions. *Dimensions of Critical Care Nursing, 25*(3), 137–142. Evidence Level IV: Nonexperimental Study.

Edmonds, C. R., Liguori, G. A., & Stanton, M. A. (2005). Two cases of a wrong-site peripheral nerve block and a process to prevent this complication. *Regional Anesthesia and Pain Medicine, 30*(1), 99–103. Evidence Level V: Case Report.

Eldridge, N. E., Woods, S. S., Bonello, R. S., Clutter, K., Ellingson, L., Harris, M. A., et al. (2006). Using the six sigma process to implement the Centers for Disease Control and Prevention Guideline for Hand Hygiene in four intensive care units. *Journal of General Internal Medicine, 21*(Suppl. 2), S35–S42. Evidence Level V: Review.

Eveillard, M., Pisante, L., Mangeol, A., Dolo, E., Guet, L., Huang, M., et al. (1998). Specific features of nosocomial infections in the elderly at a general hospital center: Five surveys of annual prevalence. *Pathologie-biologie 46*(10), 741–749. Evidence Level IV: Nonexperimental Study.

Eveillard, M., Quenon, J. L., Rufat, P., Mangeol, A., & Fauvelle, F. (2001). Association between hospital-acquired infections and patients' transfers. *Infection Control & Hospital Epidemiology, 22*(11), 693–696. Evidence Level IV: Nonexperimental Study.

Faulkner, M. (2001). A measure of patient empowerment in hospital environments catering for older people. *Journal of Advanced Nursing, 34*(5), 676–686. Evidence Level III: Quasi-experimental Study.

Fernandez, R. S., & Griffiths, R. D. (2006). Duration of short-term indwelling catheters: A systematic review of the evidence. *Journal of Wound, Ostomy, & Continence Nursing, 33*(2), 145–155. Evidence Level I: Systematic Review.

Fick, D. M., Agostini, J. V., & Inouye, S. K. (2002). Delirium superimposed on dementia: A systematic review. *Journal of the American Geriatrics Society, 50*(10), 1723–1732. Evidence Level I: Systematic Review.

Finn, K. M. (2003). Hospital-acquired acute renal failure: What hospitalists need to know. *Journal of Clinical Outcomes Management, 10*(4), 214–223. Evidence Level V: Case Study.

Foreman, M. D., Wakefield, B., Culp, K., & Milisen, K. (2001). Delirium in elderly patients: An overview of the state of the science. *Journal of Gerontological Nursing, 27*(4), 12–20.

Forster, A. J., Asmis, T. R., Clark, H. D., Al Saied, G., Code, C. C., Caughey, S. C., et al. (2004). Ottawa hospital patient-safety study: Incidence and timing of adverse events in patients admitted to a Canadian teaching hospital. *Canadian Medical Association Journal, 170*(8), 1235–1240. Evidence Level IV: Nonexperimental Study.

Forster, A. J., Clark, H. D., Menard, A., Dupuis, N., Chernish, R., Chandok, N., et al. (2004). Adverse events among medical patients after discharge from hospital. *Canadian Medical Association Journal, 170*(3), 345–349. Evidence Level IV: Nonexperimental Study.

Foust, J. B., Naylor, M. D., Boling, P. A., & Cappuzzo, K. A. (2005). Opportunities for improving post-hospital home medication management among older adults. *Home Health Care Services Quarterly, 24*(1/2), 101–122. Evidence Level V: Narrative Literature Review.

Frazier, S. C. (2005). Geropharmacology. Health outcomes and polypharmacy in elderly individuals: An integrated literature review. *Journal of Gerontological Nursing, 31*(9), 4–11. Evidence Level I: Systematic Review.

Gandhi, T. K., Weingart, S. N., Borus, J., Seger, A. C., Peterson, J., Burdick, E., et al. (2003). *Adverse drug events in ambulatory care, 348*(16), 1556–1564. Evidence Level IV: Nonexperimental Study.

Garcia-Rodriguez, J. F., Trobo, A. R., Garcia, M. V. L., Martinez, M. J. C., Millan, C. P., Vazquez, M. C., et al. (2006). The effect of performance feedback on wound infection rate in abdominal hysterectomy. *American Journal of Infection Control, 34*(4), 182–187. Level IV: Nonexperimental Study.

Gastmeier, P., Brauer, H., Forster, D., Dietz, E., Daschner, F., & Ruden, H. (2002). A quality management project in 8 selected hospitals to reduce nosocomial infections: A prospective, controlled study. *Infection Control & Hospital Epidemiology, 23*(2), 91–97. Evidence Level II: Individual Experimental Study.

Gentry, H., & Cope, S. (2005). Using silver to reduce catheter-associated urinary tract infections. *Nursing Standard, 19*(50), 51–54. Evidence Level III: Quasi-experimental Study.

Giraud, T., Dhainaut, J. F., Vaxelaire, J. F., Joseph, T., Journois, D., Bleichner, G., et al. (1993). Iatrogenic complications in adult intensive care units: A prospective two-center study. *Critical Care Medicine, 21*(1), 40–51. Evidence Level IV: Prospective Observational Study.

Gnass, S. A., Barboza, L., Bilicich, D., Angeloro, P., Treiyer, W., Grenovero, S., et al. (2004). Prevention of central venous catheter-related bloodstream infections using nontechnologic strategies. *Infection Control & Hospital Epidemiology, 25*(8), 675–677. Evidence Level IV: Nonexperimental Study.

Goetz, A. M., Kedzuf, S., Wagener, M., & Muder, R. R. (1999). Feedback to nursing staff as an intervention to reduce catheter-associated urinary tract infections. *American Journal of Infection Control, 27*(5), 402–404. Evidence Level III: Quasi-experimental Study.

Golliot, F., Astagneau, P., Cassou, B., Okra, N., Rothan-Tondeur, M., & Brucker, G. (2001). Nosocomial infections in geriatric long term care and rehabilitation facilities: Exploration in the development of a risk index for epidemiological surveillance. *Infection Control & Hospital Epidemiology, 22*(12), 746–753. Evidence Level IV: Nonexperimental Study.

Green, C. F., Mottram, D., Rowe, P. H., & Pirmohamed, M. (2000). Adverse drug reactions as a cause of admission to an acute medical assessment unit: A pilot study. *Journal of Clinical Pharmacy & Therapeutics, 25*(5), 355. Evidence Level IV: Prospective Cohort Study.

Grey, N. J., & Perdrizet, G. A. (2004). Reduction of nosocomial infections in the surgical intensive-care unit by strict glycemic control. *Endocrine Practice, 10* (Suppl. 2), 46–52. Evidence Level II: Individual Experimental Study.

Griffiths, R., & Fernandez, R. (2005). Policies for the removal of short-term indwelling catheters. *Cochrane Database of Systematic Reviews, 21*(1), CD004011. Evidence Level I: Systematic Review.

Hafner, J. W., Jr., Belknap, S. M., Squillante, M. D., & Bucheit, K. A. (2002). Adverse drug events in emergency department patients. *Annals of Emergency Medicine, 39*(3), 258–267. Evidence Level IV: Nonexperimental Study.

Hahler, B. (2006). Surgical wound dehiscence. *Medical—Surgical Nursing, 15*(5), 296–300; Quiz 301. Evidence Level V: Review.

Haley, R. W., Culver, D. H., White, J. W., Morgan, W. M., Emori, T. G., Munn, V. P., et al. (1985). The efficacy of infection surveillance and control programs in preventing nosocomial infections in U.S. hospitals. *American Journal of Epidemiology, 121*(2), 182–205. Evidence Level I: Nonexperimental Study.

Halwani, M., Solaymani-Dodaran, M., Grundmann, H., Coupland, C., & Slack, R. (2006). Cross-transmission of nosocomial pathogens in an adult intensive care unit: Incidence and risk factors. *Journal of Hospital Infection, 63*(1), 39–46. Level IV: Nonexperimental study.

Harman, J. S., Brown, E. L., Have, T. T., Mulsant, B. H., Brown, G., & Bruce, M. L. (2002). Primary care physicians' attitude toward diagnosis and treatment of late-life depression. *CNS Spectrums, 7*(11), 784–790. Evidence Level IV: Nonexperimental Study.

Hart, B., Birkas, J., Lachmann, M., & Saunders, L. (2002). Promoting positive outcomes for elderly persons in the hospital: Prevention and risk factor modification. *American Association of critical care Nurses [AACN] Clinical Issues, 13*(1), 22–33. Evidence Level V: Review.

Hazelett, S. E., Tsai, M., Gareri, M., & Allen, K. (2006). The association between indwelling urinary catheter use in the elderly and urinary tract infection in acute care. *BioMed Central Geriatrics, 6*, 15. Evidence Level IV: Nonexperimental Study.

Health Grades, Inc. (2004). Patient safety in American hospitals. Retrieved March 26, 2007, from http://www.healthgrades.com/media/english/pdf/HG_Patient_Safety_Study_Final.pdf. Evidence Level IV: Nonexperimental Study.

Hibbard, J. H., Peters, E., Slovic, P., & Tusler, M. (2005). Can patients be part of the solution? Views on their role in preventing medical errors. *Medical Care Research and Review, 62*(5), 601–616. Evidence Level IV: Nonexperimental Study.

Hollenbeak, C. S., Lave, J. R., Zeddies, T., Qanfen, P., Roland, C. E., & Sun, E. F. (2006). Factors associated with risk of surgical wound infections. *American Journal of Medical Quality, 21*(6), 29S–34S. Evidence Level IV: Nonexperimental Study.

Hsieh, H. Y., & Tuite, P. K. (2006). Prevention of ventilator-associated pneumonia: What nurses can do. *Dimensions in Critical Care Nursing, 25*(5), 205–208. Evidence Level V: Review.

Huang, W. C., Wann, S. R., Lin, S. L., Kunin, C. M., Kung, M. H., Lin, C. H., et al. (2004). Catheter-associated urinary tract infections in intensive care units can be reduced by prompting physicians to remove unnecessary catheters. *Infection Control & Hospital Epidemiology, 25*(11), 974–978. Evidence Level III: Quasi-experimental Study.

Hughes, R. G., & Clancy, C. M. (2005). Working conditions that support patient safety. *Journal of Nursing Care Quality, 20*(4), 289–292. Evidence Level V: Review.

Hugonnet, S., Chevrolet, J. C., & Pittet, D. (2007). The effect of workload on infection risk in critically ill patients. *Critical Care Medicine, 35*(1), 76–81. Evidence Level IV: Nonexperimental Study.

Hunsaker, D. M., & Hunsaker, J. C., III. (2002). Therapy-related care coronary deaths: Two case reports of rare asphyxial deaths in patients under supervised care. *American Journal of Forensic Medicine & Pathology, 23*(2), 149–154. Evidence Level V: Case Report.

Hussain, M., Oppenheim, B. A, O'Neill, P., Trembath, C., Morris, J., & Horan, M. A. (1996). Prospective survey of the incidence, risk factors, and outcome of hospital-acquired infections in the elderly. *The Journal of Hospital Infection, 32*(2),117–126. Evidence Level IV: Prospective Observational Study.

Hwang, R. W., & Herndon, J. H. (2007). The business case for patient safety. *Clinical Orthopedics and Related Research, 457*, 21–34. Evidence Level V: Review.

Imai, S., Tamada, T., Gyoten, M., Yamashita, T., & Kajihara, Y. (2004). Iatrogenic venous air embolism caused by CT injector from a risk management point of view. *Radiation Medicine, 22*(4), 269–271. Evidence Level V: Review.

Inouye, S. K. (2004). A practical program for preventing delirium in hospitalized elderly patients. *Cleveland Clinic Journal of Medicine, 71*(11), 890–896. Evidence Level VI: Expert Opinion.

Inouye, S. K., Bogardus, S. T., Jr., Charpentier, P.A., Leo-Summers, L., Acampora, D., Holford, T. R., et al. (1999). A multicomponent intervention to prevent delirium in hospitalized older patients. *New England Journal of Medicine, 340*(9),669–676. Evidence Level II: Single Experimental Study.

Inouye, S. K., Bogardus, S. T., Jr., Williams, C. S., Leo-Summers, L., & Agostini, J. V. (2003). The role of adherence on the effectiveness of nonpharmacologic interventions: Evidence from the delirium prevention trial. *Archives of Internal Medicine*, April 28, *163*(8), 958–964. Evidence Level III: Quasi-experimental Study.

Institute of Medicine (IOM]) (2001). Crossing the quality chasm: A new health system for the 21st century. Washington, DC: National Academy Press. Evidence Level I: Systematic Review.

Jacelon, C. (1999). Preventing cascade iatrogenesis in hospitalized elders: An important role for nurses. *Journal of Gerontological Nursing, 25*(10), 27–33. Evidence Level V: Narrative Literature Review.

Johnson, J. R., Kuskowski, M. A., & Wilt, T. J. (2006). Systematic review: Antimicrobial urinary catheters to prevent catheter-associated urinary tract infection in hospitalized patients. *Annals of Internal Medicine, 144*(2), 116–126. Evidence Level I: Systematic Review.

Johnstone, M. J., & Kanitsaki, O. (2006). The moral imperative of designating patient safety and quality care as a national nursing research priority. *Collegian, 13*(1), 5–9. Evidence Level V: Review.

Kaiser Family Foundation, Agency for Health Care Quality and Research, & Harvard School of Public Health (2004). National survey on consumers' experiences with patient safety and quality information. Retrieved April 25, 2007, from http://www.kff.org/kaiserpolls/pomr111704pkg.cfm. Evidence Level IV: Nonexperimental Study.

Kane, R. L. (2002). Clinical challenges in the care of frail older persons. *Aging Clinical & Experimental Research, 14*(4), 300–306. Evidence Level V: Literature Review.

Kenny, T. (1990). Erosion of individuality in care of elderly people in hospital: An alternative approach. *Journal of Advanced Nursing, 15*(5), 571–576. Evidence Level V: Review.

Kirkland, K. B., Briggs, J. P., Trivette, S. L., Wilkinson, W. E., & Sexton, D. J. (1999). The impact of surgical-site infections in the 1990s: Attributable mortality, excess length of hospitalization, and extra costs. *Infection Control & Hospital Epidemiology, 20*(11), 725–730. Evidence Level III: Quasi-experimental Study.

Kohn, L., Corrigan, J., & Donaldson, M. (Eds.) (1999). To Err Is Human: Building a safer health system. Institute of Medicine. Washington, DC: National Academy Press. Evidence Level I: Systematic Review.

Koppel, R., Metlay, J. P., Cohen, A., Abaluck, B., Localio, A. R., Kimmel, S. E., et al. (2005). The role of computerized physician order entry systems in facilitating medication errors. *Journal of the American Medical Association, 293*(10), 1197–1203. Evidence Level IV: Qualitative and Quantitative Survey, Focus Groups.

Kuzel, A. J., Woolf, S. H., Gilchrist, V. J., Engel, J. D., LaVeist, T. A., Vincent, C., et al. (2004). Patient reports of preventable problems and harms in primary health care. *Family Medicine, 2*(4), 333–340. Evidence Level IV: Qualitative Narrative Review.

Lacko, L. A., Dellasega, C., Salerno, F. A., Singer, H., DeLucca, J., & Rothenberger, C. (2000). The role of the advanced practice nurse in facilitating a clinical research study. Screening for delirium. *Clinical Nurse Specialist, 14*(3), 110–115.

Lazarou, J., Pomeranz, B. H., & Corey, P. N. (1998). Incidence of adverse drug reactions in hospitalized patients: A meta-analysis of perspective studies. *Journal of the American Medical Association, 279*(15), 1200–1205. Evidence Level I: Systematic Review.

Leape, L. L. (2000). Can we make health care safe? In *Reducing medical errors and improving patient safety: Success stories from the front lines of medicine*, S. Findlay (ed). Washington, DC: National Coalition on Health Care and Institute for Healthcare Improvement. Evidence Level VI: Expert Opinion. Retrieved on June 7, 2007 from http://www.wkkf.org/DesktopModules/WKF.00_DmaSupport/ViewDoc.aspx?LanguageID=0&CID=229&ListID=28&ItemID=1622840&fld=PDFFile.

Leape, L. L. (2005a). Five years after *To Err Is Human*: What have we learned? *Journal of the American Medical Association, 293*, 2384–2390. Evidence Level V: Review.

Leape, L. L. (2005b). Ethical issues in patient safety. *Thoracic Surgery Clinics. 15*(4), 493–501. Evidence level VI: Expert Opinion

Lee, V., Fletcher, K., Westley, C., & Fankhauser, K. A. (2004). Competent to care: Strategies to assist staff in caring for elders. *Medical–Surgical Nursing, 13*(5), 281–288; Quiz 289. Evidence Level V: Program Evaluation.

Lefevre, F., Feinglass, J., Soglin, L., Yamold, P., Martin, G., & Webster, J. (1992). Iatrogenic complications in high risk elderly patients. *Archives of Internal Medicine, 152*, 2074–2080. Evidence Level IV: Nonexperimental Study.

Lehmann, L. S., Puopolo, A. L., Shaykevich, S., & Brennan, T. A. (2005). Iatrogenic events resulting in intensive care admission: Frequency, cause, and disclosure to patients and institutions. *American Journal of Medicine, 118*(4), 409–413. Evidence Level IV: Nonexperimental Study.

Lovheim, H., Sandman, P. O., Kallin, K., Karlsson, S., & Gustafson, Y. (2006). Poor staff awareness of analgesic treatment jeopardizes adequate pain control in the care of older people. *Age & Ageing, 35*(3), 257–261. Evidence Level IV: Nonexperimental Study.

Luther, K. M., Maguire, L., Mazabob, J., Sexton, J., Heimreich, R., & Thomas, E. (2002). Engaging nurses in patient safety. *Critical Care Nursing Clinics of North America*, *14*(4), 341–346. Evidence Level III: Quasi-Experimental Study.

Mayo, N. E., Wood-Dauphinee, S., Gayton, D., & Scott, S. C. (1997). Nonmedical bed-days for stroke patients admitted to acute care hospitals in Montreal, Canada. *Stroke*, *28*(3), 543–549. Evidence Level IV: Nonexperimental Study.

McDonnell, P. J. (2002). Hospital admissions resulting from preventable adverse drug reactions. *Annals of Pharmacotherapy*, *37*(2), 303–304. Evidence Level IV: Nonexperimental Study.

McDowell, J. A., Mion, L. C., Lydon, T. J., & Inouye, S. K. (1998). A nonpharmacologic sleep protocol for hospitalized older patients. *Journal of the American Geriatrics Society*, *46*(6), 700–705. Evidence Level III: Quasi-Experimental Study.

Meade, C. M., Bursell, A. L., & Ketelson, L. (2006). Effects of nursing rounds on patient call light use, satisfaction, and safety. *American Journal of Nursing*, *106*(9), 58–70. Evidence Level III: Quasi-Experimental Study.

Milisen, K., Lemiengre, J., Braes, T., & Foreman, M. D. (2005). Multicomponent intervention strategies for managing delirium in hospitalized older people: Systematic review. *Journal of Advanced Nursing*, *52*(1), 79–90. Evidence Level I: Systematic Review.

Morris, A. H. (2004). Iatrogenic illness: A call for decision support tools to reduce unnecessary variation. *Quality & Safety in Health Care*, *13*(1) 80–81. Evidence Level V: Review.

Naylor, M. D. (2004). Transitional care for older adults: A cost-effective model. *Leonard David Institute [LDI] Issue Brief*, *9*(6), 1–4. Retrieved May 4, 2007, from http://www.upenn.edu/ldi/issuebrief9_6.pdf. Evidence Level V: Narrative Review.

Neufeld, R. R., Libow, L. S., Foley, W. J., Dunbar, J. M., Cohen, C., & Breuer, B. (1999). Restraint reduction reduces serious injuries among nursing home residents. *Journal of the American Geriatrics Society*, *47*(10), 1202–1207. Evidence Level IV: Nonexperimental Study.

Nicolle, L. E. (2005). Catheter-related urinary tract infection. *Drugs Aging*, *22*(8), 627–639. Evidence Level V: Review.

Olde-Rikkert, M. G., Rigaud, A. S., van Hoeyweghen, R. J., & de Graaf, J. (2003). Geriatric syndromes: Medical misnomer or progress in geriatrics? *The Netherlands Journal of Medicine*, *61*(3), 83–87. Evidence Level V: Review.

Page, A. (Ed.) (2004). Keeping patients safe: Transforming the work environment of nurses. Washington, DC: National Academies Press. Evidence Level I: Systematic Review.

Parke, B., Ross, D., & Moss, L. (2003). Creating a cultural shift: A gerontological enrichment program for acute care. *Journal for Nurses in Staff Development*, *19*(6), 305–312. Evidence Level V: Case Report.

Petersen, L. A., Orav, E. J., Teich, J. M., O'Neil, A. C., & Brennan, T. A. (1998). Using a computerized sign-out program to improve continuity of inpatient care and prevent adverse events. *Joint Commission Journal on Quality Improvement*, *24*(2), 77–87. Evidence Level III: Quasi-Experimental Study.

Pirret, A. M. (2003). A preoperative scoring system to identify patients requiring postoperative high dependency care. *Intensive Critical Care Nursing*, *19*(5), 267–275. Evidence Level III: Quasi-Experimental Study.

Potts, S., Feinglass, J., Lefevere, F., Kadah, H., Branson, C., & Webster, J. (1993). A quality-of-care analysis of cascade iatrogenesis in frail elderly hospital patients. *Quality Review Bulletin*, *19*(6), 199–205. Evidence Level IV: Nonexperimental Study.

Quinn, M. M., & Mannion, J. (2005). Improving patient safety using interactive, evidence-based decision support tools. *The Joint Commission Journal on Quality & Patient Safety*, *31*(12), 678–683. Evidence Level III: Quasi-Experimental Study.

Rich, M. W., Shah, A. S., Vinson, J. M., Freedland, K. E., Kuru, T., & Sperry, J. C. (1996). Iatrogenic congestive heart failure in older adults: Clinical course and prognosis. *Journal of the American Geriatrics Society*, *44*, 638–643. Evidence Level IV: Nonexperimental Study.

Richards, M. J., Edwards, J. R., Culver, D. H., & Gaynes, R. P. (1999). Nosocomial infections in the medical intensive care units in the United States: National nosocomial infections surveillance system. *Critical Care Medicine*, *27*(5), 887–892. Evidence Level IV: Nonexperimental Study.

Robinson, C. L. (2007). Relieving pain in the elderly. *Health Progress*, *88*(1), 48–53, 70. Evidence Level V: Narrative Review.

Rosenthal, V. D., Guzman, S., & Safdar, N. (2004). Effect of education and performance feedback on rates of catheter-associated urinary tract infection in intensive care units in Argentina. *Infection Control & Hospital Epidemiology, 25*(1), 47–50. Evidence Level III: Quasi-Experimental Study.

Rosenthal, V. D., Maki, D. G., Salomao, R., Moreno, C. A., Mehta, Y., Higuera, F., et al., & International Nosocomial Infection Control Consortium (2006). Device-associated nosocomial infections in 55 intensive care units of 8 developing countries. *Annals of Internal Medicine, 145*(8), 582–591. Evidence Level IV: Nonexperimental Study.

Rothschild, J. M., Landrigan, C. P., Cronin, J. W., Kaushal, R., Lockley, S. W., Burdick, E., et al. (2005). The Critical Care Safety Study: The incidence and nature of adverse events and serious medical errors in ICU. *Critical Care Medicine, 33*(8), 1694–1700. Evidence Level IV: Prospective Observational Study.

Rothschild, J., Bates, W., & Leape, L. L. (2000). Preventable medical injuries in older patients. *Archives of Internal Medicine, 160*(18), 2717–2728. Evidence Level V: Literature Review.

Rotter, M. L. (1998). Semmelweis' sesquicentennial: A little-noted anniversary of handwashing. *Current Opinion in Infectious Diseases, 11*(4), 457–460. Evidence Level V: Literature Review.

Rypkema, G., Adand, E., Dicke, H., Naber, T., De Weart, B., Disselhorst, L., et al. (2003). Cost-effectiveness of an interdisciplinary intervention in geriatric inpatients to prevent malnutrition. *Journal of Nutrition, Health and Aging, 8*(2), 122–127. Evidence Level III: Prospective Controlled Study.

Safran, D. G., Neuman, P., Schoen, P., Kitchman, M. S., Wilson, I. B., Cooper, B., et al. (2005). Prescription drug coverage and seniors: Findings from a 2003 national survey. Retrieved August 22, 2006, from http://content.healthaffairs.org/cgi/content/abstract/hlthaff.w5.152. Evidence Level IV: Survey.

Salgado, C. D., & Farr, B. M. (2003). Outcomes associated with vancomycin-resistant enterococci: A meta-analysis. *Infection Control & Hospital Epidemiology, 24*(9), 690–698. Evidence Level I: Systematic Review.

Schioler, T., Lipczak, H., Pedersen, B. L., Mogensen, T. S., Bech, K. B., Stockmarr, A., et al. (2001). Danish Adverse Event Study: Incidence of adverse events in hospitals. A retrospective review of medical records. *Ugeskr Laeger, 163*(39), 5370–5378. Evidence Level IV: Nonexperimental Study.

Schleder, B., Stott K., & Lloyd, R. (2002). The effect of a comprehensive oral-care protocol on patients at risk for ventilator-associated pneumonia. *Journal of Advocate Healthcare, 4*(1), 27–30. Evidence Level III: Quasi-experimental Study.

Segers, P., de Jong, A. P., Kloek, J. J., Spanjaard, L., & de Mol, B. A. J. (2006). Risk control of surgical site infection after cardiothoracic surgery. *Journal of Hospital Infection, 62*(4), 437–445. Evidence Level IV: Nonexperimental Study.

Shannon, R. P., O'Patel, B., Cummins, D., Shannon, A. H., Ganguli, G., & Lu, Y. (2006). Economics of central line associated bloodstream infections. *American Journal of Medical Quality, 21*(6) 7S–16S. Evidence Level IV: Nonexperimental Study.

Sharpe, V. A., & Faden, A. L. (1998). Medical harm: Historical, conceptual, and ethical dimensions of iatrogenic illness. Cambridge, United Kingdom: Cambridge University Press. Evidence Level VI: Expert Opinion.

Sherman, F. T. (2005). The 3 Hypos of hospitalization: Costly new forms of geriatric iatrogenesis prolong length of stay. *Geriatrics, 60*(5), 9–10. Evidence Level V: Case Report.

Sherwood, G., Thomas, E., Bennett, D. S., & Lewis, P. (2002). A teamwork model to promote patient safety in critical care. *Critical Care Nursing Clinics of North America, 14*(4), 333–340. Evidence Level V: Review.

Simmons-Trau, D., Cenek, P., Counterman, J., Hockenbury, D., & Litwiller, L. (2004). Reducing VAP in 6 sigma. *Nursing Management, 36*(6), 41–45. Evidence Level V: Review.

Singh, H., Watt, K., Veitch, R., Cantor, M., & Duerksen, D. R. (2006). Malnutrition is prevalent in hospitalized medical patients: Are housestaff identifying the malnourished patient? *Nutrition, 22*(4), 350–354. Evidence Level III: Quasi-experimental Study.

Sloss, E. M., Solomon, D. H., Shekelle, P. G., Young, R. T., Saliba, D., MacLean, C. H., et al. (2000). Selecting target conditions for quality of care improvement in vulnerable older adults. *Journal of the American Geriatrics Society,. 48*(4), 363–369 Evidence Level VI: Expert Opinion.

Smith, J. M. (2003). Indwelling catheter management: From habit-based to evidence-based practice. *Ostomy Wound Manage, 49*(12), 34–45. Evidence Level V: Review.

Starfield, B. (2000). Is U.S. health care really the best in the world? *Journal of the American Medical Association, 284*(4), 483–485. Evidence Level VI: Expert Opinion.

Steele, K., Gertman, P. M., Crescenzi, C., & Anderson, J. (1981). Iatrogenic disease on a general medical service at a university hospital. *New England Journal of Medicine, 304*(11), 638–642. Evidence Level IV: Nonexperimental Study.

Steele, K., Gertman, P., Crescenzi, C., & Anderson, J. (2004). Iatrogenic illness on a general medical service at a university hospital. *Quality and Safety in Health Care, 12*(1), 76–80. Evidence Level IV: Nonexperimental Study.

Stelfox, H. T., Palmisani, S., Scurlock, C., Orav, E. J., & Bates, D. W. (2006). The "To Err Is Human" report and patient safety literature. *Quality and Safety in Health Care, 15*(3), 174–178. Evidence Level V: Review.

Stierle, L. J., Mezey, M., Schumann, M. J., Esterson, J., Smolenski, M. C., Horsley, K. D., et al. (2006). The nurse competence in aging initiative: Encouraging expertise in the care of older adults. *American Journal of Nursing, 106*(9), 93–96. Evidence Level V: Review.

Sugarman, J., McCrory, D. C., & Hubal, R. C. (1998). Getting meaningful informed consent from older adults: A structured literature review of empirical research. *Journal of the American Geriatrics Society, 46*(4), 517–524. Level I: Systematic Review.

Thomas, E. J., & Brennan T. (2000). Incidence and types of preventable adverse events in elderly patients: Population-based review of medical records. *British Medical Journal, 18*(320) 741–744. Evidence Level IV: Nonexperimental Study.

Thomas, E. J., Studdert, D. M., Surstin, H. R., Orav, E. J., Zena, T., Williams, E. J., et al. (2000). Incidence and types of adverse events and negligent care in Utah and Colorado. *Medical Care, 38*(3), 261–271. Evidence Level IV: Nonexperimental Study.

Tolentino-DelosReyes, A. F., Ruppert, S. D., & Shiao, S. Y. (2007). Evidence-based practice: Use of the ventilator bundle to prevent ventilator-associated pneumonia. *American Journal of Critical Care, 16*(1), 20–27. Evidence Level III: Quasi-experimental Study.

Topal, J., Conklin, S., Camp, K., Morris, V., Balcezak, T., & Herbert, P. (2005). Prevention of nosocomial catheter-associated urinary tract infections through computerized feedback to physicians and a nurse-directed protocol. *American Journal of Medical Quality, 20*(3), 121–126. Evidence Level III: Quasi-experimental Study.

Tsilimingras, D., Rosen, A., & Berlowitz, D. (2003). Patient safety in geriatrics: A call for action. *Journal of Gerontology, Series A: Biological Sciences & Medical Sciences, 58*(9), M813–M819. Evidence Level V: Narrative Literature Review.

Tsuchida, T., Makimoto, K., Ohsako, S., Fujino, M., Kaneda, M., Miyazaki, T., et al. (2006). Relationship between catheter care and catheter-associated urinary tract infection at Japanese general hospitals: A prospective observational study. *International Journal of Nursing Studies* (in press). Evidence Level IV: Nonexperimental Study.

Vazquez-Aragon, P., Lizan-Garcia, M., Cascales-Sanchez, P., Villar-Canovas, M. T., & Garcia-Olmo, D. (2003). Nosocomial infection and related risk factors in a general surgery service: A prospective study. *Journal of Infection, 46*(1), 17–22. Evidence Level IV: Nonexperimental Study.

Villanueva, E. V., & Anderson, J. N. (2001). Estimates of complications of medical care in the adult U.S. population. *BioMed Central Health Services Research, 1*(1), 2. Evidence Level IV: Nonexperimental Study.

Vincent, C., Neale, G., & Woloshynowych, M. (2001). Adverse events in British hospitals: Preliminary retrospective record review. *British Medical Journal, 322*(7285), 517–519. Evidence Level IV: Nonexperimental Study.

Viney, M., Batcheller, J., Houston, S., & Belcik, K. (2006). Transforming care at the bedside: Designing new care systems in an age of complexity. *Journal of Nursing Care Quality, 21*(2), 143–150. Evidence Level V: Narrative Reports of IHI Project.

Wakefield, A., Attree, M., Braidman, I., Caroline, C., Johnson, M., & Cooke, H. (2005). Patient safety: Do nursing and medical curricula address this theme? *Nurse Educator Today, 25*(4), 333–340. Evidence Level V: Review.

Warren, D. K., Zack, J. E., Cox, M. J., Cohen, M. M., & Fraser, V. J. (2003). An educational intervention to prevent catheter-associated bloodstream infections in a nonteaching community medical center. *Critical Care Medicine, 31*(7), 1959–1963. Evidence Level III: Quasi-experimental Study.

Weitzel, T., Robinson, S., & Holmie, J. (2006). Preventing nosocomial pneumonia: Routine oral care reduced the risk of infection at one facility. *American Journal of Nursing, 106*(9), 72A–72E. Level III: Quasi-experimental Study.

Wenzel, R., & Edmond, M. (2001). The impact of hospital-acquired bloodstream infections. *Emerging Infectious Diseases Journal, 7*, 174–177. Evidence Level V: Review.

Wilson, R. M., Runciman, W. B., Gibberd, R. W., Harrison, B. T., Newby, L., & Hamilton, J. D. (1995). The quality in Australian health care study. *Medical Journal of Australia, 163*(9), 458–476. Evidence Level IV: Nonexperimental study.

Wisplinghoff, H., Bischoff, T., Tallent, S. M., Seifert, H., Wenzel, R. P., & Edmond, M. B. (2004). Nosocomial bloodstream infections in U.S. hospitals: Analysis of 23,179 cases from a prospective nationwide surveillance study. *Clinical Infectious Diseases, 39*(3), 309–317. Evidence Level IV: Nonexperimental Study.

World Health Organization (WHO). (2002). Prevention of hospital-acquired infection: A practical guide (2nd ed.). Geneva, Switzerland: WHO Press. Evidence Level I: Systematic Review.

Reducing Adverse Drug Events

12

DeAnne Zwicker
Terry Fulmer

Educational Objectives

On completion of this chapter, the reader will be able to:

1. conduct a comprehensive medication assessment

2. specify four medications or medication classes with a high potential for toxicity in older adults

3. describe five reasons that older adults experience adverse drug events

4. delineate strategies to prevent common medication-related problems in older adults

5. develop an individualized plan to promote medication safety of an older adult

Overview

Adults become increasingly susceptible to adverse drug events (ADEs) as they age. Physiological changes characteristic of aging predispose older adults to experience ADEs resulting in four times more hospitalizations in older versus younger persons. People older than 65 experience medication-related problems for seven major reasons: (1) age-related physiologic changes that result in altered pharmacokinetics (i.e., reduced ability to metabolize and excrete medications) and pharmacodynamics (i.e., changes in sensitivity to medications) (Mangoni & Jackson, 2003 [Level VI]; Rochon, 2006 [Level V]); (2) multiple

For a description of Evidence Levels cited in this chapter, see chapter 1, Developing and Evaluating Clinical Practice Guidelines, page 4

medications (i.e., polypharmacy), which are often prescribed by multiple providers (Hajjar & Kotchen, 2003 [Level IV]; Hanlon, Schmader, Ruby, & Weinberger, 2001 [Level V]); (3) incorrect doses of medications (over or under a therapeutic dosage) (Astin, Pelletier, Marie, & Haskell, 2000 [Level IV]; Doucette, McDonough, Klepser, & McCarthy, 2005 [Level V]; Hanlon, Schmader, Ruby, & Weinberger, et al., 2001 [Level V]; Sloane, Zimmerman, Brown, Ives, & Walsh, 2002 [Level II]); (4) medication consumption for the treatment of symptoms that are not disease-dependent or -specific (i.e., self-medication or prescribing cascades) (Neafsey & Shellman, 2001 [Level IV]; Rochon & Gurwitz, 1997 [Level V]); (5) iatrogenic causes such as adverse drug reactions (ADRs) including drug–drug or drug–disease interactions (Gurwitz et al., 2005 [Level II]; Hohl et al., 2005 [Level IV]; Lazarou, Pomeranz, & Corey, 1998 [Level I]; Petrone & Katz, 2005 [Level IV]; Pirmohamed et al., 2004 [Level IV]) and inappropriate prescribing for older adults (Fick et al., 2003 [Level VI]); (6) problems with medication adherence; and (7) medication errors (Doucette et al., 2005 [Level V]; National Council on Patient Information and Education (NCPIE), 1997 [Level VI]).

Background

It is estimated that the majority of adults older than 65 (79%) are taking medications, with 39% taking five or more drugs and up to 90% taking over-the-counter (OTC) drugs (Hanlon, Fillenbaum, Ruby, Gray & Bohannon, 2001 [Level V]). Other studies reported that older adults consume more than one-third of all prescription drugs and purchase 40% of all over-the-counter (OTC) medications (Besdine et al., 1998 [Level VI]; Hanlon, Fillenbaum, Ruby, Gray, & Bohannon, 2001 [Level V]; Kohn, Corrigan, & Donaldson, 2000 [Level VI]). Even if older adults are adherent with their prescribed medications, the combination with OTCs (often unreported to health care providers by older adults), herbal remedies, and dietary supplements may lead to adverse drug–disease interactions (Astin et al., 2000 [Level IV]) and drug–drug interactions (Rochon, 2006 [Level V]). Information, communication, and monitoring systems are needed to reduce if not eliminate preventable ADEs in this population.

Adverse Drug Events

An ADE is an adverse outcome that occurs during normal use of medicine, inappropriate use, inappropriate or suboptimum prescribing, poor adherence or self-medication, or harm due to a medication error. Older adults' susceptibility to ADEs is noted in the literature on iatrogenic events and medication errors (Childs, 2000; Gurwitz et al., 2003 [Level IV]; Hohl et al., 2005 [Level IV]). ADEs are an important cause of morbidity in older adults, leading to emergency room visits and hospital admissions (Budnitz et al., 2006 [Level V]). It is estimated that 35% of older persons experience ADEs, almost half of which are preventable (Safran et al., 2005 [Level IV]). Older adults are also at significant risk for further ADEs while in the hospital (Lazarou et al., 1998 [Level I]) and after discharge (Hanlon et al., 2006 [Level II]). Significant morbidity (Hanlon, Fillenbaum, Ruby, Gray, & Bohannon, 2001 [Level V]; Budnitz et al., 2006 [Level V]) and mortality are associated with ADEs, which are estimated to cost the health system approximately $75 billion to $85 billion annually (Fick et al., 2003 [Level VI]). ADEs are associated with preventable outcomes (i.e., depression, constipation, falls, immobility, confusion, hip fractures, rehospitalization, anorexia, and death) (Bootman, Harrison, & Cox, 1997 [Level VI]) and are linked to 106,000 deaths annually (Lazarou et al., 1998 [Level I]).

Iatrogenic Causes of ADEs

The term *iatrogenic*, as it relates to ADEs, means any undesirable condition in a patient occurring as the result of treatment by a health care professional, pertaining to an illness or injury resulting from a medication/drug or treatment. An iatrogenic medication event is one that is preventable, such as the wrong dose of a medication given resulting in an adverse outcome. ADRs, inappropriate prescribing of high risk medication to older adults, and medication errors are also considered preventable, or iatrogenic ADEs.

ADRs

An adverse drug reaction (ADR) is any toxic or unintended response to a medication. According to the Committee of Experts on Safe Medication Practices (COE, 2005), ADRs are ADEs that are preventable. The prevalence of ADR-related hospitalizations ranges from 5% to 35% (Gurwitz et al., 2003 [Level IV]; Kohn et al., 2000 [Level VI]). Among a community-dwelling population of older adults, 38% of ADRs were considered serious, life-threatening, or fatal; 27% were considered preventable (Gurwitz et al., 2005 [Level II]). Generalized to the current Medicare population, the ADR rate would be approximately 1.9 million per year with 180,000 characterized as life-threatening reactions. Pirmohamed et al. (2004 [Level IV]) reported that 70% of ADRs were either possibly avoidable or definitely avoidable in a study of 18,820 older adults. Twenty-nine percent of ADEs require evaluation by a physician, evaluation in the emergency room, or hospitalization for clinical management of the adverse reaction (Hohl et al., 2005 [Level IV]; Petrone & Katz, 2005 [Level IV]). A meta-analysis by Lazarou et al. (1998 [Level I]) reported that ADRs accounted for 6.7% of hospital admissions and in-hospital ADRs; when extrapolated, they would be the fourth to sixth leading cause of in-hospital mortality for all causes of death, which is a conservative estimate because it does not include ADRs related to errors, nonadherence, overdose, or therapeutic failures. Drug–drug and drug–disease interactions are the most common ADRs and often are preventable (Hansten, Horn, & Hazlet, 2001 [Level IV]; Juurlink, Mamdani, Kopp, Laupacis, & Redelmeier, 2003 [Level III]; Zhan et al., 2005 [Level IV]).

Inappropriate Medications

The Beers criteria comprise the standard by which inappropriate medications in aging persons are determined (Beers et al., 1991; Beers, 1997; Fick et al., 2003 [all Level VI], Health Benchmarks, 2005). Despite the criteria's acceptance by the medical community, as demonstrated by their wide use, many physicians and pharmacists remain unaware of the criteria or their updates. Studies indicate that clinicians in all settings (i.e., community, nursing home, emergency room, assisted living, and ambulatory care) continue to prescribe inappropriate medications with a *high* severity rating (according to the Beers criteria) to older adults (Hanlon, Fillenbaum, Schmader, Kuchibhatla, & Horner, 2000 [Level V]; Sloane, Zimmerman, Brown, Ives, & Walsh, 2002 [Level II]; Zhan et al., 2001, 2005 [both Level IV]). Approximately 23% of older adults take at least one medication on the Beers list that should be avoided (Fick et al., 2003 [Level VI]).

Medication Errors

The Institute of Medicine (IOM) reported in 1999 that almost 7,000 hospital deaths were associated with medication errors in 1993 (Kohn et al., 2000 [Level VI]). Medication errors occur frequently, yet many hospitals do not have systems in place such as automated order entry systems that are reported to decrease the number of medication errors (National Coordinating Council for Medication Errors Reporting and Prevention, 2001).

A medication error is defined by the Committee of Experts on Management of Safety and Quality in Health Care (COE, 2005) as any preventable event that may cause or lead to inappropriate medication use or patient harm while the medication is in the control of the health care professional, patient, or consumer. Such events may be related to professional practice, health care products, procedures, and systems, including prescribing; order communication; product labeling, packaging, and nomenclature; compounding, dispensing, and distribution; administration; education; and use. A large percentage of errors are due to administration of the wrong medication or the correct medication with the wrong dose or at the wrong time interval between dosing (NCPIE, 1997 [Level VI]). There are many reasons medication errors occur, including hospitals not using drug–drug interaction software; however, that discussion is beyond the scope of this chapter. Information regarding the immense literature on medication errors is provided in the Resources section of this chapter.

Nonadherence

A national survey of 17,685 Medicare beneficiaries older than 65 found that 52% do not take medications as prescribed (Safran et al., 2005 [Level IV]). Nonadherence (formerly called noncompliance) was primarily associated with a belief that the drug made them feel worse or was not helping (25%), or the cost of the medicine, resulting in a decision to skip or take a smaller dose (26%). Prescription drug coverage significantly impacted adherence, with 37% nonadherence among those without coverage compared to 22% nonadherence of beneficiaries with coverage. Nursing assessment and intervention directed at underlying nonadherence issues is important, but it is beyond the scope of this chapter. Further information sources are listed in the Resources section.

Acute care nurses are ideally positioned to identify or prevent potential ADEs in hospitalized older adults, as well as those about to be discharged, by reinforcing drug monitoring and focusing on drug–drug interactions, excess dosages (Doucet et al., 2002 [Level V]), drug–disease interactions (avoiding prescribing cascades) (Rochon, 2006 [Level V]), and avoiding inappropriate medications in aging persons (Fick et al., 2003 [Level VI]). However, to fulfill this role, nurses need a good system of communication with doctors, advance practice nurses, and pharmacists and must take a proactive role in assuring the safety of prescribing.

Assessment

Assessment Tools

Assessment tools are used to evaluate an older adult's ability to self-administer medications (i.e., functional capacity assessment) and the clinician's assessment for potential inappropriate medications, drug–drug interactions, drug–disease interactions, and assessment of renal function. Commonly used tools include the following:

- *2002 Criteria for Potentially Inappropriate Medication Use in Older Adults: Independent of Diagnoses or Condition.* Also known as the Beers Criteria. (Fick et al., 2003 [Level VI]) (Table 12.1). Used to assess medication list for medications that should generally be avoided in older adults.
- *2002 Criteria for Potentially Inappropriate Medication Use in Older Adults: Considering Diagnoses or Condition.* Also known as the Beers Criteria. (Fick et al., 2003 [Level VI]) (Table 12.2). Used to assess for the presence of medications that may interact adversely with a disease or condition a person has.
- *Drug–Drug Interactions* (Table 12.3) List of *some* common medications known to interact with other medications. This is most accurately determined by a computer/PDA program, such as the *Facts and Comparisons* PDA program to identify drug–drug and drug–disease interactions (see Resources in this chapter).
- *Cockroft-Gault Formula* (Figure 12.1) Useful for estimating creatinine clearance based on age, weight, and serum creatinine levels (Terrell, Heard, & Miller, 2006 [Level V]). A creatinine clearance of less than 50 ml/min places an older adult at risk for ADEs (Fouts, Hanlon, Pierper, Perfetto, & Feinberg, 1997]) and virtually all people older than 70 have a creatinine clearance of less than 50.
- *Functional Capacity (ADL, IADL, Mini-Cog/MMSE).* Used to assess physical and cognitive ability to self-administer medications. See chapter 3, *Assessment of Function*, and chapter 6, *Dementia*, respectively, or www.ConsultGeriRN.org.
- *Brown Bag Method* (Nathan, Goodyer, Lovejoy, & Rahid, 1999 [Level IV]). Method used to assess all medications an older adult has at home including prescriptions from all providers, OTC medications, and herbal remedies. Should be used in conjunction with a complete medication history. (See Interventions and Nursing Care Strategies in this chapter for details on taking a complete medication history and Table 12.4, which outlines medication history questions.)
- *Drugs Regimen Unassisted Grading Scale (DRUGS) Tool.* Standardized method for assessing potential medication-adherence problems. Used at transfer to other levels of care (Edelberg, Shallenberger, & Wei, 1999; Hutchinson, Jones, West, & Wei, 2006 [both Level IV]). (See the Resources section in this chapter.)

Assessment

Pharmacokinetic and Pharmacodynamic Changes with Aging

There are patterns related to aging that are important to consider prior to assessing medications in older adults (Mangoni & Jackson, 2003 [Level VI]; Rochon, 2006 [Level V]). *Pharmacokinetics* is best defined as the time course of absorption, distribution across compartments, metabolism, and excretion of drugs in the body. The metabolism and excretion of many drugs decreases and the physiologic changes of aging require dose adjustment for some drugs (Merck Manual, 2005 [Level VI]). Pharmacodynamics is defined as the response of the body to the drug, which is affected by receptor binding, post-receptor effects, and chemical interactions (Merck Manual, 2005 [Level VI]). Pharmacodynamic problems occur when two drugs act at the same or interrelated receptor sites, resulting in additive, synergistic, or antagonistic effects. Many interactions of drugs are multifactorial, however, with a sequence of events that are both pharmacokinetic and pharmacodynamic (Spina & Scordo, 2002 [Level VI]).The following are age-related changes in pharmaco-kinetics and -dynamics in older persons:

- Changes in drug *absorption* (i.e., increased gastric pH and decreased gastrointestinal motility in an absorptive surface) once thought to be due mainly to aging changes are more recently thought to be due at least in some part to underlying disease states rather than normal aging changes (Mangoni & Jackson, 2003 [Level VI]). There may be, however, a change of absorption rate in persons taking multiple medications—for example, fluorquinolones taken with iron may impair absorption (Semla & Rochon, 2004 [Level VI]).
- Drug *distribution* changes associated with aging include decreased cardiac output, reduced total body water, decreased serum albumin (which is more likely to be related to malnutrition or acute illness than aging), and increased body fat. Reduced total body water creates a potential for higher serum drug levels due to a low volume of distribution and occurs with water-soluble drugs (i.e., hydrophilic) such as alcohol or lithium. Decreased serum albumin results in higher unbound drug levels with protein-bound drugs such as warfarin, phenytoin, salicylic acid, and diazepam. Lipophilic drugs (e.g., long-acting benzodiazepines) are stored in the body fat of older persons and slowly leach out, resulting in increased half-life and resulting in the drug staying around longer.
- A significant change in *drug metabolism* is reduction in the cytochrome p-450 enzyme system, which affects metabolism of many drugs cleared by this enzyme system (Mangoni & Jackson, 2003 [Level VI]; Merck Manual, 2005 [Level VI]; Tune, 2001 [Level V]). Many classes of drugs are cleared by the p-450 system, including cardiovascular drugs, analgesics, NSAIDs, antibiotics, diuretics, psychoactive drugs, and others (Merck Manual, 2005 [Level VI]). (For a list drugs cleared by this enzyme system, see the Merck Manual online at http://www.merck.com/mmpe/sec20/ch306/ch306b.html.) Metabolism may be affected by disease states common in older individuals (e.g., thyroid disease, congestive heart failure, and cancer) or can be a result of drug-induced metabolic changes as well

12.1

Cockroft-Gault
Formula for
Estimation of
Creatinine
Clearance (CrCl)

Formula for Men:

CrCl in milliliters per minute* =

$$\frac{(140 - \text{age in years}) (\text{weight in kilograms})}{72 (\text{serum creatinine in milligrams per deciliter})}$$

Formula for Women: *Use above formula and multiply by 0.85.

(Mangoni & Jackson, 2003 [Level VI]). Several drugs are cleared by multi-stage hepatic metabolism (nonsynthetic and synthetic reactions), which is more likely to be prolonged in older persons. However, age does not greatly affect clearance of drugs that are metabolized by glucuronic acid conjugation (Merck Manual, 2005 [Level VI]). Conjugation is an important mechanism for the rapid inactivation and extensive removal of drugs from the body; therefore, it has major significance in the toxic effects of drugs. The capacity for conjugation of some drugs is large, but with others, saturation may occur with over-dosage or even high therapeutic doses (Prescott, 1994). Some drugs undergo hepatic metabolism, then renal clearance. Drugs such as diazepam have enormously longer half-lives in older adults because both systems are impaired.

- *Elimination or clearance* of medications from the body may be slowed due to decline in glomerular filtration rate, renal tubular secretion, and renal blood flow that naturally decreases with age (Semla & Rochon, 2004 [Level VI]). A decrease in glomerular filtration is usually not accompanied by an increase in serum creatinine due to decreasing lean muscle mass with age and subsequent decline in creatinine production. Therefore, serum creatinine is not an accurate measure of renal function in the elderly. Instead, assessment of renal function using the Cockroft-Gault formula (see Figure 12.1) should be calculated prior to initiation of renal-clearing medications (Mangoni & Jackson, 2003; Semla & Rochon, 2004 [both Level VI]).

Beers Criteria

In 1999, the Centers for Medicare & Medicaid Services (CMS) incorporated the Beers criteria (Beers et al., 1991; Beers, 1997 (Fick et al., 2003) [all Level VI]) into regulatory guidelines in long-term care. Long term care facilities can be cited if any of the drugs on the list are prescribed. The Joint Commission on Accreditation of Health Care Organizations (JCAHO) also adopted the criteria as a potential sentinel event (2007 [Level VI]) in hospitals. Many insurance providers have also incorporated the Beers criteria into quality indicators for older adults (e.g., Health Benchmarks, 2005).

Although the Beers criteria for inappropriate medications are an excellent guideline for assessing *potential* inappropriate medications, they need to be used in conjunction with patient-centered care (Swagerty & Brickley, 2005 [Level VI]). A joint position statement of the American Medical Directors Association (AMDA) and American Society of Consulting Pharmacists (ASCP) points out that the Beers criteria are based on consensus data (i.e., lower level of evidence) rather than on higher levels of evidence such as systematic reviews or randomized controlled trials.

The Beers criteria address two key areas: (1) medications or medication classes that should generally be avoided in people 65 and older; and (2) medications that should be avoided in persons older than 65 with specific medical conditions. A severity rating of *high* or *low* is given to each medication based on its potential negative impact on older adults. The most recent criteria, updated in 2003 by Fick et al., identifies 48 medications or classes that should generally be avoided in people older than 65, as well as 20 specific medications that should not be used in the presence of specific conditions (Fick et al., 2003 [Level VI]) (see Tables 12.1 and 12.2).

Several studies link medications on the inappropriate list to poor health outcomes. Fick and colleagues (2003 [Level VI]) reported that ambulatory older adults who were prescribed medications from the Beers list were more likely be hospitalized or evaluated in an emergency room than those not taking such medications. Another study reports a positive association between potentially inappropriate drug-prescribing (as defined by the Beers criteria) and ADRs in first-visit elderly outpatients (Chang et al., 2005 [Level IV]; Fu, Liu, & Christensen, 2002 [Level V]). These findings not only support the use of the Beers criteria in assessing the appropriateness of medications in the older *outpatient* population but also support the criteria's effectiveness in preventing hospitalizations due to ADRs in these settings. Although these findings cannot be generalized to acute care, acute care nurses (and other members of the health care team) need to be proactive at discharge of older adults by implementing strategies to reduce ADEs and ADRs that lead to rehospitalization of older adults transitioning to other care levels. A prospective observational study of 18,820 older patients found that 1,225 admissions were related to an ADR, a prevalence of 6.5%, after the ADR directly lead to admission in 80% of cases (Pirmohamed et al., 2004 [Level IV]).

Assessment for Adverse Drug Reactions (ADRs)

ADRs occur due to the number of medications taken by older persons and their concomitant medical conditions. The severity of adverse reactions increases in older adults due to age-related changes in pharmacokinetics and pharmacodynamics. Assessment for potential drug–disease and drug–drug interactions must be considered before initiating medications in the elderly. The most preventable ADRs in the *outpatient* setting are cardiovascular medications followed by diuretics, nonopioid analgesics, hypoglycemics, and anticoagulants (Gurwitz et al., 2003 [Level IV]). Gurwitz and colleagues (2005 [Level II]) reported that the

12.1 2002 Criteria for Potentially Inappropriate Medication Use in Older Adults: Independent of Diagnoses or Condition

Drug	Concern	Severity Rating (High or Low)
Propoxyphene (Darvon) and combination products (Darvon with ASA, Darvon-N, and Darvocet-N)	Offers few analgesic advantages over acetaminophen, yet has the adverse, effects of other narcotic drugs.	Low
Indomethacin (Indocin and Indocin SR)	Of all available nonsteroidal antiinflammatory drugs, this drug produces the most CNS adverse effects.	High
Pentazocine (Talwin)	Narcotic analgesic that causes more CNS adverse effects, including confusion and hallucinations, more commonly than other narcotic drugs. Additionally, it is a mixed agonist and antagonist.	High
Trimethobenzamide (Tigan)	One of the least effective antiemetic drugs, yet it can cause extrapyramidal adverse effects.	High
Muscle relaxants and antispasmodics: methocarbamol (Robaxin), carisoprodol (Soma), chlorzoxazone (Paraflex), metaxalone (Skelaxin), cyclobenzaprine (Flexeril), and oxybutynin (Ditropan). Do not consider the extended-release Ditropan XL.	Most muscle relaxants and antispasmodic drugs are poorly tolerated by elderly patients because these cause anticholinergic adverse effects, sedation, and weakness. Additionally, their effectiveness at doses tolerated by elderly patients is questionable.	High
Flurazepam (Dalmane)	This benzodiazepine hypnotic has an extremely long half-life in elderly patients (often days), producing prolonged sedation and increasing the incidence of falls and fracture. Medium- or short-acting benzodiazepines are preferable.	High

2002 Criteria for Potentially Inappropriate Medication Use in Older Adults: Independent of Diagnoses or Condition

12.1

Drug	Concern	Severity Rating (High or Low)
Amitriptyline (Elavil), chlordiazepoxide-amitriptyline (Limbitrol), and perphenazine-amitriptyline (Triavil)	Because of its strong anticholinergic and sedation properties, amitriptyline is rarely the antidepressant of choice for elderly patients.	High
Doxepin (Sinequan)	Because of its strong anticholinergic and sedating properties, doxepin is rarely the antidepressant of choice for elderly patients.	High
Meprobamate (Miltown and Equanil)	This is a highly addictive and sedating anxiolytic. Those using meprobamate for prolonged periods may become addicted and may need to be withdrawn slowly.	High
Doses of short-acting benzodiazepines: doses greater than lorazepam (Ativan) 3 mg; oxazepam (Serax) 60 mg; alprazolam (Xanax) 2 mg; temazepam (Restoril) 15 mg; and triazolam (Halcion) 0.25 mg	Because of increased sensitivity to benzoadiazepines in elderly patients, smaller doses may be effective as well as safer. Total daily doses should rarely exceed the suggested maximums.	High
Long-acting benzodiazepines: chlordiazepoxide (Librium), chlordiazepoxide-amitriptyline (Limbitrol), clidinium-chlordiazepoxide (Librax), diazepam (Valium), quazepam (Doral), halazepam (Paxipam), and chlorazepate (Tranxene)	These drugs have a long half-life in elderly patients (often several days), producing prolonged sedation and increasing the risk of falls and fractures. Short- and intermediate-acting benzodiazepines are preferred if a benzodiazepine is required.	High
Disopyramide (Norpace and Norpace CR)	Of all antiarrhythmic drugs, this is the most potent negative inotrope and therefore may induce heart failure in elderly patients. It is also strongly anticholinergic. Other antiarrhythmic drugs should be used.	High

12.1 (continued)

Drug	Concern	Severity Rating (High or Low)
Digoxin (Lanoxin) (should not exceed >0.125 mg/d except when treating atrial arrhythmias)	Decreased renal clearance may lead to increased risk of toxic effects.	Low
Short-acting dipyridamole (Persantine). Do not consider the long-acting dipyridamole (which has better properties than the short-acting in older adults) except for patients with artificial heart valves.	May cause orthostatic hypotension.	Low
Methyldopa (Aldomet) and methyldopa-hydrochlorothiazide (Aldoril)	May cause bradycardia and exacerbate depression in elderly patients.	High
Reserpine at doses >0.25 mg	May induce depression, impotence, sedation, and orthostatic hypotension.	Low
Chlorpropamide (Diabinese)	It has a prolonged half-life in elderly patients and could cause prolonged. hypoglycemia. Additionally, it is the only oral hypoglycemic agent that causes SIADH.	High
Gastrointestinal antispasmodic drugs: dicyclomine (Bentyl), hyoscyamine (Levsin and Levsinex), propantheline (Pro-Banthine), belladonna alkaloids (Donnatal and others), and clidinium-chlordiazepoxide (Librax)	GI antispasmodic drugs are highly anticholinergic and have uncertain effectiveness. These drugs should be avoided (especially for long-term use).	High
Anticholinergics and antihistamines: chlorpheniramine (Chlor-Trimeton), diphenhydramine (Benadryl), hydroxyzine (Vistaril and Atarax), cyproheptadine (Periactin), promethazine (Phenergan), tripelennamine, dexchlorpheniramine (Polaramine)	*All* nonprescription (OTCs) and many prescription antihistamines may have potent anticholinergic properties. Nonanticholinergic antihistamines are preferred in elderly patients when treating allergic reactions.	High

12.1 2002 Criteria for Potentially Inappropriate Medication Use in Older Adults: Independent of Diagnoses or Condition

Drug	Concern	Severity Rating (High or Low)
Diphenhydramine (Benadryl)	May cause confusion and sedation. Should not be used as a hypnotic, and when used to treat emergency allergic reactions, it should be used in the smallest possible dose.	High
Ergot mesyloids (Hydergine) and cyclandelate (Cyclospasmol)	Have not been shown to be effective in the doses studied.	Low
Ferrous sulfate >325 mg/d	Doses >325 mg/d do not dramatically increase the amount absorbed but greatly increase the incidence of constipation.	Low
All barbiturates (except phenobarbital) except when used to control seizures	Are highly addictive and cause more adverse effects than most sedative or hypnotic drugs in elderly patients.	High
Meperidine (Demerol)	Not an effective oral analgesic in doses commonly used. May cause confusion and has many disadvantages to other narcotic drugs.	High
Ticlopidine (Ticlid)	Has been shown to be no better than aspirin in preventing clotting and may be considerably more toxic. Safer, more effective alternatives exist.	High
Ketorolac (Toradol)	Immediate and long-term use should be avoided in older persons because a significant number have asymptomatic GI pathologic conditions.	High
Amphetamines and anorexic agents	These drugs have potential for causing dependence, hypertension, angina, and myocardial infarction.	High

12.1 (continued)

Drug	Concern	Severity Rating (High or Low)
Long-term use of full-dosage, longer half-life, non–COX-selective NSAIDs: naproxen (Naprosyn, Avaprox, and Aleve), oxaprozin (Daypro), and piroxicam (Feldene)	Have the potential to produce GI bleeding, renal failure, high blood pressure, and heart failure.	High
Daily fluoxetine (Prozac)	Long half-life of drug and risk of producing excessive CNS stimulation, sleep disturbances, and increasing agitation. Safer alternatives exist.	High
Long-term use of stimulant laxatives: bisacodyl (Dulcolax), cascara sagrada, and Neoloid except in the presence of opiate analgesic use	May exacerbate bowel dysfunction.	High
Amiodarone (Cordarone)	Associated with QT interval problems and risk of provoking *torsades de pointes*. Lack of efficacy in older adults.	High
Orphenadrine (Norflex)	Causes more sedation and anticholinergic adverse effects than safer alternatives.	High
Guanethidine (Ismelin)	May cause orthostatic hypotension. Safer alternatives exist.	High
Guanadrel (Hylorel)	May cause orthostatic hypotension.	High
Cyclandelate (Cyclospasmol)	Lack of efficacy.	Low
Isoxsurpine (Vasodilan)	Lack of efficacy.	Low
Nitrofurantoin (Macrodantin)	Potential for renal impairment. Safer alternatives available.	High
Doxazosin (Cardura)	Potential for hypotension, dry mouth, and urinary problems.	Low

2002 Criteria for Potentially Inappropriate Medication Use in Older Adults: Independent of Diagnoses or Condition

Drug	Concern	Severity Rating (High or Low)
Methyltestosterone (Android, Virilon, and Testrad)	Potential for prostatic hypertrophy and cardiac problems.	High
Thioridazine (Mellaril)	Greater potential for CNS and extrapyramidal adverse effects.	High
Mesoridazine (Serentil)	CNS and extrapyramidal adverse effects.	High
Short-acting nifedipine (Procardia and Adalat)	Potential for hypotension and constipation.	High
Clonidine (Catapres)	Potential for orthostatic hypotension and CNS adverse effects.	Low
Mineral oil	Potential for aspiration and adverse effects. Safer alternatives available.	High
Cimetidine (Tagamet)	CNS adverse effects including confusion.	Low
Ethacrynic acid (Edecrin)	Potential for hypertension and fluid imbalances. Safer alternatives available.	Low
Desiccated thyroid	Concerns about cardiac effects. Safer alternatives available.	High
Amphetamines (excluding methylphenidate hydrochloride and anorexics)	CNS stimulant adverse effects.	High
Estrogens only (oral)	Evidence of the carcinogenic (breast and endometrial cancer) potential of these agents and lack of cardio-protective effect in older women.	Low

Abbreviations: CNS: central nervous system; COX: cyclooxygenase; GI: gastrointestinal; NSAIDs: nonsteroidal anti-inflammatory drugs; SIADH: syndrome of inappropriate antidiuretic hormone secretion.

Reprinted with permission: Fick, D. M., Cooper, F. W., Wade, W. E., Waller, J. L., Maclean, J. R., & Beers, M. H. (2003). Updating the Beers criteria for potentially inappropriate medication use in older adults. *Archives of Internal Medicine, 163*(22), 2716–2724. Evidence Level VI: Expert Opinion.

12.2 2002 Criteria for Potentially Inappropriate Medication Use in Older Adults: Considering Diagnoses or Condition

Disease or Condition	Drug	Concern	Severity Rating (High or Low)
Heart failure	Disopyramide (Norpace), and high-sodium-content drugs (sodium and sodium salts [alginate bicarbonate, biphosphate, citrate, phosphate, salicylate, and sulfate])	Negative inotropic effect. Potential to promote fluid retention and exacerbation of heart failure.	High
Hypertension	Phenylpropanolamine hydrochloride (removed from the market in 2001), OTC pseudoephedrine (sudafed), diet pills, and amphetamines	May produce elevation of blood pressure secondary to sympathomimetic activity.	High
Gastric or duodenal ulcers	NSAIDs and aspirin (>325 mg) (COX2 inhibitors excluded)	May exacerbate existing ulcers or produce new or additional ulcers.	High
Seizures or epilepsy	Clozapine (Clozaril), chlorpromazine (Thorazine), thioridazine (Mellaril), and thiothixene (Navane)	May lower seizure thresholds.	High
Blood clotting disorders or receiving anticoagulant therapy	Aspirin, NSAIDs, dipyridamole (Persantin), ticlopidine (Ticlid), and clopidogrel (Plavix)	May prolong clotting time and elevate INR values or inhibit platelet aggregation, resulting in an increased potential for bleeding.	High
Bladder outflow obstruction	Anticholinergics and antihistamines, gastrointestinal antispasmodics, muscle relaxants, oxybutynin (Ditropan), flavoxate (Urispas), anticholinergics, antidepressants, decongestants, and tolterodine (Detrol)	May decrease urinary flow, leading to urinary retention.	High

	2002 Criteria for Potentially Inappropriate Medication Use in Older Adults: Considering Diagnoses or Condition		
Disease or Condition	Drug	Concern	Severity Rating (High or Low)
Stress incontinence	α-blockers (Doxazosin, Prazosin, and Terazosin), anticholinergics, tricyclic antidepressants (imipramine hydrochloride, doxepin hydrochloride, and amitriptyline hydrochloride), and long-acting benzodiazepines	May produce polyuria and worsening of incontinence.	High
Arrhythmias	Tricyclic antidepressants (imipramine hydrochloride, doxepin hydrochloride, and amitriptyline hydrochloride)	Concern due to proarrhythmic effects and ability to produce QT interval changes.	High
Insomnia	Decongestants, theophylline (Theodur), methylphenidate (Ritalin), MAOIs, and amphetamines	Concern due to CNS stimulant effects.	High
Parkinson's disease	Metoclopramide (Reglan), conventional antipsychotics, and tacrine (Cognex)	Concern due to their antidopaminergic and cholinergic effects.	High
Cognitive impairment	Barbiturates, anticholinergics, antispasmodics, and muscle relaxants. CNS stimulants: dextroAmphetamine (Adderall), methylphenidate (Ritalin), methamphetamine (Desoxyn), and pemolin	Concern due to CNS-altering effects.	High

12.2

12.2 (continued)

Disease or Condition	Drug	Concern	Severity Rating (High or Low)
Depression	Long-term benzodiazepine use. Sympatholytic agents: methyldopa (Aldomet), reserpine, and guanethidine (Ismelin)	May produce or exacerbate depression.	High
Anorexia and malnutrition	CNS stimulants: Dextroamphetamine (Adderall), methylphenidate (Ritalin), methamphetamine (Desoxyn), pemolin, and fluoxetine (Prozac)	Concern due to appetite-suppressing effects.	High
Syncope or falls	Short- to intermediate-acting benzodiazepine and tricyclic antidepressants (imipramine hydrochloride, doxepin hydrochloride, and amitriptyline hydrochloride)	May produce ataxia, impaired psychomotor function, syncope, and additional falls.	High
SIADH/ hyponatremia	SSRIs: fluoxetine (Prozac), citalopram (Celexa), fluvoxamine (Luvox), paroxetine (Paxil), and sertraline (Zoloft)	May exacerbate or cause SIADH.	Low
Seizure disorder	Bupropion (Wellbutrin)	May lower seizure threshold.	High
Obesity	Olanzapine (Zyprexa)	May stimulate appetite and increase weight gain.	Low

12.2 2002 Criteria for Potentially Inappropriate Medication Use in Older Adults: Considering Diagnoses or Condition

Disease or Condition	Drug	Concern	Severity Rating (High or Low)
COPD	Long-acting benzodiazepines: chlordiazepoxide (Librium), chlordiazepoxide-amitriptyline (Limbitrol), clidinium-chlordiazepoxide (Librax), diazepam (Valium), quazepam (Doral), halazepam (Paxipam), and chlorazepate (Tranxene). β-blockers: propranolol	CNS adverse effects. May induce respiratory depression. May exacerbate or cause respiratory depression.	High
Chronic constipation	Calcium channel blockers, anticholinergics, and tricyclic antidepressant (imipramine hydrochloride, doxepin hydrochloride, and amitriptyline hydrochloride)	May exacerbate constipation.	Low

Abbreviations: CNS: central nervous system; COPD: chronic obstructive pulmonary disease; INR: international normalized ratio; MAOIs: monoamine oxidase inhibitors; NSAIDs: nonsteroidal anti-inflammatory drugs; SIADH: syndrome of inappropriate antidiuretic hormone; SSRIs: selective serotonin reuptake inhibitors.

largest number of preventable ADRs occurred at the prescribing or monitoring stages and included wrong drug choices or dosages, inadequate patient education, or a clinically important drug–drug interaction. Monitoring for errors includes inadequate lab evaluation of a drug and failure to respond to signs, symptoms (including atypical symptoms), or abnormal lab levels indicative of toxicity. Assessing lab values and appropriateness of drugs and doses when orders are written and monitoring for signs and symptoms of toxicity comprise an important role for nurses in preventing ADRs in the hospital setting. These researchers suggest provider education and system interventions in health care settings to reduce ADRs.

Drug-Drug Interactions

Concurrent use of more than one drug simultaneously can result in serious toxicities in older adults resulting in synergistic effects, additive effects, or antagonistic effects. For example, concurrent use of any two of the following drugs: antiparkinson drugs, tricyclic antidepressants such as amitriptyline, antipsychotics (e.g., haldol), anti-arrhythmics (e.g., disopyramide), and OTC antihistamines (e.g., diphenhydramine, chlorpheniramine) may cause or worsen dry mouth, gum disease, blurred vision, constipation, urinary retention, and/or delirium (Merck Manual, 2005 [Level VI]).

Little is known about the epidemiology of drug–drug interactions in clinical practice (Juurlink et al., 2003 [Level III]); however, studies indicate that drug–drug interactions are a common cause of predictable ADEs (Hansten, Horn, & Hazlet, 2001 [Level IV]). A case-control study conducted by Juurlink and colleagues (2003 [Level III]) reported that drug–drug interactions resulted in serious adverse events among several classes of medications. Of 179,986 older patients treated with glyburide along with cotrimoxazole, 909 patients became hypoglycemic, 12 patients died, and no control subjects experienced hypoglycemia. Of 231,257 patients, 1,051 were admitted due to dioxin toxicity and 33 died while hospitalized. Those with digoxin toxicity were 13 times more likely to have received clarithromycin 1 week prior to hospitalization, which suggests that avoidance of concomitant use of digoxin and clarithromycin may have prevented the digoxin toxicity. In the same study, concomitant prescribing of ACE inhibitors and potassium-sparing diuretics 1 week before admission were observed in 622,285 older persons. The researchers estimated that 7.8% of hospitalizations for hyperkalemia could have been prevented if addition of potassium-sparing diuretics had been avoided (Juurlink et al., 2003 [Level III]). In a retrospective review of the National Hospital Ambulatory Medical Care Survey (NHAMCS), Zhan and colleagues (2005 [Level IV]) reported that older adults with two or more prescriptions had at least one inappropriate drug–drug combination present, and 6.6% of patients on warfarin were prescribed a drug with a potentially harmful interaction. Some other common drug–drug interactions are shown in Table 12.3.

Interactions with OTCs and Herbal Remedies

Interactions with herbal remedies and OTC medications, often overlooked, must also be assessed because older adults commonly use these remedies, consuming 40% of all OTCs (Astin et al., 2000 [Level IV]; Kohn, Corrigan, & Donaldson, 2000 [Level VI]). Hanlon, Fillenbaum, Ruby, Gray, and Bohannon (2001 [Level V]) reported that community-dwelling older adults in the United States consume approximately 1.8 OTC medications per day. Use varies somewhat with geographic area and ethnicity; highest use is in the Midwest and Whites with the lowest use among Hispanic persons. The most common OTC classes used

12.3   Examples of Common Drug–Drug Interactions

Drug 1	Drug 2	Interaction	Adverse Effect(ds)
Warfarin (Coumadin)	Diltiazem[1] Verapamil[1] Metronidazole[1,5]	Inhibits drug metabolism	↑ anticoagulation; potential bleeding
Warfarin	NSAID* [4,5]	NSAID ↓ prostaglandin	GI bleeding
	ASA[4]	Increases GI erosion; ↓ platelet aggregation	GI bleeding
	Sulfa drugs[5]	Unknown	↑ effects of warfarin, potential GI bleeding
	Macrolides	Inhibits metabolism and clearance	↑ effects of warfarin, potential GI bleeding
	Acetaminophen[5] combined with narcotic Fluconazole[5] Cipro[4] Biaxin[4]	↑ INR	Bleeding
Digoxin	Amiodorone[1,4]	↓ renal or nonrenal clearance of Digoxin	Digoxin toxicity
	Clarithromycin[1,4]	Inhibits renal clearance of Digoxin	Digoxin toxicity
	Verapamil[1,4]	↓ cardiac impulse conduction & muscle contraction	Potential bradycardia or heart block
Levothyroxine T$_4$	Calcium carbonate[1]	L-thyroxine absorbs calcium carbonate in acidic environment	Reduced absorption of L-thyroxin
Glyburide	Co-trimoxazole[4]	Potentiates effect of sulfonylureas	Hypoglycemia

	12.3	**(continued)**	
Drug 1	**Drug 2**	**Interaction**	**Adverse Effect(ds)**
Ace inhibitors	Potassium-sparing[4] diuretics[4]	Unknown	Life-threatening hyperkalemia
Diuretic	NSAID[*,1]	↓ renal perfusion	Renal impairment
Phenytoin[4] (Dilantin)	cimetidine, erythromycin, clarithromycin, fluconazole	Not specified	Increases levels of phenytoin[4] within 1 week
Theophylline	Quinolones	↓ liver metabolism of Theophylline	Theophylline toxicity

Notes: There are many other common drug–drug interactions; this table is not intended to be all-inclusive. Use of computer devices is typically the best method for determining drug–drug interactions (see Resources).
*NSAID = non-steroidal anti-inflammatory agents: prescription and over-the-counter such as toradol or ibuprofen, respectively.
Source: Adapted from:
[1] Beers, M. & Berkow, R. (2000). *The Merck Manual of Geriatric Clinical Pharmacology,* 3rd edition. NJ: Merck Research Laboratory. [Level VI].
[2] Jurrlink, Mamdani, Kopp, Laupacis, & Redelmeier (2003). Drug–drug interactions among elderly patients hospitalized for drug toxicity. *Journal of the American Medical Association, 289*(13), 1652–1658. [Level III].
[3] Tatro, D. S., ed. (2001). Drug interactions in *Facts in Facts and Comparisons.* St. Louis, MO.
[4] Feldstein et al. (2006). Reducing warfarin medication interactions. *Archives of Internal Medicine, 166,* 1009–1015. [Level III].
[5] Ament, P. W., Bertolino, J. G., & Liszewski, J. L. (2000). Clinical pharmacology: Clinically significant drug interactions. *American Family Physician, 61,* 1745–1754. Evidence Level VI: Expert Opinion.

are analgesics, laxatives, and nutritional supplements. Herbal or dietary supplement usage (e.g., ginseng, ginkgo biloba extract, and glucosamine) is on the rise among older adults, increasing from 14% in 1998 to 26% in 2002 (Kaufman, Kelly, Rosenberg, Anderson, & Mitchell, 2002; Kelly et al., 2005 [both Level IV]). Use of St. John's Wart and Echinacea are on the rise and may have now topped the list. OTC and herbal supplements are typically not reported to medical providers because most consumers do not consider them medication (Astin et al., 2000 [Level IV]); the implications for unidentified drug–drug and drug–disease interactions with OTCs and herbal remedies are astounding.

Medication Adherence

As individuals age, they may encounter difficulties that decrease their ability to adhere to medication regimens (e.g., vision impairment, arthritis, economics). Medication adherence with older adults is complex and needs careful nursing assessment. There are a number of ways to assess for potential adherence-related problems (Bergman-Evans, 2006 [Level V]; Edelberg et al., 1999 [Level IV]), as well as to ascertain adherence (Fulmer, Kim, Montgomery, & Lyder, 2000; Rohay, Dunbar-Jacob, Sereika, Kwoh, & Burke, 1996). An array of devices can assist in enhancing adherence behavior (Fulmer et al., 1999; Haynes et al., 2005 [Level V]) (see the Resources section in this chapter for further information).

Reconciliation of Medications

Poor communication of medical information at transition points of care (i.e., at admission, transfer, and discharge) often results in medication errors, but appropriate strategies can reduce the likelihood of errors (Santell, 2006 [Level VI]). Unfortunately an effective means of communicating drug therapies to other levels of care upon discharge from the hospital has not been established across the continuum (Nickerson, MacKinnon, Roberts, & Saulnier, 2005 [Level II]). MR described in the literature is performed by pharmacists (Gleason et al., 2004; Nickerson et al., 2005 [Level II]). However, MR can be performed by a nurse-collaborative team, including pharmacist consultation (Doucette et al., 2005 [Level V]) or a computer-based program(s); however, studies to date are equivocal on the use of computer-based programs for reconciliation. The MR process includes comparison of medications on admission and transfer documents with medication orders at time of admission and time of transfer to other units or discharge to other levels of care. Barriers for nurses performing MR reported in one study included lack of confidence in existing institutional safety systems, inconsistent practices (whether or not pharmacists are consulted), lack of communication between health professionals, and staffing concerns (MR is time-consuming) (Chevalier, Parker, MacKinnon, & Sketris, 2006 [Level V]). The Brown Bag method can be used for corroborating medications (Nathan et al., 1999 [Level IV]) with community dwelling older adults, when used in conjunction with a good medication admission history (Table 12.4). At discharge, the pharmacist has been involved (or can assist nurses or the care team) in identifying problems with drug therapy and communicating with the community pharmacy, medical provider, or admitting staff at the transitional site of care (Hanlon, Fillenbaum, Ruby, Gray, & Bohannon, 2001 [Level V]; Nickerson et al., 2005 [Level II]). A systematic review of multiple randomized controlled trials (RCTs) by Hanlon, Lindblad, and Gray (2004 [Level I]) included many health care settings (all studies were RCTs: five in the home-health setting, three at hospital discharge with home follow-up, three clinic-based, one in the community-pharmacy setting, and two in long-term care) where clinical pharmacist interventions showed a considerable reduction in drug-related problems as well as reduced morbidity, mortality, and health care costs. Many hospital pharmacies are now linked electronically to health care providers and/or local pharmacies but studies are lacking. Discharge education and counseling to patients including assessment of factors that might affect adherence have been shown to reduce ADEs (Nickerson et al., 2005 [Level II]).

12.4 Complete Medication History*

Date performed _____

Patient Name _____

Medication allergies and type of reaction (e.g., PCN: hives)

Prescription medications – list all including dose, frequency, and route administered
Specifically ask about eye drops, topical creams, B12 injections or other injections (if
    given at home or at medical office, how often).

Over-the-Counter Medications (OTCs)
How often do you exceed the recommended dose on package?
Do you read the labels? Why or why not?
Do you ask a pharmacist or your provider about interactions with your prescriptions?
Ask specifically about:

Pain relievers
What have you tried, what works what does not? What pain do you take it for? How often?
Allergy medications – when do you take them year round? What season? Or When
    symptoms develop?
Sinus congestion/cold or cough medications (combined products with more than one
    ingredient? If so, list ingredients)
Heart burn medications, how often?
Diarrhea or constipation treatments, how often?
Sleeping medications Ask specifically diphenhydramine (Benadryl)
Eye drops – how often what do you take them for?
Herbal remedies (orally or as a tea)

- ginkgo biloba
- ginseng
- glucosamine
- St. John's Wart
- Echinacea

Nutritional Supplements
Ask how often?
Ask specifically about:
Calcium with Vitamin D, Vitamin E, C, or B's
Mega Vitamins
Protein supplements such as Ensure, Boost
Vitamin Drinks

12.4   Complete Medication History

Medications that have been stopped and why? (Did you discontinue or did provider? Why?)

Alcohol (Ask about type/amount per day)

Smoking (what smokes and how much, e.g., cigarettes #packs per day, how many years)

Past or Annual Immunizations, date last received each
Pneumonia vaccine
Flu Vaccine
Other

Regular lab tests – performed to evaluate medications or medication side effects,
    e.g., potassium level, INR, digoxin level, liver toxicity, renal function, blood counts etc.

Use of Memory Aides – reminders to take medications, e.g., pill dispenser box

* Use Brown Bag Method in conjunction with Medication history (see assessment tools).

High Risk Medications

Many studies have revealed common high risk medications in older adults. Nurses should become familiar with high risk medications and medication classes prescribed for older adults in order to aid in preventing ADEs. Many tools are available for nurses to use to assess for high risk medications (i.e., Beers criteria) and for potential drug–drug, drug–disease, or drug–herbal interactions. Common high risk medications are discussed in the following sections.

Warfarin

Warfarin is among the highest risk medications taken by older persons; however, with proper monitoring, the risk of potential adverse sequelae can be significantly reduced. In a prospective study, Hanlon and colleagues (2006 [Level II]) found that warfarin and benzodiazepines were independent risk factors for ADRs, that ADRs are very common in frail elderly adults after hospitalization, and that polypharmacy and warfarin use consistently increase the risk of ADRs. Gaddis and colleagues (2002 [Level IV]) reported that digoxin and warfarin were the greatest source of drug interactions among 200 outpatients. A prospective observational study of 18,820 patients found that the drugs most commonly implicated in causing hospitalization due to ADRs included low-dose aspirin, diuretics, warfarin, and nonsteroidal anti-inflammatory drugs (NSAIDs), with the most common reaction being GI bleeding (Pirmohamed et al., 2004 [Level IV]). In a study of 808 frail older adults discharged from 11 Veteran Affairs hospitals to outpatient care, 33% had one or more ADRs for a rate of 1.92 per 1,000 person-days of follow-up and the rate for preventable ADRs being 0.71 per 1,000 person-days of follow-up. Independent risk factors for all ADRs were number of medications, use of warfarin, and (marginally) the use of benzo-diazepines (Hanlon et al., 2006 [Level II]). Although herbal remedies are commonly used, 58% of older persons do not report use of herbal supplements (Astin et al., 2000 [Level IV]); herbal remedies (e.g., Ginkgo biloba and garlic) interact with warfarin to augment its anticoagulant effect and may lead to serious bleeding problems (Miller, 1998 [Level V]). It is imperative to identify older adults on warfarin who fall or are at risk for falling (see chapter 9, *Preventing Falls in Acute Care*) because their risk of serious injury increases when they are taking warfarin. Nurses must be vigilant in monitoring for potential drug interactions & reactions due to warfarin.

Antihypertensive Agents

Hypertension affects approximately two-thirds of individuals older than 65 but only 27% of people have adequate control. Physiological changes of aging can produce changes in the pharmacokinetics and pharmacodynamics of cardio-vascular drugs in older persons (Nolan & Marcus, 2000 [Level VII]). The anti-hypertensives, as a class, tend to produce various unintended effects, including orthostatic hypotension (associated with diuretics and alpha-blockers), sedation and depression (associated with some beta-blockers), confusion (associated with alpha-blockers), impotence and constipation (associated with verapamil, a calcium channel blocker). Comprehensive and ongoing assessment for potential adverse effects (e.g., routinely checking orthostatic blood pressure) is key to monitoring drug efficacy while an older person is hospitalized. Older persons may also be taught to monitor their blood pressure and orthostatics at home or in other levels of care.

Dose for dose, water-soluble compounds are more potent in aging persons, whereas fat-soluble drugs can be expected to have an extended half-life. Because of changes in fat/lean body mass that characterize the aging process, older adults may require fat soluble beta-blocker dosing intervals to be increased. Fat soluble beta-blockers may be preferable in some cases, such as using pro-pranolol for tremors. Additionally, changes in central penetration of the drug that occurs as a result of age-related changes decreases the integrity of the blood-brain barrier and may predispose older adults to untoward experiences with alpha agonists as well. Many antihypertensives have a tendency to cause depression; persons on lipophilic beta-blockers in particular should be monitored for depression using a standard scale such as the GDS (see chapter 5, *Depression*).

Orthostatic hypotension is a serious problem that can affect older adults on continuous antihypertensive therapy. Sustained treatment renders them more susceptible to diuretic-induced dehydration and orthostatic changes. Orthostasis may also be due to concomitant illness (e.g., infection). The known sequelae of orthostatic hypotension in older adults include falls—true trauma and a medical emergency in physically frail or functionally compromised older adults. Orthostatic hypotension is an independent risk factor for recurrent falls in nursing home residents (Ooi, Hossain, & Lipsitz, 2000 [Level II]).

Psychoactive Drugs

Mental disorders are not a part of normal aging. Nearly 20% of people older than 55 experience mental disorders, with the most common prevalence (in order) being anxiety, severe cognitive impairment, and mood disorders. Mental disorders are under-reported and suicide rates are highest among older adults compared to younger adults. Adults older than 85 have the highest suicide rates of all—more than twice the national rate. (American Association of Geriatric Psychiatrists, 2004 [Level VI]).

In the face of prevailing clinical norms, it is recommended that sedative-hypnotic use for older adults be generally used sparingly and with intense monitoring. Gray and colleagues (2006 [Level II]) reported, in a prospective study of 9,093 patients, that older adults who take benzodiazepines (BZDs) are at greater risk for mobility problems and ADL disability, and that short-acting BZDs do not appear to improve safety benefits over long-acting agents. The likelihood of falls with fractures is more than twice as high for the long-acting BZDs than short-acting agents (Ray, Thapa, & Gideon, 2000 [Level II]). Likewise, Tamblyn and colleagues (2005 [Level II]) report 17.7% of older persons given at least one prescription for BZDs at hospital discharge (greatest risk was with higher dose BZDs) were treated for at least one injury on a follow-up visit, of which fractures were the most common. Over-sedation, respiratory depression, confusion, and other alterations in cognitive capacity, as well as falls, are frequently associated with sedative-hypnotic drug use.

In addition to the sedative-hypnotic class, psychoactive medications include antidepressants (e.g., tricyclics, selective serotonin reuptake inhibitors [SSRIs]), anxiolytics agents (e.g., diazepam, lorazepam), antipsychotics (previously referred to as neuroleptics), mood-stabilizing compounds (e.g., lithium), and psychoactive stimulants. Mood stabilizers and psychoactive stimulants are known to have a relatively narrow therapeutic window even in fully functional, younger adults. Lithium, in particular, requires close monitoring of levels and signs of toxicity in older adults; it also interacts with many other drugs. Psychoactive compounds are most frequently prescribed for agitated behaviors, to stabilize mood, and for therapeutic effects in clinical depression. Older adults are at risk because of changes in absorption, metabolism, distribution, and excretion of both parent drug and psychoactive metabolites. Some unintended interactions may be prevented if age-related changes are considered and careful surveillance is part of routine care.

The half-life of psychoactive drugs is prolonged in older adults and, in general, this class of drugs must be used with extreme caution to avoid inducing delirium, falls, and other traumatic events. Psychotropic medications are associated with an increased risk for falls. A significant correlation was made between falls and psychotropic medications in a meta-analysis of studies in people older than 60 (Leipzig, Cumming, & Tinetti, 1999 [Level I]). Although antianxiety agents, such as the BZDs and sedative-hypnotics, are generally over-prescribed for older adults, the antidepressants are generally considered to be under-prescribed. It is estimated that almost 15% of older persons living in the community, 5% in primary care, and 15% to 25% in nursing homes have significant depressive symptoms (Spina & Scordo, 2002 [Level VI]).

A major deterrent to antidepressant pharmacotherapy in this population has been the high incidence of anticholinergic side effects that occur with administration of tricyclic antidepressants. Anticholinergic side effects such as dry mouth, blurred vision, urinary retention (particularly in the presence of prostatic enlargement), cognitive alterations, cardiotoxicity, and constipation signal to the vigilant clinician that the antidepressant profile needs to be reevaluated and adjusted. Tricyclic antidepressant medications with low anticholinergic profiles include desipramine, nortriptyline, and trazadone; however, the tricyclic class should now be avoided in the elderly because the SSRIs are generally much safer.

The SSRIs, as a class of antidepressants, have strikingly different side effects than other antidepressants. This class does not cause cardiotoxicity or orthostatic hypotension and does not have anticholinergic effects, except for paroxetine, which may have mild anticholinergic effects in some elders (Salzman, 1998). In general, these drugs tend to be a better choice of antidepressants in older adults. The most common side effects are GI related (i.e., nausea, anorexia), which may be ameliorated by starting with a low dose (half that for younger adults; e.g., fluoxetine 5 mg) and slowly increasing (e.g., to 10 mg) after 1 week. A serious but uncommon sequelae of SSRIs is serotonin syndrome, which may occur if more than one antidepressant is prescribed with an SSRI or with concurrent use of St. John's Wort, a commonly self-administered OTC herbal remedy for depression.

The antipsychotics are often considered first-line pharmacotherapeutic interventions for people older than 65 presenting with agitation and behavioral problems associated with dementia (Kindermann, Dolder, Bailey, Katz, & Jeste, 2002 [Level V]). Most are not U.S. Food and Drug Administration (FDA)–approved for such use and data on their effectiveness for such purposes are lacking. Antipsychotics must be used with extreme caution in this population, largely because of the potential for development of abnormal and often irreversible involuntary movements (e.g., extrapyramidal symptoms) associated with their administration. The newer antipsychotics present a much lower risk of extrapyramidal movement disorders than conventional antipsychotics. Unlike conventional antipsychotics, the newer atypical ones (e.g., clozapine, risperidone, olanzapine, and quetiapine) apparently provide several advantages with respect to both efficacy and safety. In 2004, the FDA issued a warning against off-label use of antipsychotics for dementia-related psychotic symptoms due to potential adverse effects. The American Association of Geriatric Psychiatrists (AAGP) does not support the FDA decision and states, "the available evidence of short-term trials conducted in nursing home patients suggests that risperidone and olanzapine may be beneficial for some of the noncognitive [behavioral] symptoms but the decision must be based on individual circumstances" (AAGP, 2005, p. 1). Recent data from the Centers for Medicare and Medicaid (CMS) indicate that newer atypical antipsychotic medications, compared to older antipsychotics, do not appear to be associated with an increased risk of ventricular arrhythmias or cardiac arrest (Liperoti et al., 2005 [Level III]). Psychotropic medications are associated with an increased risk for falls, particularly in the long term care setting (Gurwitz et al., 2005 [Level II]). Drug–drug interactions with antipsychotics are common. Finkel (2004 [Level VI]) is a good resource for drug interactions associated with antipsychotics.

Anticholinergics

Medications with high anticholinergic properties must be used with great caution in older adults due to adverse effects such as inability to concentrate to frank delirium, agitation, hallucinations, blurred vision, slowed GI motility, decreased secretions, urinary retention, and constipation (Spina & Scordo, 2002 [Level VI]; Terrell Heard, K., & Miller, 2006; Tune, 2001 [both Level V]). Urinary retention, resulting from an anticholinergic, can be a lethal side effect in a male with benign prostatic hypertrophy (BPH) and a history of UTIs; urosepsis and death may result. Catterson and colleagues (1997) discuss the vicious cycle of treatment and/or iatrogenesis that may occur with administration of anticholinergic drugs. An illustrative example is an older adult with dementia and BPH who is administered diphenhydramine (i.e., Benadryl) for sleep and who is also taking oxybutinin (i.e., Ditropan), both of which have anticholinergic properties. The additive effects of the two medications may lead to urinary retention and agitation, which may in turn lead to treatment of the agitation with antipsychotics (which also have anticholinergic effects) and exacerbate the problem and cascade of events further. Rochon and colleagues (2006) refer to this as the "prescribing cascade."

Anticholinergic properties occur not only in antidepressant and antipsychotic medications, as previously mentioned, but are also properties of most OTC antihistamines and sleep aids, intestinal and bladder relaxants, corticosteroids, antihypertensives, anti-arrythmics, and other cardiovascular drugs and some antibiotics. See Tune (2001 [Level V]) for a complete list of medications with anticholinergic effects. Additionally, syncopal events and falls are common sequelae of high anticholinergic drug use, again resulting in increased morbidity and mortality in older adults.

Cardiotonics

Digoxin is useful in treating congestive heart failure (CHF) due to *systolic* dysfunction in the elderly, but it is not the recommended treatment for CHF from underlying *diastolic* dysfunction in older adults. Digoxin toxicity occurs more frequently in older adults, presents atypically, and may result in death. Juurlink and colleagues (2003 [Level III]) reported that about 2.3% of cases of digoxin toxicity could have been prevented in hospitalized older adults. Ahmed, Allman, and DeLong (2002 [Evidence Level III]) reported that digoxin is often prescribed inappropriately in hospital patients. Classic symptoms of digoxin toxicity (i.e., nausea, anorexia, visual disturbance) may occur; however, symptomatic cardiac disturbance and arrhythmias are more common in the elderly and are not often thought to be due to digoxin toxicity. Older adults may experience toxicity symptoms even with normal plasma levels of digoxin (Flaherty, Perry, Lynchard, & Morley, 2000). Many older people will have some reduction in renal function with aging; therefore, monitoring for symptoms, especially atypical symptoms of digoxin toxicity, and for renal function and potassium levels is important.

Particular caution must be exercised when digoxin is prescribed with diuretics; this combination can cause hypokalemia and exacerbate renal impairment, which can potentiate digoxin toxicity. Because the therapeutic window for digoxin is narrow and because it is water-soluble (e.g., the drug has a smaller volume of distribution and thus higher plasma concentration), correct and safe dosing of older adults is challenging. The maximum recommended dose in older persons for treating heart failure is 0.125 milligram (Beers, 1997; Fick et al., 2003 [Level VI]); doses for treating atrial fibrillation may be higher. Digoxin binds to protein and because many debilitated older adults have low serum albumin levels, higher plasma levels and digoxin toxicity may result.

Despite the recommendation that ACE inhibitors (ACEI) should be prescribed for all patients with heart failure due to left ventricular/systolic dysfunction and who have normal renal function (Jones, 2000; Packer et al., 1999 [Level II]), Sloane and colleagues (2002 [Level II]) found that 62% of adults in assisted living residences (n = 2014) were not on an ACE inhibitor. Monitoring of renal function and serum potassium should continue as the ACEI dose is titrated up. Rarely do older patients on an ACE inhibitor need potassium supplementation, the combination of which can be lethal. Juurlink and colleagues (2003 [Level III]) reported that 523 of 1,222,093 patients on ACE inhibitors were hospitalized with hyperkalemia; of these patients, 21 died while in the hospital.

OTCs

Self-medication with OTC medications, herbal remedies, and dietary supplements may lead to adverse drug–disease interactions (Astin et al., 2000 [Level IV]) and drug–drug interactions (Rochon, 2006). Neafsey and Shellman (2001 [Level IV]) found that 86% of a sample of 168 older adults attending a hypertension clinic reported at least two or more self-medication practices that could result in an adverse drug interaction. In the United States, community-dwelling older adults take about as many OTC drugs as prescription drugs; among the OTC medications, analgesics, laxatives, and nutritional supplements are utilized most frequently (Hanlon, Schmader, Ruby, & Weinberger, 2001 [Level V]). Salicylates, such as aspirin, are a significant concern with regard to ADRs in older people. In a study of 18,820 patients, Pirmohamed et al. (2004 [Level IV]) found that 18% of all ADR hospital admissions were aspirin-related and lowdose aspirin was implicated most often. ASA in combination with alcohol, because of its water solubility, can worsen age-related renal insufficiency and chronic salicylate intoxication can result. Cold remedies that include alcohol are a significant source of drug potentiation in aging adults. Indeed, alcohol consumption is frequently omitted from history-taking of older adults even though it interacts with OTC and prescription medications in frank and subtle ways to produce unintended drug harm.

The OTCs most commonly implicated in hospital admissions are low dose aspirin and NSAIDs (Pirmohamed et al., 2004 [Level IV]). The FDA has been evaluating OTC ingredients and labeling of OTCs; however, it is a long-range project and yet to be seen if the FDA will be more specific as to safety issues that relate to older adults. Astin and colleagues (2000 [Level IV]) reported that 24% of seniors use herbal remedies (the most common being ginkgo biloba and garlic) and 58% did not report usage to their primary provider. Gingko biloba and garlic interact with warfarin to augment its anticoagulant effect and may lead to bleeding (Miller, 1998 [Level V]); the potential adverse consequences left unaddressed are significant.

Interventions and Nursing Care Strategies

Comprehensive Medication Assessment and Management

Medication management begins with a thorough drug history and medication assessment obtained from an older adult or a reliable informant. Medication history errors occur in up to 67% of patients at the time of admission to the hospital and increase up to 83% when nonprescription drugs were included (Tam et al., 2005 [Level I]), suggesting, by the authors, a need for a systematic approach to accurate medication histories at the time of admission. No studies provide a systematic approach to history taking, although specific aspects of the medication history and assessment includes the following evidence-based activities:

- Obtain a *complete medical history* and validate that the medication history is true (Lau, Florax, Porsius, & De Boer, 2000 [Level IV]) ascertaining the numbers and types of medications typically consumed, as well as an estimate of how long the older adult has been taking the drug.
- Nathan and colleagues (1999 [Level IV]) recommend that older adults bring all their medications to the provider/hospital/other health care setting (using the Brown Bag method, this requires bringing all prescription, OTC, and herbal remedies in a brown bag) in order to document medication types, instructions for self-administration, dates, and duration of the drug regimen. This method fosters identification of multiple prescribers and dispensing pharmacies and can signal polypharmacy and/or possible substance abuse, particularly with regard to analgesics, anxiolytics, and sedative-hypnotics.
- Focused questions by the clinician should address nicotine and alcohol use, as well as vitamins, herbal remedies, and OTC medications that are routinely used (Astin et al., 2000; Lau et al., 2000 [both Level IV]). This information should be included in the medication profile. (See Table 12.4 for a suggested medication history.) Little information is available about medication history-taking or even education of pharmacists regarding medication history interviews (Ellington et al., 2002).
- Ask detailed questions about OTC and "recreational" drugs, alcohol use, and herbal or other folk remedies. Be specific about the actual amount and under what circumstances these substances are used. Accurate information can help explain symptoms that otherwise may not make sense. Evaluate for duplicate medications, which often occurs due to unrecognized trade names versus generic names and OTCs with the same active ingredients in them (e.g., acetaminophen) (Astin et al., 2000 [Level IV]).
- Perform *medication reconciliation* to verify actual medication regimen at hospital admission and discharge (Gleason et al., 2004 [Level IV];

Nickerson et al., 2005 [Level II]) and across the continuum of care (Nickerson et al., 2005 [Level II]). The eighth goal of the Joint Commission on Accreditation of Health Care Organizations (JCAHO) mandates medication reconciliation across practice sites requiring an accurate and complete reconciliation of medications across the continuum. The intent of this standard is to ensure that when a person moves from one "setting, service, practitioner, or level of care within or outside the organization," a complete current list of medications will be communicated to the next provider or service and be reconciled (compared) at the new setting, service practitioner, or level of care (JCAHO, 2006, 2007; Tangalos & Zarowitz, 2006 [both Level VI]).

- Monitor new symptoms and consider the likelihood of their being due to an ADR (Petrone & Katz, 2005 [Level IV]; Rochon, 2006 [Level V]) prior to requesting a new medication to treat symptoms; avoid the prescribing cascade.

- Attempt a trial of nonpharmacological interventions/treatments prior to requesting medication for new symptoms. Nurses often make these recommendations when notifying primary providers for a new problem/symptom.

- Continually monitor for possible toxicity to those drugs with high prevalence of toxicity (see high risk medications section in this chapter). PDA technology can help nurses assess high risk medications such as *Facts and Comparisons* (see Resources section in this book).

- When falls occur, always consider medications as a source. Particularly consider recently added medications that are high risk for causing falls, such as diuretics (see chapter 9, *Preventing Falls in Acute Care*).

- Nurses need to collaborate with the interdisciplinary team to effect change in reducing the numbers of ADEs and ADRs, many of which are preventable (Hanlon, et al., 2001 [Level V]). Although many studies describe and recommend an interdisciplinary approach as the best method for improving drug-treatment outcomes (Lam & Ruby, 2005; Williams, et al., 2004 [both Level II]), most do not delineate the specific role or function of the individual team members (other than the pharmacist making recommendations to the physician), nor do they measure outcomes of the team. Some recommendations to consider for an interdisciplinary approach include a medication care team (i.e., nurses, pharmacist, primary physician, social worker) with specific functions assigned to review medications at admission and discharge utilizing evidence-based recommendations. The following list of discharge interventions may be performed by various team members, such as:
  - Reminder systems may be instituted by pharmacists in collaboration with nurses as reported effective by Muir, Sanders, Wilkinson, & Schmader (2001 [Level III]). A visual intervention (medication grid) was delivered to physicians to see if it could reduce medication-regimen complexity. Researchers reported that this simple intervention had a significant impact on medication-regimen complexity in older adults. The pharmacist may also review (preferably using a computer-based program) the medication list at admission, when new medications are added, and prior to discharge for potential drug–drug

interactions, drug–disease interactions, and/or inappropriate medications for older adults. In a study by Simon et al. (2006 [Level II]), age-specific alerts sustained the effectiveness of drug-specific alerts to reduce potentially inappropriate prescribing in older people, resulting in a considerably decreased burden of the alerts. Computerized medication order entry has the potential to prevent an estimated 84% of dose, frequency, and route errors. Anywhere from 28% to 95% of ADEs can be prevented by reducing medication errors through computerized monitoring systems (AHRQ, 2001 [Level I]). A study in ambulatory care using a quasi-experimental design found that medication interaction alerts modestly reduced the frequency of coprescribing of interacting medications; however, the study concluded additional efforts would be required to further reduce rates of inappropriate prescribing of warfarin with interacting drugs (Feldstein et al., 2006 [Level III]). The pharmacist may also function as the communicator of the hospital drug regimen to the community pharmacy, primary care provider, and/or other levels of care.

- The social worker may review issues at home such as access to medications, cost, caregiver support, and barriers to discharge interventions.

- Nurses and other interdisciplinary members need to be proactive participants in reducing rehospitalization related to ADEs and implement discharge education and counseling to patients, including:

  - *Assess abilities and limitations* such as functional ability, including the ability to read the medication label, open the medication container, and consume or self-administer the prescribed medication as intended (see chapter 3, *Assessment of Function*, and chapter 4, *Assessing Cognitive Function*) (Curry, Walker, Hogstel, & Burns, 2005 [Level VI]). The care plan should address actual and potential problems and the need for reassessment at regular intervals and after major medical events (e.g., CVA or delirium).

  - *Devices to accommodate* some impairments or barriers may be recommended. For example, tamper-proof lids are often difficult for elders to remove, particularly if there are arthritic changes. A simple request to the pharmacist to provide a non-childproof lid may improve the safe and effective use of a prescribed medication.

  - *Assess cognitive and affective status* to ensure that memory problems or vegetative symptoms associated with depression are not interfering with the safe use of prescription drugs (see chapter 4, *Assessing Cognitive Function*, and chapter 5, *Depression*).

  - *Assess health literacy* (Curry et al., 2005 [Level VI]). Query whether the older person understands what the drug is to be used for, how often it is to be taken, circumstances of ingestion (e.g., with food), and other aspects of drug self-administration that signal intelligent drug use; use the DRUGS tool (Edelberg et al., 1999 [Level IV]; Hutchison, Jones, West, & Wei, 2006 [Level IV]).

  - *Assess for ability to recognize generic* versus brand name medication and their use (Curry et al., 2005 [Level VI]). Ask the older adult to describe circumstances in which the medication was not used or was used differently than prescribed. If the older adult cannot describe medication use, consider removing the drug or provide written instruction for the home (Muir et al., 2001 [Level III]).

- *Assess beliefs, concerns, and problems* related to the medication regimen. Ask the older adult if she or he believes that the drug is actually doing what it is intended to do. If the medication is not useful, not creating symptom relief, or causing adverse effects, consider removing it or replacing it with a more acceptable substitute.

- *Discuss the impact of medication expenses.* Many medications, particularly those that are new to the market, can be prohibitively expensive, particularly for people on fixed incomes. Discuss the influence of television ads. Ask the older adult what concerns they have about the costs and risks of administration (Curry et al., 2005 [Level VI]). Also discuss Medicare part D concerns and confusion. Where economic problems are identified, generic drugs and other avenues should be explored to manage the cost issue.

- *Consider instrumental issues* related to drug use, such as availability of family members or other social supports to facilitate medication adherence, and who monitors the need to change specific medications dictated by third-party reimbursement and medication coverage plans. It is particularly important with Medicare Part D coverage to ensure that those enrolled understand that after a certain dollar amount is reached, the older adult will the be required to pay full price for prescriptions, called the "doughnut hole."

- *Assess factors that might affect adherence* (Nickerson et al., 2005 [Level II]). See the Resources section for literature on adherence.

- Patients should be given the *necessary information* and the opportunity to exercise the degree of control they choose over health care decisions that affect them and the necessary information to effectuate this. Patients who are informed and are involved in decision making are less likely to make decisions that may lead to ADRs, such as abruptly discontinuing a medication that should be tapered off slowly (National Coordinating Council for Medication Errors Reporting and Prevention, 2001).

Conclusion

Nurses have the unique opportunity to intervene and to reduce ADEs in older adults in the hospital setting and at transition to other levels of care. Traditionally, focused on "caring," nurses have taken the lead in implementing preventive strategies on behalf of the patient. While acute care nurses are not typically prescribers unless they are advanced practice nurses (APNs) with prescriptive authority, they have always reviewed and confirmed medication orders, carried them out, and alerted the primary provider of concerns and problems with medications; nurses have always ensured a culture of safety and must continue to be proactive in doing so. Nurses are also responsible for identifying wrong drugs, dosages, and so on prior to administering them. Given that nurses are at the bedside 24/7, they can make medication suggestions to prescribers based on their holistic knowledge of the patient and recognition of new symptoms. Nurses are in a pivotal position to reduce ADEs in older persons at discharge as well. Nurses are the primary source for providing discharge education and counseling to older adults at discharge; therefore, they play a key role in preventing medication-related consequences after discharge, including prevention of rehospitalization due to medication-related problems. Consulting with experts on the interdisciplinary team and/or use of computer programs can facilitate provision of discharge information.

Case Study and Discussion

Mr. R., a 72-year-old retired college professor, is admitted to your preoperative surgery unit for a TURP with a 24-hour anticipated stay. He also has a history of recurrent UTIs and is admitted with a temperature of 102°F. He says he feels confused today and isn't sure why he is here. He is a widower with two children and three grown grandchildren; the closest relative lives 200 miles away. Mr. R. has a history of Parkinson's disease, osteoarthritis, BPH, constipation, and recent elevated blood pressure readings. On your admission history, you ask Mr. R. about OTCs and herbal remedies. You learn he has been taking Ibuprofen 400 mg four times per day for unrelieved osteoarthritis (OA) pain during the past 2 weeks, as well as Benadryl 25 mg to help him "sleep with the pain" and OTC glucosamine. He also admits to taking Gingko biloba because, he says, "I'm worried about becoming senile from the Parkinson's."

Because Mr. R. has a history of significant BPH and is scheduled for TURP, you take a look at his medication list and medical conditions. He is taking Sinemet, Benadryl, and Vicodin but unclear of dosages. You look up the medications on your PDA and learn that the three medications taken together can have an additive effect and cause urinary retention, placing Mr. R. at risk for urosepsis. You quickly notify the on-call resident of Mr. R.'s fever and signs of delirium (confusion) (which could indicate impending urosepsis) and inform her about what you know about the medication interactions and Mr. R.'s history. You recommend a stat urinalysis with culture (along with his preoperative lab work). He is admitted to the medical surgical floor instead of to surgery that day. Intravenous fluids and the first dose of antibiotics are initiated after the U/A is collected; his surgery is delayed until his fever and UTI are resolved. You make a note on his discharge/care planning form to educate Mr. R. regarding:

- Benadryl is not recommended in older adults; particularly in combination with the other meds he is taking, Sinemet and Vicodin (a smooth muscle relaxant which may cause constipation and urinary retention), which may have led to acute urinary retention as well as constipation. If he requires Vicodin (or other narcotic analgesia) for

- pain, he will need increased fluids, dietary modification, and possibly Lactulose (i.e., an osmotic laxative) to prevent/treat constipation.
- Recent high blood pressure readings may be related to NSAID (i.e., Ibuprofen) use. Recommend discontinuance of NSAIDs and monitor B/P off them during hospitalization. Inform him that OA is not inflammatory, and NSAIDs are not recommended for OA and are high risk for adverse effects in older adults. Also consider a consultation with the pain service.
- Educate about the risks of self-medication with OTCs and recommend consultation with primary provider and/or pharmacist before purchasing OTCs, including herbal remedies. Recommend a complete medication history once confusion (delirium) clears.
- Nurses on the other levels of care (e.g., pre- and post-op) need to be informed of the need for ongoing monitoring of his mental status for delirium (see chapter 7, *Delirium: Prevention, Early Recognition, and Treatment*), blood pressure (due to recent high readings), and pain-related to OA as well as post-op pain.

Acknowledgment

We would like to acknowledge and thank Mark Beers, MD, for his thoughtful review of this chapter.

Resources

High Risk Medications in Aging

Beers Criteria

Fick et al. (2003). Beers Criteria of Potentially Inappropriate Medications. *Archives of Internal Medicine*, available online at http://archinte.ama-assn.org/cgi/content/full/163/22/2716

Warfarin

Feldstein, A. C., Smith, D. H., Perrin, N., Yang, X., Simon, S. R., & Krall, M., et al. (2006). Reducing warfarin medication interactions: An interrupted time series evaluation. *Archives of Internal Medicine, 166*(9), 1009–1015. Evidence Level III: Quasi-experimental Study.

Medications in Older Adults

PDF File: Assessment for High Risk Medications. Retrieved September 28, 2006, from http://www.ConsultGeriRN.org.

Anticholinerics

Tune, L. E. (2001). Anticholinergic effects of medication in elderly patients. *Journal of Clinical Psychiatry, 62* (Suppl. 21), 11–14. Evidence Level V: Review.

Drug–Drug Interactions with Antipsychotics

Finkel, S. (2004 [Level VI]). Pharmacology of antipsychotics in the elderly: A focus on atypicals. *Journal American Geriatrics Society, 5:* (Suppl.), 258–265.

Ventricular Arrhythmias and MI Associated with Antipsychotics

Liperoti, R., Gambassi, G., Lapane, K. L., Chiang, C., Pedone, C., Mor, V., et al. (2005). Conventional and atypical antipsychotics and the risk of hospitalization for ventricular arrhythmias or cardiac arrest. *Archives of Internal Medicine, 165*(6), 696–701. [Level III].

Common Drug–Drug Interactions (see PDA materials also)

Ament, P. W., Bertolino, J. G., & Liszewski, J. L. (2000). Clinical pharmacology: Clinically significant drug interactions. *American Family Physician, 61*, 1745–1754. Evidence Level VI: Expert Opinion.

Pain

Hutt, E., Pepper, G. A., Vojir, C., Fink, R., & Jones, K. R. (2006). Assessing the appropriateness of pain-medication prescribing practices in nursing homes. *Journal of American Geriatrics Society, 54*(2), 231–239.

Medication/Medical Error Prevention

National Coordination Council for Medication Error Prevention. *Medication Error Reporting and Prevention information.* Retrieved September 26, 2006, from http://www.nccmerp.org/councilRecs.html

Joanna Briggs Institute (2006). Strategies to reduce medication errors with reference to older adults. *Nursing Standard, 20*(41), 53–57. Review Article. The primary references on which this information is based are available online via Blackwell Synergy at www.blackwell-synergy.com, and to members of the institute via the Web site: www.joannabriggs.edu.au. Evidence Level I: Systematic Review.

Preventing Medication Errors: Quality Chasm Series (2007). Board on Health Care Services (HCS). Retrieved September 28, 2006, from http://www.nap.edu/nap-cgi/skimit.cgi?isbn=0309101476&chap=127-134.

Institute for Healthcare Improvement. *Patient Safety Related to Medications in the Hospital.* Accessed on April 30, 2007. http://www.ihi.org/IHI/Topics/PatientSafety/MedicationSystems/ImprovementStories/FSHighAlertMedsHeightenedVigilance.htm

Santell, J. P., & Hicks, R. W. (2005). *Medication errors involving geriatric patients. Joint Commission Journal on Quality & Patient.* Safety, 32(4), 225–229.

Practice Guidelines

Geriatric Nursing Protocols. Web site provides various geriatric-specific protocols as well as tools and resources, including *Medications in Older Adults* from a multitude of geriatric experts across the country. Retrieved September 29, 2005, from www.ConsultGeriRN.org now available at hartfordIGN.org

University of Iowa Gerontological Nursing Interventions Research Center, Research Dissemination Core–Academic Institution (October 2004). *Improving medication management for older adult clients.* 55 pages. NGC: 003993.

Retrieved September 28, 2006, from the National Guideline Clearinghouse (NGC) at www.guideline.gov.

American Society of Health System Pharmacists (ASHP) (1995). *Preventing Medication Errors in Hospitals.* Retrieved September 28, 2006, from http://www.ashp.org/bestpractices/MedMis/MedMis_Gdl_ADR.pdf

ASHP Guidelines on Adverse Drug Monitoring and Reporting

American Society of Health System Pharmacists (ASHP). Access at http://www.ashp.org/bestpractices/MedMis/MedMis_Gdl_Hosp.pdf

Herbal Remedies

Drug–drug, drug–dietary supplement, and drug–citrus fruit and other food interactions—what have we learned? *Journal of Clinical Pharmacology,* June 2004. Access at *www.jclinpharm.org*

Drug interactions with herbal products & grapefruit juice: A conference report, *Clinical Pharmacology & Therapeutics,* January 2004. Access at *www.ascpt.org*

Assessment Tools

Dietary Supplement Intake Form; includes drug interactions. American Academy of Orthopedic Surgeons. Patient Safety Checklists. Access at http://www3.aaos.org/safety/dietary.pdf

Drugs Regimen Unassisted Grading Scale (DRUGS) Tool (Edelberg et al., 1999; Hutchison et al., 2006 [both Level IV]). Retrieved September 28, 2006, from http://www.fda.gov/medwatch/safety/2006/safety06.htm#chronological \

Medication Management Tool. Bergmen-Evans, B. (2004). Used to assess several domains of ability to manage medications independently. Access (order at) research-disemination-core@uiowa.edu or telephone 319-384-4429.

Medication Adherence

Haynes, R. B., Yao, X., Degani, A., Kripalani, S., Garg, A., & McDonald, H. P. (2005). Interventions for enhancing medication compliance. *Cochrane Database of Systematic Reviews* 2007, Issue 1. Accessed January 30, 2007, at www.mrw.interscience.wiley.com/cochrane/clsysrev/articles/CD000011/frame.html

Continuing Education on Medication Adherence. Foody, J. (2006). Medical adherence: America's other drug problem. Medscape, LLC. Accessed January 4, 2007, at www.medscape.som/viewprogram/6450_pnt

JCAHO Standards

Traynor, K. (2006). Four JCAHO medication management standards to change July 1. *American Journal of Health-System Pharmacy, 63*(13), 1210–1212. Evidence Level VI: Expert Opinion.

JCAHO Patient Safety Goals Related to Medications (2007)

http://www.jointcommission.org/PatientSafety/NationalPatientSafetyGoals/

JCAHO High Alert Meds

Sentinel event information related to High Alert Medications. http://www.jointcommission.org/SentinelEvents/SentinelEventAlert/sea_11.htm

PDA Resources

Facts and Comparisons

Drug information including drug–drug and drug–disease interactions for your handheld. Access/order at http://pdacortex.pdaorder.com/pdaorder/-/-/item?oec-catalog-item-id=1377

The Medical Letter's Handbook of Adverse Drug Interactions

Access at http://www.medicalletter.org/
Free demo at: http://medlet-best.securesites.com/html/software_desc2.htm

The Medical Letter on Drugs and Therapeutics

Handbook of Adverse Drug Interactions (manual); Adverse Drug Interactions Program (software, Internet). Software searches for interactions between 2 and up to 25 drugs. 1000 Main Street New Rochelle, NY 10801-7537 E-mail: custserv@themedicalletter.org

Box 12.1

Nursing Standard of Practice Protocol: Reducing Adverse Drug Events in Older Adults

I. **GOAL:** Reduce adverse drug events in older adults.

II. **OVERVIEW:** Adverse drug events, whether from drug–drug or drug–disease interactions, inappropriate prescribing, poor adherence, or medication errors, lead to serious or potentially fatal outcomes for older adults. More than half of adverse drug events may be preventable (NCC MERP, 2001[Level VI]; Rochon, 2006 [Level V]; Safran et al., 2005 [Level IV]).

III. BACKGROUND

    A. Definitions
        1. *Adverse Drug Event (ADE)*: Injury occurring during the patient's drug therapy, whether resulting from appropriate care or from unsuitable or suboptimum care. Includes ADEs during normal use of medicine and any harm secondary to a medication error. ADEs can have different outcomes: worsening of existing pathology or lack of expected health-status improvement (COE, 2005; p. 1).
        2. *Iatrogenic ADEs*: Any undesirable condition in a patient occurring as the result of treatment by a health care professional; pertaining to an illness or injury resulting from a medication or drug.
        3. *Adverse drug reaction (ADR)*: Any noxious or unintended and undesired effect of a drug that occurs at normal human doses for prophylaxis, diagnosis, or therapy. According to Committee

of Experts on Safe Medication Practices, ADEs are preventable (COE, 2005; p. 2), including medical errors and nonadherence.

4. *Medication nonadherance*: The number of doses not taken or taken incorrectly that jeopardizes the patient's therapeutic outcome (NCPIE, 1997 [Level VI]).

5. *Drug–drug interactions*: Changes in a drug's effects by another drug taken during the same period. The interactions are basically pharmacokinetic or pharmacodynamic (Merck Manual of Diagnosis and Therapy, 2005 [Level VI]).

6. *Drug–disease interactions*: Undesired drug effects (exacerbation of a disease or condition by a drug) that occur in patients with certain disease states (e.g., beta-blocker given to patient with depression, worsens the depression chospasm).

7. *Pharmacokinetics*: The time course of absorption, distribution across compartments, metabolism, and excretion of drugs in the body. The metabolism and excretion of many drugs decrease and the physiological changes of aging require dosage adjustment for some drugs (Merck Manual, 2005 [Level VI]).

8. *Pharmacodynamics*: The response of the body to the drug, which is affected by receptor binding, postreceptor effects, and chemical interactions (Merck Manual, 2005 [Level VI]). Pharmacodynamic problems occur when two drugs act at the same or interrelated receptor sites, resulting in additive, synergistic, or antagonistic effects. The effects of two or more drugs together can be either *additive* (combination of drugs "add up" to increase effect), *synergistic* (one agent magnifies the effect of the other), or *antagonistic* (one medication inhibits the effect of the other).

9. *Medication Reconciliation*: the process of comparing a patient's medication orders to all of the medications that the person has been taking (Santell, 2006 [Level VI]).

B. Epidemiology

1. It is estimated that the majority of older adults older than 65 (79%) are on medications, with 39% taking five or more prescription drugs and up to 90% taking over-the-counter drugs (Hanlon et al., 2001a [Level V]). People older than 65 consume more than one-third of all prescription drugs and purchase 40% of all over-the-counter medicines (Kohn et al., 2000 [Level VI]).

2. In a large study of women 65 years of age and older, 12% took 10 or more medications and 23% took at least five prescribed medications (Kaufman et al., 2002 [Level IV]).

3. An estimated 35% of older persons experience ADEs and almost half of these are preventable (Safran et al., 2005 [Level IV]).

4. Prevalence of ADR-related hospitalizations ranges from 5% to 35% (Gurwitz et al., 2003 [Level IV]).

5. Serious ADRs that occur during hospitalization are at 6.7% and, when extrapolated, are the fourth to sixth leading cause of in-hospital mortality for all causes of death and likely an

underestimate because ADRs related to nonadherence or errors in administration therapeutic failures are not included (Lazarou et al., 1998 [Level I]).

6. ADEs are estimated to cost the health care system $75 billion to $85 billion annually (Fick et al., 2003 [Level VI]) and result in 106,000 deaths annually (Lazarou et al, 1998; [Level I]).

C. Etiology

Adults become increasingly susceptible to ADEs as they age. Physiological changes characteristic of aging predispose older adults to experience ADEs resulting in four times more hospitalizations in older versus younger persons. People older than 65 experience medication-related problems for seven major reasons:

1. Age-related physiologic changes that result in altered pharmacokinetics and pharmacodynamics (Mangoni & Jackson, 2003 [Level VI]; Rochon, 2006 [Level V]).

2. Multiple medications (i.e., polypharmacy) that are often prescribed by multiple providers (Hanlon, Schmader, Ruby, & Weinberger, 2001 [Level V]; Hajjar & Kotchen, 2003 [Level IV])

3. Incorrect doses of medications (over or under a therapeutic dosage) (Astin et al., 2000 [Level IV]; Hanlon, Schmader, Ruby, & Weinberger, 2001 [Level V]; Sloane et al., 2002 [Level II]).

4. Medication consumption for the treatment of symptoms that are not disease-dependent or specific (i.e., self-medication or prescribing cascades) (Neafsey & Shellman, 2001 [Level IV]; Rochon & Gurwitz, 1997 [Level V]).

5. Iatrogenic causes such as:
   a. ADRs: drug–drug or drug–disease interactions (Gurwitz et al., 2005 [Level II]; Hohl et al., 2005 [Level IV]; Lazarou et al., 1998 [Level I]; Petrone & Katz, 2005 [Level IV])
   b. Inappropriate prescribing for older adults (Fick et al., 2003 [Level VI])

6. Problems with medication adherence (Fulmer et al., 1999 (Level VI]), Haynes et al., 2005 [Level V]).

7. Medication errors (Doucette et al., 2005 [Level V]; National Council on Patient Information and Education (NCPIE), 1997 [Level VI]).

IV. ASSESSMENT TOOLS AND STRATEGIES

A. Assessment Tools

1. Use appropriate assessment tools as indicated for each individual's needs and specific setting:
   a. Beers Criteria: 2002 Criteria for Potentially Inappropriate Medication Use in Older Adults: Independent (see Table 12.1). 2002 Criteria for Potentially Inappropriate Medication Use in Older Adults: Considering Diagnoses or Condition (see Table 12.2) (Fick et al., 2003 [Level VI]).

  b. Common Drug–Drug Interactions (see Table 12.3). List of some commonly known interactions.
  c. Cockroft-Gault Formula: to estimate renal function (see Figure 12.1).
  d. Functional Capacity (ADL, IADL, Mini-Cog, or MMSE). See chapter 3, *Assessment of Function*, and chapter 4, *Assessing Cognitive Function*.
  e. Brown Bag Method (Nathan et al., 1999 [Level IV]). Method used to assess all medications an older adult has at home, including prescriptions from all providers, OTC medications, and herbal remedies (all medications are to be brought in a "brown bag"). Should be used in conjunction with a complete medication history (see Table 12.4).
  f. Drugs Regimen Unassisted Grading Scale (DRUGS) Tool. Assessment of self-administration ability (Edelberg, Shallenberger, & Wei, 1999 [Level IV]; Hutchinson, Jones, West, & Wei, 2006 [both level IV]). Typically used at time of transfer to other levels of care (see Resources section).
B. Assessment Strategies
  1. Comprehensive medication assessment should be performed at admission, discharge, and intervals in between (Petrone & Katz, 2005 [Level IV]; Shekelle et al., 2001). Obtain a detailed medication history and confirm its accuracy (Lau et al., 2000 [Level IV]); Tam et al., 2005 [Level I], detailing the type and amount of prescriptions, OTCs, vitamins, supplements, and herbal remedies (Hanlon et al., 2001a [Level V]; Kaufman et al., 2002 [Level IV]), alcohol and illicit drugs, using appropriate assessment tool (e.g., Brown Bag method) (Nathan et al., 1999 [Level IV]).
  2. Assess renal function using Cockroft-Gault formula for assessing renal function prior to administering renal-clearing drugs (see Figure 12.1).
  3. Reconciliation of medications ordered at admission and at discharge in consultation with a pharmacist (Gleason et al., 2004 [Level IV]; Santell, 2006 [Level VI]), geriatric expert, or computer-based program (Joanna Briggs Institute, 2006 [Level I]; Feldman, McDonald, Rosati, Murtaugh, Kovner, et al., 2006 [Level IV]).
  4. Review medication list using Beers criteria for potentially inappropriate medications, particularly those with *high severity* and for potential drug–drug and drug–disease interactions (see Tables 12.1 and 12.2) (Fick et al., 2003 [Level VI]; Zhan et al., 2005 [Level IV]).
  5. At discharge from hospital, use appropriate tools to assess individual's ability to self-administer medications:
    a. Assess functional capacity: ADLs, IADLs, Mini-Cog. See chapter 3, *Assessment of Function*, and chapter 4, *Assessing Cognitive Function*.

b. Assess individuals (at admission or initial encounter and at discharge) who administer their own medicines with DRUGS tool to identify potential areas of self-administration difficulty (see Resources) (Edelberg et al., 1999; Edelberg, Shallenberger, Hausdorff, & Wei, 2000; Hutchinson, Jones, West, & Wei, 2006 [all Level IV]).

V. INTERVENTIONS AND NURSING CARE STRATEGIES

A. Reducing ADEs (during and posthospitalization)
   1. *Patient empowerment.* Patients should be given the necessary information and the opportunity to exercise the degree of control they choose over health care decisions that affect them. If patients are involved in decision making, they are less likely to make decisions that may lead to ADRs (NCC MERP, 2001 [Level VI]), such as abruptly discontinuing a medication that should be tapered off. (Preventing Medication Errors: Quality Chasm Series (2007) [Level VI]).
   2. *Comprehensive Medication Assessment* on admission as indicated in assessment (see Table 12.4).
   3. *Collaborate with the interdisciplinary team* to effect change in reducing the numbers of ADEs and ADRs, many of which are preventable (Hanlon, Schmader, Ruby, & Weinberger, 2001 [Level V]).
   4. *Prescribing Principles.* Monitoring for appropriate prescribing and alerting the prescriber to potential problem areas helps reduce medication-related problems. Prescribing a medication is multifaceted: deciding that a drug is truly indicated; choosing the best drug; determining appropriate dose for the individual; monitoring for toxicity and effectiveness; and seeking consultation when necessary (Rochon, 2006 [Level V]). These principles support recommendations to:
      a. *Reduce the dose.* "Start Low and Go Slow," or give the lowest possible dose when starting a medication and slow upward titration to obtain clinical benefit; many ADEs are dose-related (Petrone & Katz, 2005 [Level IV]; Rochon, 2006 [Level V]). Primary provider should be notified if the dosage ordered is higher than the recommended starting dose (e.g., digoxin maximum dose ≤ 0.125 mg for treatment of CHF) (Fick et al., 2003 [Level VI]).
      b. *Discontinue unnecessary therapy.* Prescribers are often reluctant to stop medications, especially if they did not initiate the treatment. This practice increases the risk for an adverse event (Rochon, 2006 [Level V]).
      c. *Attempt a trial of nonpharmacological interventions/treatments* prior to requesting medication for new symptoms (Rochon, 2006 [Level V]).

d. *Recommend safer drugs.* Avoid drugs that are likely to be associated with adverse outcomes (review Beers Criteria) (Petrone & Katz, 2005 [Level IV]).

e. *Assess renal function* using Cockroft-Gault formula (for renally cleared drugs) to determine accurate dosage prior to prescribing such as many routinely prescribed IV antibiotics. Dosage recommendations are available based on this formula in PDR and other common prescribing resources.

f. *Optimize drug regimen.* When prescribing medications, the focus should be on risk versus benefit where the expected health benefit (e.g., relief of agitation in dementia with psychosis) exceeds the expected negative consequences (e.g., morbidity and mortality from falls that result in hip fracture) (Leipzig et al., 1999 [Level I]; Ooi et al., 2000 [Level II]).

g. *Initiation of new medication.* Assess for potential drug–disease and drug–drug interactions and correct dosages, the most common causes of ADRs, before starting new drugs (Doucet et al., 2002 [Level V]; NCC MERP, 2001 [Level VI]; Petrone & Katz, 2005 [Level IV]).

h. *Avoid the prescribing cascade.* Avoid the prescribing cascade by *first* considering a new symptom as being a consequence of a current medication prior to adding a new medication (Rochon, 2006 [Level V]; Rochon & Gurwitz, 1997 [Level V]).

i. *Avoid inappropriate medications in older persons.* Review criteria for potentially inappropriate medications (see Table 12.1) or drug–disease interactions (see Table 12.2) and potential drug–drug interactions (see Table 12.3) (Fick et al., 2006 [Level VI]).

B. Specific interventions for prevention of Iatrogenic Adverse Drug Reactions (in hospital and after discharge)

1. Consider any new symptom as a possible ADR before requesting/administering new medication for the symptom, avoiding the prescribing cascade (example in context) (Gurwitz et al., 2003 [Level IV]).

2. Monitor medication orders for wrong drug choices (high risk inappropriate medications, drug–disease and drug–drug interactions), wrong dosages, or administration errors (Doucette et al. 2005 [Level V]; Gurwitz et al., 2003 [Level IV]; Hanlon et al., 1997 [Level IV]). Consider use of technological handheld devices such as PDA for quick access to Beers criteria, drug–drug or drug–disease interactions, and geriatric assessment tools (see www.ConsultGeriRN.org and Resources section of this chapter).

3. Improve prescribing practices by documenting indication for initiation of new drug therapy, maintaining a current medication list, documenting response to therapy, as well as the need for ongoing treatment (Knight & Avorn, 2001 [Level VI]; Merle, Laroche,

Dantoine, & Charmes, 2005 [Level VI]) and evaluating co-morbidities (Merle et al., 2005 [Level VI]).

4. Institutional implementation of computer-assisted technology for medication order entry: has the potential to prevent an estimated 84% of dose, frequency, and route errors; and from 28% to 95% of ADEs can be prevented by reducing medication errors through computerized monitoring systems (AHRQ, 2001 [Level I]). Identifying and reporting of ADRs can also be performed using computer-assisted National Surveillance system. Institutions must facilitate a culture of safety to reduce ADRs/ADEs.

C. Interventions at Discharge

1. *Reconciliation* of medications at discharge (Gleason et al., 2004 [Level IV]; Nickerson et al., 2005 [Level II]; JCAHO, 2006, 2007 [Level VI]) helps to reduce ADR/ADEs and therefore rehospitalization.

2. *Assess abilities and limitations* and health literacy in self-administration of medications using appropriate tools at discharge (Curry et al., 2005 [Level VI]) and recognize that self-administration and nonadherence can induce ADRs (Merle et al., 2005 [Level VI]).

3. *Assess for adherence* issues that may develop after discharge, which can help to reduce ADEs (Nickerson et al., 2005 [Level II]) and rehospitalization (Bergman-Evans, 2006; Edelberg et al., 1999 [Level IV]; Fulmer et al., 2000). Recommend devices that can assist in enhancing adherence behavior (Fulmer et al., 1999) and interventions to address cost and other adherence issues.

4. *Patient/Caregiver Education*. Provide patient and caregiver education using relevant nursing content and principles (Curry et al., 2005 [Level VI]) including assessment of factors that might affect adherence. Nurses are the primary source for providing education to patients at discharge; therefore, their role is key to preventing medication-related consequences after hospitalization, including rehospitalization. Discharge education and counseling includes:

a. Education tailored to the age group and needs of the individual (Bergman-Evans, 2006)

b. Educate the patient/caregiver about benefits and risks (Shekelle et al., 2001) and potential medication side effects (Rochon, 2006 [Level V]).

c. Teach safe medication management (Curry et al., 2005 [Level VI]).

d. Consider an interactive computer program (Personal Education Program [PEP]) designed for the learning styles and psychomotor skills of older adults to teach about potential drug interactions that can result from self-medication with OTC agents and alcohol (Neafsey, Strickler, Shellman, & Chartier, 2002 [Level II]).

VI. EXPECTED OUTCOMES

A. Patients will:
1. Experience fewer iatrogenic outcomes from medication-related events.
2. Understand their medication regimens upon discharge from the hospital.
B. Health care providers will:
1. Use a range of interventions to prevent, alleviate, or ameliorate medication problems with older adults.
2. Improve prescribing practices by documenting indication for initiation of new drug therapy, maintaining a current medication list, documenting response to therapy, as well as the need for ongoing treatment (Knight & Avorn, 2001 [Level VI]).
3. Evaluate nature and origins of medication-related problems in a timely manner.
4. Increase their knowledge about medication safety in older adults.
5. Increase referrals to appropriate practitioners (e.g., geriatrician, geriatric/gerontological or psychiatric clinical nurse specialist, nurse practitioner, or consultation-liaison service).
C. Institution will:
1. Provide education to health care providers regarding prevention, identification, and reporting of ADRs (Gurwitz et al., 2003 [Level IV]).
2. Make information on ADRs accessible to patients (Gurwitz et al., 2003 [Level IV]).
3. Enhance surveillance and reporting of ADRs using a National Surveillance system (Gurwitz et al., 2003 [Level IV]; JCAHO, 2007 [Level VI]). Consider use of computerized physician ordering system (Gurwitz et al., 2003 [Level IV]; Joanna Briggs Institute, 2006 [Level I]).
4. Track and report morbidity and mortality due to medication-related problems.
5. Provide a system for medication reconciliation and follow-up its effectiveness with regard to rehospitalization rates due to ADRs.
6. Review for careful documentation of iatrogenic medication and other iatrogenic events for CQI.
7. Provide ongoing education related to safe medication management for physicians and staff.

VII. FOLLOW-UP

A. Health care providers will:
1. Provide consistent and appropriate care and follow-up in presence of a medication-related problem.

2. Evaluate with physical exam and laboratory tests (as appropriate) on regular basis to ensure that the older adult is responding to therapy as expected (Edelberg et al., 2000 [Level IV]).

B. Institutions will:

1. Provide ongoing assessment of staff competence in assessing and intervening for prevention of ADEs.
2. Embed reduction of ADEs in the culture of safety.

VIII. RELEVANT PRACTICE GUIDELINES

A. Bergman-Evans, B. (2004). Improving medication management for older adult clients. Iowa City, IA: University of Iowa Gerontological Nursing Interventions Research Center, Research Dissemination Core; 2004 Oct. [Level I]. Available at www.guideline.gov; NGC Guideline # 003993.
B. Health Care Association of New Jersey (HCANJ). (2006). Medication management guideline. Hamilton, NJ: Health Care Association of New Jersey (HCANJ); Available at www.guideline.gov. Note: Geared for posthospital institutions for adult patients.

References

Agency for Healthcare Research and Quality (AHRQ) (March 2001). *Reducing and preventing adverse drug events to decrease hospital costs*. Research in Action, Issue 1. AHRQ Publication #01-0020. Agency for Healthcare Research and Quality, Rockville, MD. Retrieved September 28, 2006, from http://www.ahrq.gov/qual/aderia/aderia.htm. Evidence Level I: Systematically Reviewed Clinical Practice Guideline(CPG).

Ahmed, A., Allman, R. M., & DeLong, J. F. (2002). Inappropriate use of digoxin in older hospitalized heart failure patients. *Journals of Gerontology Series A-Biological Sciences & Medical Sciences, 57*(2), M138–M143. Evidence Level III: Case Control Study.

Ament, P. W., Bertolino, J. G., & Liszewski, J. L. (2000). Clinical pharmacology: clinically significant drug interactions. *American Family Physician. 61*, 1745–1754. Evidence Level VI: Expert Opinion.

American Association of Geriatric Psychiatrists (AAGP) (2005). *Comment on the U.S. Food and Drug Administration's (FDA) advisory on off-label use of atypical antipsychotics in the elderly*. Retrieved September 22, 2006, from http://www.aagponline.org/prof/antipsychstat_0705.asp

Astin, J. A., Pelletier, K. R., Marie, A., & Haskell, W. L. (2000). Complementary and alternative medicine use among elderly persons: One-year analysis of a Blue Shield Medicare supplement. *Journals of Gerontology Series A-Biological Sciences & Medical Sciences, 55A*, M4–M9. Evidence Level IV: Survey.

Beers, M. H. (1997). Explicit criteria for determining potentially inappropriate medication use by the elderly: An update. *Archives of Internal Medicine, 157*, 1531–1536. Evidence Level VI: Expert Opinion Based on Review.

Beers, M. H., Ouslander, J. G., Fingold, S. F., Morgenstern, H., Reuben, D. B., Rogers, W., et al. (1992). Inappropriate medication prescribing in skilled nursing facilities. *Annals of Internal Medicine, 117*, 684–689.

Beers, M. H., Ouslander, J. G., Rollingher, I., Reuben, D. B., Brooks, J., & Beck, J. C. (1991). Explicit criteria for determining inappropriate medication use in nursing home residents. *Archives of Internal Medicine, 151*, 1825–1832. Evidence Level VI: Expert Opinion Based on Review.

Bergman-Evans, B. (2004). *Improving medication management for older adult clients* Evidence-Based Guideline. Iowa City, IA: University of Iowa Gerontological Nursing Intervention Research Center (GNIRC). Evidence Level I: Systematically Reviewed Clinical Practice Guideline (CPG).

Bergman-Evans, B. (2006). AIDES to improving medication adherence in older adults. *Geriatric Nursing, 27*(3), 174–182. Evidence Level V: Review.

Besdine, R., Beers, M., Bootman, Fulmer, T., Gerbino, P., & Manasse, H., et al. (1998). *When medicine hurts instead of helps: Preventing medication problems in older persons.* Washington, DC: Alliance for Aging Research. Evidence Level VI: Expert Consensus.

Bootman, J. L., Harrison, D. L., & Cox, E. (1997). The health care cost of drug-related morbidity and mortality in nursing facilities. *Archives of Internal Medicine, 157*(18), 2089–2096. Evidence Level VI: Expert Opinion.

Budnitz, D. S., Pollock, D. A., Weidenbach, K. N., Mendelsohn, A. B., Schroeder, T. J., & Annest, J. L. (2006). National surveillance of emergency department visits for outpatient adverse drug events. *Journal of the American Medial Association, 296*(15), 1858–1866. Evidence Level V: Observational Study.

Catterson, M. L., Preskorn, S. H., & Martin, R. L. (1997). Pharmacodynamic and pharmacokinetic considerations in geriatric psychopharmacology. The Psychiatric Clinics of North America, *20*(1), 205–218.

Chang, C. M., Liu, P. Y., Yang, Y. H., Yang, Y. C., Wu, C. F., & Lu, F. H. (2005). Use of the Beers criteria to predict adverse drug reactions among first-visit elderly outpatients. *Pharmacotherapy, 25*(6), 831–838. Evidence Level IV: Nonexperimental Study.

Chevalier, B. A., Parker, D. S., MacKinnon, N. J., & Sketris, I. (2006). Nurses' perceptions of medication safety and medication reconciliation practices. *Canadian Journal of Nursing Leadership, 19*(3): 61–72. Evidence Level IV: Nonexperimental Study.

Childs, N. (2000). IOM report spurs patient safety activity on Capitol Hill. *Provider, 26*(2), 10–11.

Committee of Experts (COE) on Safe Medication Practices (2005). *Glossary of terms related to patient and medication safety.* Retrieved September 1, 2006, from http://www.who.int/patientsafety/highlights/COE_patient_and_medication_safety_gl.pdf.

Curry, L. C., Walker, C., Hogstel, M. O., & Burns, P. (2005). Teaching older adults to self-manage medications: Preventing adverse drug reactions. *Journal Gerontological Nursing, 31*(4), 32–42. Evidence Level VI: Expert Opinion.

Doucet, J., Jego, A., Noel, D., Geffroy, C. E., Capet, C., Coquard, A., et al. (2002). Preventable and non-preventable risk factors for adverse drug events related to hospital admission in the elderly: A prospective study. *Clinical Drug Investigations, 22*, 385–392. Evidence Level V: Review.

Doucette, W. R., McDonough, R. P., Klepser, E., & McCarthy, R. (2005). Comprehensive medication therapy management: Identifying and resolving drug-related issues in a community pharmacy. *Clinical Therapeutics, 27*(7), 1104–1111. Evidence Level V: Observational Study.

Edelberg, H. K., Shallenberger, E., Hausdorff, J. M., & Wei, J. Y. (2000). One-year follow-up of medication management capacity in highly functioning older adults. *Journal of Gerontology: Medical Sciences, 55a*, M550–M553. Evidence Level IV: Nonexperimental Study.

Edelberg, H. K., Shallenberger, E., & Wei, J. Y. (1999). Medication management capacity in highly functioning community-dwelling older adults: Detection of early deficits. *Journal American Geriatrics Society, 47*, 592–596. Evidence Level IV: Cohort Study.

Ellington, A. M., Barrnett, C. W., Johnson, D. R., & Nykamp, D. (2002). Current methods used to teach the medication history interview to doctor of pharmacy students. *American Journal of Pharmaceutical Education, 66*, 103–107.

Feldman, P. H., McDonald, M., Rosati, R. J., Murtaugh, C., Kovner, C., Goldberg, J. D., et al. (2006). Exploring the utility of automated drug alerts in home health care. *Journal for Healthcare Quality, 28*(1), 29–40. Evidence Level IV: Nonexperimental Study.

Feldstein, A. C., Smith, D. H., Yahg, X., Simon, S. R., Krall, M., Sittig, D. F., et al. (2006). Reducing warfarin medication interactions. *Archives of Internal Medicine, 166*, 1009–1015. Evidence Level III: Quasi-experimental Study.

Fick, D. M., Cooper, F. W., Wade, W. E., Waller, J. L., Maclean, J. R., & Beers, M. H. (2003). Updating the Beers criteria for potentially inappropriate medication use in older adults. *Archives of Internal Medicine, 163*(22), 2716–2724. Evidence Level VI: Expert Opinion Based on Review.

Finkel, S. (2004). Pharmacology of antipsychotics in the elderly: A focus on atypicals. *Journal of American Geriatrics Society, 52* (Suppl.), 258–265. Evidence Level VI: Expert Opinion.

Flaherty, J. H., Perry, H. M., Lynchard, G. S., & Morley, J. E. (2000). Polypharmacy and hospitalization among older home care patients. *Journal of Gerontology Series A, Biological Sciences and Medical Sciences, 55*(10), M554–M559.

Fouts, M., Hanlon, J., Pierper, C., Perfetto, E., & Feinberg, J. (1997). Identification of elderly nursing facility residents at high risk for drug-related problems. *The Consultant Pharmacist, 12*, 1103–1111. Level VI: Expert Opinion.

Fu, A. Z., Liu, G. G., & Christensen, D. B. (2004). Inappropriate medication use and health outcomes in the elderly. *Journal of the American Geriatrics Society, 52*(11), 1934–1939. Level IV: Nonexperimental Study.

Fulmer, T. T., Feldman, P. H., Kim, T. S., Carty, B., Beers, M., Molina, M., et al. (1999). Enhanced medication compliance. *Journal of Gerontological Nursing, 24*, 6–14. Level VI: Expert Opinion.

Fulmer, T., Kim, T. S., Montgomery, K., & Lyder, C. (2000). What the literature tells us about the complexity of medication compliance in the elderly. *Generations, 24*(4), 43–48. Level V: Review.

Gaddis, G. M., Holt, T. R., & Woods, M. (2002). Drug interactions in at-risk emergency department patients. *Academic Emergency Medicine, 9*(11), 1162–1167. Evidence Level IV: Nonexperimental Study.

Gleason, K. M., Groszek, J. M., Sullivan, C., Rooney, D., Barnard, C., & Noskin, G. A. (2004). Reconciliation of discrepancies in medication histories and admission orders of newly hospitalized patients. *American Journal of Health-System Pharmacists, 61*, 1689–1695. Evidence Level IV: Nonexperimental Study.

Gray, S. L., LaCroix, A. Z., Hanlon, J. T., Penninx, B. W., Bough, D. K., Leveille, S.G., et al. (2006). Benzodiazepine use and physical disability in community-dwelling older adults. *Journal of the American Geriatrics Society, 54*(2), 224–230. Evidence Level II: Single Experimental Study.

Gurwitz, J. H., Field, T. S., Avorn, J., McCormick, D., Jain, S., Eckler, M., et al. (2005). The incidence of adverse drug events in two large academic long-term care facilities. *American Journal of Medicine, 118*, 251–268. Evidence Level II: Single Experimental Study.

Gurwitz, J. H., Field, T. S., Harrold, L. R., Rothschild, J., Debellis, K., Seger, A. C., et al. (2003). Incidence and preventability of adverse drug events among older persons in the ambulatory setting. *Journal of the American Medical Association, 289*(9), 1107–1116. Evidence Level IV: Cohort Study, Retrospective Review.

Hajjar, I., & Kotchen, T. A. (2003). Trends in prevalence, awareness, treatment and control of hypertension in the United States, 1998–2000. *Journal of the American Medical Association, 290*, 199–206. Evidence Level IV: Nonexperimental Study/Survey.

Hanlon, J. T., Fillenbaum, G. G., Ruby, C. M., Gray, S., & Bohannon, A. (2001). Epidemiology of over-the-counter drug use in community-dwelling elderly. *United States perspective. Drugs & Aging, 18*(2), 123–131. Evidence Level V: Literature Review.

Hanlon, J. T., Fillenbaum, G. G., Schmader, K. E., Kuchibhatla, M., & Horner, R. D. (2000). Inappropriate drug use among community-dwelling elderly. *Pharmacotherapy, 20*, 575–582. Evidence Level V: Review.

Hanlon, J. T., Lindblad, C. I., & Gray, S. L. (2004). Can clinical pharmacy services have a positive impact on drug-related problems and health outcomes in community-based older adults? *American Journal Geriatric Pharmacotherapy, 2*(1), 3–13. Evidence Level I: Systematic Review.

Hanlon, J. T., Pieper, C. F., Hajjar, E. R., Sloane, R. J., Lindbald, C. I., Ruby, C. M., et al. (2006). Incidence and predictors of all and preventable adverse drug reactions in frail elderly persons after hospital stay. *Journals of Gerontology Series A-Biological Sciences & Medical Sciences, 61A*(5), 511–515. Evidence Level II: Single Experimental Study.

Hanlon, J. T., Schmader, K. E., Koronkowski, M. J., Weinberger, M., Landsman, P. B., Samsa, G. P., et al. (1997). Adverse drug events in high risk older outpatients. *Journal of the American Geriatrics Society, 45*, 945–958. Evidence Level IV: Cohort Study.

Hanlon, J. T., Schmader, K. E., Ruby, C. M., & Weinberger, M. (2001). Suboptimal prescribing in older inpatients and outpatients. *Journal of the American Geriatrics Society, 49*(2), 200–209. Evidence Level V: Review.

Hansten, P. D., Horn, J. R., & Hazlet, T. K. (2001). Operational classification of drug interactions. *Journal of the American Pharmaceutical Association, 41*(2), 161–165. Evidence Level IV: Nonexperimental Study.

Haynes, R. B., Yao, X., Degani, A., Kripalani, S., Garg, A., & McDonald, H. P. (2005). Interventions for enhancing medication adherence. *Cochrane Database of Systematic Reviews* 2007, Issue 1. Retrieved January 30, 2007, from www.mrw.interscience.wiley.com/cochrane/clsysrev/articles/CD000011/frame.html Evidence Level V: Review.

Health Benchmarks (2005). *Appropriate medication use in the elderly (drugs that should be avoided)*. Retrieved August 8, 2006, from http://www.bcbsil.com/provider/pdf/appro_med_elderly1.pdf#search=%22health%20benchmarks%2C%20appropriate%20medications%2C%20BCBS%22.

Hohl, C. M., Robitaille, C., Lord, V., Dankoff, J., Colacone, A., Pham, L., et al. (2005). Emergency physician recognition of adverse drug-related events in elder patients presenting to an emergency department. *Academic Emergency Medicine, 12*(3), 197–205. Evidence Level IV: Nonexperimental study.

Hutchison, L. C., Jones, S. K., West, D. S., & Wei, J. Y. (2006). Assessment of medication management by community living elderly persons with two standardized assessment tools: A cross-sectional study. *American Journal of Geriatric Pharmacotherapy, 4*(2), 144–153. Evidence Level IV: Nonexperimental study.

Joanna Briggs Institute. (2006). Strategies to reduce medication errors with reference to older adults. *Nursing Standard, 20*(41), 53–57. Evidence Level I: Systematic Review.

Joint Commission on Accreditation of Health Care Organizations (JCAHO). (2007). National Patient Safety Recommendations, Goal # 8: Medication Reconciliation, Evidence Level VI: Expert Opinion. Retrieved March 22, 2007, from www.jointcommission.org/PatientSafety/NationalPatientSafetyGoals/

Joint Commission on Accreditation of Health Care Organizations (JCAHO). (2006). Sentinel Events Alert: Using Medication Reconciliation to Prevent Errors an addendum to Alert #35. Evidence Level VI: Expert Opinion. Retrieved March 22, 2007, from http://www.jointcommission.org/SentinelEvents/SentinelEventAlert/sea_35.htm.

Juurlink, D. N., Mamdani, M., Kopp, A., Laupacis, A., & Redelmeier, D. A. (2003). Drug–drug interactions among elderly patients hospitalized for drug toxicity. *Journal of the American Medical Association, 289*(13), 1652–1658. Evidence Level III: Quasi-experimental Study.

Kaufman, D. W., Kelly, K. P., Rosenberg, L., Anderson, T. E., & Mitchell, A. A. (2002). Recent patterns of medication use in the ambulatory adult population in the United States. *The Sloane Survey. Journal of the American Medical Association, 287*, 377–344. Evidence Level IV: Nonexperimental Study.

Kelly, J. P., Kaufman, D. W., Kelley, K., Rosenberg, L., Anderson, T. E., & Mitchell, A. A. (2005). Recent trends in use of herbal and other natural products. *Archives of Internal Medicine, 165*, 281. Evidence Level IV: Nonexperimental Study.

Kindermann, S. S., Dolder, C. R., Bailey, A., Katz, I. R., & Jeste, D. V. (2002). Pharmacological treatment of psychosis and agitation in elderly patients with dementia: Four decades of experience. *Drugs and Aging, 19*, 257–276. Evidence Level V: Review.

Knight, E. L., & Avorn, J. (2006). Quality indicators for appropriate medication use in vulnerable elders. *Annals of Internal Medicine, 135*, 703. Accessed November 1, 2006, from http://www.rand.org/pubs/reprints/RP1134/index.html. Evidence Level VI: Expert Opinion.

Kohn, L., Corrigan, J., & Donaldson, M. (2000). *to err is human: Building a safer health system*. Washington, DC: National Academy Press. Evidence Level VI: Expert Opinion.

Lam, S., & Ruby, C. M. (2005). Impact of an interdisciplinary team on drug therapy outcomes in a geriatric clinic. *American Journal of Health-System Pharmacists, 62*(6), 626–629. Evidence Level II: Single Experimental Study.

Lau, H. S., Florax, C., Porsius, A. J., & De Boer, A. (2000). The completeness of medication histories in hospital medical records of patients admitted to general internal medicine wards. *British Journal of Clinical Pharmacology, 49*, 597–603. Evidence Level IV: Nonexperimental Study.

Lazarou, J., Pomeranz, B. H., & Corey, P. N. (1998). Incidence of adverse drug reactions in hospitalized patients: A meta-analysis of prospective studies. *Journal American Medical Association, 279*(15), 1200–1205. Evidence Level I: Meta-analysis/Systematic Review.

Leipzig, R. M., Cumming, R. G., & Tinetti, M. E. (1999). Drugs and falls in older people: A systematic review and meta-analysis. *Journal of the American Geriatrics Society, 47*, 30. Evidence Level I: Meta-analysis/Systematic Review.

Liperoti, R., Gambassi, G., Lapane, K. L., Chiang, C., Pedone, C., Mor, V., et al. (2005). Conventional and atypical antipsychotics and the risk of hospitalization for ventricular arrhythmias or cardiac arrest. *Archives of Internal Medicine, 165*(6), 696–701. Evidence Level III: Matched Case Control Study.

Liu, G. G., & Christensen, D. B. (2002). The continuing challenge of inappropriate prescribing in the elderly: An update of the evidence. *Journal of the American Pharmaceutical Association, 42*(6), 847–857. Evidence Level V: Review.

Mangoni, A. A., & Jackson, S. H. D. (2003). Age-related changes in pharmacokinetics and phamacodynamics: Basic principles and practical applications. *British Journal of Clinical Pharmacology, 57*(1), 6–14. Evidence Level VI: Expert Opinion.

Merck Manual Professional (2005). *Drug therapy in the elderly*. In Clinical Pharmacology (section). Retrieved September 29, 2006, from http://www.merck.com/mmpe/sec20/ch306/ch306a.html. Evidence Level VI: Expert Opinion.

Merle, L., Laroche, M., Dantoine, T., & Charmes, J. P. (2005). Predicting and preventing adverse drug reactions in the very old. *Drugs and Aging, 22*(5), 375–392. Evidence Level VI: Expert Opinion.

Miller, L. G. (1998). Herbal medicinals: Selected clinical considerations. Focusing on known or potential drug–herb interactions. *Archives of Internal Medicine, 158*(20), 2200–2211. Evidence Level V: Review.

Muir, A. J., Sanders, L. L., Wilkinson, W. E., & Schmader, K. (2001). Reducing medication regimen complexity: A controlled trial. *Journal of General Internal Medicine, 16*(2), 77–82. Evidence Level III: Quasi-experimental Study.

Nathan, A., Goodyer, L., Lovejoy, A., & Rahid, A. (1999). "Brown bag" method review as a means of optimizing patients' use of medication and of identifying potential clinical problems. *Family Practice, 16*(3), 278–182. Evidence Level IV: Nonexperimental Study.

National Coordinating Council for Medication Errors Reporting and Prevention (2001). *Taxonomy of medication errors*. Retrieved September 1, 2006, from http://www.nccmerp.org/pdf/taxo2001-07-31.pdf. Evidence Level VI: Expert Opinion.

National Council on Patient Information and Education (NCPIE) (1997). *The other drug problem: Statistics on medicine use and compliance*. Retrieved November 1, 2006, from http://www.medscape.com/viewarticle/406691_print. Evidence Level VI: Expert Opinion.

Neafsey, P. J., & Shellman, J. (2001). Adverse self-medication practices of older adults with hypertension attending blood pressure clinics: Adverse self-medication practices. *Internet Journal of Advanced Nursing Practice, 5*(1),15. Evidence Level IV: Nonexperimental Study.

Neafsey, P. J., Strickler, Z., Shellman, J., & Chartier, V. (2002). An interactive technology approach to educate older adults about drug interactions arising from over-the-counter self-medication practices. *Public Health Nursing, 19*(4), 255–262. Evidence Level II: Single Experimental Study.

Nickerson, A., MacKinnon, N. J., Roberts, N., & Saulnier, L. (2005). Drug-therapy problems, inconsistencies, and omissions identified duration medication reconciliation and seamless care services. *Healthcare Quarterly, 8* (special issue), 65–72. Evidence Level II: Single Experimental Study/RCT.

Nolan, P. E., Jr., & Marcus, F. I. (2000). Cardiovascular drug use in the elderly. *American Journal of Geriatric Cardiology, 9*(3), 127–129. Evidence Level VI: Expert Opinion.

Ooi, W. L., Hossain, M., & Lipsitz, L. S. (2000). The association between orthostatic hypotension and recurrent falls in nursing home residents. *American Journal of Medicine, 108*(2), 106–111. Evidence Level II: Single Experimental Study.

Packer, M., Pooler-Wilson, P. A., Armstrong, P. W., Cleland, J. G., Horowitz, J. D., Massie, B. M., et al. (1999). Comparative effects of low and high doses of angiotensin converting enzyme inhibition, lisinopril, on morbidity and mortality in chronic heart failure. *ATLAS Study Group*, 2312–2318. Evidence Level II: Single Experimental Study/RCT.

Petrone, K., & Katz, P. (2005). Approaches to appropriate drug prescribing for the older adult. *Primary Care Clinics in Office Practice, 32*, 755–775. Evidence IV: Nonexperimental Study.

Pirmohamed, M., James, S., Meakin, S., Green, C., Scott, A. K., Walley, T. J., et al. (2004). Adverse drug reactions as cause of admission to hospital: Prospective analysis of 18,820 patients.

British Medical Journal, 329(7456), 15–19. Evidence Level IV: Prospective Observational Study.

Prescott, P. F. (1994). Drug conjugation in clinical toxicology. *Biochemical Society Transactions, 12*(1), 96–99.

Ray, W. A., Thapa, P. B., & Gideon, P. (2000). Benzodiazepines and the risk of falls in nursing home residents. *Journal of the American Geriatrics Society, 48*(6), 682–685.

Rochon, P. A. (2006). *Drug prescribing for older adults.* Retrieved September 15, 2006, from http://www.utdol.com/utd/store/index.do Evidence Level V: Literature Review.

Rochon, P. A., & Gurwitz, J. H. (1997). Optimising drug treatment for elderly people: The prescribing cascade. *British Medical Journal, 315,* 1096–1099. Evidence Level V: Review.

Rohay, J., Dunbar-Jacob, J., Sereika, S., Kwoh, K., & Burke, L. E. (1996). The impact of method of calculation of electronically monitored adherence data. *Controlled Clinical Trials, 17*(82S–83S), A76.

Safran, D. G., Neuman, P., Schoen, C., Kitchman, M. S., Wilson, I. B., Cooper, B., et al. (2005). *Prescription drug coverage and seniors: Findings from a 2003 national survey.* Retrieved August 22, 2006, from http://content.healthaffairs.org/cgi/content/abstract/hlthaff.w5.152. Evidence Level IV: Survey/Nonexperimental Study.

Salzman, C. (1998). *Clinical geriatric pharmacology.* Baltimore, MD: Williams & Wilkins.

Santell, J. P. (2006). Reconciliation failures lead to medication errors. *Joint Commission Journal on Quality & Patient Safety, 32*(4), 225–229.

Semla, T., & Rochon, P. (2004). Pharmacotherapy. In E. L. Cobbs & E. H. Duthie (Eds.), *Geriatrics review syllabus: A core curriculum in geriatric medicine* (5th ed.). Malden, MA: Blackwell Publishing. Level of Evidence VI: Expert Opinion.

Shekelle, P. G., MacLean, C. H., Morton, S. C., & Wegner, N. S. (2001). ACOVE quality indicators. *Annals of Internal Medicine, 135,* 653–667.

Simon, S. R., Smith, D. H., Feldstein, A. C., Perrin, N., Yang, X., Zhou, Y., et al. (2006). Computerized prescribing alerts and group academic detailing to reduce the use of potentially inappropriate medications in older people. *Journal of the American Geriatrics Society, 54*(6), 963–968. Evidence Level II: RCT.

Sloane, P. D., Zimmerman, S., Brown, L. C., Ives, T. J., & Walsh, J. F. (2002). Inappropriate medication prescribing in residential care/assisted living facilities. *Journal of the American Geriatrics Society, 50,* 1001–1011. Evidence Level II: Single Experimental Study.

Spina, E., & Scordo, M. G. (2002). Clinically significant drug interactions with antidepressants in the elderly. *Drugs Aging, 19,* 299–320. Evidence Level VI: Opinion.

Surgeon General's Report (1999). *Older adults and mental health.* Retrieved September 22, 2006, from http://www.surgeongeneral.gov/library/mentalhealth/chapter5/sec1.html

Swagerty, D., & Brickley, R. (2005). American Medical Directors Association and American Society of Consultant Pharmacists joint position statement on the Beers list of potentially inappropriate medications in older adults. *Journal of American Medical Directors Association, 6*(1), 80–86. Evidence Level VI: Expert Opinion.

Tam, V. C., Knowler, S. R.., Cornish, P. L., Fine, N., Marchesano, R., & Etchells, E. E. (2005). Frequency, type and clinical importance of medication history errors at admission to hospital: A systematic review. *Canadian Medical Association Journal, 173*(5): 510–515. Evidence Level I: Systematic Review.

Tamblyn, R., Abrahamowicz, M., Berger, R., McLeod, P., & Bartlett, G. (2005). A 5-year prospective assessment of the risk associated with individual benzodiazepine and doses in new elderly users. *Journal of the American Geriatrics Society, 53,* 233–341. Evidence Level II: Single Experimental.

Tangalos, E. G., & Zarowitz, B. J. (2006). Medication management in the elderly. *Annals of Long-Term Care, 14*(8), 27–31. Evidence Level VI: Journal Article.

Terrell, K. M., Heard, K., & Miller, D. K. (2006). Prescribing to older ED patients. *American Journal of Emergency Medicine, 24*(4), 468–478. Evidence Level V: Review.

Tune, L. E. (2001). Anticholinergic effects of medication in elderly patients. *Journal of Clinical Psychiatry, 62* (Suppl. 21), 11–14. Evidence Level V: Review.

Williams, M. E., Pulliam, C. C., Hunter, R., Johnson, T. M., Owens, J. E., Kincaid, J., et al. (2004). The short-term effect of interdisciplinary medication review on function and cost in ambulatory elderly people. *Journal of the American Geriatrics Society, 52*(1), 93–98. Level of Evidence II: RCT/Single Experimental Study.

Zhan, C., Correa-de-Araujo, R., Bierman, A. S., Sangl, J., Miller, M. R., Wickizer, S. W., et al. (2005). Suboptimal prescribing in elderly outpatients: Potentially harmful drug–drug interactions and drug–disease interactions. *Journal of the American Geriatrics Society, 53,* 262–267. Evidence Level IV: Nonexperimental Study.

Zhan, C., Sangl, J., Bierman, A. S., Miller, M. R., Friedman, B., & Wickizer, S. W., et al. (2001). Potentially inappropriate medication use in the community-dwelling elderly: Findings from the 1996 expenditure panel survey. *Journal of the American Medical Association, 286*(22), 2823–2829. Evidence Level IV: Retrospective Analysis of Survey.

Urinary Incontinence

13

Annemarie
Dowling-Castronovo
Christine Bradway

Educational Objectives

At the completion of this chapter, the reader should be able to:

1. discuss transient and established etiologies of urinary incontinence (UI)

2. describe the core components of a nursing assessment for UI in hospitalized older adults

3. discuss the importance of nurse collaboration within the interdisciplinary team in an effort to best assess and document type of UI

4. develop an individualized plan of care for an older adult with UI

5. list limited indications for indwelling catheter use

Overview

Persistent myths regarding urinary incontinence (UI) among lay and health care providers are captured by the axiom: "You are born wearing diapers ... you die wearing diapers." Despite evidence supporting UI management strategies (Fantl et al., 1996 [Level I]); International Consultation on Incontinence (ICI), 2000 [Level VI]), nursing staff and laypersons often use containment strategies, such as diapers, to manage UI. Individuals with UI erroneously believe that containing UI is a normal consequence of aging (Bush, Castellucci, & Phillips 2001 [Level IV]; Dowd, 1991 [Level IV]; Kinchen et al., 2003 [Level IV]; Milne, 2000

For a description of Evidence Levels cited in this chapter, see chapter 1, Developing and Evaluating Clinical Practice Guidelines, page 4

309

[Level IV]; Mitteness, 1987a, 1987b [Level VI]). In addition, incontinent persons feel that UI is a personal problem, it is difficult to talk about (Bush et al., 2001 [Level IV]), and prefer self-help strategies rather than seeking professional advice (Milne, 2000 [Level IV]). Personal care strategies are often the result of information gained through lay media and personal contacts, not necessarily from health care professionals (Cochran, 2000 [Level VI]; Jeter & Wagner, 1990 [Level IV]; Miller, Brown, Smith, & Chiarelli, 2003 [Level IV]; Milne, 2000 [Level IV]). Therefore, attitudes and beliefs regarding UI are important for nurses to consider in an effort to best assess and manage UI.

UI affects more than 17 million adults in the United States and is most often defined as the involuntary loss of urine sufficient to be a problem (Fantl et al., 1996 [Level I]; National Association for Continence, 1998 [Level IV]; Resnick & Ouslander, 1990 [Level VI]). Prevalence and incidence rates of UI are viewed cautiously due to inconsistencies with definitions and measurements of both these epidemiological statistics. In addition, variable or poorly articulated UI definitions (Abrams et al., 2002 [Level V]; Palmer, 1988 [Level V]), as well as underreporting and underassessment of UI (Schultz, Dickey, & Skoner, 1997 [Level IV]), can render data of questionable reliability. Prevalence of UI in community-dwelling adult populations ranges from 8% to 38% (Anger, Saigal, Litwin, & The Urologic Diseases of America Project, 2006 [Level IV]; Diokno, Brock, Brown, & Herzog, 1986 [Level IV]; Herzog & Fultz, 1990 [Level V]; Johnson et al., 1998 [Level IV]). For individuals with dementia, UI prevalence rates range from 11% to 90%; higher prevalence rates reflect institutionalized cognitively impaired older adults (Brandeis, Baumann, Hossain, Morris, & Resnick, 1997 [Level IV]; Skelly & Flint, 1995 [Level V]). Although the highest prevalence rate occurs in institutionalized older adults, 15% to 53% of homebound elderly and 10% to 42% of older adults admitted to acute care also suffer from UI (Dowd & Campbell, 1995 [Level IV]; Fantl et al., 1996 [Level I]; McDowell et al., 1999 [Level II]; Palmer, Bone, Fahey, Mamom, & Steinwachs, 1992 [Level IV]; Schultz et al., 1997 [Level IV]). For example, 36% of older hospitalized adults develop acute UI (e.g., new-onset UI, meaning that these individuals were continent on admission) (Kresevic, 1997 [Level IV]); for patients undergoing hip surgery, the incidence of acute UI is 19% to 32% (Palmer, Baumgarten, Langenberg, & Carson, 2002 [Level IV]; Palmer, Myers, & Fedenko, 1997 [Level IV]).

In addition to being a common geriatric syndrome, UI significantly affects health-related quality of life (HRQOL) (Shumaker, Wyman, Uebersax, McClish, & Fantl, 1994 [Level IV]). The consequences of UI may be characterized physically, psychosocially, and economically. An episode of urge UI occurring once weekly or more frequently is associated with falls or fracture (Brown et al., 2000a [Level IV]). Other physical consequences associated with UI include skin irritations or infections, urinary tract infections (UTIs), pressure ulcers, and limitation of functional status (Fantl et al., 1996 [Level I]; Johnson et al., 1998 [Level IV]). UI is associated with psychological distress (Bogner et al., 2002 [Level IV]) including depression, poor self-rated health, and social isolation or condition-specific functional loss (Bogner et al., 2002 [Level IV]; Fantl et al., 1996 [Level I]; Johnson et al., 1998 [Level IV]). Therefore, it is essential that nurses assess and treat UI when addressing other health problems such as depression or falls.

Although there is conflicting evidence as to UI being a predictor for nursing home placement, UI has been identified as a marker of frailty in community-dwelling older adults (Holroyd-Leduc, Mehta, & Covinsky, 2004 [Level I]). The negative psychosocial impact of UI affects not only the individual but also the family caregiver(s) (Cassells & Watt, 2004 [Level IV]). Economically, the total direct cost for all incontinent individuals is estimated to be more than $16 billion annually (Wilson, Brown, Shin, Luc, & Subak, 2001 [Level IV]; Wyman, 1997 [Level V]).

Nurses are in a key position to identify and treat UI in hospitalized older adults. This chapter reviews the etiologies and consequences of UI, with emphasis on the most common types of UI encountered in the acute care setting. Assessment parameters and care strategies for UI are highlighted and a nursing standard of practice protocol for recognizing and treating UI is presented. The protocol focuses on comprehensive assessment and management of UI for hospitalized older adults.

Assessment of The Problem

Adverse physiologic consequences of UI commonly encountered in acute care facilities include an increased potential for UTIs and indwelling catheter use, dermatitis, skin infections, and pressure ulcers (Sier, Ouslander, & Orzeck, 1987 [Level IV]). Moreover, UI that results in functional decline predisposes older individuals to complications associated with bedrest and immobility (Harper & Lyles, 1988 [Level V]).

Etiologies of Urinary Incontinence

Continence is a complex, multidimensional phenomenon influenced by anatomical, physiological, psychological, and cultural factors (Gray, 2000 [Level V]). Thus, continence requires intact lower urinary tract function; cognitive and functional ability to recognize voiding signals and use a toilet or commode; the motivation to maintain continence; and an environment that facilitates the process (Jirovec, Brink, & Wells, 1988 [Level VI]). Physiologically, continence is a result of urethral pressure being equal to or greater than bladder pressure (Hodgkinson, 1965 [Level V]), of which angulation of the urethra, supported by pelvic muscles, plays a role (DeLancy, 1994 [Level IV]). Continence also requires the ability to suppress autocontractility of the detrusor (Hodgkinson, 1965 [Level V]). Micturition (i.e., urination) involves voluntary as well as reflexive control of the bladder, urethra, detrusor muscle, and urethral sphincter. When the bladder volume reaches approximately 400 milliliters, stretch receptors in the bladder wall send a message to the brain and an impulse for voiding is sent back to the bladder. The detrusor muscle then contracts and the urethral sphincter relaxes to allow urination (Gray, Rayome, & Moore, 1995 [Level VI]). Normally, the micturition reflex can be voluntarily inhibited (at least for a time) until an individual desires to void or finds an appropriate place for voiding. UI occurs as the result of a disruption at any point during this process. For a comprehensive review, Gray (2000 [Level V]) provides a detailed analysis of voiding physiology. Common age-associated changes, including a decrease in bladder capacity, benign prostatic hyperplasia (BPH) in men, and menopausal loss of estrogen in women, can affect lower urinary tract function and predispose older individuals to UI (Bradway & Yetman, 2002 [Level VI]). Despite these aging changes, UI is not considered a normal consequence of aging.

The Agency for Healthcare Research and Quality (AHRQ) identifies two types of UI: transient (acute) and established (chronic) (Fantl et al., 1996 [Level I]).

Transient UI is characterized by the sudden onset of potentially reversible symptoms. Causes of transient UI include delirium, infections (e.g., untreated UTI), atrophic vaginitis, urethritis, pharmaceuticals, depression or other psychological disorders that affect motivation or function, excessive urine production, restricted mobility, and stool impaction or constipation (which creates additional pressure on the bladder and can cause urinary urgency and frequency). Hospitalized older adults are at risk of developing transient UI. Complicated by shorter hospital stays, these individuals may also be at risk of being discharged without resolution of transient UI and, thus, urine leakage persists and may become established UI. However, transient UI is often preventable, or at least reversible (e.g., transient UI precipitated by a UTI that resolves with successful treatment, or acute UI related to diuresis therapy for heart failure exacerbation), if the underlying cause for the UI is identified and treated (Fantl et al., 1996 [Level I]; Palmer, 1996 [Level VI]).

Kresevic (1997 [Level IV]) reported that hospitalized older adults with new-onset UI were more likely to be on bedrest, restrained, depressed, dehydrated, malnourished, and dependent in ambulation when compared to their continent counterparts. Furthermore, the relative risk of developing new-onset UI was twofold for older adults with depression (OR=2.28), malnutrition (OR=2.29), and dependent ambulation (OR=2.55). Study participants identified that being able to walk, having use of a bedpan/commode, and nursing assistance fostered continence (Kresevic, 1997). Likewise, Palmer and colleagues (2002 [Level IV]) determined that in addition to mobility dependency, other risk factors for new-onset UI, specific to a hip fracture population, included institutionalization prior to hospital, the presence of confusion preceding hip fracture, and being an African American woman.

Established UI has either a sudden or gradual onset and is often present prior to hospital admission. However, health care providers or family caregivers may discover it initially during the course of an acute illness, hospitalization, or abrupt change in environment or daily routine (Palmer, 1996 [Level VI]). Types of established UI include stress, urge, mixed, overflow, and functional.

Stress UI is defined as an involuntary loss of urine associated with activities that increase intra-abdominal pressure. Symptomatically, individuals with stress UI usually present with complaints of small amounts of daytime urine loss that occurs during physical effort or exertion (e.g., position change, coughing, sneezing) that result in increased intra-abdominal pressure. Stress UI is more common in women; however, stress UI may also be identified in men post-prostatectomy (Abrams et al., 2003 [Level V]; Fantl et al., 1996 [Level I]; Hunter, Moore, Cody, & Glazener, 2005 [Level I]).

Urge UI is characterized by an involuntary urine loss associated with a strong desire to void (i.e., urgency). Individuals with urge UI often complain of being unable to hold the urge to urinate and leak on the way to the bathroom. In addition to urgency, signs and symptoms of urge UI most often include urinary frequency, nocturia and enuresis, and UI of moderate to large amounts. Bladder changes common in aging make older adults particularly prone to this type of UI (Abrams et al., 2003 [Level V]; Fantl et al., 1996 [Level I]). An individual with an overactive bladder (OAB) may complain of urgency, with or without UI. Individuals with an OAB also may have urinary frequency and nocturia. Assessment should focus on pathologic or metabolic conditions that may explain these symptoms (Abrams et al., 2003 [Level V]).

Mixed UI is defined as involuntary urine loss as a combination of stress UI and urge UI (Fantl et al., 1996 [Level I]). Symptoms include both urge and stress UI symptoms.

Overflow UI is an involuntary loss of urine associated with over-distention of the bladder and may be caused by an under active detrusor muscle or outlet obstruction leading to over-distention of the bladder and leakage of urine. Individuals with overflow UI often describe dribbling, urinary retention or hesitancy, urine loss without a recognizable urge, an uncomfortable sensation of fullness or pressure in the lower abdomen, and incomplete bladder emptying. Clinically, suprapubic palpation may reveal a distended or painful bladder as a result of urine retention, which may be acute or chronic. A common condition associated with this type of UI is BPH. Neurological conditions such as multiple sclerosis and spinal cord injuries or diabetes mellitus (DM), which result in bladder muscle denervation, may also cause overflow UI (Abrams et al., 2003 [Level V]; Doughty, 2000 [Level VI]; Fantl et al., 1996 [Level I])

Functional UI is caused by nongenitourinary factors, such as cognitive or physical impairments, that result in an inability for the individual to be independent in voiding. For example, acutely ill hospitalized individuals may be challenged by a combination of an acute illness and environmental changes. This, in turn, makes the voiding process even more complex, resulting in a functional type of UI (Fantl et al., 1996 [Level I]).

Assessment Parameters

Nurse continence experts suggest that entry-level nurses demonstrate the ability to collect and organize data surrounding urine control and implement nursing interventions that promote continence (Jirovec, Wyman, & Wells, 1998 [Level VI]). Nurses play a critical role in the basic assessment and management of UI in hospitalized older adults. Because UI is an interdisciplinary issue, collaboration with other members of the health care team is essential. However, it is no longer sufficient for nurses to identify and document the presence of UI. According to incontinence experts, the type of UI should be determined and documented based on a careful history and focused assessment; urodynamic tests are not required as part of the initial assessment of UI (ICI, 2000 [Level VI]). Basic history and examination techniques are presented herein to assist nurses in identifying the type of UI along with a nursing standard of practice protocol (see Box 13.1) to guide UI assessment and management.

History

When a patient is admitted to the hospital, nursing history should include questions to determine if the individual has pre-existing UI or risk factors (Table 13.1) for UI. Nurses should be alert to the following UI-associated risk factors specific to the hospital setting: depression, malnourishment, dependent ambulation, being a resident in a long term care institution, confusion, and being an African American woman (Kresvic, 1997 [Level IV]; Palmer et al., 2002 [Level IV]). Therefore, nurses should screen for depression, determine body mass index (BMI), monitor albumin and total protein levels if available, consult with the dietician, and perform a validated assessment of both cognitive and functional status.

Nurses should include screening questions such as "Have you ever leaked urine? If yes, how much does it bother you?" for all older adult patients. Although not validated in the hospital setting, examples of screening instruments used in other settings include the Urinary Distress Inventory-6 (UDI-6) and the Male Urinary Distress Inventory (MUDI). The UDI-6 is a self-report symptom inventory for UI that is reliable and valid for identifying the type of established UI in community-dwelling females (Lemack & Zimmern, 1999 [Level IV]; Uebersax, Wyman, Shumaker, McClish, & Fantl, 1995 [Level IV]). The MUDI is a valid and reliable measure of urinary symptoms in the male population (Robinson & Shea, 2002 [Level IV]). Determining the degree of "bother" and the effect on HRQOL is important and should include the perspective of both the patient and caregiver or significant other. Various instruments for quantifying bother and HRQOL exist (Abrams et al., 2003 [Level V]; Bradway, 2003 [Level VI]; Robinson & Shea, 2002 [Level IV]; Shumaker et al., 1994 [Level IV]).

Historical questions should focus on the characteristics of UI: time of onset, frequency, and severity of the problem. Questions also should review past health history and address possible precipitants of UI such as coughing, uncontrollable urinary urgency, functional decline, and acute illness (e.g., UTI, hip fracture). Nurses should inquire about lower urinary tract symptoms such as nocturia, hematuria, and urinary hesitancy, as well as current management strategies for UI.

The presence and rationale for an indwelling urinary catheter should be documented. For example, Tag F315 of the U.S. Centers for Medicare and Medicaid (2005) regulate indwelling urinary catheter usage in nursing home settings.Appropriate indications in the nursing home include: (1) urinary retention unmanageable by other measures (e.g., intermittent catheterization); (2) prevention of urine contamination to stage III or IV pressure ulcers; and (3) severe impairment or terminal illness that makes changing soiled clothes and repositioning uncomfortable. Therefore, the presence of an indwelling urinary catheter without one of these appropriate indications must prompt nurses to evaluate its appropriateness and if necessary, consult with other members of the health care team with regard to discontinuing the catheter.

A bladder diary or voiding record is the clinical "gold standard" for obtaining objective information about a patient's voiding pattern, incontinent episodes, and UI severity. There are numerous voiding records available; for example, visit http://kidney.niddk.nih.gov and search for "bladder diary." Although the

13.1 Risk Factors Associated with Urinary Incontinence

Risk Factor	Source
Age	Holroyd-Leduc & Straus, 2004 [Level I]) Age was associated with Urge UI, not Stress UI
Caffeine intake	Holroyd-Leduc & Straus, 2004 [Level I])
Immobility/functional limitations	Fantl et al., 1996 [Level I] Holroyd-Leduc & Straus, 2004 [Level I] Kresvic, 1997 [Level IV]
Impaired cognition	Fantl et al., 1996 [Level I]
Medications	Fantl et al., 1996 [Level I]
Obesity	Fantl et al., 1996 [Level I] Brown et al., 1996 [Level IV]
Diuretics	Fantl et al., 1996 [Level I]
Smoking	Fantl et al., 1996 [Level I]
Fecal impaction	Fantl et al., 1996 [Level I]
Malnutrition	Kresvic, 1997 [Level IV]
Depression	Kresvic, 1997 [Level IV]
Delirium	Fantl et al., 1996 [Level I]
Pregnancy/vaginal delivery/episiotomy	Fantl et al., 1996 [Level I]) Holroyd-Leduc & Straus, 2004 [Level I]
Low fluid intake	Fantl et al., 1996 [Level I]
Environmental barriers	Fantl et al., 1996 [Level I]
High-impact physical activities	Fantl et al., 1996 [Level I]
Diabetes mellitus	Fantl et al., 1996 [Level I]) Holroyd-Leduc & Straus, 2004 [Level I]

13.1 Risk Factors Associated with Urinary Incontinence

Risk Factor	Source
Parkinson's disease	Holroyd-Leduc & Straus, 2004 [Level I]
Stroke	Fantl et al., 1996 [Level I]) Holroyd-Leduc & Straus, 2004 [Level I]) Meijer et al., 2003 [Level I]) Thomas et al., 2005 [Level I]
Chronic obstructive pulmonary disease	Dowling-Castronovo, 2004 [Level VI] Holroyd-Leduc & Straus, 2004 [Level I]
Estrogen depletion	Fantl et al., 1996 [Level I]) Holroyd-Leduc & Straus, 2004 [Level I]
Hysterectomy	Brown, Sawaya, Thom, & Grady, 2000b [Level I] Holroyd-Leduc & Straus, 2004 [Level I]
Pelvic muscle weakness	Fantl et al., 1996 [Level I]) Kegel, 1956 [Level VI] DeLanacy, 1994 [Level IV] Holroyd-Leduc & Straus, 2004 [Level I]
Childhood nocturnal enuresis	Fantl et al., 1996 [Level I])
Race	Fantl et al., 1996 [Level I] Holroyd-Leduc & Straus, 2004 [Level I]: White women having higher rates of moderate and severe UI than Black women [Level I]
Arthritis and/or back problems	Holroyd-Leduc & Straus, 2004 [Level I]
Hearing and/or visual impairment	Holroyd-Leduc & Straus, 2004 [Level I]
Prostate surgery	Hunter, Moore, Cody, & Glazener, 2004 [Level I]

7-day voiding record is the most evaluated and recommended tool used to quantify UI and identify activities associated with unwanted urine loss (Jeyaseelan, Roe, & Oldham, 2000 [Level I]), a 3-day voiding record has been recommended as more feasible in outpatient and long term care settings (Fantl et al., 1996 [Level I]; ICI, 2000 [Level VI]). A voiding record completed for even 1 day may help identify patients with bladder dysfunction or those requiring further referral. Advanced practice nurses or urologic/continence specialists can assist nursing staff with interpretation and offer suggestions regarding nursing interventions based on information from the voiding record.

Comprehensive Assessment

A wide variety of medications can adversely affect continence. Diuretics are the most commonly known class of medications that contribute to UI due to polyuria, frequency, and urgency. Anticholinergics may cause mental status changes, urinary retention with or without overflow incontinence, and stool impaction. Various psychotropic medications (e.g., tricyclic antidepressants, antipsychotics, sedative-hypnotics) have anticholinergic effects, contribute to immobility, cause sedation and possibly delirium—each of which negatively affects bladder control. Alpha-adrenergic blockers may cause urethral relaxation whereas alpha-adrenergic agonists may cause urinary retention. Calcium channel blockers also may cause urinary retention (Kane, Ouslander, & Abrass, 2004 [Level VI]).

Nurses should document all over-the-counter (OTC), herbal, and prescription medications on admission. Additionally, nurses must closely scrutinize new medications as possible causes if UI suddenly develops during a patient's hospital stay. Medications that may contribute to iatrogenic (i.e., hospital-caused) UI include diuretics and sedative-hypnotics. Essentially, when a hospitalized patient develops transient UI, the nurse must ask the question: Could a new medication be affecting this patient's bladder control? If the answer is yes, then the nurse reviews this finding with the prescribing practitioner to learn if the contributing medication may be discontinued or modified.

Important components of a comprehensive examination include abdominal, genital, rectal, and skin examinations. In particular, the abdominal examination should assess for suprapubic distention indicative of urinary retention. Inspection of male and female genitalia can be completed during bathing or as part of the skin assessment. The nurse should observe the patient for signs of perineal irritation, lesions, or discharge. In women, a Valsalva maneuver (if not medically contraindicated) or voluntary cough may identify pelvic prolapse (e.g., cystocele, rectocele, uterine prolapse) or stress UI as a result of increased intra-abdominal pressure with bearing down (Burns, 2000 [Level VI]). Postmenopausal women are especially prone to atrophic vaginitis. Significant findings for atrophic vaginitis include perineal inflammation, tenderness (and, on occasion, trauma as a result of touch), and thin, pale genitalia tissues. During the genitalia examination, patients should be instructed to cough to determine if there is urine leakage, again caused by increased intra-abdominal pressure, which may be attributed to stress UI. Digital rectal and skin examinations are essential in identifying transient causes of UI such as constipation, fecal impaction, and the presence of fungal rashes. The "anal wink" (i.e., contraction of

13.1

Post Void Residual (PVR)

Instruct the patient to void. Post-void (ideally within 15 minutes or less) measure the residual urine remaining in the bladder by either:

- Bladder Sonography (Scan)

    Noninvasive ultrasound of the suprapubic area identifies the residual amount of urine, or

- Sterile catheterization

A PVR of greater than 100cc is considered abnormal and requires further evaluation by a urology specialist

Adapted from Shinopulos (2000 [Level VI])

the external anal sphincter) indicates intact sacral nerve routes and is assessed by lightly stroking the circumanal skin. Absence of the "anal wink" may suggest sphincter denervation (Burns, 2000 [Level VI]) and risk for stress UI. In men, the prostate gland should be palpated during the rectal examination because BPH contributes to urge or overflow UI. A normal prostate gland is symmetrically heart-shaped, about the size of a large chestnut, and often described as "rubbery" or similar to the tip of the nose. When enlarged, as with BPH, the examiner may palpate symmetrical enlargement. Pain on palpation or asymmetrical borders may be indicative of prostatitis or prostate cancer, respectively (Gray & Haas, 2000 [Level VI]).

In some cases, diagnostic testing may provide additional information. The most common diagnostic testing includes urinalysis, urine culture and sensitivity, and postvoid residual urine (PVR) (ICI, 2000 [Level VI]). Urinalysis and urine cultures are used to identify the presence of a UTI and bacterial agent responsible, which may contribute to acute UI. When dealing with a suspected UTI in a patient with an indwelling urinary catheter, change the entire system (Wound Ostomy Continence Nurse's Society, 1996 [Level VI]) prior to obtaining a urine specimen. A measurement of PVR may reveal incomplete bladder emptying. Two ways to accurately evaluate PVR are bladder sonography and catheter insertion after the patient has voided (Figure 13.1). An additional diagnostic test such as a simple bedside urodynamic test, which provides information regarding detrusor activity, may be warranted in some cases (Burns, 2000; Weiss, 1998 [both Level VI]).

A simple bedside urodynamic test is most likely to be performed by an advance practice nurse or physician. It is done after a PVR has been performed and measured via the sterile catheterization method. After the bladder is emptied, the catheter is maintained in the bladder. A 50 mL syringe (without plunger) is connected to the catheter, with the center of the syringe in alignment with the symphysis pubis. Sterile water is then instilled to fill the bladder. The fluid level is monitored for evidence of bladder contractions, which are reflected in movement of the fluid level. Urge UI is likely if severe urgency or bladder contractions are noted at less than 300 mL (Weiss, 1998 [Level VI]).

Functional, environmental, and mental status assessments are essential components of the UI evaluation in older adults. Nurses should observe the patient voiding, assess mobility, note any use of assistive devices, and identify any obstacles that interfere with appropriate use of toilets or toilet substitutes, such as a bedside commode.

Interventions and Care Strategies

Palmer's conceptual model for continence management stresses the need for public education (1996 [Level VI]). Evidence demonstrates that hospital nurses lack the knowledge necessary for evidence-based incontinence care (Connor & Kooker, 1998 [Level IV]; Cooper & Watt, 2003 [Level IV]); therefore, adapting this for the acute care environment includes staff education. A brief unit-based in-service followed by patient rounds may be instrumental in identifying patients at risk for UI and those actually experiencing UI. The North American Nursing Diagnosis Association (NANDA), Nursing Interventions Classifications (NIC), and Nursing Outcomes Classification (NOC) provide structure for planning and evaluating UI assessment and management (Johnson, Bulechek, McCloskey-Dochterman, Maas, & Moorhead, 2001 [Level VI]). However, there is no structured guidance for the assessment and management of transient UI. Nurses are likely to be the first to identify and perhaps prevent transient UI. Research is needed to understand the role nurses play in preventing UI (Sampselle, Palmer, Boyington, O'Dell, & Wooldridge, 2004 [Level VI]).

Treating Transient and Functional Causes of UI

First, transient causes of UI should be investigated, identified, and treated. Individuals with a history of established UI should have usual voiding routines and continence strategies immediately incorporated into the acute care plan, whenever possible. Nurses play an essential role in the initiation of discharge planning and patient or caregiver teaching regarding all aspects of UI. Teaching and discharge planning should begin at admission as appropriate, reviewed continually, and revised as necessary.

The environment is vital in managing UI, particularly functional UI. Incontinent older adults are often dependent on adaptive devices (e.g., walker) or caregivers for assistance with voiding, making them "dependently continent." Call bells should be identified and within easy reach. If limited mobility is anticipated, nursing staff should consider using an elevated toilet or commode seat, male or female urinal, or bedpan. Nurses should obtain referrals to physical and occupational therapy for ambulation aids, gait training, further assessment of activities of daily living (ADLs) associated with continence, and improved muscle strength. Physical and chemical restraints should be avoided, including side rails (see case studies). Patients should be encouraged and assisted to void before leaving the unit for tests (Fantl et al., 1996 [Level I]; Jirovec, 2000 [Level VI]; Jirovec et al., 1988 [Level VI]; Palmer, 1996 [Level VI]).

Toileting programs (e.g., individualized, scheduled toileting programs; prompted voiding) have varied success rates (Colling, Ouslander, Hadley, Eisch, & Campbell, 1992 [Level II]; Eustice, Roe, & Paterson, 2005 [Level I];

Ostaszkiewicz, Johnston, & Roe, 2005 [Level I]). A voiding record is essential for developing an individualized scheduled toileting program, which mimics the patient's normal voiding patterns and requires continual assessment and re-evaluation for successful outcomes. For example, if the initial scheduled toileting time is set for 8 a.m., yet at 6:30 a.m. the patient consistently attempts to independently void or is noted to be incontinent, then the toileting time should be adjusted to 6 a.m. Prompted voiding requires the caregiver to ask if the patient needs to void, offer assistance, and then offer praise for successful voiding (Eustice et al., 2005 [Level I]; Jirovec, 2000 [Level VI]; Ostaszkiewicz et al., 2005 [Level I]).

Healthy Bladder Behavior Skills

Traditionally, nursing interventions for UI focus on containment strategies by means of receptacles (e.g., bedpan, urinal, commode, urinary catheters) or by various absorbent products (e.g., sanitary napkin, adult diaper, incontinent pad) (Harmer & Henderson, 1955; Henderson & Nite, 1978). Various treatments beyond containment strategies include dietary management; pelvic floor muscle exercises (PFMEs), also known as Kegel exercises (Kegel, 1956 [Level VI]); urge inhibition and bladder training (retraining) strategies; toileting programs (e.g., individualized, scheduled toileting programs, prompted voiding); pharmacological therapy; and surgical options (Fantl et al., 1996 [Level I]). These treatments (excluding pharmacological and surgical options) are viewed as healthy bladder behavior skills (HBBS). Although the recommendation is to offer HBBS to all older adults with UI (Fantl et al., 1996 [Level I]; ICI, 2000 [Level VI]); Teunissen, deJonge, van Weel, & Lagro-Janssen, 2004 [Level I]), it is unclear how to best incorporate HBBS in the care of hospitalized older adults. Despite the fact that contemporary nursing-practice textbooks list and describe HBBS as nursing interventions (Kozier, Erb, Berman, & Snyder, 2004; Taylor, Lillis, & LeMone, 2005 [both Level VI]), many of these interventions have not been adequately examined in the acute care setting, and nurses do not routinely implement these interventions in the acute care setting (Bayliss, Salter, & Locke, 2003; Schnelle et al., 2003; Watson, Brink, Zimmer, & Mayer, 2003 [all Level IV]). Recall, under-reporting, and under-assessment are barriers to optimally addressing UI in the hospital setting, as reflected in the study by Schultz and colleagues (1997 [Level IV]), which reported that only 0.1% of medical records captured the problem of UI present at the time of hospital admission. Accurate assessment and identification of type of UI is needed before care strategies are initiated.

Prior to instituting HBBS, nurses need to assess the motivation of a patient, informal caregiver, and nursing staff because behavior modification is a premise of HBBS (Palmer, 2004 [Level VI]). Examples of dietary management strategies include avoiding certain foods and beverages known to be bladder irritants such as caffeine, acidic foods or fluids, and NutraSweet® (Gray & Haas, 2000 [Level VI]). Some individuals with a BMI greater than 27 may benefit from a weight-loss program. For example, in one study, a weight loss of 5% to 10% significantly decreased UI episodes for some obese women (Subak et al., 2005 [Level II]).

If not contraindicated, the nurse recommends adequate fluid intake, specifically water, and an increased intake of dietary fiber to maintain bowel regularity.

It is important to work closely with older adults who fear that unwanted urine loss is a result of increased fluid intake. Education should focus on the adverse consequence of inadequate fluid intake, such as volume depletion and potential for dehydration, and that too little fluid intake may result in concentrated urine, which, in turn, may cause increased bladder contractions and increased feelings of urinary urgency. Lastly, to manage and limit nocturia, patients may be advised to limit fluid intake a few hours before bedtime (Doughty, 2000 [Level VI]; Fantl et al., 1996 [Level I]; ICI, 2000 [Level VI]). In the hospital setting, nurses must note the schedule of diuretics. For example, many institutions schedule every 12-hour diuretic dose times at 10 a.m. and 10 p.m. For some patients, it will be extremely important that nurses navigate organizational processes to reschedule diuretic doses to alternate times, such as 6 a.m. and 6 p.m. This simple strategy may decrease nocturia, which, in turn, will likely decrease risk for falls. Research that examines which UI interventions best modify fall risk is needed (Wolf, Riolo, & Ouslander, 2000 [Level VI]).

PFMEs are better than no treatment for stress and urge UI (Bo, Talseth, & Holme, 1999 [Level II]; Flynn, Cell, & Luisi, 1994 [Level IV]; Hay-Smith & Dumoulin, 2006 [Level I]; Holroyd-Leduc & Straus, 2004 [Level I]. PFME holds promise for the primary prevention of UI but requires additional research (Hay-Smith, Herbison, & Morkved, 2002 [Level I]). PFMEs were developed to augment the strength, endurance, and coordination of the pelvic muscles, which play a role in maintaining continence. Integrating PFMEs into the plan of care requires an assessment of the patient's baseline understanding of PFMEs to identify knowledge deficits. Ideally, PFMEs are taught during a vaginal or rectal examination when the clinician manually assists the patient to identify the pelvic muscles by instructing the patient to squeeze around the gloved examination finger. This method allows for performance appraisal (Hay-Smith et al., 2002 [Level I]). Alternately, PFMEs may be verbally taught by instructing the patient to gently squeeze or contract the rectal or vaginal muscle. Either teaching method includes instructions to not squeeze the stomach, buttocks, or thigh muscles (because this only increases intra-abdominal pressure) but rather to isolate the contraction of the pelvic muscles. Preferably, each exercise should consist of contracting for 10 seconds and relaxing for 10 seconds. Some patients may need to start with 3 or 5 seconds and then increase as their muscle gets stronger. There is no set "exercise dose" (DuMoulin, Hammers, Paulus, Berendsen, & Halfens, 2005 [Level I]); however, it is usual practice to recommend 15 PFMEs three times per day. Patients may notice improvement in 2 to 4 weeks but not immediately. Nurses should reinforce compliance and other HBBS and initiate a referral for discharge follow-up with a continence specialist, if available (Bradway, Hernly, & the NICHE faculty, 1999a [Level VI]).

Urge inhibition is based on behavioral theory and is another recommended HBBS for treatment of urge UI (ICI, 2000 [Level VI]; Teunissen et al., 2004 [Level I]), although the mechanism of how urge inhibition works is not well understood (Gray, 2005 [Level VI]; Smith, 2000 [Level VI]). Urge inhibition includes distraction techniques (e.g., reciting a favorite poem or song), relaxation techniques, and rapid PFMEs, with the goal being to suppress the urge to void until desirable (Smith, 2000 [Level VI]).

Bladder training (retraining) is another behavioral technique used to treat urge UI (ICI, 2000 [Level VI]; Teunissen et al., 2004 [Level I]) and OAB and is often used in conjunction with urge-inhibition techniques. Bladder training re-quires a baseline bladder diary to determine the timing of voids and UI episodes. If urinary frequency is present, the patient is instructed to lengthen the time be-tween voids in an effort to retrain the bladder. When a strong urge to void occurs, the patient is instructed to use urge-inhibition techniques to suppress urinary urgency. For example, if the patient is not in a position to empty the bladder in a socially appropriate manner, the nurse instructs the patient to quickly squeeze and relax pelvic-floor muscles several times to suppress the urge to void. This technique is sometimes referred to as "quick flicks" (Gray, 2005 [Level VI]). Relaxation and distraction and urge-inhibition techniques are also beneficial during bladder training.

In some instances (e.g., for patients experiencing incomplete bladder emp-tying or overflow UI), patients and staff can use the Crede's maneuver (i.e., deep suprapubic palpation). The Crede's maneuver is used with caution and re-quires manual compression over the suprapubic area during bladder emptying. The Crede's maneuver should be avoided if vesicoureteral reflux (i.e., abnor-mal flow of urine from the bladder back up the ureters) or overactive sphincter mechanisms are suspected because it may dangerously elevate pressure within the bladder (Doughty, 2000 [Level VI]). In some cases, instructing patients to double void (i.e., after an initial void, instruct the patient to stand or reposition for a second void) also facilitates bladder emptying.

Additional Nursing Interventions

Despite the promise of antiseptic urinary catheters (Brosnahan & Kent, 2004 [Level I]), indwelling urinary catheters should be avoided as a treatment for UI. Dowd and Campbell (1995 [Level IV]) discovered a UTI incidence of 10% associated with indwelling catheter use. They suggest that unintended infec-tions may have increased length of hospital stay and decreased opportunities for nursing staff to identify incontinence as a problem. In addition, a European study of 141 hospitals demonstrated that catheter-associated UTI was present in more than 60% of nosocomial UTI cases (Bouza et al., 2001 [Level IV]). The Wound Ostomy Continence Nurses Society (1996 [Level VI]) recommends specific indications for indwelling catheter use, including severe acute illness, urinary retention uncontrollable by other interventions (including medication management and sterile intermittent catheterization), and UI management for patients with Stage III–IV pressure ulcers of the trunk, such the sacral or ischial areas. (see chapter 11, *Iatrogenesis: The Nurse's Role in Preventing Patient Harm*)

Sterile intermittent catheterization may result in a lower incidence of infec-tion (Saint et al., 2006 [Level II]; Terpenning, Allada, & Kauffaman, 1989 [Level IV]; Warren, 1997 [Level VI]) and may be a feasible alternative to placement of an indwelling urinary catheter for managing urinary retention with or without overflow UI. Decisions regarding catheterization require careful consideration of the benefits and burdens associated with use because it has long been docu-mented that indwelling urinary catheters are positively associated with bacturia, UTIs, uricemia, urethral erosion, and death (LeBlanc & Christensen, 2005 [Level V]; Madigan & Neff, 2003 [Level I]; Wong, 1981 [Level VI]; Zimakoff, Stickler, Pontoppidan, & Larsen, 1996 [Level IV]). One study reported the unjustified use of indwelling urinary catheters in 21% of cases; moreover, continued catheterization was unjustified 47% of the time (Jain, Parada, & Smith 1995 [Level IV]). Strategies to reduce UTIs associated with indwelling urinary catheter use in hospital settings include protocols that provide indications for appropriate indwelling urinary catheter use and for discontinuing indwelling urinary catheters (Reilly et al. 2006 [Level V]). When an indwelling urinary catheter is indicated, it is recommended that (1) the smallest lumen size catheter be used; (2) sterile water is used to inflate the catheter balloon and balloon volume is assessed every 2 weeks or as clinically indicated; and, (3) the catheter is secured to the patient's thigh. No evidence supports routine collection of urine or routine timing of catheter changes (The Society of Urologic Nurses and Associates, 2005 [Level VI]).

Although a causal link between UI and skin breakdown has not been adequately supported, maintaining skin integrity is a goal of nursing care. Decomposition of urinary urea by microorganisms releases ammonia and forms ammonium hydroxide, an alkali. This alkali makes the protective "acid mantle" of the skin vulnerable and jeopardizes skin integrity. If UI episodes persist despite management strategies, perineal skin care interventions should focus on maintaining the integrity of the protective acid mantle of the skin (Ersser, Getliffe, Voegeli, & Regan, 2005 [Level I]). Although absorbent products are commonly used for UI containment, there is little evidence available to guide product selection and no evidence of how absorbent products may interact with the acid mantle. Pertaining to reusable versus disposable absorbent products, there is no demonstrable risk of cross-infection with reusable absorbent products when appropriate laundering protocols are followed, and there are no clear cost savings with using one versus the other. However, it is reported that the use of diapers is significantly associated with an increased risk for infection (Zimakoff et al., 1996 [Level IV]). Although bed pads contain urine, consumer satisfaction is questionable, and there are no studies on the use of chair pads. Essentially, there is no clear evidence to suggest one absorbent product being superior to another. However, the evidence does support pilot testing of absorbent products according to individual circumstances, including patient, family, and institutional preferences (Dunn, Kowanko, Patersonk, & Pretty, 2002 [Level I]).

Case Studies and Discussion

CASE #1

A student nurse received a report on Mr. G., an 86-year-old man with a history of Alzheimer's dementia who is hospitalized for delirium. The nurse was told that Mr. G. was "pleasantly confused," required full assistance with personal care, and spent most of the day in a Geri-chair. The student nurse performed an assessment that revealed the following:

Patient sleeping in bed with all siderails up, call bell within reach, no urinal in sight. PMH-CAD, Mild HTN, Mild osteoarthritis

PSH: None

Medications: diphenhydramine (Benadryl) 25mg PRN for sleep, enalapril (Vasotec) 5mg PO OD for HTN, MVI 1 tab PO OD, donepezil (Aricept) 10 mg PO OD for Alzheimer's dementia, Vitamin E 400iu PO BID supplement for Alzheimer's dementia

VS: 114/60, 72, 14, 98.0F

Alert and oriented to self; sleepy; no focal deficits

Heart Rate: Regular

Breath sounds clear, slightly decreased at the bases

Abdomen: +BS in all quadrants, soft, nontender, no suprapubic tenderness; left quadrant slightly dull to percussion; no palpable masses

Dry adult diaper in place

The student nurse learns from the patient's wife (i.e., the primary care provider at home) that the patient has experienced occasional urinary leaking in the past but not to the extent of needing "diapers." He has a history of chronic constipation. With the nursing instructor's guidance, the student nurse assisted Mr. G. to a dangling position at the side of the bed. After assessing and evaluating that the patient's muscular strength was strong, ambulation was attempted. The patient ambulated to the bathroom, the adult diaper was removed, and Mr. G. was prompted to void. He successfully voided and had a bowel movement. He proceeded to wash his hands and returned to the bedside chair (not the Geri-chair) and enjoyed breakfast. The adult diaper was left off during the time the student nurse was there to assist him. During this time, Mr. G. made one attempt to initiate voiding and was successfully assisted by the student nurse.

The importance of ongoing nursing assessment was stressed as being vital to quality of care. Had the student nurse just transferred the patient to the Geri-chair, he may not have effectively emptied his bowel and bladder. Mr. G.'s constipation was addressed by providing appropriate fluid and fiber intake and by continuing with an individualized toilet schedule as tolerated. The avoidance of diphenhydramine for the elderly was also discussed because it is known to cause anticholinergic effects including urinary retention. Diphenhydramine raises concerns about sedation as well, which may alter Mr. G.'s response to the need to void.

Evidence suggests that prompted voiding and individualized toileting schedules reduce the number of UI episodes (Eustice et al., 2005 [Level I]; Ostaszkiewicz et al., 2005 [Level I]). In addition, prompted voiding in cognitively impaired long term care residents has demonstrated an increase in self-initiative toileting activities (Holroyd-Leduc & Straus, 2004 [Level I]). However, these strategies have not been studied in the hospital setting. Despite this lack of evidence, Case Study #1 demonstrates that these nursing interventions may also be beneficial for acutely hospitalized older adults.

CASE #2

Ms. W. is a 92-year-old patient hospitalized for an exacerbation of heart failure (HF). Her past health history is also significant for DM, HTN, CAD, and osteoarthritis. Initially, Ms. W. required an indwelling urinary catheter for accurate fluid management. During that time, the staff utilized wrist restraints to prevent her from removing intravenous lines and the catheter.

Today is hospital day 5. The nurse receives the shift report that Ms. W. is ready for discharge. On assessment, the nurse finds Ms. W. lying in bed with all side rails up and the indwelling urinary catheter has not been discontinued.

Individuals with acute exacerbations of HF are at high risk for transient UI and exacerbation of established UI. In addition, these individuals are prone to postural hypotension and polypharmacy as a result of multiple co-morbid conditions, such as diabetes. During an acute hospital stay, nursing interventions should focus on diuretic management, such as attention to increased voiding needs and appropriate use of urinals, a bedside commode, or other assistive devices. Patients often require careful fluid and electrolyte management, necessitating the temporary use of an indwelling urinary catheter; however, nursing care should focus on expedient catheter removal. These interventions decrease the risk of catheter-associated UTIs or trauma that may exacerbate UI symptoms (McGann, 2000 [Level VI]).

Summary

Although acute care stays are generally short, UI is a significant health problem that should not be overlooked. Behavioral and supportive therapies and patient education should be initiated by nurses if the patient is cognitively, physically, and emotionally able to participate. Evidence from long term care and community settings suggests that nurse continence experts play an essential role in improving the quality of continence care (DuMoulin et al., 2005 [Level I]; McDowell et al., 1999 [Level II]; Watson, 2005 [Level VI]). Therefore, if patients remain incontinent at discharge, hospital nurses have the responsibility to design a plan that includes referral to a continence nurse specialist or other continence expert for follow-up.

Other than identifying UI as a risk for falls, there are no requirements specific to UI from The Joint Commission (http://www.jointcommission.org/). Nevertheless, it is recommended that a continuous quality improvement (CQI) criterion should encompass critical elements in an effective and successful urinary continence program. For example, quality indicators for UI may include appropriate documentation of UI, if the UI is transient or established, if an indwelling urinary catheter was used during hospitalization or on discharge, and evidence of documentation of referrals. In addition, the AHRQ Guideline for UI (Fantl et al., 1996 [Level I]) or other published guidelines (e.g., those found at the National Guideline Clearinghouse http://www.guideline.gov/Compare/comparison.aspx?file=INCONTINENCE1.inc) may be used clinically and facility-wide for program development and CQI.

In summary, nurses have a significant role in improving the assessment and treatment of UI in hospitalized older adults. It is recommended that nurses are particularly vigilant for patients who are "admitted dry and become wet" during a hospitalization. These patients will particularly benefit from evidence-based assessment and management. Moreover, nurses can help to promote changes in attitudes toward UI and provide education on individual, facility-wide, community, and national levels.

Resources

Incontinence Impact Questionnaire Short Version (IIQ-7) http://www. americangeriatrics.org/education/UItool02.pdf

Urinary Distress Inventory Short Version (UDI-6) http://www.fpminstitute. com/files/pelvic-floor-distress-inventory.pdf

Wound Ostomy Continence Nurses Society 150 South Coast Highway, Suite 201 Laguna Beach, CA 92651 (888) 224-WOCN http://www.wocn.org An international society providing a source of networking and research for nurses specializing in enterostomal and continence care.

National Association for Continence (NAFC) (800) BLADDER http://www.nafc. org/ A not-for-profit organization dedicated to improving the lives of individuals with incontinence.

The John A. Hartford Institute for Geriatric Nursing http://www.ConsultGeriRN. org/ This Web site takes the reader to the "Try This" series, which includes a 2-page UI information sheet to share with hospital staff.

Society of Urologic Nurses and Associates (SUNA) National Headquarters East Holly Avenue, Box 56 Pitman, NY 08071-0056 (888) TAP-SUNA http://www. suna.org/ An international organization dedicated to nursing care of individuals with urologic disorders.

GeroNurseOnline Geriatric Resources and tools www.ConsultGeriRN. Click Resources tab in Urinary Incontinence topic.

Box 13.1

Nursing Standard of Practice Protocol: Urinary Incontinence (UI) in Older Adults Admitted to Acute Care

I. GOAL

    A. Nursing staff will utilize comprehensive assessments and implement evidence-based management strategies for patients identified with UI.

    B. Nursing staff will collaborate with interdisciplinary team members to identify and document type of UI.

    C. Patients with UI will not have UI-associated complications.

II. OVERVIEW

UI affects approximately 17 million Americans (Fantl et al., 1996 [Level I]; National Association for Continence, 1998 [Level IV]; Resnick & Ouslander, 1990 [Level VI]). More than 35% of older adults admitted to the hospital develop UI [Kresvic, 1997 [Level IV]). In addition to medications, constipation/fecal impaction, low fluid intake, environmental barriers, diabetes mellitus, and stroke (Fantl et al., 1996 [Level I]; Holroyd-Leduc & Straus, 2004 [Level I]; Meijer et al., 2003 [Level I]; Thomas et al., 2005 [Level I]), immobility, impaired cognition, malnutrition, and depression are factors specific to identifying older adults at risk for UI in the hospital setting (Kresvic, 1997 [Level IV]). Complications of UI include falls, skin irritation leading to pressure ulcers, social isolation, and depression (Bogner et al., 2002 [Level IV]; Brown et al., 2000a [Level IV]; Fantl et al., 1996 [Level I]; Johnson et al., 1998 [Level IV]). Nurses play a key role in the assessment and management of UI.

III. BACKGROUND

A. Definitions

UI is the involuntary loss of urine sufficient to be a problem (Fantl et al., 1996 [Level I]). UI may be transient (acute) or established (chronic). Types of established UI include:

1. Stress UI: defined as an involuntary loss of urine associated with activities that increase intra-abdominal pressure (Abrams et al., 2003 [Level V]; Fantl et al., 1996 [Level I]; Hunter et al., 2005 [Level I]).

2. Urge UI: characterized by an involuntary urine loss associated with a strong desire to void (urgency) (Abrams et al., 2003 [Level V]; Fantl et al., 1996 [Level I]). An individual with an overactive bladder (OAB) may complain of urinary urgency, with or without UI (Abrams et al., 2003 [Level V]).

3. Mixed UI: usually defined as a combination of Stress UI and Urge UI.

4. Overflow UI: an involuntary loss of urine associated with over-distention of the bladder and may be caused by an under-active detrusor muscle or outlet obstruction leading to over-distention of the bladder and overflow of urine (Abrams et al., 2003 [Level V]; Doughty, 2000 [Level VI]; Fantl et al., 1996 [Level I]).

5. Functional UI: caused by nongenitourinary factors, such as cognitive or physical impairments that result in an inability for the individual to be independent in voiding (Fantl et al., 1996 [Level I]).

B. Epidemiology

UI affects approximately 17 million Americans (Fantl et al., 1996 [Level I]; National Association for Continence, 1998 [Level IV]; Resnick & Ouslander, 1990 [Level VI]). UI studies specific to the hospital setting demonstrate that UI is present in 10% to 42% of older adults (Dowd & Campbell, 1995 [Level IV]; Fantl et al., 1996 [Level I]; Palmer et al., 1992 [Level IV]; Schultz et al., 1997 [Level IV]). New-onset UI was identified in 35% of one patient sample (Kresvic, 1997 [Level IV]). Therefore, it is essential to assess for UI and implement a protocol that offers evidence-based management strategies.

IV. Parameters of Assessment

A. Document the presence/absence of UI for all patients on admission (ICI, 2000 [Level VI]).
B. Document the presence/absence of an indwelling urinary catheter.
   1. Determine appropriate indwelling catheter use: severely ill patients, patient with Stage III–IV pressure ulcers of the trunk, urinary retention unresolved by other interventions (Wound Ostomy Continence Nurse's Society, 1996 [Level VI]).
C. For patients with presence of UI:
   The nurse collaborates with interdisciplinary team members to:
   1. Determine whether the UI is transient, established (Stress/Urge/ Mixed/Overflow/Functional), or both and document (Fantl et al., 1996 [Level I]; ICI, 2000 [Level VI]); Johnson et al., 2001 [Level VI]).
   2. Identify and document the possible etiologies of the UI (Fantl et al., 1996 [Level I]; ICI, 2000 [Level VI]).

V. Nursing Care Strategies

A. General principles that apply to prevention and management of *all* forms of UI:
   1. Identify and treat causes of transient UI (ICI, 2000 [Level VI]).
   2. Identify and continue successful prehospital management strategies for established UI.
   3. Develop an individualized plan of care using data obtained from the history and physical examination and in collaboration with other team members.
   4. Avoid medications that may contribute to UI (Kane et al., 2004 [Level VI]).
   5. Avoid indwelling urinary catheters whenever possible to avoid risk for UTI (Dowd & Campbell, 1995 [Level IV]; Bouza et al., 2001 [Level IV]; Madigan & Neff, 2003 [Level I]; Zimakoff et al., 1996 [Level IV]; & Wong, 1981 [Level VI]).
   6. Monitor fluid intake and maintain an appropriate hydration schedule.
   7. Limit dietary bladder irritants (Gray & Haas, 2000 Level VI]).
   8. Consider adding weight loss as a long-term goal in discharge planning for those with a BMI greater than 27 (Subak et al., 2005 [Level II]).
   9. Modify the environment to facilitate continence (Fantl et al., 1996 [Level I]; Jirovec, 2000 [Level VI]; Palmer, 1996 [Level VI]).

10. Provide patients with usual undergarments in expectation of continence, if possible.
11. Prevent skin breakdown by providing immediate cleansing after an incontinent episode and utilizing barrier ointments (Ersser et al., 2005 [Level I]).
12. Pilot test absorbent products to best meet patient, staff, and institutional preferences (Dunn et al., 2002 [Level I]), bearing in mind that diapers have been associated with UTIs (Zimakoff et al., 1996 [Level IV]).

B. Strategies for specific problems:

Stress UI:
1. Teach PFMEs (Bo et al., 1999 [Level II]; Hay-Smith & Dumoulin, 2006 [Level I]; ICI, 2000 [Level VI]).
2. Provide toileting assistance and bladder training PRN (ICI, 2000 [Level VI]).
3. Consider referral to other team members if pharmacological or surgical therapies are warranted.

Urge UI:
1. Implement bladder training (retraining) (ICI, 2000 [Level VI]; Teunissen et al., 2004 [Level I]).
2. If patient is cognitively intact and is motivated, provide information on urge inhibition (Gray, 2005 [Level VI]; Smith, 2000 [Level VI]).
3. Teach PFMEs to be used in conjunction with #1 (Flynn et al., 1994 [Level IV]).
4. Collaborate with prescribing team members if pharmacologic therapy is warranted.
5. Initiate referrals for those patients who do not respond to the previous steps.

Overflow UI:
1. Allow sufficient time for voiding.
2. Discuss with interdisciplinary team the need for determining a post-void residual (PVR) (ICI, 2000 [Level VI]; Shinoplous, 2000 [Level VI]; Weiss, 1998 [Level VI]) (see Figure 13.1).
3. Instruct patients in double voiding and Crede's maneuver (Dougherty, 2000 [Level VI]).
4. Sterile intermittent is preferred over indwelling catheterization (Saint et al., 2006 [Level II]; Terpenning et al., 1989 [Level IV]; Warren, 1997 [Level VI]) PRN.
5. Initiate referrals to other team members for those patients requiring pharmacological or surgical intervention.

Functional UI:
1. Provide individualized, scheduled toileting or prompted voiding (Eustice et al., 2005 [Level I]; Jirovec, 2000 [Level VI]; Ostaszkiewicz et al., 2005 [Level I]).
2. Provide adequate fluid intake.
3. Refer for physical and occupational therapy PRN.

4. Modify environment to maximize independence with continence (Fantl et al., 1996 [Level I]; Jirovec, 2000 [Level VI]; Jirovec, Brink, & Wells, 1988 [Level VI]); Palmer, 1996 [Level VI]).

VI. Evaluation of Expected Outcomes

A. Patients:
  1. Will have fewer or no episodes of UI or complications associated with UI.
B. Nurses:
  1. Will document assessment of continence status at admission and throughout hospital stay. If UI is identified, document and determine type of UI.
  2. Will use interdisciplinary expertise and interventions to assess and manage UI during hospitalization.
  3. Will include UI in discharge planning needs and refer PRN.
C. Institution:
  1. Incidence and prevalence of transient UI will decrease.
  2. Hospital policies will require assessment and documentation of continence status.
  3. Will provide access to AHRQ Guidelines for Managing Acute and Chronic UI.
  4. Staff will receive administrative support and ongoing education regarding assessment and management of UI.

VII. Follow-up Monitoring of Condition

A. Provide patient/caregiver discharge teaching regarding outpatient referral and management.
B. Incorporate continuous quality improvement (CQI) criteria into existing program.
C. Identify areas for improvement and enlist multidisciplinary assistance in devising strategies for improvement

VIII. Relevant Practice Guidelines

National Guideline Clearinghouse Guideline Synthesis: (updated 2007). Evaluation and management of urinary incontinence. http://www.guideline.gov/Compare/comparison.aspx?file= INCONTINENCE1.inc

References

Abrams, P., Cardozo, L., Fall, M., Griffiths, D., Rosier, P., Ulmsten, U., et al. (2002). The standardization of terminology of lower urinary tract function: Report from the standardization subcommittee of the International Continence Society. *Urology, 61,* 37–49. Evidence Level V: Narrative Literature Review.

Anger, J. T., Saigal, C. S., Litwin, M. S., & The Urologic Diseases of America Project (2006). The prevalence of urinary incontinence among community-dwelling adult women: Results from the national health and nutrition examination survey. *The Journal of Urology, 175*(2), 601–604. Evidence Level IV: Nonexperimental Study.

Bayliss, V., Salter, L., & Locke, R. (2003). Pathways for continence care: An audit to assess how they are used. *British Journal of Nursing, 12*, 857–863. Evidence Level IV: Nonexperimental Study.

Bo, K., Talseth, T., & Holme, I. (1999). Single-blind, randomized controlled trial of pelvic floor exercises, electrical stimulation, vaginal cones, and no treatment in management of genuine stress incontinence. *British Medical Journal, 318*, 487–493. Evidence Level II: RCT.

Bogner, H. R., Gallo, J. J., Sammel, M. D., Ford, D. E., Armenian, H. K., & Eaton, W. W. (2002). Urinary incontinence and psychological distress in community-dwelling older adults. *Journal of the American Geriatrics Society, 50*, 489–495. Evidence Level IV: Nonexperimental Study.

Bouza, E., San Juan, R., Munoz, P., Voss, A., Kluytmans, J., & Cooperative Group of the European Study Group on Nosocomial Infections (2001). A European perspective on nosocomial urinary tract infections II: Report on incidence, clinical characteristics and outcome (ESGNI-004 study). *Clinical Microbiology & Infection, 7*(10), 532–542. Evidence Level IV: Nonexperimental Study.

Bradway, C. (2003). Urinary incontinence among older women: Measurement of the effect on health-related quality of life. *Journal of Gerontological Nursing, 29*(7), 13–19. Evidence Level VI: Journal Article.

Bradway, C., Hernley, S., & the NICHE Faculty (1999a). Urinary incontinence in older persons. In I. Abraham, M. M. Bottrell, T. Fulmer, & M. D. Mezey (Eds.), *Geriatric nursing protocols for best practice* (pp. 41–49). New York: Springer Publishing Company. Evidence Level VI: Expert Opinion.

Bradway, C., Hernely, S., & the NICHE Faculty (1999b). Urinary incontinence in older adults admitted to acute care. *Geriatric Nursing, 19*(2), 98–102. Evidence Level VI: Expert Opinion.

Bradway, C., & Yetman, G. (2002). Genitourinary problems. In V. T. Cotter & N. E. Strumpf (Eds.), *Advanced practice nursing with older adults: Clinical guidelines*. (pp. 83–102). McGraw-Hill: New York. Evidence Level VI: Expert Opinion.

Brandeis, G. H., Baumann, M. M., Hossain, M., Morris, J. N., & Resnick, N. M. (1997). The prevalence of potentially remediable urinary incontinence in frail older people: A study using the minimum data set. *Journal of the American Geriatrics Society, 45*, 179–184. Evidence Level IV: Nonexperimental Study.

Brosnahan, J. E., & Kent, B. (2004). Short-term indwelling catheters (a systematic review) evidence for a primary nursing decision. *Worldviews on Evidence-Based Nursing, 1*(4), 228. Evidence Level I: Systematic Review.

Brown, J. S., Sawaya, G., Thom, D. H., & Grady, D. (2000b). Hysterectomy and urinary incontinence: A systematic review. *The Lancet, 356*, 535–539. Evidence Level I: Systematic Review.

Brown, J. S., Seeley, D. G., Fong, J., Black, D. M., Ensrud, K. E., & Grady, D. (1996). Urinary incontinence in older women: Who is at risk? *Obstetrics and Gynecology, 87*, 715–721. Evidence Level IV: Nonexperimental Study.

Brown, J. S., Vittinghoff, E., Wyman, J. F., Stone, K. L., Nevitt, M. C., Ensrud, K. E., et al. (2000a). Urinary incontinence: Does it increase risk for falls and fractures? *Journal of the American Geriatrics Society, 48*, 721–725. Evidence Level IV: Nonexperimental Study.

Burns, P. A. (2000). Stress urinary incontinence. In D. B. Doughty (Ed.), *Urinary & fecal incontinence nursing management* (2nd ed., pp. 63–89). St. Louis, MO: Mosby. Evidence Level VI: Expert Opinion.

Bush, T. A., Castellucci, D. T., & Phillips, C. (2001). Exploring women's beliefs regarding urinary incontinence. *Urologic Nursing, 21*, 211–218. Evidence Level IV: Nonexperimental Study.

Cassells, C., & Watt, E. (2004). The impact of incontinence on older spousal caregivers. *Journal of Advanced Nursing, 42*, 607–616. Evidence Level IV: Nonexperimental Study.

Centers for Medicare & Medicaid Services (CMS), Department of Health & Human Services (DHHS). CMS Manual System Publication 100–107. State Operations Provider Certification. June 28, 2005. F 315 Urinary Incontinence. Retrieved March 27, 2007, from http://www.cms.hhs.gov/transmittals/downloads/R8SOM.pdf. Evidence Level VI: Regulatory Opinion.

Cochran, A. (2000). Don't ask, don't tell: The incontinence conspiracy. *Manage Care Quarterly*, *8*(1), 44–52. Evidence Level VI: Journal Article.

Colling, J., Ouslander, J., Hadley, B. J., Eisch, J., & Campbell, E. (1992). The effects of patterned urge-response toileting (PURT) on urinary incontinence among nursing home residents. *Journal of the American Geriatrics Society*, *40*(2), 135–141. Evidence Level II: RCT Experimental Study.

Connor, P. A., & Kooker, B. M. (1996). Nurses' knowledge, attitudes, and practices in managing urinary incontinence in the acute care setting. *MEDSURG Nursing*, *5*(2), 87–92 (note that article continues on p. 117). Evidence Level IV: Nonexperimental Study.

Cooper, G., & Watt, E. (2003). An exploration of acute care nurses' approach to assessment and management of people with urinary incontinence. *Journal of Wound, Ostomy, and Continence Nursing*, *30*, 305–313. Evidence Level IV: Nonexperimental Study.

DeLancey, J. O. L. (1994). Structural support of the urethra as it relates to stress urinary incontinence: The hammock hypothesis. *American Journal of Obstetrics and Gynecology*, *170*, 1713–1723. Evidence Level IV: Nonexperimental Study.

Diokno, A. C., Brock, B. M., Brown, M. B., & Herzog, A. R. (1986). Prevalence of urinary incontinence and other urological symptoms in the noninstitutionalized elderly. *Journal of Urology*, *136*(5), 1022–1025. Evidence Level IV: Nonexperimental Study.

Doughty, D. B. (2000). Retention with overflow. In D. B. Doughty (Ed.), *Urinary & fecal incontinence nursing management* (2nd ed., pp. 159–180). St. Louis, MO: Mosby. Evidence Level VI: Expert Opinion.

Dowd, T. (1991). Discovering older women's experience of urinary incontinence. *Research in Nursing and Health*, *14*, 179–186. Level Evidence IV: Nonexperimental Study.

Dowd, T. T., & Campbell, J. M. (1995). Urinary incontinence in an acute care setting. *Urologic Nursing*, *15*, 82–85. Evidence Level IV: Nonexperimental Study.

Dowling-Castronovo, A. (2004). Urinary incontinence: An exploration of the relationship between age, COPD, and obesity. Unpublished analysis. Evidence Level VI: Expert Opinion.

DuMoulin, M. F. M. T., Hammers, J. P. H., Paulus, A., Berendsen, C., & Halfens, R. (2005). The role of the nurse in community continence care: A systematic review. *International Journal of Nursing Studies*, *42*, 479–492. Evidence Level I: Systematic Review.

Dunn, S., Kowanko, I., Patersonk, J., & Pretty, L. (2002). Systematic review of the effectiveness of urinary continence products. *Journal of WOCN*, *29*(3), 129–142. Evidence Level I: Systematic Review.

Ersser, S. J., Getliffe, K., Voegeli, D., & Regan, S. (2005). A critical review of the inter-relationship between skin vulnerability and urinary incontinence and related nursing intervention. *International Journal of Nursing Studies*, *42*, 823–835. Evidence Level I: Systematic Review.

Eustice, S., Roe, B., & Paterson, J. (2005). Prompted voiding for the management of urinary incontinence in adults. *The Cochrane Database of Systematic Reviews*, Issue 2. Art. No.: CD002113. DOI: 10.1002/14651858.DC002113. Evidence Level I: Systematic Review.

Fantl, A., Newman, D. K., Colling, J., DeLancey, J. O. L., Keeys, C., & Loughery, R. (1996). *Urinary incontinence in adults: Acute and chronic management*. Agency for Health Care Policy and Research, Publication No. 92-0047: Rockville, MD. Evidence Level I: CPCG Based on Systematic Review.

Flynn, L., Cell, P., & Luisi, E. (1994). Effectiveness of pelvic muscle exercises in reducing urge incontinence among community-residing elders. *Journal of Gerontological Nursing*, *20*(5), 23–27. Evidence Level IV: Nonexperimental Study.

Gray, M. (2005). Assessment and management of urinary incontinence. *The Nurse Practitioner*, *30*(7), 32–41. Evidence Level VI: Journal Article.

Gray, M. I. (2000). Physiology of voiding. In D. B. Dougherty (Ed.), *Urinary and fecal incontinence. Nursing management* (2nd ed.). St. Louis, MO: Mosby. Evidence Level V: Review.

Gray, M. L., & Haas, J. (2000). Assessment of the patient with urinary incontinence. In D. B. Dougherty (Ed.), *Urinary and fecal incontinence: Nursing management* (2nd ed.). St. Louis, MO: Mosby. Evidence Level VI: Expert Opinion.

Gray, M., Rayome, R., & Moore, K. (1995). The urethral sphincter: An update. *Urologic Nursing*, *15*, 40–53. Evidence Level VI: Journal Article.

Harmer, B., & Henderson, V. (1955), *Textbook of the principles and practice of nursing* (5th Ed.). New York: Macmillan Publishing Co.

Harper, C. M., & Lyles, Y. M. (1988). Physiology and complications of bed rest. *Journal of the American Geriatrics Society, 36*, 1047–1054. Evidence Level V: Narrative Literature Review.

Hay-Smith, E. J. C., & Dumoulin, C. (2006). Pelvic floor muscle training versus no treatment, or inactive control treatments, for urinary incontinence in women. *The Cochrane Database of Systematic Reviews*, Issue 1. Art. No.: CD005654. DOI: 10.1002/14651858.CD005654. Level Evidence I: Systematic Review.

Hay-Smith, J., Herbison, P., & Morkved, S. (2002). Physical therapies for prevention of urinary and faecal incontinence in adults (review). *The Cochrane Database of Systematic Reviews*, Issue 2. Art. No.: CD003191. DOI: 10.1002/14651858.CD003191. Level Evidence I: Systematic Review.

Henderson, V., & Nite, G. (1978). *Principles and practice of nursing* (6th ed.). New York: Macmillan Publishing Co., Inc.

Herzog, A. R., & Fultz, N. (1990). Prevalence and incidence of urinary incontinence in community-dwelling populations. *Journal of the American Geriatrics Society, 38*, 273–281. Evidence Level V: Narrative Literature Review.

Hodgkinson, C. P. (1965). Stress urinary incontinence in the female. *Surgery, Gynecology & Obstetrics, 120*, 595–613. Evidence Level V: Narrative Literature Review.

Holroyd-Leduc, J. M., Mehta, K. M., & Covinsky, K. E. (2004). Urinary incontinence: An association with death, nursing home admission, and functional decline. *Journal of the American Geriatrics Society, 52*, 712–718. Evidence Level I: Systematic Review.

Holroyd-Leduc, J., M., & Straus, S. E. (2004). Management of urinary incontinence in women. *Journal of the American Medical Association: Scientific Review, 291*(8), 986–995. Evidence Level I: Systematic Review.

Hunter, K. F., Moore, K. N., Cody, D. J., & Glazener, M. A. (2005). Conservative management for postprostatectomy urinary incontinence. *The Cochrane Database of Systematic Reviews*, Issue 2. No.: CD001843.pub2. DOI: 10.1002/14651858.CD001843.pub2. Evidence Level I: Systematic Review.

International Consultation on Incontinence (ICI) (2000). Assessment and treatment of urinary incontinence. *Lancet, 355*, 2153–2158. Evidence Level VI: Respected Experts.

Jain, P., Parada, J. P., & Smith, L. G. (1995). Overuse of the indwelling urinary tract catheter in hospitalized medical patients. *Archives of Internal Medicine, 155*(13), 1425–1429. Evidence Level IV: Nonexperimental Study.

Jeter, K. F., & Wagner, D. B. (1990). Incontinence in the American home. *Journal of the American Geriatrics Society, 38*(3), 379–383. Evidence Level IV: Nonexperimental Study.

Jeyaseelan, S. M., Roe, B. H., & Oldham, J. A. (2000). The use of frequency/volume charts to assess urinary incontinence. *Physical Therapy Reviews, 5*(3), 141–146. Evidence Level I: Systematic Review.

Jirovec, M. M. (2000). Functional incontinence. In D. B. Dougherty (Ed.), "Urinary & fecal incontinence nursing management (2nd ed., pp. 145–157). St. Louis: Mosby. Evidence Level VI: Expert Opinion.

Jirovec, M. M., Brink, C. A., & Wells, T. J. (1988). Nursing assessments in the inpatient geriatric population. *Nursing Clinics of North America, 23*, 219–230. Evidence Level VI: Journal Article.

Jirovec, M. M., Wyman, J. F., & Wells, T. J. (1998). Addressing urinary incontinence with educational continence-care competencies. *Image: The Journal of Nursing Scholarship, 30*, 375–378. Evidence Level VI: Journal Article.

Johnson, M., Bulechek, G., McCloskey-Dochterman, J., Maas, M., & Moorhead, S. (2001). *Nursing Diagnoses, Outcomes, and Interventions: NANDA, NOC, and NIC Linkages*. St. Louis, MO: Mosby. Evidence Level VI: Expert Opinion.

Johnson, T. M., Kincade, J. E., Shulamit, L., Busby-Whitehead, J., Hertz-Picciotto, I., & DeFriese, G. H. (1998). The association of urinary incontinence with poor self-related health. *Journal of the American Geriatrics Society, 46*, 693–699. Evidence Level IV: Nonexperimental Study.

Kane, R., Ouslander, J., & Abrass, I. (2004). *Essentials of clinical geriatrics* (5th ed.). New York: McGraw-Hill. Evidence Level VI: Expert Opinion.

Kegel, A. H. (1956). Stress incontinence of urine in women: Physiologic treatment. *International College of Surgeons, 25*, 487–499. Evidence Level VI: Expert Opinion.

Kinchen, K., Burgio, K., Diokno, A., Fultz, N. H., Bump, R., & Obenchain, R. (2003). Factors associated with women's decisions to seek treatment for urinary incontinence. *Journal of Women's Health, 12,* 687–697. Evidence Level IV: Nonexperimental Study.

Kozier, B., Erb, G., Berman, A., & Snyder, S. (2004). *Fundamentals of nursing concepts, process, and practice* (7th ed.). Upper Saddle River, NJ: Prentice Hall. Evidence Level VI: Expert Opinion.

Kresvic, D. M. (1997). New-onset urinary incontinence among hospitalized elders. Doctoral dissertation, Case Western Reserve University, 1997, UMI No. 9810934. Evidence Level IV: Nonexperimental Study.

LeBlanc, K., & Christensen, D. (2005). Addressing the challenge of providing nursing care for elderly men suffering from urethral erosion. *Journal of Wound, Ostomy Nurses Society, 32*(2), 131–134. Evidence Level V: Case Report.

Lemack, G. E., & Zimmern, P. E. (1999). Predictability of urodynamic findings based on the Urogenital Distress Inventory-6 questionnaire. *Urology, 54,* 461–466. Evidence Level IV: Nonexperimental Study.

Madigan, E., & Neff, F. F. (2003). Care of patients with long-term indwelling urinary catheters. *Online Journal of Issues in Nursing, 8*(3). Retrieved February 6, 2007, from http://www.nursingworld.org/ojin/hirsh/topic2/tpc2_1.htm. Evidence Level I: Systematic Review.

McDowell, B. J., Engberg, S., Sereika, S., Donovan, N., Jubeck, M. E., Weber, E., et al. (1999). Effectiveness of behavioral therapy to treat incontinence in homebound older adults. *Journal of the American Geriatrics Society, 47,* 309–318. Evidence Level II: Single RCT.

McGann, P. (2000). Co-morbidity in heart failure in the elderly. *Clinical Geriatric Medicine, 16,* 631–648. Evidence Level VI: Journal Article.

Meijer, R., Ihnenfeldt, D. S., de Groot, I. J. M., van Limbeek, J., Vermeulen, M., & de Haan, R. J. (2003). Prognostic factors for ambulation and activities of daily living in the subacute phase after stroke. A systematic review of the literature. *Clinical Rehabilitation, 17,* 119–129. Evidence Level I: Systematic Review.

Miller, Y. D., Brown, W. J., Smith, N., & Chiarelli, P. (2003). Managing urinary incontinence across the lifespan. *International Journal of Behavioral Medicine, 10*(2), 143–162. Evidence Level IV: Nonexperimental Study.

Milne, J. (2000). The impact of information on health behaviors of older adults with urinary incontinence. *Clinical Nursing Research, 9,* 161–176. Evidence Level IV: Nonexperimental Study.

Mitteness, L. S. (1987a). The management of urinary incontinence by community-living elderly. *The Gerontologist, 27*(2), 185–193. Evidence Level IV: Nonexperimental Study.

Mitteness, L. S. (1987b). So what do you expect when you're 85?: Urinary incontinence in late life. In J. A. Roth & P. Conrad (Eds.), *Research in the sociology of health care, Vol. 6* (pp. 177–219). Greenwich, CT: JAI Press, Inc. Evidence Level IV: Nonexperimental Study.

National Association for Continence (December 4, 1998). *Release of findings from consumer survey on urinary incontinence: Dissatisfaction with treatment continues to rise.* Spartansburg, SC: Author. Evidence Level IV: Nonexperimental Study.

Ostaszkiewicz, J., Johnston, L., & Roe, B. (2004). Timed voiding for the management of urinary incontinence in adults. *The Cochrane Database of Systematic Reviews (Protocol),* Issue Art. No.: CD002802. DOI: 10.1002/14651858. CD002802.pub2. Evidence Level I: Systematic Review.

Palmer, M. H. (1988). Urinary incontinence: The magnitude of the problem. *Nursing Clinics of North America, 23*(1), 139–157. Evidence Level V: Literature Review.

Palmer, M. H. (1996). *Urinary continence: Assessment and promotion.* Gaithersburg, MD: Aspen. Evidence Level VI: Expert Opinion.

Palmer, M. H. (2004). Use of health behavior change theories to guide urinary incontinence research. *Nursing Research, 53*(6S), S49–S55. Evidence Level VI: Journal Article.

Palmer, M., Baumgarten, M., Langenberg, P., & Carson, J. L. (2002). Risk factors for hospital-acquired incontinence in elderly female hip-fracture patients. *Journal of Gerontology, 10,* M672–M677. Evidence Level IV: Nonexperimental Study.

Palmer, M. H., Bone, L. R., Fahey, M., Mamom, J., & Steinwachs, D. (1992). Detecting urinary incontinence in older adults during hospitalization. *Applied Nursing Research, 5,* 174–180. Evidence Level IV: Nonexperimental Study.

Palmer, M. H., Myers, A. H., & Fedenko, K. M. (1997). Urinary continence changes after hip-fracture repair. *Clinical Nursing Research, 6*, 8–24. Evidence Level IV: Nonexperimental Study.

Reilly, L., Sullivan, P., Ninni, S., Fochesto, D., Williams, K., & Fetherman, B. (2006). Reducing Foley catheter device days in an intensive care unit: Using the evidence to change practice. *Advanced Critical Care, 17*(3), 272–283. Evidence Level V: Program Evaluation Data.

Resnick, N. M., & Ouslander, J. G. (1990). Urinary incontinence: Where do we stand and where do we go from here. *Journal of the American Geriatrics Society, 38*, 264–265. Evidence Level VI: Journal Article.

Robinson, J. P., & Shea, J. A. (2002). Development and testing of a measure of health-related quality of life for men with urinary incontinence. *Journal of the American Geriatrics Society, 50*, 935–945. Evidence Level IV: Nonexperimental Study.

Saint, S., Kaufman, S. R., Rogers, M. A. M., Baker, P. D., Ossenkop, K., & Lipsky, B. A. (2006). Condom versus indwelling urinary catheters: A randomized trial. *Journal of the American Geriatrics Society, 54*, 1055–1061. Evidence Level II: RCT Experimental Study.

Sampselle, C. M. (1999). Pelvic-floor muscle training was the most effective conservative treatment for genuine stress urinary incontinence. *Evidence-Based Obstetrics & Gynecology, 1*, 113. Evidence Level VI: Journal Article/Expert Opinion.

Sampselle, C. M., Palmer, M. H., Boyington, A. R., O'Dell, K. K., & Wooldridge, L. (2004). Prevention of urinary incontinence in adults. *Nursing Research, 53*, S61–S67. Evidence Level VI: Journal Article.

Schnelle, J. F., Cadogoan, M. P., Grbic, D., Bates-Jensen, B. M., Osterweil, D., Yoshii, J., et al. (2003). A standardized quality assessment system to evaluate incontinence in the nursing home. *Journal of the American Geriatrics Society, 51*, 1754–1761. Evidence Level IV: Nonexperimental Study.

Schultz, A., Dickey, G., & Skoner, M. (1997). Self-report of incontinence in acute care. *Urologic Nursing, 17*(1), 23–28. Evidence Level IV: Nonexperimental Study.

Shinopulos, N. (2000). Bedside urodynamic studies: Simple testing for urinary incontinence. *Nurse Practitioner, 25*(6), 19–25. Level Evidence VI: Expert Opinion.

Shumaker, S. A., Wyman, J. F., Uebersax, J. S., McClish, D., & Fantl, J. A. (1994). Health-related quality of life measures for women with urinary incontinence: The Incontinence Impact Questionnaire and the Urogenital Distress Inventory: Continence Program in Women (CPW). *Quality of Life Research, 3*, 291–306. Evidence Level IV: Nonexperimental Study.

Sier, H., Ouslander, J., & Orzeck, S. (1987). Urinary incontinence among geriatric patients in the acute care hospital. *Journal of the American Medical Association, 257*, 1767–1771. Evidence Level IV: Nonexperimental Study.

Skelly, J., & Flint, A. (1995). Urinary incontinence associated with dementia. *Journal of the American Geriatrics Society, 43*, 286–294. Evidence Level V: Literature Review.

Smith, D. A. (2000). Urge incontinence. In D. B. Dougherty (Ed.), *Urinary & fecal incontinence nursing management* (2nd ed., pp. 91–104). Mosby, MO: St. Louis. Evidence Level VI: Expert Opinion.

Subak, L. L., Whitcomb, E., Hui, S., Saxton, J., Vittinghoff, E., & Brown, J. S. (2005). Weight loss: A novel and effective treatment for urinary incontinence. *The Journal of Urology, 174*, 190–195. Evidence Level II: RCT.

Taylor, C., Lillis, C., & LeMone, P. (2005). *Fundamentals of nursing: The art and science of nursing care* (5th ed.). New York: Lippincott Williams & Wilkins. Evidence Level VI: Expert Opinion.

Terpenning, M. S., Allada, R., & Kauffaman, C. A. (1989). Intermittent urethral catheterization in the elderly. *Journal of the American Geriatrics Society, 37*, 411–416. Evidence Level IV: Nonexperimental Study.

Teunissen, T. A. M., deJonge, A., van Weel, C., & Lagro-Janssen, A. L. M. (2004). Treating urinary incontinence in the elderly: Conservative measures that work: a systematic review. *The Journal of Family Practice, 53*(1), 25–32. Evidence Level I: Systematic Review.

The Society of Urologic Nurses and Associates (SUNA) (2005). Clinical Practice Guideline: Care of the patient with an indwelling catheter. *Urologic Nursing, 26*(1), 80–81. Also available at http://www.medscape.com/viewarticle/525695. Level VI: Expert Opinion.

Thomas, L. H., Barrett, J., Cross, S., French, B., Leathley, M., Sutton, C., et al. (2005). Prevention and treatment of urinary incontinence after stroke in adults. *The Cochrane Database of*

Systematic Reviews, Issue 3. Art. No.: CD004462.pub2. DOI: 10.1002/14651858.CD004462. pub2. Evidence Level I: Systematic Review.

Uebersax, J. S., Wyman, J. F., Shumaker, S. A., McClish, D. K., & Fantl, J. A. (1995). Short forms to assess life quality and symptom distress for urinary incontinence in women: The Incontinence Impact Questionnaire and the Urogenital Distress Inventory. *Neurourology and Urodynamics, 14*, 131–139. Evidence Level IV: Nonexperimental Study.

Warren, J. W. (1997). Catheter-associated urinary tract infections. *Infectious Disease Clinics of North America, 11*(3), 609–622. Level VI: Journal Article.

Watson, N. M. (2005). Advancing quality of urinary incontinence evaluation and treatment in nursing homes through translational research. *Worldviews on Evidence-Based Nursing, 1*(Sl): S21–S25. Evidence Level VI: Journal Article

Watson, N. M., Brink, C. A., Zimmer, J. G., & Mayer, R. D. (2003). Use of the Agency for Health Care Policy and Research Urinary Incontinence Guideline in nursing homes. *Journal of the American Geriatrics Society, 51*, 1779–1786. Evidence Level IV: Nonexperimental Study.

Weiss, B. D. (1998). Diagnostic evaluation of urinary incontinence in geriatric patients. *American Family Physician, 57*(11). Retrieved February 6, 2007, from http://www.aafp.org/afp/980600ap/weiss.html. Evidence Level VI: Journal Article.

Wilson, L., Brown, J. S., Shin, G. P., Luc, K. O., & Suback, L. L. (2001). Annual direct cost of urinary incontinence. *Obstetrics and Gynecology, 98*(3), 398–406. Evidence Level IV: Nonexperimental.

Wolf, S. L., Riolo, L., & Ouslander, J. G. (2000). Urge incontinence and the risk of falling in older women. *Journal of the American Geriatrics Society, 48*, 847–848. Evidence Level VI: Respected Experts.

Wong, E. S. (1981). Guidelines for preventing catheter-associated urinary tract infections. *Centers for Disease Control.* Retrieved February 6, 2007, from http://www.cdc.gov/ncidod/dhqp/gl_catheter_assoc.html. Evidence Level VI: Expert Opinion.

Wound Ostomy Continence Nurse's Society (1996). Indwelling Catheter Fact Sheet. Retrieved February 6, 2007, from http://www.wocn.org/publications/facts/pdf/C_INDCAT.pdf. Evidence Level VI: Expert Opinion.

Wyman, J. F. (1997). The "costs" of urinary incontinence. *European Urology, 32* (Suppl.), 13–19. Evidence Level V: Literature Review.

Zimakoff, J., Stickler, D. J., Pontoppidan, B., & Larsen, S. O. (1996). Bladder management and urinary tract infections in Danish hospitals, nursing homes, and home care: A national prevalence study. *Infection Control and Hospital Epidemiology, 17*, 215–221. Evidence Level IV: Nonexperimental Study.

Mealtime Difficulties

14

Elaine J. Amella

Educational Objectives

On completion of this chapter, the reader should be able to:

1. assess older adults for critical issues related to performance at mealtimes: physical and cognitive functioning, resistance to eating, cultural/religious factors

2. modify the mealtime environment to one that promotes adequate intake and normalizes social interaction

3. educate staff and caregivers to provide individualized assistance at meals while preserving the independence and dignity of the person being assisted

Overview

Most health professionals realize the critical role nutrition plays in maintaining health and function in older adults; however, issues surrounding the ingestion of food may be ignored. An older adult's capacity to consume calories may rest on more than the correct mixture of macro- and micro-nutrients, but how, when, where, and with whom meals are taken may have a very strong influence. Factors that comprise the mealtime experience may be especially decisive when an

For a description of Evidence Levels cited in this chapter, see chapter 1, Developing and Evaluating Clinical Practice Guidelines, page 4

individual's mental status is compromised and/or acute disease is present. This chapter reviews issues that can lead to mealtime difficulties for older adults and presents evidence-based strategies to resolve them.

Background

Although maintenance of good nutrition is important throughout the life span, it is critical during older age, especially if chronic illness is present. A focus of *Healthy People* 2010 (U.S. Department of Health and Human Services [USDHHS], 2000) addresses the need to reduce chronic illness related to nutrition with objectives related to diabetes and heart disease; increasing the number of older adults who achieve a healthy weight; and increasing food security—that is, having adequate access and finances to acquire a healthy diet. Of the top ten causes of death (Minino, Heron, & Smith, 2006), a lifetime of good nutrition would positively improve nine causes: heart disease, cancer, stroke, chronic lower respiratory disease, diabetes, Alzheimer's disease, influenza/ pneumonia, nephritic syndrome/nephritis, and septicemia, with accidents (fifth in order) being the outlier (National Center for Health Statistics, 2006). Thus, a focus on nutrition is certainly warranted in the older population; however, one area that may be overlooked as a cause for nutritional problems is the process of how older people choose, prepare, serve, and ingest food, or how others do it for them—the phenomenon of meals. *Meal* is defined as "the food served and eaten, especially at one of the customary, regular occasions for taking food during the day, as breakfast, lunch, or supper; one of these regular occasions or times for eating food" (Flexner & Hauck, 1987, p. 1191). Meals are custom-driven and contextually based; even the time that food is eaten and what is eaten at each meal can be dictated by culture and habit.

Numerous cultural and religious rituals influence the way that food is consumed; thus, the meaning of food and the way it is shared often supplant the nutritional value of the calories consumed by individuals. Therefore, examining mealtime and food as merely an exercise necessary to acquire needed nutrients misses the critical social aspect of meals. However, persons entrusted with serving or assisting with meals often frame meals only in the context of nutritional requirements, examining those requirements only when an individual experiences unplanned outcomes, such as weight loss or gain. The professional nurse has historically played a critical role in the interdisciplinary team to assess and manage problems with nutrition and hydration for older adults; however, little attention has been paid to the context of meals and how food and fluid are presented in a manner that is in keeping with the ideals of individualized care.

Assessment of Problem

A standardized assessment instrument that evaluates nutrition, such as the Mini Nutritional Assessment (MNA®), which has been validated and is used widely in the community, institution, and acute care setting, has only one question that even indirectly deals with meals: "How many full meals does the patient eat daily?" The individual is then asked: "Do you normally eat breakfast, lunch, and dinner?" The following definition of a full meal is given: A full meal is defined as an eating occasion when the patient "sits down" to eat and consumes more than two items/dishes (Guigoz, Vellas, & Garry, 1997; MNA, 2005 [Level III]). An alternative assessment instrument that has been used exclusively in the community, SCREEN II, shows strong psychometrics but does not address contextual issues (Keller, Goy, & Kane, 2005 [Level III]). Assessment of the entire process of mealtimes has been compartmentalized by instruments to examine behavior of persons with dementia when being assisted (Edinburgh Feeding in Dementia Questionnaire [EdFED-Q], Watson, 1996 [Level III]); food complaints (Minimum Data Set, item K.4.a, Centers for Medicare & Medicaid [CMS], 2006); oral movements (Scale of Oral Functions in Feeding, Stratton, 1981 [Level III]); identifying feeding and mealtime behaviors (Screening Tool of Feeding Problems [STEP], Kuhn & Matson, 2002 [Level IV]); and functional ability during meals (Eating Behavior Scale; Tulley, Matrakas, Muir, & Musallam, 1997 [Level IV]). Although the MDS item is the mostly widely used because it administered to all residents of nursing homes in the United States, it was found to be inaccurate in 32% of cases (Simmons, Lim, & Schnelle, 2002 [Level IV]). Watson's EdFED-Q is the most widely tested in nursing home and community settings and has strong psychometrics: the ability to correctly measure what it is supposed to and to be consistent over time with different raters. Older adults should also be assessed for intake; the Meal Portion method has been shown as a valid method to estimate calories and protein when comparing estimates by various providers and weighing (Berrut et al., 2002 [Level III]). The Meal Portion method directs the person assisting at meals to break each food item served into quarters and record whether 0, 1/4, 1/2, or the whole portion is consumed. Then, using the meal recipes, total calories and nutrients consumed can be calculated. Notable among all these instruments, however, is lack of attention to the context of meals—that is, attributes of the setting and the persons who are assisting with meals. (See "Mealtime Difficulties" at www.ConsultGeriRN.org for MNA and EdFed. Also see the Resources in this chapter for more information on these and other assessment tools.)

As an individual ages, the likelihood of functional impairment increases. With increased frailty, loss of function follows a predictable pattern, with the ability to feed oneself the last activity of daily living (ADL) to be lost (Katz, Ford, Moskowitz, Jackson, & Jaffe, 1963 [Level IV]). The most recent national data on disability showed that 19.7% of all older adults (i.e., 65 years and older) are chronically disabled, with 3.1% of those living in the community requiring assistance with five to six ADLs (Federal Interagency Forum on Aging-Related Statistics, 2006 [Level IV]). Although self-feeding must be promoted for all persons for as long as possible, techniques for promotion of independence at mealtimes are often not used by both formal and informal caregivers, which reinforces dependence. Assessment of capacity for self-feeding is essential to promote independence and integrity at meals; referral to an occupational therapist is essential (see also chapter 3, *Assessment of Function*).

Different religious beliefs may have strict requirements for preparation and blessing of food before it can be consumed (Bermudez & Tucker, 2004 [Level IV]). Individuals who follow dietary restrictions for religious reasons may not eat when religious rules have not been observed. In general, most cultures promote the washing of hands before meals; this may not be offered in institutional settings. Older adults who have serious chronic illness should be consulted regarding preferences for food and fluid intake. If it is not already documented in an advance directive, they should be asked about their wishes regarding treatment with artificial nutrition and hydration. If an older adult loses the capacity for decision making, the proxy for health care decisions should be consulted rather than the provider assuming responsibility for the management of nutritional care (see chapter 23, *Health Care Decision Making*, and chapter 24, *Advance Directives*).

Interventions and Care Strategies

Nutritional Health

Assessment and management of nutritional health is discussed in chapter 15, *Nutrition*; therefore, the reader is referred to that chapter. However, professional nurses are reminded that nutritional health is best assessed and managed through an interdisciplinary approach because it is a multifaceted issue. Minimally, the dietician, provider (e.g., physician, nurse practitioner), dentist, speech and language pathologist, occupational therapist, and patient/caregiver should be consulted when designing a nutritional plan of care.

Cognitive Impairments

Cognitive deficits impair the ability to eat and drink. People with severe cognitive impairments may develop refuse-like or aversive behavior that affect their ability to be assisted at meals (Amella, 2002 [Level IV]). Watson (1996) developed a psychometrically sound instrument, the ED-FedQ, to measure the declining ability to consume food offered related to resistance. Nurses can use the principles of this instrument to determine the stage of resistive eating behavior. In the earlier stages, more active behaviors are displayed (e.g., the individual pushes food away or turns his or her head away from the feeder). In later stages, passive behaviors occur, as the patient does not swallow and allows food to fall from his or her mouth. In late-stage dementia, a primitive and less forceful swallow pattern may develop. The upper airway is not well protected, making the use of bottle or syringe-type feeding not only undignified but also ineffective and unsafe. (See the Resources section for access to this tool.)

Increasing Intake

Obesity is a growing problem among older adults (Centers for Disease Control and Prevention [CDC], 2003 [Level V]); however, inadequate intake resulting in undernutrition continues to be a principal concern for clinicians caring for older adults. Several factors have been shown to influence intake, including psychosocial causes and context (i.e., where they ate and with whom). Eating alone or without social engagement decreases intake (Beck & Ovesen, 2003 [Level IV]) along with feeling anxious, mildly depressed, and angry (Paquet,

St. Arnaud-McKenzie, Kergoat, Ferland, & Dube, 2003 [Level IV]). Taylore and Barr report that eating smaller, more frequent meals increases intake of fluids; however, it does not increase food intake (2006 [Level IV]), nor does an exercise and scheduled toileting program (Simmons & Schnelle, 2004 [Level III]). Eating in the dining room increased total consumption of calories but did not influence intake of protein, nor did it influence weight gain (Wright, Hickson, & Frost, 2006 [Level III]). Keller (2006 [Level IV]) reported that a Meals on Wheels program increased intake as well as decreased self-reported depression.

Feeding Assistance and Staff Training

Lack of staff assistance and inadequate education of caregivers who are responsible for delivering, serving, and actively assisting at meals have been shown to place institutionalized older residents at risk for mealtime problems. Mealtimes are one of the most time-consuming ADLs and is unfortunately not reimbursed at the required levels. Simmons and Schnelle (2006 [Level IV]) reported in an observational study that residents with low intake required 35 to 40 minutes of staff assistance despite their level of dependency, which does not reflect the current level of federal funding for this ADL. This issue of reimbursed staff time to assist with eating may be linked to other institutional findings, such as less consumption of food by nursing home residents who ate in bed, with staffing levels the most powerful predictor of time in bed (Bates-Jensen, Schnelle, Alessi, Al Samarri, & Levy-Storm 2004 [Level IV]). When surveyed, nursing assistants and licensed nurses identified lack of time and training, as well as "working short staffed," as being related to residents not receiving enough food (Crogan, Shutz, Adams, & Massey, 2001 [Level IV]). Strategies that produced better mealtime outcomes included "meal rounds" by a dietician and food-service supervisors working with unit staff, which allowed for early identification of residents at risk for nutritional problems and early intervention, especially those with dysphagia and those needing assistance at meals (Keller, Gibbs-Ward, Randall-Simpson, Bocock, & Dimou, 2006 [Level IV]). When nursing assistants were trained in feeding skills and the residents they assisted using those improved strategies were then evaluated using the EdFED-Q, the residents receiving the new strategies had better eating behavior and were given more time to eat (Chang & Lin, 2005 [Level IV]).

Environment and Interaction

Because of the strong social and cultural components of eating, where one dines is sometimes as important as what one eats. Nurses should simply ask themselves, "Would I want to eat my next meal where this person is eating?" If the answer is no, then steps should be taken to improve the dining environment. Small changes in the dining environment may make large improvements in a patient's capacity and motivation to eat or be fed. Unfortunately, in institutions, the mealtime experience is often determined more by the living arrangements rather than individual needs (Synder & Fjellstrom, 2005 [Level IV]).

Gibbs-Ward and Keller (2005 [Level IV]) reiterated this theme in their grounded-theory approach to discovering what made mealtimes better, finding that several factors emerged as critical to older adults: each mealtime was seen as a unique process; residents are central to the process through their actions, not only at meals but also during the time surrounding meals, such as socializing while waiting; and internal and external influences affect meals, with the ideal being individualized care. The individualized nature of meals was reflected in interviews with nursing home residents who described the meaning of food and food service during their lifetime and how that changed once they were institutionalized. These interviews reflected themes of Remembering our Roots, Relating to Others, and Giving Life, with residents yearning for personalized attention to preferences and sharing traditional foods (Evans, Crogan, & Shultz, 2005 [Level IV]). When attempting to quantify "appetite," Wikby and Fagerskiold (2004 [Level IV]) found that internal factors such as mood and personal values, as well as external factors regarding the food, environment, and social interactions, directly affected appetite for residents. External factors such as decreased noise, increased lighting, and relaxing music at meals positively influenced residents' mealtime behavior (Hick-Moore, 2005 [Level III]; McDaniel, Hunt, Hackes, & Pope, 2001 [Level III]). Using contrasting colors (foreground/ background) in tableware and tablecloths and placing dishes in similar positions may help persons with low vision be more independent (Ellexson, 2004 [Level VI]. Proper positioning using an appropriate, supportive chair promotes good eating posture (Rappl & Jones, 2000 [Level V]). Family dining was shown to be an effective way to increase body weight and fine motor function in a randomized control trial involving 178 residents (Nijs, deGraaf, Kok, & vanStaveren, 2006 [Level II]) and modestly improved communication among residents with dementia during meals (Altus, Engelman, & Mathews, 2002 [Level III]). Denmark has modified the living environment within its nursing homes to a "stay-and-living environment," where meals are eaten in small groups—much like family dining, residents assist in choosing the menu and take part in meal preparation (Kofod & Birkemose, 2004 [Level IV]). Results of this change in mealtime patterns in four homes were mixed: the Body Mass Index (BMI) was similar to national norms for the institutionalized age; the attempts at increased socialization and control over food preparation and menu made little difference to those older adults interviewed, whereas the staff believed that conditions were much improved. The researchers felt that in this altered context, it was still the staff responsibility to create the ambience of shared meals within an institution (Kofod & Birkemose, 2004 [Level IV]). Unfortunately, nurses may be unaware of the lack of social interaction between residents and staff, and this time may become bereft of former patterns that gave meaning to meals for residents (Pearson, Fitzgerald, & Nay, 2003 [Level IV]; Stabell, Eide, Solheim, Solberg, & Rustoen, 2004 [Level IV]). Above all, dining is a shared experience. Successful completion of the meal is dependent on who assists or feeds the patient and the interpersonal process that person uses to interact with the patient (Amella, 2002, 1999 [both Level IV]). Caregivers who are able to let the patient set the tempo of the meal and allow others to make choices will be more effectual in increasing intake. These studies point to a need to individualize mealtimes for people in institutions, and the responsibility for assuring that that occurs rests with a sensitive and well-trained staff.

Case Study and Discussion

Mrs. Simpson is an 84-year-old female who is admitted to a short-stay skilled nursing unit within a hospital with the following diagnoses: poorly controlled Type II diabetes, heart failure (Stage C), and moderate-stage dementia with deterioration in mental status since admission. Her medications now include a short-acting oral antidiabetic agent that is given at mealtimes (i.e., repaglidine), loop diuretic, ACE inhibitor (i.e., fosinopril), beta-blocker (i.e., bisoprolol), and aldosterone antagonist (i.e., spironolactone). Medications can cause a decrease in appetite, so Mrs. Simpson needs to have a side-effect profile for all drugs developed by the pharmacologist. Mrs. Simpson's appetite declined while hospitalized and she experience two episodes of hypoglycemia when she received her oral agent at breakfast and then did not eat well at lunch and supper. Since then she was placed on repaglinide. She was placed on this short-stay unit before returning to her daughter's home so that a plan of care could be developed for a safe discharge. The staff notes that Mrs. Simpson tires easily when seated in a chair, so they have been serving her meals in bed. Her tolerance for any exercise is decreasing as she becomes more deconditioned. Additionally, since admission, she is more agitated at night and has been getting out of bed calling for her daughter. During the day, she sleeps and thus shows even less interest in eating. The physician is considering inserting a PEG tube until her medical condition stabilizes. Mrs. Simpson is a member of the Seventh Day Adventist church.

Mrs. Simpson has several issues that require close monitoring, first of which are her two severe chronic illnesses: diabetes and heart failure. Both conditions must be medically managed before discharge can be attempted. However, those illnesses in conjunction with her dementia are causing her to have unmet nutritional needs that could be addressed by careful assessment and interventions.

Initially, the nurse should observe Mrs. Simpson during each meal during the course of the day, noting whether her capacity to eat fluctuates across the day and if she would benefit from progressive assistance. Because she has dementia, the nurse can quantify her mealtime behaviors with the EdFED-Q to see if she is resisting meals or is unable to complete the process of ingestion without regular cues and prompts. Consultation with the entire health care team, including the provider, speech and language pathologist, dietician, dentist, occupational therapist, clergy, and social worker, is warranted to assure that any unmet needs are addressed, such as adequacy of diet; problems with food consistency and swallowing; requirements for adaptive equipment; a vegetarian diet that adheres to her religious tenets, with increased whole grains, fruits, and water instead of fruit juice; adequate oral health; and assistants who are knowledgeable about the effects of her illness.

Daily activities could be structured so that Mrs. Simpson is allowed to rest before meals and then is assisted to get out of bed while she eats. Aides to eating might include playing her favorite music and having someone present to assist if her strength wanes and to provide pleasant social interaction. Staff assisting should be alert for signs of dysphagia such as regular attempts to "clear" the throat or small coughs. When directly assisting, staff needs to follow Mrs. Simpson's tempo and not rush her. Using the evaluation from the EdFED-Q, the staff member can offer cues and prompts when needed. Encouraging family members to visit and eat with Mrs. Simpson may normalize the meal if there is not excessive distraction or noise. Other staff should also avoid performing tasks in the room while Mrs. Simpson is eating.

With more attention paid to the environment, the interaction, the varying need for assistance based on the patient's need at the time, and resolution of her medical problems, Mrs. Simpson's intake begins to improve. The family and church members bring foods she once enjoyed, and they are more confident they can manage her mealtimes and nutritional problems at home. The consultation order for a PEG tube is rescinded.

Summary

Inadequate use of evidence-based interventions as well as a lack of tested "bundled programs" that address multiple issues confronted during meals (e.g., staff, environment, food preferences) make recommendations difficult. The studies to date have methodological flaws and do not account for confounding factors that may alter results, as noted by Watson and Green (2006 [Level I]) in the only systematic review published on studies concerning feeding and dementia published between 1993 and 2003. As such, health professionals are left to examine trends across several studies and to note that certain interventions seem to make a difference in some settings: family-style dining, music at meals, and staff interaction with older adults made a difference in various outcomes, some of which were not robust. Clearly, a diagnosis based on careful assessment using instruments normed to this population, an interdisciplinary plan of care based on the lifelong preferences and patterns of the patient and the family, and the thoughtful training of caregivers, as well as allowing them adequate time to assist at meals, should be heartily recommended.

Resources

Assessment Tools MNA® *Mini-Nutritional Assessment* (2005). Retrieved January 20, 2007, from http://www.mna-elderly.com

Edinburgh Feeding in Dementia Questionnaire Watson, R. (1996). The Mokken scaling procedure (MSP) applied to the measurement of feeding difficulty in elderly people with dementia. *International Journal of Nursing Studies*, 33, 385–393.

To obtain copies for the SCREEN, contact: Dr. Heather Keller Family Relations & Applied Nutrition, University of Guelph hkeller@uoguelph.ca

Box 14.1

Nursing Standard of Practice Protocol: Assessment and Management of Mealtime Difficulties

I. GOAL: To maintain or improve nutritional intake at meals and provide a quality mealtime experience that fosters dignity and pleasure in eating, as well as respecting cultural and personal preferences, for as long as possible.

II. OVERVIEW
Guiding Principles

A. The adequate intake of nutrients is necessary to maintain physical and emotional health.
B. Mealtime is an opportunity not only to ingest nutrients but also to maintain critical social aspects of life.
C. The social components of meals will be observed, including mealtime rituals, cultural norms, and food preferences.
D. Persons will be encouraged and assisted to self-feed for as long as possible.
E. Persons dependent in eating will be assisted with dignity.
F. End-of-life decisions by the individual or his or her proxy regarding the provision or termination of food and fluid will be respected.
G. The quality of mealtime is an indicator of quality of life and care of an individual.

III. BACKGROUND

A. Definitions
   1. *Feeding* is "the process of getting the food from the plate to the mouth. It is a primitive sense without concern for social niceties" (Katz, Downs, Cash, & Grotz, 1970, p. 21).
   2. *Eating* is "the ability to transfer food from plate to stomach through the mouth" (Katz et al., 1970, p. 21). Eating involves the ability to recognize food, the ability to transfer food to the mouth, and the phases of swallowing.
   3. *Anorexia* is characterized by a refusal to maintain a minimally normal body weight (American Psychiatric Association, 1994, p. 539). May have physiological basis in the elderly.
   4. *Dehydration* is "a fluid imbalance caused by too little fluid taken in or too much fluid lost or both" (Weinberg & Minaker, 1995, p. 1552).
   5. *Dysphagia* is "an abnormality in the transfer of a bolus from the mouth to the stomach" (Groher, 1997, p. 1).

6. *Apraxia* is an inability to carry out voluntary muscular activities related to neuromuscular damage. As it relates to eating and feeding, it involves loss of the voluntary stages of swallowing or the manipulation of eating utensils.
7. *Agnosia* is the inability to recognize familiar items when sensory cuing is limited.

B. Etiology

Mealtime difficulties can have multiple causes from both physiological and psychological origins. Health professionals need to consider multiple etiologies and not assume that difficulties are related only to increased confusion from a cognitive decline.

1. Cognitive/neurological: Parkinson's disease; amyotrophic lateral sclerosis; dementia, especially Alzheimer's disease; stroke
2. Psychological: depression
3. Iatrogenic: lack of adaptive equipment; use of physical restraints that limit ability to move, position, or self-feed; improper chair or table surface or discrepancy of chair to table height; use of wheelchair in lieu of table chair; use of disposable dinnerware, especially for patients with cognitive or neuromuscular impairments

VI. PARAMETERS OF ASSESSMENT

A. Assessment of Older Adult and Caregivers
1. Rituals used before meals (e.g., handwashing and toilet use); dressing for dinner.
2. Blessings of food or grace, if appropriate.
3. Religious rites or prohibitions observed in preparation of food or before meal begins (e.g., Muslim, Jewish, and Seventh-Day Adventist; consult with pastoral counselor, if available).
4. Cultural or special cues: family history, especially rituals surrounding meals.
5. Preferences as to end-of-life decisions regarding withdrawal or administration of food and fluid in the face of incapacity, or request of designated health proxy; ethicist or social worker may facilitate process.

B. Assessment Instruments:
1. EdFED-Q for persons with moderate to late-stage dementia (Watson, 1996 [Level III]).
2. Katz Index of ADL for functional status (Katz et al., 1970 [Level III]).
3. Food diary/Meal Portion method (Berrut et al., 2002 [Level III]).

V. NURSING INTERVENTIONS

A. Environment
1. Dining or patient room: encourage older adult to eat in dining room to increase intake (Bates-Jensen et al., 2004 [Level IV]),

personalize dining room, no treatments or other activities occurring during meals, no distractions.

2. Tableware: use of standard dinnerware (e.g., china, glasses, cup and saucer, flatware, tablecloth, napkin) versus disposable tableware and bibs.

3. Furniture: older adult seated in stable arm chair; table-appropriate height versus eating in wheelchair or in bed (Rappl & Jones, 2000 [Level V]).

4. Noise level: environmental noise from music, caregivers, and television is minimal (McDaniel et al., 2001 [Level III]); personal conversation between patient and caregiver is encouraged.

5. Music: pleasant, preferred by patient (Hick-Moore, 2005 [Level III]; Watson & Green, 2006 [Level I]).

6. Light: adequate and nonglare-producing versus dark, shadowy, or glaring (McDaniel et al., 2001 [Level III]).

7. Contrasting background/foreground: use contrasting background and foreground colors with minimal design to aid persons with decreased vision (Ellexson, 2004 [Level IV]).

8. Odor: food prepared in area adjacent to or in dining area to stimulate appetite (Amella, 2004 [Level V]).

9. Adaptive equipment: available, appropriate, and clean; caregivers and/or older adult knowledgeable in use; occupational therapist assists in evaluation.

B. Caregiver/Staffing
1. Provide an adequate number of well-trained staff (Chang & Lin, 2005 [Level IV]; Crogan et al., 2001 [Level IV]).

2. Deliver an individualized approach to meals (Gibbs-Ward & Keller, 2005 [Level IV]; Synder & Fjellstrom, 2005 [Level IV]) including choice of food, tempo of assistance.

3. Position of caregiver relative to elder: eye contact; seating so caregiver faces elder patient in same plane (Amella, 2004 [Level V]).

4. Cueing: caregiver cues elder whenever possible with words or gestures (Simmons & Schnelle, 2006 [Level IV]).

5. Self-feeding: encouragement to self-feed with multiple methods versus assisted feeding to minimize time (Simmons & Schnelle, 2006 [Level IV]).

6. Mealtime rounds: interdisciplinary team to examine multifaceted process of meal service, environment, and individual preferences (Keller et al., 2006 [Level IV]).

VI. EVALUATION/EXPECTED OUTCOMES

A. Individual
1. Corrective and supportive strategies reflected in plan of care.
2. Quality of life issues emphasized in maintaining social aspects of dining.

3. Culture, personal preferences, and end-of-life decisions regarding nutrition respected.

B. Health Care Provider

1. System disruptions at mealtimes minimized.
2. Family and staff informed and educated to patient's special needs to promote safe and effective meals.
3. Maintenance of normal meals and adequate intake for the patient reflected in care plan.
4. Competence in diet assessment; knowledge of and sensitivity to cultural norms and preferences for mealtimes reflected in care plan.

C. Institution

1. Documentation of nutritional status and eating and feeding behavior meets expected standard.
2. Alterations in nutritional status, eating and feeding behaviors assessed and addressed in a timely manner.
3. Involvement of interdisciplinary team (geriatrician, advanced practice nurse [NP/CNS], dietitian, speech therapist, dentist, occupational therapist, social worker, pastoral counselor, ethicist) appropriate and timely.
4. Nutritional, eating, and/or feeding problems modified to respect individual preferences and cultural norms.
5. Adequate number of well-trained staff who are committed to delivering knowledgeable and individualized care.

VII. FOLLOW-UP MONITORING

A. Providers' competency to monitor eating and feeding behaviors.
B. Documentation of eating and feeding behaviors.
C. Documentation of care strategies and follow-up of alterations in nutritional status and eating and feeding behaviors.
D. Documentation of staffing and staff education; availability of supportive interdisciplinary team.

References

Altus, D. E., Engelman, K. K., & Mathews, R. M. (2002). Using family-style meals to increase participation and communication in persons with dementia. *Journal of Gerontological Nursing, 28*(9), 47–53. Evidence Level III: Quasi-experimental Study.

Amella, E. J. (1999). Factors influencing the amount of food consumed by nursing home residents with dementia. *Journal of the American Geriatrics Society, 47,* 879–885. Evidence Level IV: Nonexperimental Study.

Amella, E. J. (2002). Resistance at mealtimes for persons with dementia. *Journal of Nutrition, Health and Aging, 6*(2), 117–122. Evidence Level IV: Nonexperimental Study.

Amella, E. J. (2004). Feeding and hydration issues for older adults with dementia. *Nursing Clinics of North America, 39*(3), 607–623. Evidence Level V: Narrative Review.

American Psychiatric Association (1994). *Diagnostic and statistical manual of mental disorders* (4th ed.). Washington, DC: Author.

Bates-Jensen, B. M., Schnelle, J. F., Alessi, C. A., Al Samarri, N. R., & Levy-Storm, L. (2004). The effects of staffing on in-bed times of nursing home residents. *Journal of the American Geriatrics Society, 52*(6), 931–938. Evidence Level IV: Nonexperimental Study.

Beck, A. M., & Ovesen, L. (2003). Influence of social engagement and dining location on nutrtitional intake and body mass index of old nursing home residents. *Journal of Nutrition for the Elderly, 22*(4), 1–11. Evidence Level IV: Nonexperimental Study.

Bermudez, O. I., & Tucker, K. L. (2004). Cultural aspects of food choices in various communities of elders. *Generations, 28*(3), 22–27. Evidence Level IV: Nonexperimental Study.

Berrut, G., Favreau, A. M., Dizo, E., Tharreau, B., Poupin, C., & Gueringuili, M. (2002). Estimation of calorie and protein intake in aged patients: Validation of a method based on meal portions consumed. *Journals of Gerontology: Medical Science, 57*(1), M52–M56. Evidence Level III: Quasi-experimental Study.

Centers for Disease Control and Prevention (CDC) (2003). Public health and aging: Trends in aging—United States and worldwide. *Morbidity & Mortality Weekly Report, 52*(06), 101–106. Evidence Level V: Program Evaluation.

Centers for Medicare and Medicaid Services (CMS) (2006). *Minimum Data Set (MDS), Version 2.0.* Retrieved January 20, 2007, from http://www.cms.hhs.gov/NursingHomeQualityInits/downloads/MDS20MDSAllForms.pdf

Chang, C., & Lin, L. (2005). Effects of a feeding skills training program on nursing assistants and dementia patients. *Journal of Clinical Nursing, 14*(10), 1185–1192. Evidence Level IV: Nonexperimental Study.

Crogan, N. L., Shultz, J. A., Adams, C. E., & Massey, L. K. (2001). Barriers to nutrition care for nursing home residents. *Journal of Gerontological Nursing, 27*(12), 25–31. Evidence Level IV: Nonexperimental Study.

Ellexson, M. T. (2004). Access to participation: Occupational therapy and low vision. *Topics in Geriatric Rehabilitation, 20*(3), 154–172. Evidence Level IV: Nonexperimental Study.

Evans, B. C., Crogan, N. L., & Shultz, J. A. (2005). Innovations in long term care: The meaning of mealtimes: Connections to the social world of nursing homes. *Journal of Gerontological Nursing, 31*(2), 11–17. Evidence Level IV: Nonexperimental study.

Federal Interagency Forum on Aging-Related Statistics (2006). Older Americans update 2006: Key indicators of well-being. Retrieved January 21, 2007, from http://agingstats.gov/update2006/default.htm

Flexner, S. B., & Hauck, L. C. (Eds.) (1987). *The random house dictionary of the english language* (2nd ed., Unabridged). New York: Random House.

Gibbs-Ward, A. J., & Keller, H. H. (2005). Mealtimes as active processes in long term care. *Canadian Journal of Dietetic Practice and Research, 66*(1), 5–11. Evidence Level IV: Nonexperimental Study.

Groher, M. E. (1997). *Dysphagia: Diagnosis and management* (3rd ed.). Boston: Butterworth-Heinemann.

Guigoz, Y., Vellas, B., & Garry, P. J. (1997). Mini-Nutritional Assessment: A practical assessment tool for grading the nutritional state of elderly patients. In B. J. Vellas, P. J. Garry, & J. L. Albarede. (Eds.), *Facts, research and interventions in geriatrics: Nutrition in the elderly* (3rd ed., pp. 15–60). Evidence Level III: Quasi-experimental Study.

Hick-Moore, S. L. (2005). Relaxing music at mealtime in nursing homes: Effect on agitated patients with dementia. *Journal of Gerontological Nursing, 31*(12), 26–32. Evidence Level III: Quasi-experimental Study.

Katz, S., Downs, T. D., Cash, H. R., & Grotz, R. C. (1970). Progress in the development of the Index of ADL. *The Gerontologist, 10*(1), 20–30. Evidence Level IV: Quasi-experimental Study.

Katz, S., Ford, A. B., Moskowitz, R. W., Jackson, B. A., & Jaffe, M. W. (1963). The Index of ADL: A standardized measure of biological and psychological function. *Journal of the American Medical Association, 185*, 915–919. Evidence Level IV: Nonexperimental Study.

Keller, H. H. (2006). Meal programs improve nutritional risk: A longitudinal analysis of community-living seniors. *Journal of the American Dietetic Association, 106*(7), 1042–1048. Evidence Level IV: Nonexperimental Study.

Keller, H. H., Gibbs-Ward, A., Randall-Simpson, J., Bocock, M. A., & Dimou, E. (2006). Meal rounds: An essential aspect of quality nutrition services in long term care. *Journal of the American Medical Directors Association, 7*, 40–45. Evidence Level IV: Nonexperimental Study.

Keller, H. H., Goy, R., & Kane, S. L. (2005). Validity and reliability of SCREEN II (Seniors in the community: Risk evaluation for eating and nutrition, Version II). *European Journal of Clinical Nutrition, 59*(10), 1149–1157. Evidence Level III: Quasi-experimental Study.

Kofod, J., & Birkemose, A. (2004). Meals in nursing homes. *Scandinavian Journal of Caring Sciences, 18,* 128–134. Evidence Level IV: Nonexperimental Study.

Kuhn, D. E., & Matson, J. L. (2002). A validity study of the Screening Tool of Feeding Problems (STEP). *Journal of Intellectual & Developmental Disability, 27*(3), 161–167. Evidence Level IV: Nonexperimental Study.

McDaniel, J. H., Hunt, A., Hackes, B., & Pope, J. F. (2001). Impact of dining room environment on nutritional intake of Alzheimer's residents: A case study. *American Journal of Alzheimer's Disease and Other Dementias, 16*(5), 297–302. Evidence Level III: Quasi-experimental Study.

Minino, A. M., Heron, M. P., & Smith, B. L. (2006). Death: Preliminary data for 2004. In *National Vital Statistics Reports, 15*(19). Hyattsville, MD: National Center for Health Statistics.

MNA® *Mini-Nutritional Assessment* (2005). Retrieved January 20, 2007, from http://www.mna-elderly.com. Evidence Level III: Quasi-experimental Study.

National Center for Health Statistics (2006). *Deaths – Leading Causes*. Retrieved February 17, 2007, from http://www.cdc.gov/nchs/fastats/lcod.htm.

Nijs, K. A., deGraaf, C., Kok, F. J., & vanStaveren, W. A. (2006). Effect of family-style meals on quality of life, physical performance, and body weight of nursing home residents: Cluster randomized controlled trial. *British Medical Journal, 332*(7551), 1180–1184. Evidence Level II: RCT.

Paquet, C., St. Arnaud-McKenzie, D., Kergoat, M. J., Ferland, G., & Dube, L. (2003). Direct and indirect effects of everyday emotions on food intake of elderly patients in institutions. *The Journals of Gerontology: Medical Sciences, 58*(2), 153–158. Evidence Level IV: Nonexperimental Study.

Pearson, A., Fitzgerald, M., & Nay, R. (2003). Mealtimes in nursing homes. The role of nursing staff. *Journal of Gerontological Nursing, 29*(6), 40–47. Evidence Level IV: Nonexperimental Study.

Rappl, L., & Jones, D. A. (2000). Seating evaluation: Special problems and interventions for older adults. *Topics in Geriatric Rehabilitation, 16*(2), 63–72. Evidence Level V: Case Report.

Simmons, S. F., Lim, B., & Schnelle, J. F. (2002). Accuracy of minimum data set in identifying residents at risk for undernutrition: Oral intake and food complaints. *Journal of the American Medical Directors Association, 3*(3), 140–145. Evidence Level IV: Nonexperimental Study.

Simmons, S. F., & Schnelle, J. F. (2004). Effects of exercise and scheduled-toileting interventions on appetite and constipation in nursing home residents. *The Journal of Nutrition, Health & Aging, 8*(2), 116–121. Evidence Level III: Quasi-experimental Study.

Simmons, S. F., & Schnelle, J. F. (2006). Feeding assistance needs of long-stay nursing home residents and staff time to provide care. *Journal of the American Geriatric Society, 54*(6), 919–924. Evidence Level IV: Nonexperimental Study.

Stabell, A., Eide, H., Solheim, G. A., Solberg, K. N., & Rustoen, T. (2004). Nursing home residents' dependence and independence. *Journal of Clinical Nursing, 13*(6), 677–686. Evidence Level IV: Nonexperimental Study.

Stratton, M. (1981). Behavioral assessment scale of oral functions in feeding. *The American Journal of Occupational Therapy, 35*(11), 719–721. Evidence Level III: Quasi-experimental Study.

Synder, Y. M., & Fjellstrom, C. (2005). Food provision and meal situation in elderly care: Outcomes in different social contexts. *Journal of Nutrition and Dietetics, 18*(1), 45–52. Evidence Level IV: Nonexperimental Study.

Taylore, K. A., & Barr, S. I. (2006). Provision of small, frequent meals does not improve energy intake of elderly residents with dysphagia who live in extended-care facilities. *Journal of the American Dietetic Association, 106*(7), 1115–1118. Evidence Level IV: Nonexperimental Study.

Tulley, M. W., Matrakas, K. L., Muir, J., & Musallam, K. (1997). The Eating Behavior Scale: A simple method of assessing functional ability in patients with Alzheimer's Disease. *Journal of Gerontological Nursing, 23*(7), 9–15. Evidence Level IV: Nonexperimental Study.

U.S. Department of Health and Human Services (USDHHS) (2000). *Healthy People 2010* (Online). Retrieved from http://www.health.gov/healthypeople

Watson, R. (1996). The Mokken Scaling Procedure (MSP) applied to the measurement of feeding difficulty in elderly people with dementia. *International Journal of Nursing Studies, 33,* 385–393. Evidence Level III: Quasi-experimental Study.

Watson, R., & Green, S. M. (2006). Feeding and dementia: A systematic literature review. *Journal of Advanced Nursing, 54*(1), 86–94. Evidence Level I: Systematic Review.

Weinberg, A. D., & Minaker, K. L. (1995). Dehydration: Evaluation and management in older adults. Council on Scientific Affairs, American Medical Association. *Journal of the American Medical Association, 274*(19), 1552–1556.

Wikby, K., & Fagerskiold, A. (2004). The willingness to eat. *Scandinavian Journal of Caring Sciences, 18*(2), 120–127. Evidence Level IV: Nonexperimental Study.

Wright, L., Hickson, M., & Frost, G. (2006). Eating together is important: Using a dining room in an acute elderly medical ward increases energy intake. *Journal of Human Nutrition and Dietetics, 19*(1), 23–26. Evidence Level III: Quasi-experimental Study.

Nutrition

15

Rose Ann
DiMaria-Ghalili

Educational Objectives

At the completion of this chapter, the reader should be able to:

1. recognize factors that place an older adult at risk for malnutrition

2. discuss methods to screen and assess nutritional status in an older adult

3. utilize appropriate nursing interventions in a hospitalized older adult who is either at risk for malnutrition or has malnutrition

Overview

Nutritional status is the balance of nutrient intake, physiological demands, and metabolic rate (DiMaria-Ghalili, 2002 [Level IV]). Nutrition-related conditions in older adults include obesity and malnutrition. Recent data from the Health of the United States indicate that of the older adults sampled, 71% of women and 76% of men aged 65 to 74 and 60% of women and 67% of men aged 75 and older have a body mass index (BMI) greater than or equal 25 and are considered overweight (National Center for Health Statistics, 2005 [Level V]). Although obesity is a problem in older adults, malnutrition is of greater concern because

For a description of Evidence Levels cited in this chapter, see chapter 1, Developing and Evaluating Clinical Practice Guidelines, page 4

it can often be unrecognizable and impacts morbidity, mortality, and quality of life (Chen, Schilling, & Lyder, 2001 [Level V]). Malnutrition is also a precursor for frailty in older adults. Malnutrition in the elderly is defined as "faulty or inadequate nutritional status; undernourishment characterized by insufficient dietary intake, poor appetite, muscle wasting, and weight loss" (Chen et al., 2001 [Level V]). In older adults, malnutrition exists along the continuum of care (Furman, 2006 [Level VI]) because the prevalence of malnutrition is found in older adults in the community, acute care, and long term care settings. Older adults admitted to acute care settings from either the community or long term care settings may already be malnourished or may be at risk for the development of malnutrition during hospitalization. Therefore, it is imperative that acute care nurses carefully assess and monitor the nutritional status of older adults to identify the risk factors for malnutrition so that appropriate interventions are instituted in a timely fashion. The focus of this geronursing protocol is aimed at the discussion of nutrition in aging as it relates to risk factors, implications, and interventions for malnutrition in older adults. See standard of practice protocol Box 15.1.

Background and Statement of Problem

In the United States, 40% to 60% of hospitalized older adults are malnourished or at risk for malnutrition (Nutrition Screening Initiative, 2002 [Level V]). Malnutrition is also a global problem for the elderly in industrialized nations. For example, one in every five older adults admitted to the hospital in England was found to be malnourished (The Malnutrition Prevalence Group, 2000 [Level IV]). The major type of malnutrition in the elderly is protein-energy under nutrition, which is characterized by the presence of clinical (i.e., physical signs such as wasting, low BMI) and biochemical (i.e., albumin or other serum protein) evidence of insufficient intake (Beers, 2005 [Level VI]). Marasmus and kwashiorkor are two forms of protein-energy under nutrition. Marasmus is characterized by a marked depletion of muscle mass and fat stores; however, visceral protein levels and organ function are normal (Beers, 2005 [Level VI], Chen et al., 2001 [Level V]). Marasmic individuals look malnourished and cachetic and often have a history of weight loss. However, they have adapted to decreased nutrient intake and may be able to function fairly well unless exposed to additional metabolic stress. Due to their limited nutritional reserve, they can rapidly develop hypoalbuminemic malnutrition. Kwashiorkor is referred to more commonly as hypoalbuminemic malnutrition and is characterized by a loss of visceral protein (e.g., albumin, transferring, and prealbumin) and is often associated with edema. Patients with hypoalbuminemic malnutrition may look well nourished and not report a history of weight loss. This type of malnutrition typically develops when there is inadequate protein intake relative to the body's needs during a hypermetabolic state, such as in injury, infection, and draining wounds.

The risk factors for malnutrition in older adults are multifactorial and include dietary, economic, psychosocial, and physiological factors (DiMaria-Ghalili & Amella, 2005 [Level VI]). Dietary factors include little or no appetite (Carlsson, Tidermark, Ponzer, Soderqvist, & Cederholm, 2005 [Level II]; Reuben, Hirsch, Zhou, & Greendale, 2005 [Level II]; Saletti et al., 2005

[Level IV]), problems with eating or swallowing, eating inadequate servings of nutrients (Margetts, Thompson, Elia, & Jackson, 2003 [Level IV]), and eating fewer than two meals a day (Saletti et al., 2005 [Level IV]). Limited income may cause restriction in the number of meals or dietary quality of meals eaten per day (Souter & Keller, 2002 [Level IV]). Isolation is also a risk factor because older adults who live alone may lose their desire to cook due to loneliness, and appetite often decreases after the loss of a spouse (Shahar, 2001 [Level IV]). Impairment in functional status can place the elderly at risk for malnutrition because adequate functioning is needed to secure and prepare food. Difficulty in cooking is related to disabilities (Souter & Keller, 2002 [Level IV]) and disabilities can hinder the ability to prepare or ingest food (Saletti et al., 2005 [Level IV]). Chronic conditions can negatively influence nutritional intake (Margetts et al., 2003) as can cognitive impairment (Kagansky et al., 2005 [Level IV]). Psychological factors are known risk factors for malnutrition. For example, depression is related to unintentional weight loss (Morley, 2001 [Level V]; Thomas et al., 2002 [Level IV]). Furthermore, poor oral health (Saletti et al., 2005 [Level IV]) and xerostomia (i.e., dry mouth due to decreased saliva) can impair the ability to lubricate, masticate, and swallow food (Saletti et al., 2005). Antidepressants, antihypertensives, and bronchodilators can contribute to xerostomia (DiMaria-Ghalili & Amella, 2005 [Level VI]). Change in taste (e.g., from medications, nutrient deficiencies, or tastebud atrophy) can also alter nutritional intake (DiMaria-Ghalili & Amella, 2005).

Body composition changes in normal aging include increase in body fat, including visceral fat stores (Hughes et al., 2004 [Level IV]), and a decrease in lean body mass (Janssen, Heymsfield, Allison, Kotler, & Ross, 2002 [Level IV]). Furthermore, the low skeletal muscle mass associated with aging is related to functional impairment and physical disability (Janssen, Heymsfield, & Ross, 2002 [Level IV]).

The impact of malnutrition on the health of hospitalized older adults is well documented. In this population, malnutrition is related to prolonged hospital stay (Pichard et al., 2004 [Level IV]), increased risk for poor health status, recent hospitalization, and institutionalization (Margetts et al., 2003 [Level IV]). Additionally, low Mini Nutritional Assessment (MNA) scores are predictors of prolonged hospital stays and mortality (Kagansky et al., 2005 [Level IV]).

Assessment of Problem

Areas of nutritional status assessment in hospitalized older adults should focus on identification of malnutrition and risk factors for malnutrition. The MNA (Guigoz, Lauque, & Vellas, 2002 [Level V]) is a comprehensive two-level tool that can be used to screen and assess an older hospitalized patient for malnutrition by evaluating the presence of risk factors for malnutrition in this age group. The validity and reliability of the MNA for use in hospitalized older adults is well documented (Salva et al., 2004 [Level V]). If a patient scores less than 11 on the screen, then the assessment section should be completed in order to compute the Malnutrition Indicator Score. The screening section of the MNA is easy to administer and consists of six questions. The assessment section requires measurement of mid-arm muscle circumference and calf circumference. Although these anthropometric measurements are relatively easy to obtain using a tape measure, nurses may first require training in these procedures prior to incorporating the MNA as part of a routine nursing assessment. Protocols should be established to identify interventions to be implemented once the screening and assessment data are obtained, including consultation with a dietitian. (See www.ConsultGeriRN.org, *Assessing nutrition in older adults* [PDF file] for MNA, Nutrition topic; and Resources in this chapter.)

Additional assessment strategies include proper measurement of height and weight and a detailed weight history. Height should always be directly measured and never recorded via patient self-report. An alternative way to measuring standing height is knee-height (Salva et al., 2004 [Level V]). Knee-height calipers are relatively inexpensive to purchase and can be used for many patients. To obtain a knee-height measure, the patient must be supine and the left knee positioned at a 90-degree angle. Using the calipers, the measurement is taken from the heel to the anterior surface of thigh. Estimated height is then made by using the following formulas (Rombeau, Caldwell, Forlaw, & Guenter, 1989 [Level VI]):

$$\text{Men (cm)} = 6,419 - (0.04 \times \text{age}) + (2.02 \times \text{knee height in cm})$$

$$\text{Women (cm)} = 84.88 - (0.24 \times \text{age}) + (1.83 \times \text{knee height in cm})$$

Because this method to measure height in older adults is not frequently used in clinical practice, nurses would require training in the use of knee-height calipers. A calorie count or dietary intake analysis is a good way to quantify the type and amount of nutrients ingested during hospitalization (DiMaria-Ghalili & Amella, 2005 [Level VI]). Laboratory indicators of nutritional status include measures of visceral proteins such as serum albumin, transferrin, and prealbumin (DiMaria-Ghalili & Amella, 2005 [Level VI]). However, these visceral proteins are also negative acute-phase reactants and are decreased during a stressed state, limiting the ability to predict malnutrition in an acutely ill hospitalized patient. Nonetheless, albumin is a strong prognostic marker for morbidity and mortality in older hospitalized patients (Sullivan, Roberson, & Bopp, 2005 [Level IV]).

Interventions and Care Strategies

The nursing interventions outlined in the protocol focus on enhancing or promoting nutritional intake and range in complexity, from basic fundamental nursing care strategies to the administration of artificial nutrition via parenteral or enteral routes. Prior to initiating targeted nutritional interventions in a hospitalized older adult, it must first be determined if the older adult can't eat, shouldn't eat, or won't eat (American Society for Parenteral and Enteral Nutrition, 2002). One factor to consider is whether the gastrointestinal tract (starting with the mouth) is working properly without any functional, mechanical, or physiological alterations that would limit the ability to adequately ingest, digest, and/or absorb food. Also, it needs to be determined whether older adults have any chronic or acute health condition in which the normal intake of food is contraindicated or are they simply not eating or is their appetite decreased? If the gastrointestinal tract is functional and can be used to provide nutrients, then nutritional interventions should be targeted at promoting adequate oral intake.

Nursing care strategies focus on ways to increase food intake as well as ways to enhance and manage the environment to promote increased food intake. When functional or mechanical factors limit the ability to take in nutrients, nurses should obtain interdisciplinary consultations from speech therapists, occupational therapists, physical therapists, psychiatrists, and/or dietitians to collaborate on strategies that would enhance the ability of older adults to feed themselves or to eat. Oral nutritional supplementation has been shown to improve nutritional status in malnourished hospitalized older patients (Milne, Avenell, & Potter, 2006 [Level I]) and should be considered in those who are malnourished or at risk for malnutrition. When used, oral liquid nutritional supplements should be given at least 60 minutes prior to meals (Wilson, Purushothaman, & Morley, 2002 [Level IV]). Specialized nutritional support should be reserved for select situations. If the provision of nutrients via the gastrointestinal tract is contraindicated, then parenteral nutrition via the central or peripheral route should be initiated (American Society for Parenteral and Enteral Nutrition, 2002). If the gastrointestinal tract can be utilized, then nutrients should be delivered via enteral tube feeding (American Society for Parenteral and Enteral Nutrition, 2002). The exact location of the tube and type of feeding tube inserted depend on the disease state, length of time tube feeding is required, and risk for aspiration. Patients started on specialized nutritional support should be routinely reassessed for its continued need and transitioned to oral feeding when feasible. Also, advance directives, if not completed, should be addressed prior to initiating specialized nutritional support (see chapter 23, *Health Care Decision Making*, and chapter 24, *Advance Directives*).

Case Study and Discussion

Mrs. V. H. is a 75-year-old female admitted to the hospital with a myocardial infarction and is on a telemetry unit for further workup prior to coronary artery bypass grafting surgery. On admission, her standing height is 5 feet 8 inches and she weighs 140 pounds. Her BMI is 21.33. Her past medical history is significant for osteoarthritis. She describes herself as generally in good health up until she was admitted to the hospital. Medications include 400 mg of ibuprofen q 6 hours, prn. Mrs. V. H. is the primary caregiver for her 80-year-old husband, who has altered cognitive functioning and is bedridden after a stroke 3 years ago. She administers her husband's gastrostomy tube feedings and turns and positions her husband to prevent decubitus ulcers. She receives assistance from three times a week when a home health aide visits for 4 hours each visit. During this time, she is able to go shopping and run errands. She complained of being tired and lacking energy prior to admission. Her weight history is significant for a 10-pound weight loss in the past 3 months. Mrs. V. H. said she started taking oral energy drinks because she was often too tired to cook a complete dinner for herself and lacked energy and was concerned about weight loss. She reported regaining 2 pounds after taking three cans of an oral nutritional supplement per day for about 4 weeks. She reported having more strength after regaining some of her weight back. Although she is married and lives with her husband, she is isolated because she does not have any social support systems on which to rely. Her only living relative is a cousin who is 70 years old, lives 60 miles away, and visits twice a month. During the assessment, Mrs. V. H. continually complained of being physically exhausted from caring for her husband at home and being too tired to eat or cook a nutritious meal for herself. She is worried about how she will care for her husband upon discharge from surgery and hopes that she can recover in the same nursing home to which her husband was admitted.

Although Mrs. V. H. does not have any chronic conditions or functional limitations that may place her at risk for malnutrition, her social history is significant for risk. As the sole caregiver for her disabled husband, she is isolated and tired and has a decreased appetite. She reports a history of unintentional loss of 10 pounds in 3 months. Her MNA score of 7 is based on moderate loss of appetite, weight loss greater that 6.6 pounds during the last 3 months, goes out, has suffered an acute disease, no psychological problems, and has a BMI of 21.33. Because her score is below 11, she is at risk or malnutrition, and a complete assessment level of the MNA is performed. Her total MNA assessment score is 17.5, based on an assessment score of 10.5 and a screening score of 7.0, indicating that she is at risk for malnutrition. Her serum albumin on admission is within normal limits. Although she is on a regular diet, she only takes in about 50% of her meals. Oral nutritional supplements are ordered twice daily between meals. Consultations are obtained from the social worker, dietitian, and physical therapist.

Conclusion

Hospitalized older adults are at risk for malnutrition. Nurses should carefully assess and monitor the nutritional status of older hospitalized patients so that appropriate nutrition-related interventions can be implemented in a timely fashion.

Acknowledgment

This work is based on the geriatric nursing protocol series. See www.ConsultGeriRN.org, Nutrition topic.

Resources

American Dietetic Association

- White Paper: Public Policy Strategies for Nutrition and Aging
  http://www.eatright.org/cps/rde/xchg/ada/hs.xsl/advocacy_2849_ENU_
  HTML.htm
- Position Statement: Nutrition Across the Spectrum of Aging
  http://www.eatright.org/cps/rde/xchg/ada/hs.xsl/advocacy_1735_ENU_
  HTML.htm
- Position Statement: Liberalized Diets for Older Adults in Long Term Care
  http://www.eatright.org/ada/files/Liberalizednp.pdf

Drug–Nutrient Interactions

- U.S. Food and Drug Administration, National Consumers League
  http://vm.cfsan.fda.gov/~lrd/fdinter.html
- National Institutes of Health Clinical Center: Drug Nutrient Interactions
  http://clinicalcenter.nih.gov/ccc/patient_education/drug_nutrient/

Mini-Nutritional Assessment http://www.mna-elderly.com/
Nutrition in the Elderly http://www.ConsultGeriRN.org
Knee-Height Measurement Florida International University's long term
   care Institute Resource Materials http://www.fiu.edu/%7Enutreldr/
   LTC_Institute/materials/LTC_Products.htm#7

Regulatory/Authoritative Web Sites

- American Geriatrics Society
  http://www.americangeriatrics.org
- American Medical Directors Association: Resource Library
  http://www.amda.com/library/
- Centers for Medicare and Medicaid Services
  http://www.medicare.gov/Nursing/Campaigns/NutriCareAlerts.asp
- Practicing Physician Education in Geriatrics
  http://www.gericareonline.net/
- National Conference of Gerontological Nurse Practitioners: Home Page
  http://www.ncgnp.org
- National Gerontological Nursing Association: Home Page
  http://www.ngna.org/
- National Institutes of Health
  http://www.nlm.nih.gov/medlineplus/nutritionforseniors.html
- The Gerontological Society of America: Home Page
  http://www.geron.org/
- U.S. Department of Health and Human Services: Home Page
  http://www.hhs.gov/

Box 15.1

Nursing Standard of Practice Protocol: Nutrition in Aging

I. **GOAL:** Improvement in indicators of nutritional status in order to optimize functional status and general well-being and promote positive nutritional status.

II. **OVERVIEW:** Older adults are at risk for malnutrition, with 40% to 60% of hospitalized older adults malnourished or at risk for malnutrition.

III. **BACKGROUND**

   A. Definitions:
     1. *Malnutrition*: Any disorder of nutritional status, including disorders resulting from a deficiency of nutrient intake, impaired nutrient metabolism, or overnutrition.
     2. *Protein-energy under-nutrition*: The presence of clinical (i.e., physical signs such as wasting, low body mass index [BMI]) and biochemical (i.e., albumin or other serum protein) evidence of insufficient intake.
   B. Etiology and/or Epidemiology. Older adults are at risk for undernutrition due to dietary, economic, psychosocial, and physiological factors (DiMaria-Ghalili & Amella, 2005 [Level VI]).
     1. Dietary intake
       a. Little or no appetite (Carlsson et al., 2005 [Level II]; Reuben et al., 2005 [Level II]; Saletti et al., 2005 [Level IV])
       b. Problems with eating or swallowing (Margetts et al., 2003 [Level IV])
       c. Eating inadequate servings of nutrients (Margetts et al., 2003 [Level IV])
       d. Eating fewer than two meals a day (Saletti et al., 2005 [Level IV])
     2. Limited income may cause restriction in the number of meals eaten per day or dietary quality of meals eaten (Souter & Keller, 2002 [Level IV])
     3. Isolation
       a. Older adults who live alone may lose desire to cook because of loneliness (Shahar, 2001 [Level IV]).
       b. Appetite of widows decreases (Shahar, 2001 [Level IV]).
       c. Difficulty cooking due to disabilities (Souter & Keller, 2002 [Level IV]).
       d. Lack of access to transportation to buy food (DiMaria & Amella, 2005 [Level VI]).

4. Chronic Illness
   a. Chronic conditions can affect intake (Margetts et al., 2003 [Level IV]).
   b. Disability can hinder ability to prepare or ingest food (Saletti et al., 2005 [Level IV]).
   c. Depression can cause decreased appetite (Thomas et al., 2002 [Level IV]; Morley, 2001 [Level V]).
   d. Poor oral health (e.g., cavities, gum disease, and missing teeth) and xerostomia, or dry mouth, impairs ability to lubricate, masticate, and swallow food (Saletti et al., 2005 [Level IV]).
   e. Antidepressants, antihypertensives, and bronchodilators can contribute to xerostomia (dry mouth) (DiMaria-Ghalili & Amella, 2005 [Level VI]).
5. Physiological changes
   a. Decrease in lean body mass and redistribution of fat around internal organs lead to decreased caloric requirements (Hughes et al., 2004 [Level IV]; Janssen et al., 2002 [Level IV]).
   b. Change in taste (from medications, nutrient deficiencies, or tastebud atrophy) can also alter nutritional status (DiMaria-Ghalili & Amella, 2005 [Level VI]).

VI. PARAMETERS OF ASSESSMENT

A. General: During routine nursing assessment, any alterations in general assessment parameters that influence intake, absorption, or digestion of nutrients should be further assessed to determine if an older adult is as nutritional risk. These parameters include the following:
   1. Subjective assessment, including present history, assessment of symptoms, past medical and surgical history, and co-morbidities (University of Texas, School of Nursing, 2006, guideline)
   2. Social history(University of Texas, School of Nursing, 2006, guideline).
   3. Drug–nutrient interactions: Drugs can modify the nutrient needs and metabolism of older people. Restrictive diets, malnutrition, changes in eating patterns, alcoholism, and chronic disease with long-term drug treatment are some of the risk factors in elderly that place them at risk for drug–nutrient interactions (Boullata, 2004 [Level VI]). The U.S. Food and Drug Administration and National Institutes for Health have Internet resources for common drug–nutrient interactions.
   4. Functional limitations (Salva et al., 2004 [Level V]).
   5. Psychological status (Salva et al., 2004 [Level V]).
   6. Objective assessment: physical examination with emphasis on oral exam (see chapter 17, *Oral Health Care*), loss of subcutaneous fat, muscle wasting, BMI (University of Texas, School of Nursing, 2006, guideline) and dysphagia.

B. Dietary Intake: in-depth assessment of dietary intake during hospitalization may be documented with a 3-day calorie count (dietary intake analysis) (DiMaria-Ghalili & Amella, 2005 [Level VI]).

C. Risk Assessment Tool: The MNA should be administered to determine if an older hospitalized patient is either at risk for malnutrition or has malnutrition. The MNA determines risk based on food intake, mobility, BMI, history of weight loss, psychological stress, or acute disease and dementia or other psychological conditions. If the score is 11 points or less, the in-depth MNA assessment should be administered (DiMaria-Ghalili & Amella, 2005 [Level VI]; Salva et al., 2004 [Level V]). See the Resources section for the MNA tool or www.ConsultGeriRN.org, Nutrition topic.

D. Anthropometry
   1. Obtain an accurate weight and height through direct measurement. Do not rely on patient recall. If patient cannot stand erect to measure height, then knee-height measurements should be taken to estimate height using special knee-height calipers. Height should never be estimated or recalled, due to shortening of the spine with advanced age; self-reported height may be off by as many as 2.4 cm (DiMaria-Ghalili & Amella, 2005 [Level VI]; Salva et al., 2004 [Level V]).
   2. Weight history: A detailed weight history should be obtained along with current weight. Detailed history should include a history of weight loss, whether the weight loss was intentional or unintentional, and during what period. A loss of 10 pounds during a 6-month period, whether intentional or unintentional, is a critical indicator for further assessment (DiMaria-Ghalili & Amella, 2005 [Level VI]; National Collaborating Centre for Acute Care, 2005, guideline).
   3. Calculate BMI to determine if weight for height is within the normal range of 22–27. A BMI below 22 is a sign of under-nutrition. (National Collaborating Centre for Acute Care, 2005, guideline; Nutrition Screening Initiative, 2002 [Level V]).

E. Visceral Proteins. Serum albumin, transferrin, and prealbumin are visceral proteins commonly used to assess and monitor nutritional status (DiMaria-Ghalili & Amella, 2005 [Level VI]). However, these proteins are negative acute-phase reactants; therefore, during a stress state, production is usually decreased. In an older hospitalized patient, albumin levels may be a better indicator of prognosis than nutritional status (Sullivan et al., 2005 [Level IV]).

V. NURSING CARE STRATEGIES
(DiMaria-Ghalili & Amella, 2005 [Level VI]
A. Collaboration
   1. Refer to dietitian if patient is at risk for or has under-nutrition.

2. Consult with pharmacist to review patient's medications for possible drug–nutrient interactions.
3. Consult with a multidisciplinary team specializing in nutrition.
4. Consult with social worker, occupational therapist, and speech therapist as appropriate.

B. Alleviate Dry Mouth
1. Avoid caffeine; alcohol; tobacco; and dry, bulky, spicy, salty, or highly acidic foods.
2. If patient does not have dementia or swallowing difficulties, offer sugarless hard candy or chewing gum to stimulate saliva.
3. Keep lips moist with petroleum jelly.
4. Encourage frequent sips of water.

C. Maintain adequate nutritional intake:
1. Daily requirements for healthy older adults include 30 kcal per kg of body weight and 0.8 to 1 g/kg of protein per day, with no more than 30% of calories from fat. Caloric, carbohydrate, protein, and fat requirements may differ depending on degree of malnutrition and physiological stress.

D. Improve oral intake
1. Mealtime rounds to determine how much food is consumed and whether assistance is needed.
2. Limit staff breaks to before or after patient mealtimes to ensure adequate staff are available to help with meals.
3. Encourage family members to visit at mealtimes.
4. Ask family to bring favorite foods from home when appropriate.
5. Ask about and honor patient food preferences.
6. Suggest small frequent meals with adequate nutrients to help patients regain or maintain weight.
7. Provide nutritious snacks.
8. Help patient with mouth care and placement of dentures before food is served.

E. Provide conducive environment for meals
1. Remove bedpans, urinals, and emesis basin from room before mealtime.
2. Administer analgesics and antiemetics on a schedule that will diminish the likelihood of pain or nausea during mealtimes.
3. Serve meals to patients in a chair if they can get out of bed and remain seated.
4. Create a more relaxed atmosphere by sitting at the patient's eye level and making eye contact during feeding.
5. Order a late food tray or keep food warm if patients are not in their room during mealtime.
6. Do not interrupt patients for round and nonurgent procedures during mealtimes.

F. Specialized nutritional support (American Society for Parenteral and Enteral Nutrition, 2002, guidelines)

    1. Start specialized nutritional support when a patient cannot, should not, or will not eat adequately and if the benefits of nutrition outweigh the associated risks.

    2. Prior to initiation of specialized nutritional support, review the patient's advanced directives regarding the use of artificial nutrition and hydration.

G. Provide oral supplements

    1. Supplements should not replace meals but rather be provided between meals but not within the hour preceding a meal and at bedtime (Wilson et al., 2002 [Level IV]). See National Collaborating Centre for Acute Care Clinical Guideline (2006) for algorithm for use of oral supplements.

H. N.P.O. orders

    1. Schedule older adults for test or procedures early in the day to decrease the length of time they are not allowed to eat and drink.

    2. If testing late in the day is inevitable, ask physician whether the patient can have an early breakfast.

    3. See American Society of Anesthesiologists practice guideline regarding recommended length of time patients should be kept n.p.o. for elective surgical procedures.

VI. EVALUATION AND EXPECTED OUTCOMES

A. Patient:

    1. Will experience improvement in indicators of nutritional status.

    2. Will improve functional status and general well-being.

B. Provider:

    1. Should ensure that care provides food and fluid of adequate quantity and quality in an environment conducive to eating, with appropriate support (e.g., modified eating aids) for people who can potentially chew and swallow but are unable to feed themselves (National Collaborating Center for Acute Care, 2006).

    2. Should continue to reassess patients who are malnourished or at risk for malnutrition (National Collaborating Center for Acute Care, 2006).

    3. Should monitor for refeeding syndrome (National Collaborating Center for Acute Care, 2006).

C. Institution:

    1. Will ensure that all health care professionals who are directly involved in patient care receive education and training on the importance of providing adequate nutrition (National Collaborating Center for Acute Care, 2006).

D. QA/QI

    1. Establish QA/QI measures surrounding nutritional management in aging patients.

E. Educational

    1. Provider education and training includes the following:

a. nutritional needs and indications for nutrition support
b. options for nutrition support (oral, enteral, and parenteral)
c. ethical and legal concepts
d. potential risks and benfits
e. when and where to seek expert advice
f. (National Collaborating Center for Acute Care, 2006)
2. Patient and/or caregiver education includes how to maintain or improve nutritional status, as well as how to administer, when appropriate, oral liquid supplements, enteral tube feeding, or parenteral nutrition.

VII. FOLLOW-UP MONITORING
(National Collaborating Centre for Acute Care, 2006)
A. Monitor for gradual increase in weight over time.
   1. Weigh patient weekly to monitor trends in weight.
   2. Daily weights are useful for monitoring fluid status.
B. Monitor and assess for refeeding syndrome.
   1. Carefully monitor and assess patients the first week of aggressive nutritional repletion.
   2. Assess and correct the following electrolyte abnormalities: Hypophosphatemia, hypokalemia, hypomagnesemia, hyperglycemia, and hypoglycemia.
   3. Assess fluid status with daily weights and strict intake and output.
   4. Assess for congestive heart failure in patients with respiratory or cardiac difficulties.
   5. Ensure caloric goals will be reached slowly during 3 to 4 days to avoid refeeding syndrome when repletion of nutritional status is warranted.
   6. Be aware that refeeding syndrome is not exclusive to patients started on aggressive artificial nutrition but may also be found in elderly individuals with chronic co-morbid medical conditions and poor nutrient intake started with aggressive nutritional repletion via oral intake.

VIII. RELEVANT GUIDELINES

A. American Society of Anesthesiologists (1999). Practice guidelines for preoperative fasting and the use of pharmacologic agents to reduce the risk of pulmonary aspiration: Application to health patients undergoing elective procedures. *Anesthesiology, 90,* 896–905.
B. National Collaborating Centre for Acute Care (2006). *Nutrition support in adults: Oral nutrition support, enteral tube feeding and parenteral nutrition.* London, UK: National Institute for Health and Clinical Excellence (NICE). Clinical guideline no. 32. Electronic

copies: Available in PDF format from that National Institutes for Health and Clinical Excellence (NICE) Web site.

C. American Society for Parenteral and Enteral Nutrition (2002). Guidelines for the use of parenteral and enteral nutrition in adult and pediatric patients. *Journal of Parenteral and Enteral Nutrition, 26,* 1SA–138SA. (Note: These guidelines are undergoing revision.)

D. University of Texas, School of Nursing (2006). *Unintentional weight loss in the elderly.* Austin, TX: University of Texas, School of Nursing. (Note: These guidelines are located at www.guidelines.gov. However, the companion document with full bibliography is not in the public domain.)

References

American Society for Parenteral and Enteral Nutrition (2002). Guidelines for the use of parenteral and enteral nutrition in adult and pediatric patients. *Journal of Parenteral and Enteral Nutrition, 26,* 1SA–138SA.

Beers, M. H. (Ed.) (2005). Protein-energy under-nutrition. *The Merck manual of geriatrics* (3rd ed.) Retrieved June 20, 2005, from http://www.merck.com/mrkshared/mmg/sec8/ch61/ch61a.jsp. Evidence Level VI: Expert Opinion.

Boullata, J. (2004) Drug–nutrient interactions. In P.H. Worthington (Ed.), *Practical aspects of nutritional support: An advanced practice guide* (pp. 431–454). Philadelphia: Saunders. Evidence Level VI: Expert Opinion.

Carlsson, P., Tidermark, J., Ponzer, S., Soderqvist, A., & Cederholm, T. (2005). Food habits and appetite of elderly women at the time of a femoral neck fracture and after nutritional and anabolic support. *Journal of Human Nutrition and Dietetics, 18,* 117–120. Evidence Level II: Individual Experimental Study.

Chen, C., Schilling, L. S., & Lyder, C. H. (2001). A concept analysis of malnutrition in the elderly. *Journal of Advanced Nursing, 36,* 131–142. Evidence Level V: Narrative Literature Review.

DiMaria-Ghalili, R. A. (2002). Changes in nutritional status and postoperative outcomes in elderly CABG patients. *Biological Research for Nursing, 4,* 73–84. Evidence Level IV: Nonexperimental Study.

DiMaria-Ghalili, R. A., & Amella, E. (2005). Nutrition in older adults. *American Journal of Nursing, 105*(3), 40–51. Evidence Level VI: Expert Opinion.

Furman, E. F. (2006). Under-nutrition in older adults across the continuum of care: Nutritional assessment, barriers, and interventions. *Journal of Gerontological Nursing, 32*(1), 22–27. Evidence Level VI: Expert Opinion.

Guigoz, Y., Lauque, S., & Vellas, B. J. (2002). Identifying the elderly at risk for malnutrition: The Mini Nutritional Assessment. *Clinics in Geriatric Medicine, 18,* 737–757. Evidence Level V: Narrative Literature Review.

Hughes, V. A., Roubenoff, R., Wood, M., Frontera, W. R., Evans, W. J., & Fiatorone-Singh, M. A. (2004). Anthropometric assessment of 10-year changes in body composition in the elderly. *American Journal of Clinical Nutrition, 80,* 475–482. Evidence Level IV: Nonexperimental Study.

Janssen, I., Heymsfield, S. B., Allison, D. B., Kotler, D. P., & Ross, R. (2002). Body mass index and waist circumference independently contribute to the prediction of nonabdominal, abdominal, subcutaneous, and visceral fat. *American Journal of Clinical Nutrition, 75,* 683–688. Evidence Level IV: Nonexperimental Study.

Janssen, I., Heymsfield, S. B., & Ross, R. (2002). Low relative skeletal muscle mass (sarcopenia) in older persons is associated with functional impairment and physical disability. *Journal of the American Geriatrics Society, 50,* 889–896. Evidence Level IV: Nonexperimental Study.

Kagansky, N., Berner, Y., Koren-Morag, N., Perelman, L., Knobler, H., & Levy, S. (2005). Poor nutritional habits are predictors of poor outcome in very old hospitalized patients. *American Journal of Clinical Nutrition, 82*, 784–791. Evidence Level IV: Nonexperimental Study.

Margetts, B. M., Thompson, R. L., Elia, M., & Jackson, A. A. (2003). Prevalence of risk of undernutrition is associated with poor health status in older people in the UK. *European Journal of Clinical Nutrition, 57*, 69–74. Evidence Level IV: Nonexperimental Study.

Milne, A. C., Avenell, A., & Potter, J. (2006). Meta-analysis: Protein and energy supplementation in older people. *Annals of Internal Medicine, 144*, 37–48. Evidence Level I: Meta-analysis.

Morley, J. E. (2001). Anorexia, sarcopenia, and aging. *Nutrition, 17*(7–8), 660–663. Evidence Level V: Narrative Literature Review.

National Center for Health Statistics (2005). *Health, United States, 2005, with chartbook on trends in the health of Americans.* Hyattsville, MD.

National Collaborating Centre for Acute Care (2006). *Nutrition support in adults: Oral nutrition support, enteral tube feeding and parenteral nutrition.* London, UK: National Institute for Health and Clinical Excellence (NICE). Clinical guideline no. 32. Electronic copies: Available in PDF format from that National Institutes for Health and Clinical Excellence (NICE) Web site.

Nutrition Screening Initiative (2002). *Nutrition state of principle, 2002.* Retrieved August 1, 2004, from http:/www.eatright.org/Public/Files/nutrition(1).pdf. Evidence Level V: Review.

Pichard, C., Kyle, U. G., Morabia, A., Perrier, A., Vermuelen, B., & Unger, P. L. (2004). Nutritional assessment: Lean body mass depletion at hospital admission is associated with an increased length of stay. *American Journal of Clinical Nutrition, 79*, 613–618. Evidence Level IV: Nonexperimental Study.

Reuben, D. B., Hirsch, S. H., Zhou, K., & Greendale, G. A. (2005). The effects of megestrol acetate suspension for elderly patients with reduced appetite after hospitalization: A phase II randomized clinical trial. *Journal of the American Geriatrics Society, 53*, 970–975. Evidence Level II: Individual Experimental Study.

Rombeau, J. L, Caldwell, M. D., Forlaw, L., & Guenter, P. (1989). *Atlas of nutritional support techniques.* Boston: Little, Brown and Company. Evidence Level VI: Expert Opinion.

Saletti, A., Johansson, L., Yifter-Lindgren, E., Wissing, U., Osterberg, K., & Cederholm, T. (2005). Nutritional status and a 3-year follow-up in elderly receiving support at home. *Gerontology, 51*, 192–198. Evidence Level IV: Nonexperimental Study.

Salva, A., Corman, B., Andrieu, S., Salas, J., Vellas, B., and the International Association of Gerontology/International Academy of Nutrition and Aging (IAG/IANA) Task Force (2004). Minimum data set for nutritional intervention studies in elderly people. *Journal of Gerontology: Medical Sciences, 59A*, 724–729. Evidence Level V: Narrative Literature Review.

Shahar, D. R. (2001). The effect of widowhood on weight change, dietary intake, and eating behavior in the elderly population. *Journal of Aging and Health, 13*, 189–199. Evidence Level IV: Nonexperimental Study.

Souter, S., & Keller, C. (2002). Food choice in the rural-dwelling older adult. *Southern Online Journal of Nursing Research, 5*(3). Retrieved August 1, 2004, from http://www.snrs.org/members/SOJNR_articles/iss05vol03.pdf. Evidence Level IV: Nonexperimental Study.

Sullivan, D. H., Roberson, P. K., & Bopp, M. M. (2005). Hypoalbuminemia 3 months after hospital discharge: Significance for long-term survival. *Journal of the American Geriatrics Society, 53*, 1222–1226. Evidence Level IV: Nonexperimental Study.

The Malnutrition Prevalence Group (2000). Prevalence of malnutrition on admission to four hospitals in England. *Clinical Nutrition, 19*, 191–195. Evidence Level IV: Nonexperimental Study.

Thomas, D. R., Zdrowski, C. D., Wilson, M, Conright, K. C., Lewis, C., Tariq, S., et al. (2002). Malnutrition in subacute care. *American Journal of Clinical Nutrition, 75*, 308–313. Evidence Level IV: Nonexperimental Study.

Wilson, M. G., Purushothaman, R., & Morley, J. E. (2002). The effect of liquid dietary supplements on energy intake in the elderly. *American Journal of Clinical Nutrition, 75*, 944–947. Evidence Level IV: Nonexperimental Study.

Managing Oral Hydration

16

Janet C. Mentes

Educational Objectives

After completion of this chapter, the reader will be able to:

1. describe older adults at risk for dehydration

2. identify keys aspects of a hydration assessment

3. list specific interventions to promote hydration in older adults across care settings

4. identify outcomes of a hydration-management program

Overview

A recent study using markers (i.e., serum sodium, osmolality, and BUN/creatinine ratio) for dehydration and volume depletion from the Established Populations for Epidemiologic Studies of the Elderly (EPESE) found that the prevalence for these conditions in community-dwelling elders could range from 0.5%

For a description of Evidence Levels cited in this chapter, see chapter 1,
Developing and Evaluating Clinical Practice Guidelines, page 4

NOTE: Portions of this chapter were adapted with permission from J. C. Mentes and the Iowa Veterans Affairs Nursing Research Consortium (2004). Evidence-based protocol: Hydration management. In M.G. Titler (Series Ed.), Series on evidence-based practice for older adults. Iowa City, IA: University of Iowa College of Nursing Gerontological Nursing Interventions Research Center, Research Translation and Dissemination Core.

to 60% depending on the markers used (Stookey, Pieper, & Cohen, 2005 [Level IV]). Another study of dehydration in older adults found that 48% of elders presenting with dehydration at an ER unit were from the community (Bennett, Thomas, & Riegel, 2004 [Level IV]). Maintaining adequate fluid balance is an essential component of health across the life span; older adults are more vulnerable to shifts in water balance—both over-hydration and dehydration—because of age-related changes and increased likelihood that they have several medical conditions. Dehydration is the more frequent occurrence in elders (Warren et al., 1994 [Level IV]; Xiao, Barber, & Campbell, 2004 [Level IV]). In fact, avoidable hospitalizations for dehydration in older adults have increased by 40% from 1990 to 2000, at a cost of 1.14 billion dollars (Xiao et al., 2004 [Level IV]).

Consequences of dehydration can cause further morbidity, including constipation, increased falls, medication toxicity, increased infections (i.e., urinary and respiratory) (Mukand, Cai, Zielinski, Danish, & Berman, 2003 [Level IV]), and decreased risk of bladder cancer in men (Michaud et al., 1999 [Level IV]). High daily intakes of water (i.e., five or more 8-ounce glasses) compared with low intakes (two or fewer glasses), but not other types of fluid, were associated with decreased fatal coronary heart disease in middle-aged and older adults (Chan, Knutsen, Blix, Lee, & Fraser, 2002 [Level IV]). Finally, consuming 16 ounces of tepid water before a meal significantly increased healing time, especially for pressure ulcers, and decreased likelihood of delirium (Mentes & Culp, 2003 [Level III]; Weinberg, Minaker, & The Council on Scientific Affairs, AMA,1995 [Level I]). Dehydration in elders with multiple co-morbid conditions can precipitate an emergency hospitalization and increase the risk for repeated hospitalizations (Gordon, An, Hayward, & Williams, 1998 [Level IV]; Xiao et al., 2004 [Level IV]). The most serious consequence of dehydration is an increased 1-year mortality rate, which was documented in 50% of older Medicare beneficiaries admitted for a hospitalization with a primary or secondary diagnosis of dehydration (Warren et al., 1994 [Level IV]).

Conversely, adequate fluid consumption has been associated with decreased falls, decreased constipation, and decreased use of laxatives (Robinson & Rosher, 2002 [Level IV]). Adequate hydration may have even more far-reaching positive effects, such as better rehabilitation outcomes in older orthopedic patients (Mukand et al., 2003 [Level IV]) and improved postprandial orthostatic hypotension in older individuals with autonomic failure (Shannon et al., 2002 [Level IV]).

Oral hydration of older adults is particularly complex for various reasons. In this chapter, issues of age-related changes, risk factors, assessment measures, and nursing strategies for effective interventions for dehydration are addressed.

Background and Statement of Problem

Water is an essential component of body composition. Intricate cellular functions, such as gene expression, protein synthesis, and uptake and metabolism of nutrients, are affected by hydration status. Organ systems, specifically the cardiovascular and renal systems, are particularly vulnerable to fluctuating levels of hydration (Metheny, 2000 [Level VI]).

Fluid is found in different compartments in the body. Two basic compartments are the intracellular, or water within the cell, and extracellular, or water outside the cells. The extracellular compartment can be further categorized into the interstitial compartment, or the water between cells, and the intravascular compartment, or fluid in the blood vessels. Of course, when thinking about where water can be found in the body, it is realized that water serves as a solvent for many essential elements, such as the electrolytes sodium, potassium, and others. Fluid with these elements moves between the compartments in an orchestrated manner, guided by electrochemical forces that are exerted by electrolytes, by large molecules such as glucose, and by the colloidal osmotic pressure of proteins contained in the blood. Cellular factors, such as cell permeability and transport of elements and nutrients across this membrane, also contribute to the pattern of fluid distribution in the body. Therefore, hydration problems rarely involve body water alone but rather are a water and electrolyte problem (Metheny, 2000 [Level VI]).

Older individuals are at increased risk for hydration problems for various reasons. First, as individual's age, total body water decreases from 50%–70% to 40%–50% of body weight. For example, a female weighing 60 kg (132 pounds) at age 35 with 55%, or 33 kg, of body weight as water would have significantly less body weight as water at age 75, assuming that she weighed the same and that only 45%, or 27 kg, was water (Metheny, 2000 [Level VI]). Second, older individuals tend to lose muscle cells, which increases the proportion of fat cells to muscle cells. Fat cells are known to contain less water than muscle cells, which decreases overall intracellular fluids (Metheny, 2000 [Level VI]). Third, the risk of hydration problems is further increased with another age-related change involving the hormonally regulated thirst mechanism. Although not completely understood, elderly individuals do not experience thirst as intensely as younger individuals; in fact, their thirst is not proportional to metabolic needs in response to dehydrating conditions (Kenney & Chiu, 2001 [Level V]; Mack et al., 1994 [Level III]; Miescher & Fortney, 1989 [Level III]; Phillips et al., 1984 [Level III]; Phillips, Bretherton, Johnson, & Gray, 1991 [Level III]). Therefore, a major hydration management mechanism is impaired with age. Fourth, renal efficiency as measured by creatinine clearance decreases with age. In studying healthy older adults who had no renal or urinary tract disease, were normotensive, and did not use diuretics or antihypertensive drugs, Lindeman and colleagues (1985 [Level IV]) found that creatinine clearance decreased on average by 0.75 mL/min per year starting at age 40. It is important to note that one-third of study participants had no decrease in renal function. However, in general, older individuals lose their water reserves through loss of fluid-rich muscle cells, impaired renal conservation of water, and decreased fluid replacement due to lack of thirst. Finally, myriad other clinical factors that are more likely to occur as one ages but are not a direct effect of aging also contribute to increased risk, including cardiovascular disease, diabetes, multiple medical problems, malnutrition, and medication usage.

Definitions

Hydration Management

Hydration management is the promotion of adequate fluid balance that prevents complications resulting from abnormal or undesired fluid levels (see both Fluid Management and Fluid Monitoring nursing interventions in McCloskey-Dochterman & Bulechek, 2004, pp. 348–349, 352).

Dehydration

Dehydration is depletion in total body water content due to pathologic fluid losses, diminished water intake, or a combination of both. It results in hypernatremia (greater than 145mEq/L) in the extracellular fluid compartment, which draws water from the intracellular fluids. The water loss is shared by all body-fluid compartments and relatively little reduction in extracellular fluids occurs. Thus, circulation is not compromised unless the loss is very large. This is also known as intracellular or hypernatremic dehydration (Na^+ greater than or equal to145mEq/L).

Volume Depletion

Dehydration and volume depletion are often used synonymously to refer to dehydration; however, there are differences in symptoms and in emergency management between the two conditions. *Volume depletion* is the loss of both sodium and water with greater losses of sodium resulting in extracellular fluid loss and a reduction in intravascular volume (Mange et al., 1997 [Level V]). Major causes of volume depletion include blood loss, diarrhea, and vomiting, with individuals experiencing lightheadedness and orthostatic blood pressure changes.

Risk Factors for Dehydration

Community-Dwelling Elders

From findings of two recent studies, healthy community-dwelling older adults have no apparent changes in hydration status (Bossingham, Carnell, & Campbell, 2005 [Level II]; Morgan, Masterson, Fahlman, Topp, & Boardley, 2003 [Level IV]). Bossingham and colleagues (2005 [Level II]) studied older and younger adults using a controlled diet study. Total water intake, water output, and markers of hydration status (i.e., specific gravity and plasma osmolality) were not different between younger and older adults and fell within accepted clinical ranges. They did find normal age-related changes in body composition, specifically decreased fat-free body mass. Morgan and colleagues (2003 [Level IV]) also found that older adults who fasted for 12 hours exhibited normal values for the clinical markers of hydration, including specific gravity, serum osmolality, serum sodium, hematocrit, and hemoglobin. Only urine osmolality values were higher than normal.

These studies suggest an important consideration for risk of dehydration. Older adults, under normal conditions, maintain adequate hydration; however, when stressed by physical or emotional illness, surgery, or trauma, they are at increased risk for dehydration (Bossingham et al., 2005 [Level II]; Luckey & Parsa, 2003 [Level IV]; Morgan et al., 2003 [Level IV]). Therefore, a change in health status in a healthy older adult is an important risk factor for dehydration.

Institutionalized Older Adults

Risk for dehydration in ill or frail older adults across care settings has been more frequently studied. Although there is no one outstanding risk factor for dehydration, age, gender, ethnicity, class and number of medications taken, level of ADL dependency, presence of cognitive impairment, presence of medical conditions such as infectious processes, and a prior history of dehydration all have been associated with dehydration in older adults (Mentes & The Iowa Veterans Affairs Nursing Research Consortium, 2004 [Level I]).

Increasing age is associated with increased likelihood of dehydration (Ciccone, Allegra, Cochrane, Cody, & Roche, 1998 [Level IV]; Lavisso-Mourey, Johnson, & Stolley, 1988 [Level IV]; Warren et al., 1994 [Level IV]). Ciccone and colleagues (1998 [Level IV]) found that adults 85 years and older were three times more likely to have a diagnosis of dehydration on admission to an emergency department than adults ages 65 to 74 years. Older African American adults have higher prevalence rates of dehydration on hospitalization than White adults (Lancaster, Smicklas-Wright, Heller, Ahern, & Jensen, 2003 [Level IV]; Warren et al., 1994 [Level IV]). Female gender has been associated with risk for dehydration in nursing home residents (Lavisso-Mourey et al., 1988 [Level IV]); however, male hospitalized patients had an increased risk for dehydration (Warren et al., 1994 [Level IV]) and, more recently, no gender differences were detected in a large database study (Xiao et al., 2004 [Level IV]).

In general, individuals in long term care (LTC) settings are considered at increased risk, with one-third of residents experiencing a dehydration episode in a 6-month period (Mentes, 2006a [Level IV]). Specific factors that have been studied in LTC residents include the following:

- older than 85 years of age (Gaspar, 1999 [Level IV]; Lavisso-Mourey et al., 1988 [Level IV])
- female (Gaspar, 1988 [Level IV]; Lavisso-Mourey et al., 1988 [Level IV])
- functionally semidependent (e.g., those individuals who are cognitively unaware of their needs yet have mobility and those who are physically unable to meet their needs but who can express them) (Gaspar, 1988 [Level IV])
- functionally more independent (Gaspar, 1999 [Level IV]; Mentes & Culp, 2003 [Level III])
- semidependent with eating (Gaspar, 1999 [Level IV])
- Alzheimer's disease or other dementias (Albert, Nakra, Grossberg, & Caminal, 1989; 1993 [both Level III])
- four or more chronic conditions (Lavisso-Mourey et al., 1988 [Level IV])
- more than four medications (Lavisso-Mourey et al., 1988 [Level IV])
- fever (Pals et al., 1995 [Level IV]; Weinberg et al., 1994 [Level IV])

- few fluid ingestion opportunities (Gaspar, 1988; 1999 [both Level IV])
- inadequate nutrient intake (Gaspar, 1999 [Level IV])
- inadequate staff and professional supervision (Kayser-Jones, Schell, Porter, Barbaccia, & Shaw, 1999 [Level IV])

Special Populations

Several groups of patients, based on medical diagnosis, are at increased risk for dehydration, including chronically mentally ill, surgical, stroke, and end-of-life (EOL) patients.

Chronically Mentally Ill Patients

Special consideration should be given to chronic mentally ill elders (e.g., individuals with schizophrenia, bipolar disorder, obsessive-compulsive disorder) because they may be at risk for hydration problems. Their antipsychotic medications may blunt their thirst response and put them at increased risk in hot weather for dehydration and heat stroke (Batscha, 1997 [Level V]). In addition, even small increases in their antipsychotic medications may predispose them to neuroleptic malignant syndrome (NMS), of which hyperthermia and dehydration are prominent features (Bristow & Kohen, 1996 [Level V]; Jacobs, 1996 [Level V]; Sadev, Mason, & Hadzi-Pavlovic, 1997 [Level V]). In these individuals, risks for over-hydration stem from a combination of the drying side effects of prescribed psychotropic medications and the individual's compulsive behaviors that result in excessive fluid intake (Cosgray, Davidhizar, Giger, & Kreisl, 1993 [Level V]).

Stroke Patients

There is increasing evidence that people who suffer from dysphagia as a result of stroke are at increased risk for dehydration (Whelan, 2001 [Level II]). This appears to be related not only to the dysphagia resulting from the stroke but also the poor palatability of the thickened fluids offered to patients to prevent aspiration.

Surgical Patients

Prolonged nothing by month (NPO) status prior to elective surgery has been linked to increased risk of dehydration and adverse effects such as, thirst, hunger, irritability, headache, hypovolemia, and hypoglycemia in surgical patients (Smith, Vallance, & Slater, 1997 [Level II]; Yogendran, Asokumar, Cheng, & Chung, 1995 [Level II]). Crenshaw and Winslow have found that despite the formulation of national fasting guidelines (available at www.asahq.org/publicationsAndServices/NPO.pdf), patients were still being instructed to fast too long prior to surgery (Crenshaw & Winslow, 2002 [Level IV]). In fact, patients may safely consume clear liquids up to 2 hours prior to elective surgery using general anesthesia, regional anesthesia, or sedation anesthesia.

EOL Patients

Maintaining or withholding fluids at the end of life remains a controversial issue. Proponents suggest that dehydration in the terminally ill patient is not painful and lessens other noxious symptoms of terminal illness, such as excessive pulmonary secretions, nausea, edema, and pain (i.e., dehydration acts as a natural anesthetic) (Dalal & Bruera, 2004 [Level I]). Opponents to this position suggest that associated symptoms of dehydration, such as acute confusion and delirium, are stressful and reduce the quality of life for a terminally ill elder (Bruera, Belzile, Wantantabe, & Fainsinger, 1996 [Level IV]).

Most research has been done with terminally ill cancer patients and has examined discomforts of dehydration, including thirst, dry mouth, and agitated delirium. However, research has not demonstrated a link between biochemical markers of dehydration and these various symptoms in terminally ill patients (Burge, 1993 [Level IV]; Ellershaw, Sutliffe, & Saunders, 1995 [Level IV]; Morita, Tei, Tsunoda, Inoue, & Chihara, 2001 [Level IV]). It is suggested that several confounding factors influence the uncomfortable dehydration-like symptoms that accompany the end of life, including use and dosage of opiates, type and location of cancer, hyperosmolality, stomatitis, and oral breathing (Morita et al., 2001 [Level IV]). On the other hand, Bruera et al. (1996 [Level IV]) have determined that small amounts of fluids delivered subcutaneously via hypodermoclysis plus opioid rotation were effective in decreasing delirium and antipsychotic use and did not cause edema in terminally ill patients. Therefore, it is recommended that maintaining or withholding fluids at the end of life is an individual decision that should be based on the etiology of illness, use of medications, presence of delirium, and family and patient preferences (Dalal & Bruera, 2004 [Level I]; Morita et al., 2001 [Level IV]).

Assessment of Hydration Status

Hydration Habits

Hydration habits may indicate level of risk for dehydration in older adults. Some hydration habits may have developed during a lifetime and others are adaptations to current health status. Four major categories of hydration habits in nursing home residents have been identified (Mentes, 2006a [Level IV]). The categories include those elders who "can drink," "can't drink," "won't drink," and those who are at the "end of life." For example, older adults who "can drink" are those who are functionally capable of accessing and consuming fluids but who may not know what is an adequate intake or may forget to drink secondary to cognitive impairment. Elders who "can't drink" are those who are physically incapable of accessing or safely consuming fluids related to physical frailty or difficulty swallowing Elders who "won't drink" are those who are capable of consuming fluids safely but who do not because of concerns about being able to reach the toilet with or without assistance or who relate that they have never consumed many fluids. Elders who are terminally ill comprise the EOL category. Understanding hydration habits of older adults can help nurses to plan appropriate interventions to improve or ensure adequate intake (Mentes, 2006a [Level IV]).

Indicators of Hydration Status

A priority for nursing, regardless of clinical setting, is the prevention of dehydration. Unfortunately, many of the standard tests for detection of dehydration only confirm a diagnosis of dehydration after it is too late to prevent the episode. In fast-paced nursing environments, it is difficult to monitor the fluid intake of all older patients. Although controversial, the use of urine color and specific gravity has been shown to be a reliable indicator of hydration status (not dehydration) in older individuals in nursing homes and a Veterans Administration Medical Center with adequate renal function (Culp, Mentes, & Wakefield, 2003; Mentes, Wakefield, & Culp, 2006 [both Level IV]). Specifically, the use of urine color, as measured by a urine color chart, can be helpful in monitoring hydration status (Armstrong et al., 1994 [Level IV]; Mentes & The Iowa Veterans Affairs Nursing Research Consortium, 2004 [Level I]). The urine color chart has eight standardized colors ranging from pale straw (number 1) to greenish brown (number 8), approximating urine specific gravities of 1.003 to 1.029 (Armstrong et al., 1994 [Level IV]). The color chart is most effective when an individual's average urine color is calculated during several days for an individual referent value. If an older person's urine becomes darker from his or her average color, further assessment into recent intake and health status can be conducted and fluids can be adjusted to improve hydration status before dehydration occurs. Limitations in using urine indices to estimate specific gravity include (1) certain medications and foods can discolor the urine (Wakefield, Mentes, Diggelmann, & Culp, 2002 [Level IV]; Mentes, 2006a [Level IV]); (2) people must be able to give a urine specimen for a color evaluation; and (3) best results in the use of urine color as an indicator have been documented in older adults with adequate renal function (Mentes et al., 2006 [Level IV]).

Bioelectrical impedance analysis (BIA) is a measurement that has been used mostly in the fitness industry to estimate body composition, including body mass index (BMI), total body water (TBW), and intracellular and extracellular water. Several nursing studies have used impedance measurements to estimate TBW, intracellular and extracellular water (Culp, Mentes, & Wakefield, 2003 [Level IV]; Culp et al., 2004 [Level II]). Although mostly used in research, BIA is a noninvasive, reliable method to estimate body water (Ritz, 2001 [Level IV]). Because TBW is weight and body composition dependent, this measure is best used after a baseline value of TBW, intracellular, and extracellular fluid in liters has been documented, then deviations from the individual baseline can be noted.

Dehydration

Dehydration is the loss of body water from intracellular and interstitial fluid compartments that is associated with hypertonicity (Mange et al., 1997 [Level V]). Therefore, the most reliable indicators of dehydration are elevated serum sodium, serum osmolality, and BUN/creatinine ratio (Table 16.1). The most common clinical assessments of dehydration include the presence of dry oral mucous membranes, tongue furrows, decreased saliva, sunken eyes, decreased urine output, upper-body weakness, and a rapid pulse (Gross et al., 1992 [Level IV]). Decreased axillary sweat production as a clinical sign of dehydration has produced contradictory results, making it an unreliable

16.1	Approximate Ranges of Laboratory Tests for Hydration Status	
	Value Ranges for	
Test	Impending Dehydration	Dehydration
BUN/creatinine ratio	20–24	>25
Serum osmolality	normal 280–300 mmol/kg	>300 mmol/kg
Serum sodium		>150 meq/L
Urine osmolality		>1,050 mmol/kg
Urine specific gravity	1.020–1.029	>1.029
Urine color	dark yellow	greenish-brown
Amount of urine	800–1,200 cc/day	<800 cc/day

Armstrong et al., 1994, 1998; Mentes, Culp, & Wakefield, 2006 [all Level IV]; Metheny, 2000 [Level VI]; Wakefield et al., 2002; Wallach, 2000 [both Level IV].

Source: Adapted with permission from J. C. Mentes and The Iowa Veterans Affairs Nursing Research Consortium (2004). Evidence-based protocol: Hydration management. In M. G. Titler (Series ed.), *Series on evidence-based practice for older adults.* Iowa City, IA: The University of Iowa College of Nursing Gerontological Nursing Interventions Research Center, Research Translation and Dissemination Core.

indicator of dehydration (Eaton, Bannister, Mulley, & Connolly, 1994; Gross et al., 1992 [both Level IV]). Assessment of sternal skin turgor as a sign of dehydration has been a mainstay in nursing practice; however, it is not a reliable indicator for dehydration in older individuals because of age-related changes in skin elasticity (Gross et al., 1994 [Level IV]).

Interventions

The hydration management intervention is an individualized daily plan to promote adequate hydration based on risk-factor identification that is derived from a comprehensive assessment. The intervention is divided into two phases: risk identification and hydration management.

Risk Identification

Based on the collected assessment data, a risk appraisal for hydration problems is completed using the Dehydration Risk Appraisal Checklist (DRAC)

16.1

Dehydration Risk Appraisal Checklist

DEHYDRATION RISK APPRAISAL CHECKLIST

Patient ID_____

The greater the number of characteristics present, the greater the risk for hydration problems. Please check all that apply.

- ☐ >85 years
- ☐ Female

- ☐ BMI <21 or >27
  [BMI = weight(kg)/height(m)^2]

Significant Health Conditions

- ☐ Dementia/ + screen for cognitive impairment
- ☐ Depression/ +screen for depression
- ☐ CVA
- ☐ Diabetes
- ☐ Urinary Incontinence

- ☐ Renal Disease
- ☐ Cardiac Arrhythmias
- ☐ Malnutrition
- ☐ History of dehydration
- ☐ History of repeated infections

Medications

- ☐ >4 medications
- ☐ Laxatives
- ☐ Steroids
- ☐ ACE Inhibitors

- ☐ Diuretics
- ☐ Psychotropics: Antipsychotics,
  Antidepressants, Anxioytics

Intake Behaviors

- ☐ Requires assistance to drink
- ☐ Has difficulty swallowing/Chokes
- ☐ Can drink independently but forgets
- ☐ Poor eater (eats <50% of food)

- ☐ Semi-dependent with feeding
- ☐ Fluid intake of <1,500ml/day
- ☐ Spills
- ☐ Receives tube feedings

Laboratory Indicators

- ☐ Urine specific gravity >1.020
- ☐ Urine Color dark yellow

- ☐ BUN/Creatinine >20:1

Reprinted with permission from J. C. Mentes and The Iowa Veterans Affairs Nursing Research Consortium (2004). Evidence-based protocol: Hydration management. In M. G. Titler (Series ed.), *Series on evidence-based practice for older adults.* Iowa City, IA: The University of Iowa College of Nursing Gerontological Nursing Interventions Research Center, Research Translation and Dissemination Core.

(Figure 16.2). The DRAC was developed from an extensive literature review of risk factors for dehydration in older adults residing in LTC settings. The original 42-item checklist has been reduced to 31 items including health conditions, medications, intake behaviors, functional status, and laboratory values that have been linked to dehydration. These items can be collected during an admission/baseline assessment and can be linked to Minimum Data Set (MDS) data. The presence of a higher number of items implies greater risk for dehydration (Mentes, 2006b [Level V]). The checklist is currently being evaluated for validity and reliability.

Hydration Management

Managing fluid intake for optimal fluid balance consists of acute management of oral intake and ongoing management of oral intake.

Acute Management of Oral Intake

Any individual who develops a fever, vomiting, diarrhea, or a nonfebrile infection should be closely monitored by implementing intake and output records and provision of additional fluids as tolerated (Weinberg et al., 1994 [Level I]). Individuals who are required to be NPO for diagnostic tests should be given special consideration to shorten the time and should be provided with adequate amounts of fluids and food when they have completed their tests. For many procedures, a 2-hour fluid fast is recommended (American Society of Anesthesiology Task Force on Preoperative Fasting, 1999 [Level I]).

Any individual who develops unexplained weight gain, pedal edema, neck-vein distension, or shortness of breath should be evaluated and closely monitored for over-hydration. Fluids should be temporarily restricted and the individual's primary care provider notified. Specific attention should be focused on individuals who have renal disease or congestive heart failure. Older adults taking selective serotonin reuptake inhibitors (SSRIs) should have their serum-sodium levels and their hydration status monitored carefully because they are at risk for hyponatremia and increasing fluid intake may aggravate an evolving hyponatremia (Movig, Leufkens, Lenderlink, & Egberts, 1992 [Level IV]).

Ongoing Management of Oral Intake

Ongoing management of oral intake consists of the following five components:

1. Calculate a daily fluid goal.
   All older adults should have an individualized fluid goal determined by a documented standard for daily fluid intake. There is preliminary evidence that the standard suggested by Skipper (1993) of 100 mL/kg for the first 10 kg of weight, 50 mL/kg for the next 10 kg, and 15 mL for remaining kg is preferred (Chidester & Spangler, 1997 [Level IV]).

   Because this standard reflects fluid from all sources, to calculate a standard for fluids alone, 75% of the total calculated from the formula can be used. This formula allows for at least 1,500 mL of fluid per day as a minimum, which has been shown to be well tolerated in older men ages 55 to 75 (Spigt,

16.2

Examples of Daily Fluid Goal

> ### *Examples*
> 70-kg (154-lb.) resident would have a fluid goal of 2,250 mL/day.
>
> 60-kg (132-lb.) resident would have a fluid goal of 2,100 mL/day.
>
> 50-kg (110-lb.) resident would have a fluid goal of 1,950 mL/day.

Knottnerus, Westerterp, Olde-Rikkert, & van Schayck, 2006 [Level II]). Other standards include the following:

- 1,600 mL per m^2 of body surface/day (Butler & Talbot, 1948 [Level VI]; Gaspar, 1988 [Level IV]) or, more recently, Gaspar (1999 [Level IV]) recommended 75% of this standard
- 30 mL/kg body weight with 1,500 mL/day minimum (Chernoff, 1994 [Level VI])
- 1 mL/kcal fluid for adults (Food and Nutrition Board, 1989 [Level VI: Expert Opinion])
- 1,600 mL/day (Hodgkinson, Evans, & Wood, 2003 [Level I])

2. Compare individual's current intake to the amount calculated from applying the standard to evaluate the individual's hydration status.
3. Provide fluids consistently throughout the day (Ferry, 2005 [Level V]).
   a. Plan fluid intake as follows: 75% to 80% delivered at meals and 20% to 25% delivered during nonmeal times, such as medication times and planned nourishment times (Simmons, Alessi, & Schnelle, 2001 [Level II]).
   b. Offer a variety of fluids, remembering the individual's previous intake pattern (Zembrzuski, 1997 [Level V]). Alcoholic beverages, which exert a diuretic effect on the patient, should not be counted toward the fluid goal. Caffeinated beverages may be counted toward the fluid goal based on individual assessment because there is evidence that in individuals who are regular users, there are no untoward effects on fluid balance and that recommendations to refrain from moderate amounts of caffeinated beverages (250 to 300 mg, equivalent of two to three cups of coffee or five to eight cups of tea) may adversely affect fluid balance in older adults (Maughan & Griffin, 2003 [Level I]).
   c. Fluid with medication administrations should be standardized to a prescribed amount (e.g., *at least* 180 mL or 6 oz.) per administration time.
4. Plan for at-risk individuals
   For residents who are at risk of under-hydration because of poor intake, the following strategies can be implemented based on time, setting, and formal or informal caregiver issues:
   a. Fluid rounds mid-morning and late afternoon, where caregiver provides additional fluids (Robinson & Rosher, 2002 [Level IV]).
   b. Provide two 8-ounce glasses of fluid in morning and evening (Robinson & Rosher, 2002 [Level IV]).

c. "Happy Hours" in the afternoon, where residents can gather together for additional fluids and socialization (Musson et al., 1990 [Level V]).

d. "Tea Time" in the afternoon, where residents come together for fluids, nourishment, and socialization (Mueller & Boisen, 1989 [Level V]).

e. Use of modified fluid containers based on resident's intake behaviors (e.g., ability to hold cup and swallow) (Mueller & Boisen, 1989 [Level V]).

f. Offer a variety of fluids and encourage ongoing intake throughout the day for cognitively impaired residents; offer fluids that resident prefers (Simmons et al., 2001 [Level II]).

5. Fluid regulation and documentation

a. Individuals who are cognitively intact, visually capable, and have adequate renal function can be taught how to regulate their intake through the use of a color chart to compare to the color of their urine (Armstrong et al., 1994 [Level IV]; Armstrong, Herrera-Soto, Hacker, Kavouras, & Maresh, 1998 [Level IV]; Mentes, Culp, & Wakefield, 2006 [Level IV]). For those individuals who are cognitively impaired, caregivers can be taught how to use the color chart.

b. Frequency of documentation of fluid intake will vary among settings and is dependent on an individual's condition. However, in most settings, at least one accurate intake and output recording should be documented, including the amount of fluid consumed, intake pattern, difficulties with consumption, and urine specific gravity and color (Mentes & The Iowa Veterans Affairs Nursing Research Consortium, 2004 [Level I]).

c. Accurate calculation of intake requires knowledge of the volumes of containers used to serve fluids, which should be posted in a prominent place on the care unit, because a study by Burns (1992 [Level IV]) suggested that nurses over- or under-estimated the volumes of common vessels.

Evaluation

Adherence to the hydration-management guideline can be monitored by the frequency of monitoring (to be determined by setting), as follows:

- Urine specific-gravity checks, preferably a morning specimen (Armstrong et al., 1994, 1998 [both Level IV]; Wakefield et al., 2002 [Level IV]). A value greater than or equal to 1.020 implies an under-hydrated state and requires further monitoring (Mentes et al., 2006 [Level IV]; Kavouras, 2002 [Level IV]).

- Urine color chart monitoring, preferably a morning specimen (Armstrong et al., 1994, 1998 [both Level IV]; Wakefield et al., 2002 [Level IV]).

- 24-hour intake recording (output recording may be added; however, in settings where individuals are incontinent of urine, an intake recording should suffice).

Expected improved health outcomes of consistent application of a hydration management plan include the following:

- maintenance of body hydration (Mentes & Culp, 2003 [Level III]; Robinson & Rosher, 2002 [Level IV]; Simmons et al., 2001 [Level II])

- decreased infections, especially urinary tract infections (McConnell, 1984 [Level III]; Mentes & Culp, 2003 [Level III]; Robinson & Rosher, 2002 [Level IV])
- improvement in urinary incontinence (Spangler, Risley, & Bilyew [Level III])
- lowered urinary pH (Hart & Adamek, 1984 [Level III])
- decreased constipation (Robinson & Rosher, 2002 [Level IV])
- decreased acute confusion (Mentes, Culp, Maas, & Rantz, 1999 [Level IV])

Case Study and Discussion

Mrs. Chung is an 87-year-old Chinese American woman who has resided in Sunny Days Assisted Living Facility for the past month. She is fiercely independent despite recently experiencing some declines in her health. Her medical diagnoses include hypertension, for which she receives atenolol 25 mg daily and enalapril 20 mg daily; status post-mild CVA with residual left-sided weakness, for which she is taking 80 mg of aspirin daily; osteoarthritis, for which she takes Tylenol extra strength twice daily; and cataracts, for which she is reluctant to have surgery. She is cognitively intact and requires only minor assistance with bathing.

Recently, Mrs. Chung has become more withdrawn and concerned about her health. Her family has noticed that she has altered some of her daily routines. For example, she has eliminated her daily tea because she finds it difficult to use the new microwave at the assisted care facility (ACF) to heat her water because of unfamiliarity. She stays in her bed much of the day, complaining that she doesn't have any energy. When questioned, she reluctantly admits that she has been having more problems with her long-standing urinary incontinence and she is afraid to leave her room because she is fearful that she won't be able to make it to a bathroom on time. Consequently, she has further restricted the amount of fluid that she consumes on a daily basis.

Mrs. Chung is at high risk for dehydration given that she has recently begun to restrict her fluids due to unfamiliarity with the microwave to heat her water for tea. Elders from different cultures may wish to have their beverages served at different temperatures. Especially when ill, ethnic elders may prefer to have warmed beverages. In addition, Mrs. Chung is "treating" her urinary incontinence by restricting her fluids, which places her at risk for dehydration and urinary tract infections. This scenario is not uncommon in older adults struggling to maintain independence. One of the major reasons for admission to a nursing home is the presence of urinary incontinence. Finally, there is some evidence that Mrs. Chung is depressed, which would also place her at risk for dehydration often secondary to decreased food and fluid intake. Additional risk factors include her age, gender, and use of an ACE-inhibitor, which acts on the renin angiotension aldosterone (RAA) system.

Interventions to prevent dehydration in Mrs. Chung would include evaluating her for a urinary tract infection and offering her an evaluation for her urinary incontinence, which could include use of medications, if indicated; use of behavioral strategies, including urge inhibition; and/or Kegel exercises. Education around the importance of maintaining adequate fluid intake to minimize urinary incontinence is indicated, which should include a discussion about the amount of daily fluids required and the provision of a graduated cup to help her ascertain appropriate amounts. Helping her simplify the use of the microwave and/or attendance at social events at the ACF where fluids are provided could be implemented. Lastly, an evaluation for depression may be indicated if the previous interventions do not improve her mood.

Conclusions

Dehydration in older adults is a costly yet preventable health problem. Best practices for hydration management have been identified primarily in the nursing home population, including providing access to fluids at all times, regularly offering fluids throughout the day, assessing fluid preferences and providing the fluid of choice, and appropriate supervision of personnel who will be providing the fluids. Access to fluids means that fasting times for older adults are limited to the shortest period, fluids are available at all times, and nursing personnel assess the ability to self-manage hydration in older individuals. Regularly offering fluids through fluid rounds, a beverage cart, or other novel means such as teatime is another principle of good hydration practices. Accommodating older peoples' preferences for type and appropriate temperature of beverage has been shown to increase fluid intake. Last, appropriate supervision of how much fluid per day is required and how assistance is given to elders who are not capable of drinking themselves to ensure that required amounts are consumed is also key in maintaining adequate hydration. The hydration practices of healthier, community-dwelling older adults is less well known and requires further study.

Box 16.1

Nursing Standard of Practice Protocol: Oral Hydration Management

I. **GOAL:** To minimize episodes of dehydration in older adults.

II. **OVERVIEW:** Maintaining adequate fluid balance is an essential component of health across the life span; older adults are more vulnerable to shifts in water balance, both over-hydration and dehydration, because of age-related changes and increased likelihood that they have several medical conditions. Dehydration is the more frequently occurring problem.

III. BACKGROUND AND STATEMENT OF PROBLEM

A. Definitions
   1. *Hydration management* is the promotion of adequate fluid balance that prevents complications resulting from abnormal or undesired fluid levels. (See both Fluid Management and Fluid Monitoring nursing interventions in McCloskey-Dochterman & Bulechek, 2004).
   2. *Dehydration* is depletion in TBW content due to pathologic fluid losses, diminished water intake, or a combination of both. It results in hypernatremia (>145 mEq/L) in the extracellular fluid compartment, which draws water from the intracellular fluids. The water loss is shared by all body fluid compartments and relatively little reduction in extracellular fluids occurs. Thus, circulation is not compromised unless the loss is very large. This is also known as intracellular dehydration or *hypernatremic dehydration* (Na $\geq$ 145 mE/L).
   3. *Volume depletion* is the loss of both sodium and water with greater losses of sodium resulting in extracellular fluid loss and a reduction in intravascular volume (Mange et al., 1997 [Level V]). Also called *hypotonic dehydration*.
B. Etiologic factors associated with dehydration
   1. Age-related changes in body composition with resulting decrease in TBW (Metheny, 2000 [Level VI]).
   2. Decreasing renal function (Lindeman et al., 1985 [Level IV])
   3. Lack of thirst (Kenney & Chiu, 2001 [Level V]; Mack et al., 1994 [Level III]; Miescher & Fortney, 1989 [Level III]; Phillips et al., 1984, 1991 [both Level III])
C. Risk Factors
   1. Individuals older than 85 (Ciccone et al., 1998 [Level IV]; Lavisso-Mourey et al., 1988 [Level IV]; Warren et al., 1994 [Level I]).
   2. Individuals who are institutionalized (Mentes, 2006a [Level IV])
   3. Individuals with ADL dependencies, specifically feeding and eating (Gaspar, 1999 [Level IV])
   4. Individuals with a diagnosis of dementia (Albert et al., 1989, 1993 [both Level III])
   5. Individuals with infections (Warren et al., 1994 [Level IV])
   6. Individuals who have had prior episodes of dehydration (Mentes, 2006a [Level IV])

IV. PARAMETERS OF ASSESSMENT

(Mentes & The Iowa Veterans Affairs Nursing Research Consortium, 2004 [Level I])
A. Health history
   1. Specific disease states: dementia, congestive heart failure, chronic renal disease, malnutrition, and psychiatric disorders such

as depression (Albert et al., 1989, 1993 [both Level III]; Warren et al., 1994 [Level IV])

2. Presence of co-morbidities: more than four chronic health conditions (Lavisso-Mourey et al., 1988 [Level IV])
3. Prescription drugs: number and types (Lavisso-Mourey et al., 1988 [Level IV])
4. Past history of dehydration, repeated infections (Mentes, 2006a [Level IV])

B. Physical Assessments (Mentes & The Iowa Veterans Affairs Nursing Research Consortium, 2004 [Level I])
   1. Vital signs
   2. Height and weight
   3. BMI
   4. Review of systems
   5. Indicators of hydration

C. Laboratory Tests
   1. Urine specific gravity (Wakefield et al., 2002; Mentes et al., 2006 [both Level IV])
   2. Urine color (Wakefield et al., 2002; Mentes et al., 2006 [both Level IV])
   3. BUN/creatinine ratio
   4. Serum sodium
   5. Serum osmolality

D. Individual fluid intake behaviors (Mentes, 2006a [Level IV])

V. NURSING CARE STRATEGIES

A. Risk Identification (Mentes & The Iowa Veterans Affairs Nursing Research Consortium, 2004 [Level I]).
   1. Identify acute situations: vomiting, diarrhea, or febrile episodes
   2. Use a tool to evaluate risk: Dehydration Appraisal Checklist

B. Acute Hydration Management
   1. Monitor input and output (Weinberg et al., 1994 [Level I]).
   2. Provide additional fluids as tolerated (Weinberg et al., 1994 [Level I]).
   3. Minimize fasting times for diagnostic and surgical procedures (American Society of Anesthesiology Task Force on Preoperative Fasting, 1999 [Level I]).

C. Ongoing Hydration Management
   1. Calculate a daily fluid goal (Mentes & The Iowa Veterans Affairs Nursing Research Consortium, 2004 [Level I]).
   2. Compare current intake to fluid goal (Mentes & The Iowa Veterans Affairs Nursing Research Consortium, 2004 [Level I]).
   3. Provide fluids consistently throughout the day (Ferry, 2005 [Level V]; Simmons et al., 2001 [Level II]).
   4. Plan for at-risk individuals
      a. Fluid rounds (Robinson & Rosher, 2002 [Level IV]).

    b. Provide two 8-oz. glasses of fluid, one in the morning and the other in the evening (Robinson & Rosher, 2002 [Level IV])

    c. "Happy Hours" to promote increased intake (Musson et al., 1990 [Level V]).

    d. "Tea time" to increase fluid intake (Mueller & Boisen, 1989 [Level V]).

    e. Offer a variety of fluids throughout the day (Simmons et al., 2001 [Level II]).

  5. Fluid regulation and documentation

    a. Teach able individuals to use a urine color chart to monitor hydration status (Armstrong et al., 1994, 1998; Mentes et al., 2006 [all Level IV]).

    b. Document a complete intake recording including hydration habits (Mentes & The Iowa Veterans Affairs Nursing Research Consortium, 2004 [Level I]).

    c. Know volumes of fluid containers to accurately calculate fluid consumption (Burns, 1992 [Level IV]; Hart & Adamek, 1984 [Level III]).

    d. d. Maintenance of body hydration (Mentes & Culp, 2003 [Level III]; Robinson & Rosher, 2002 [Level IV]; Simmons et al., 2001 [Level II]).

VI. EVALUATION AND EXPECTED OUTCOMES

A. Decreased infections, especially urinary tract infections (McConnell, 1984; Mentes & Culp, 2003; [both Level III]; Robinson & Rosher, 2002 [Level IV])

B. Improvement in urinary incontinence (Spangler et al., 1984 [Level III])

C. Normal urinary pH (Hart & Adamek, 1984 [Level III])

D. Decreased constipation (Robinson & Rosher, 2002 [Level IV])

E. Decreased acute confusion (Mentes et al., 1999 [Level IV])

VII. FOLLOW-UP MONITORING OF CONDITION

A. Urine color chart monitoring in residents with better renal function (Armstrong et al., 1994, 1998; Wakefield et al., 2002 [all Level IV]).

B. Urine specific-gravity checks (Armstrong et al., 1994, 1998; Wakefield et al., 2002 [all Level IV]).

C. 24-hour intake recording (Metheny, 2000 [Level VI]).

VIII. RELEVANT PRACTICE GUIDELINES

A. Hydration-Management Evidence-Based Protocol available from The University of Iowa College of Nursing Gerontological Nursing Interventions Research Center Research Dissemination Core. Author: Janet Mentes, revised 2004. Access at www.nursing.uiowa.edu/centers/gnirc/protocols.htm

References

Albert, S., Nakra, B., Grossberg, G., & Caminal, E. (1989). Vasopressin response to dehydration in Alzheimer's disease. *Journal of the American Geriatrics Society, 37*, 843–847. Evidence Level III: Quasi-experimental Study.

Albert, S., Nakra, B., Grossberg, G., & Caminal, E. (1993). Drinking behavior and vasopressin responses to hyperosmolality in Alzheimer's disease. *International Psychogeriatrics, 6*, 79–86. Evidence Level III: Quasi-experimental Study.

American Society of Anesthesiology Task Force on Preoperative Fasting (1999). Practice guidelines for preoperative fasting and the use of pharmacologic agents to reduce the risk of pulmonary aspiration: Application to healthy patients undergoing elective procedures. *Anesthesiology, 90*, 896–905. Level I: Systematic Review.

Armstrong, L., Herrera-Soto, J., Hacker, F., Kavouras, S., & Maresh, C. (1998). Urinary indices during dehydration, exercise, and rehydration. *International Journal of Sport Nutrition, 8*, 345–355. Evidence Level IV: Nonexperimental Study.

Armstrong, L., Maresh, C., Castellani, J., Bergeron, M., Kenefick, R., La Grasse, K., et al. (1994). Urinary indices of hydration status. *International Journal of Sport Nutrition, 4*, 265–279. Evidence Level IV: Nonexperimental Study.

Batscha, C. (1997). Heat stroke: Keeping your patients cool in the summer. *Journal of Psychosocial Nursing, 35*(7), 12–17. Evidence Level V: Case Report.

Bennett, J., Thomas, V., & Riegel, B. (2004). Unrecognized chronic dehydration in older adults: Examining prevalence rate and risk factors. *Journal of Gerontological Nursing, 30*(11), 22–28. Evidence Level IV: Nonexperimental Study.

Bossingham, M., Carnell, N., & Campbell, W. (2005). Water balance, hydration status, and fat-free mass hydration in younger and older adults. *American Journal of Clinical Nutrition, 81*, 1342–1350. Evidence Level II: Single Experimental Study.

Bristow, M., & Kohen, D. (1996). Neuroleptic malignant syndrome. *British Journal of Hospital Medicine, 55*, 517–520. Evidence Level V: Care Report.

Bruera, E., Belzile, M., Wantanabe, S., & Fainsinger, R. L. (1996). Volume of hydration in terminal cancer patients. *Supportive Care in Cancer, 4*, 147–150. Evidence Level IV: Nonexperimental Study.

Burge, F. (1993). Dehydration symptoms of palliative care cancer patients. *Journal of Pain Symptom Management, 8*, 454–464. Evidence Level IV: Nonexperimental Study.

Burns, D. (1992). Working up a thirst. *Nursing Times, 88*(62), 44–45. Evidence Level IV: Nonexperimental Study.

Butler, A. M., & Talbot, N. B. (1948). Parental fluid therapy: Estimation and provision of daily maintenance requirements. *New England Journal of Medicine, 231*, 585–590. Evidence Level VI: Expert Opinion.

Chan, J., Knutsen, S., Blix, G., Lee, J., & Fraser, G. (2002). Water, other fluids, and fatal coronary heart disease. *American Journal of Epidemiology, 155*, 827–833. Evidence Level IV: Nonexperimental Study.

Chernoff, R. (1994). Meeting the nutritional needs of the elderly in the institutional setting. *Nutrition Review, 52*(4), 132–136. Evidence Level VI: Expert Opinion.

Chidester, J., & Spangler, A. (1997). Fluid intake in the institutionalized elderly. *Journal of the American Dietetic Association, 97*, 23–28. Evidence Level IV: Nonexperimental Study.

Ciccone, A., Allegra, J. R., Cochrane, D. G., Cody, R. P., & Roche, L. M. (1998). Age-related differences in diagnoses within the elderly population. *American Journal of Emergency Medicine, 16*, 43–48. Evidence Level IV: Nonexperimental Study.

Cosgray, R., Davidhizar, R., Giger, J., & Kreisl, R. (1993). A program for water-intoxicated patients at a state hospital. *Clinical Nurse Specialist, 7*(2), 55–61. Evidence Level V: Program Evaluation.

Crenshaw, J., & Winslow, E. (2002). Preoperative fasting: Old habits die hard. *American Journal of Nursing, 102*(5), 36–44. Evidence Level IV: Nonexperimental Study.

Culp, K., Mentes, J., & Wakefield, B. (2003). Hydration and acute confusion in long term care residents. *Western Journal of Nursing Research, 25*, 251–266. Evidence Level IV: Nonexperimental Study.

Culp, K., Wakefield, B., Dyck, M., Cacchione, P., DeCrane, S., & Decker, S. (2004). Bioelectrical impedance analysis and other hydration parameters as risk factors for delirium in rural nursing home residents. *Journal of Gerontology: Medical Sciences, 59A*, 813–817. Evidence Level II: Single Experimental Study.

Dalal, S., & Bruera, E. (2004). Dehydration in cancer patients: To treat or not to treat. *Journal of Supportive Oncology, 2*, 467–487. Evidence Level I: Systematic Review.

Eaton, D., Bannister, P., Mulley, G., & Connolly, M. (1994). Axillary sweat in clinical assessment of dehydration in ill elderly patients. *British Medical Journal, 308*, 1271. Evidence Level IV: Nonexperimental Study.

Ellershaw, J., Sutcliffe, J., & Saunders, C. (1995). Dehydration and the dying patient. *Journal of Pain Symptom Management, 10*, 192–197. Evidence Level IV: Nonexperimental Study.

Ferry, M. (2005). Strategies for ensuring good hydration in the elderly. *Nutrition Reviews, 63*(6), S22–S29. Evidence Level V: Literature Review.

Food and Nutrition Board (1989). *Recommended dietary allowances* (10th ed.). Washington, DC: National Academy Press. Evidence Level VI: Expert Opinion.

Gaspar, P. (1988). What determines how much patients drink? *Geriatric Nursing, 9*(4), 221–224. Evidence Level IV: Nonexperimental Study.

Gaspar, P. (1999). Water intake of nursing home residents. *Journal of Gerontological Nursing, 25*(4), 22–29. Evidence Level IV: Nonexperimental Study.

Gordon, J., An, L., Hayward, R., & Williams, B. (1998). Initial emergency department diagnosis and return visits: Risk versus perception. *Annals of Emergency Medicine, 32*, 569–573. Evidence Level IV: Nonexperimental Study.

Gross, C., Lindquist, R., Anthony, W., Granieri, R., Allard, K., & Webster, B. (1992). Clinical indicators of dehydration severity in elderly patients. *The Journal of Emergency Medicine, 10*, 267–274. Evidence Level IV: Nonexperimental Study.

Hart, M., & Adamek, C. (1984). Do increased fluids decrease urinary stone formation? *Geriatric Nursing, 5*(6), 245–248. Evidence Level III: Quasi-experimental Study.

Hodgkinson, B., Evans, D. E., & Wood, J. (2003). Maintaining oral hydration in older adults: A systematic review. *International Journal of Nursing Practice, 9*, S19–S29. Evidence Level I: Systematic Review.

Jacobs, L. (1996). The neuroleptic malignant syndrome: Often an unrecognized geriatric problem. *Journal of the American Geriatrics Society, 44*, 474–475. Evidence Level V: Care Report.

Kavouras, S. (2002). Assessing hydration status. *Current Opinion in Clinical Nutrition and Metabolic Care, 5*, 519–524. Evidence Level IV: Nonexperimental Study.

Kayser-Jones, J., Schell, E., Porter, C., Barbaccia, J., & Shaw, H. (1999). Factors contributing to dehydration in nursing homes: Inadequate staffing and lack of professional supervision. *Journal of the American Geriatrics Society, 47*, 1187–1194. Evidence Level IV: Nonexperimental Study.

Kenney, W. L., & Chui, P. (2001). Influence of age on thirst and fluid intake. *Medicine & Science in Sports and Exercise, 33*, 1524–1532. Evidence Level V: Literature Review.

Lancaster, K. J., Smicklas-Wright, H, Heller, D.A., Ahern, F.M. & Jensen, G. (2003). Dehydration in Black and White older adults using diuretics. *Annals of Epidemiology, 13, 525–529.* Evidence Level IV: Nonexperimental Study.

Lavisso-Mourey, R., Johnson, J., & Stolley, P. (1988). Risk factors for dehydration among elderly nursing home residents. *Journal of the American Geriatrics Society, 36*, 213–218. Evidence Level IV: Nonexperimental Study.

Lindeman, R., Tobin, J., & Shock, N. (1985). Longitudinal studies on the rate of decline in renal function with age. *Journal of the American Geriatrics Society, 33*, 278–285. Evidence Level IV: Nonexperimental Study.

Luckey, A., & Parsa, C. (2003). Fluid and electrolytes in the áged. *Archives of Surgery, 138*, 1055–1060. Evidence Level IV: Nonexperimental Study.

Mack, G., Weseman, C., Langhans, G., Scherzer, H., Gillen, C., & Nadel, E. (1994). Body fluid balance in dehydrated healthy older men: Thirst and renal osmoregulation. *Journal of Applied Physiology, 76*, 1615–1623. Evidence Level III: Quasi-experimental Study.

Mange, K., Matsuura, D., Cizman, B., Soto, H., Ziyadeh, F., Goldfarb, S., et al. (1997). Language guiding therapy: The case of dehydration versus volume depletion. *Annals of Internal Medicine, 127*, 848–853. Evidence Level: V: Literature Review

Maughan, R. J., & Griffin, J. (2003). Caffeine ingestion and fluid balance: A review. *Journal of Human Nutrition and Dietetics, 16*(6), 411–420. Evidence Level I: Systematic Review.

McCloskey-Dochterman, J. C., & Bulechek, G. M. (Eds.) (2004). *Nursing Interventions Classification (NIC)* (4th ed., pp. 348–349, 352). St. Louis, MO: Mosby.

McConnell, J. (1984). Preventing urinary tract infections: Nursing measures alone reduced UTI in a nursing home. *Geriatric Nursing, 5*(8), 361–362. Level III: Quasi-experimental Study.

Mentes, J. (2006a). A typology of oral hydration problems exhibited by nursing home residents. *Journal of Gerontological Nursing, 23*(1), 13–21. Evidence Level IV: Nonexperimental Study.

Mentes, J. (2006b). Oral hydration in older adults: Greater awareness is needed in preventing, recognizing, and treating dehydration. *The American Journal of Nursing, 106*(6), 40–49. Evidence Level V: Narrative Literature Review.

Mentes, J., & Culp, K. (2003). Reducing hydration-linked events in nursing home residents. *Clinical Nursing Research, 12*, 210–225. Evidence Level III: Quasi-experimental Study.

Mentes, J., Culp, K., Maas, M., & Rantz, M. (1999). Acute confusion indicators: Risk factors and prevalence. Using MDS data. *Research in Nursing & Health, 22*, 95–105. Evidence Level IV: Nonexperimental Study.

Mentes, J. C., and The Iowa Veterans Affairs Nursing Research Consortium (2004). Evidence-based protocol: Hydration management. In M. G. Titler (Series Ed.), *Series on evidence-based practice for older adults*. Iowa City, IA: The University of Iowa College of Nursing Gerontological Nursing Interventions Research Center, Research Translation and Dissemination Core. Evidence Level I: Systematic Review.

Mentes, J., Wakefield, B., & Culp, K. (2006). Use of a urine color chart to monitor hydration status in nursing home residents. *Biological Research for Nursing, 7*, 197–203. Evidence Level IV: Nonexperimental Study.

Metheny, N. (2000). Fluid and electrolyte balance. In *Nursing considerations* (4th ed., pp. 3–12, 24–26). St. Louis, MO: Lippincott, Williams, & Wilkins. Evidence Level VI: Expert Opinion.

Michaud, D., Spiegelman, D., Clinton, S., Rimm, E., Curhan, G., Willett, W., et al. (1999). Fluid intake and the risk of bladder cancer in men. *The New England Journal of Medicine, 340*, 1390–1397. Evidence Level IV: Nonexperimental Study.

Miescher, E., & Fortney, S. (1989). Responses to dehydration and rehydration during heat exposure in young and older men. *American Journal of Physiology, 257*(26), R1050–R1056. Evidence Level III: Quasi-experimental Study.

Morgan, A., Masterson, M., Fahlman, M., Topp, R., & Boardley, D. (2003). Hydration status of community-dwelling seniors. *Aging Clinical and Experimental Research, 15*, 301–304. Evidence Level IV: Nonexperimental Study.

Morita, T., Tei, Y., Tsunoda, J., Inoue, S., & Chihara, S. (2001). Determinants of the sensation of thirst in terminally ill cancer patients. *Support Care Cancer, 9*, 177–186. Evidence Level IV: Nonexperimental Study.

Movig, K., Leufkens, H., Lenderlink, A., & Egberts, A. (1992). Serotonergic antidepressants associated with an increased risk for hyponatremia in the elderly. *European Journal of Clinical Pharmacology, 58*, 143–148. Evidence Level IV: Nonexperimental Study.

Mueller, K., & Boisen, A. (1989). Keeping your patient's water level up. *RN, 52*, 65–66, 68. Evidence Level V: Program Evaluation.

Mukand, J., Cai, C., Zielinski, A., Danish, M., & Berman, J. (2003). The effects of dehydration on rehabilitation outcomes of elderly orthopedic patients. *Archives of Physical Medicine Rehabilitation, 84*, 58–61. Evidence Level IV: Nonexperimental Study.

Musson, N., Kincaid, J., Ryan, P., Glussman, B., Varone, L., Gamarra, N., et al. (1990). Nature, nurture, nutrition: Interdisciplinary programs to address the prevention of malnutrition and dehydration. *Dysphagia, 5*, 65–101. Evidence Level V: Program Evaluation.

Pals, J., Weinberg, D., Beal, L., Levesque, P., Cunningham, T., & Minaker, K. (1995). Clinical triggers for detection of fever and dehydration: Implications for long term care nursing. *Journal of Gerontological Nursing, 21*(4), 13–19. Evidence Level IV: Nonexperimental Study.

Phillips, P., Bretherton, M., Johnston, C., & Gray, L. (1991). Reduced osmotic thirst in healthy elderly men. *American Journal of Physiology, 261*, R166–R171. Evidence Level III: Quasi-experimental Study.

Phillips, P., Rolls, B., Ledingham, J., Forsling, M., Morton, J., Crowe, M., et al. (1984). Reduced thirst after water deprivation in healthy elderly men. *New England Journal of Medicine, 311*, 753–759. Evidence Level III: Quasi-experimental Study.

Ritz, P. (2001). Bioelectrical impedance analysis estimation of water compartments in elderly diseased patients: The source study. *Journal of Gerontology Medical Sciences, 56,* M344–M348. Evidence Level IV: Nonexperimental Study.

Robinson, S., & Rosher, R. (2002). Can a beverage cart help improve hydration? *Geriatric Nursing, 23,* 208–211. Evidence Level IV: Nonexperimental Study.

Sadev, P., Mason, C., & Hadzi-Pavlovic, D. (1997). Case control study of neuroleptic malignant syndrome. *American Journal of Psychiatry, 154,* 1156–1158. Evidence Level V: Care Report.

Shannon, J., Diedrich, A., Biaggioni, I., Tank, J., Robertson, R. M., Robertson, D., et al. (2002). Water-drinking as a treatment for orthostatic syndromes. *American Journal of Medicine, 112,* 355–360. Evidence Level IV: Nonexperimental Study.

Simmons, S., Alessi, C., & Schnelle, J. (2001). An intervention to increase fluid intake in nursing home residents: Prompting and preference compliance. *Journal of the American Geriatrics Society, 49,* 926–933. Evidence Level II: Single Experimental Study.

Skipper, A. (1993). Monitoring and complications of enteral feeding. In A. Skipper (Ed.), *Dietitian's handbook of enteral and parenteral nutrition* (p. 298). Rockville, MD: Aspen Publishers.

Smith, A., Vallance, H., & Slater, R. (1997). Shorter preoperative fluid fasts reduce postoperative emesis. *British Medical Journal, 314,* 1486. Evidence Level II: Single Experimental Study.

Spangler, P., Risley, T., & Bilyew, D. (1984). The management of dehydration and incontinence in nonambulatory geriatric patients. *Journal of Applied Behavior Analysis, 17,* 397–401. Evidence Level III: Quasi-experimental Study.

Spigt, M. G., Knottnerus, J. A., Westerterp, K. R., Olde-Rikkert, M.G. M., & van Schayck, C. P. (2006). The effects of 6 months of increased water intake on blood sodium, glomerular filtration rate, blood pressure, and quality of life in elderly (aged 55–75) men. *Journal of the American Geriatrics Society, 54,* 438–443. Evidence Level II: Single Experimental Study.

Stookey, J. D., Pieper, C. F., & Cohen, H. J. (2005). Is the prevalence of dehydration among community-dwelling older adults really low? Informing the current debate over the fluid recommendation for adults aged 70+ years. *Public Health Nutrition, 8,* 1275–1285. Evidence Level IV: Nonexperimental Study.

Wakefield, B., Mentes, J., Diggelmann, L., & Culp, K. (2002). Monitoring hydration status in elderly veterans. *Western Journal of Nursing Research, 24,* 132–142. Evidence Level IV: Nonexperimental Study.

Wallach, J. (2000). *Interpretation of diagnostic tests* (7th ed., pp.135–141). Philadelphia: Lippincott, Williams & Wilkins.

Warren, J., Bacon, E., Harris, T., McBean, A., Foley, D., & Phillips, C. (1994). The burden and outcomes associated with dehydration among U.S. elderly, 1991. *American Journal of Public Health, 84,* 1265–1269. Evidence Level IV: Nonexperimental Study.

Weinberg, A., Minaker, K., & The Council on Scientific Affairs, AMA (1995). Dehydration: Evaluation and management in older adults. *Journal of the American Medical Association, 274,* 1562–1556. Evidence Level I: Systematic Review.

Weinberg, A., Pals, J., Levesque, P., Beals, L., Cunningham, T., & Minaker, K. (1994). Dehydration and death during febrile episodes in the nursing home. *Journal of the American Geriatrics Society, 42,* 968–971. Evidence Level IV: Nonexperimental Study.

Whelan, K. (2001). Inadequate fluid intakes in dysphagic acute stroke. *Clinical Nutrition, 20,* 423–428. Evidence Level II: Single Experimental Study.

Xiao, H., Barber, J., & Campbell, E. (2004). Economic burden of dehydration among hospitalized elderly patients. *American Journal of Health-System Pharmacists, 61,* 2534–2540. Evidence Level IV: Nonexperimental Study.

Yogendran, S., Asokumar, B., Cheng, D., & Chung, F. (1995). A prospective randomized double-blinded study of the effect of intravenous fluid therapy on adverse outcomes on outpatient surgery. *Anesthesia & Analgesia, 80,* 682–686. Evidence Level II: Single Experimental Study

Zembrzuski, C. (1997). A three-dimensional approach to hydration of elders: Administration, clinical staff, and in-service education. *Geriatric Nursing, 18*(1), 20–26. Evidence Level V: Program Evaluation.

Oral Health Care

17

Linda J. O'Connor

Educational Objectives

At the completion of this chapter, the reader will be able to:

1. discuss the consequences of poor oral health

2. describe a thorough oral assessment in an older adult

3. describe the oral hygiene plan of care for nonintubated older adults

4. discuss nursing interventions for oral care

Background

Poor oral health is associated with malnutrition, dehydration, brain abscesses, valvular heart disease, joint infections, cardiovascular disease, pneumonia, aspiration pneumonia, and poor glycemic control in Type I and II diabetes (Abe, Ishihara, & Okuda, 2001 [Level IV]; Coleman, 2002 [Level III]; Fowler, 2001 [Level V]; Imsand, Janssens, Auckenthaler, Mojon, & Budtz-Jorgensen, 2002 [Level V]; Mojon, 2002 [Level V]; Scannapieco, 1999 [Level V]; Taylor, Loesche,

For a description of Evidence Levels cited in this chapter, see chapter 1, Developing and Evaluating Clinical Practice Guidelines, page 4.

Adapted from L. J. O'Connor & J. A. Ship (September 2005). Oral Health Care in Aging. www.ConsultGeriRN.org

& Terpenning, 2000 [Level IV]; Terpenning et al., 2001 [Level IV]; Yoneyama et al., 2002 [Level II]). Oral health also affects nutritional status, ability to speak, self-esteem, mental wellness, and overall well-being. Despite oral health being essential to overall health status and quality of life, more than a quarter of older adults have not seen a dental professional in the past 5 years (Ship, 2002 [Level V]). Many oral diseases are not part of the natural aging process but rather side effects of medical treatment and medications.

Plaque retention is a problem in elderly people who have difficulty in mechanically removing plaque due to diminished manual dexterity, impaired vision, or chronic illness (Simons, Brailsfords, Kidd, & Beighton, 2001 [Level IV]; Simons, Kidd, & Beighton, 1999 [Level III]). The functional ability and cognitive status of older adults affect their ability to perform oral care and denture care. Lack of good oral hygiene increases the risk for development of secondary infections, extended hospital stays, and significant negative health outcomes. Multiple medications produce side effects that affect the oral cavity. Cardiac medications can cause salivary dysfunction, gingival enlargement, and lichenoid mucosal reactions (Cianco, 2004 [Level V]; Ship, 2000 [Level V]). Steroid treatment can predispose a patient to oral candidiasis, and cancer treatments can cause a plethora of oral conditions such as stomatitis, salivary hypofunction, microbial infections, and xerostomia. Xerostomia is complaints of dry mouth and objective evidence of salivary dysfunction; it is probably not the result of the aging process and therefore requires intervention and prevention. Its prevalence in the elderly is 25% to 40+ %. Some causes are multiple medications, several medical conditions, head and neck radiation, and chemotherapy.

The mouth reflects the culmination of multiple stressors over the years and, as the mouth ages, it is less able to tolerate these stressors. With an increase in chronic disease and medication usage as a person ages, the prevalence of root caries, tooth loss, oral cancers, soft-tissue lesions, and periodontal problems increases significantly (Al-Shammari, Al-Khabbaz, Al-Ansari, Neiva, & Wang, 2005; Shimazaki, Soh, Koga, Miyazaki, & Takehara, 2003 [both Level IV]). Many of the oral health problems in the elderly could be avoided with routine preventive care. Many older adults believe in the myth that a decline in their oral health is a normal part of aging.

Assessment

Physical Assessment

The promotion of oral health through assessment and good oral hygiene is an essential of nursing care. The oral assessment is part of a nurse's head-to-toe assessment of an older adult and is done on admission and at the beginning of each shift. Nurses assess the condition of the oral cavity (i.e., lips, oral mucosa, and tongue); the presence of or absence of natural teeth and/or dentures; the ability to function with or without natural teeth and/or dentures; and the patient's ability to speak, chew, and swallow. The oral cavity should be pink, moist, and intact. Natural teeth should be intact and dentures (partial or full) should fit comfortably and not be moving when the older adult is speaking.

Any abnormal findings such as dryness, swelling, sores, ulcers, bleeding, white patches, broken or decayed teeth, halitosis, ill-fitting dentures, difficulty swallowing, signs of aspiration, and pain are documented by the nurse and the health care team is informed. Poorly fitting dentures can cause ulcerations, candidiasis (i.e., oral fungal infection), masses, and denture stomatitis. Denture stomatitis presents as red, inflamed tissue beneath dentures, caused by fungal infections and insufficient oral hygiene. Some oral mucosal diseases that nurses may see are angular cheilitis (i.e., red and white cracked lesions in the corners of the mouth, caused by inflammation and a fungal infection), cicatrical pemphigoid (i.e., produces red, inflamed lesions on the gingival, palate, tongue, and cheek tissues), lichen planus (i.e., most common form presents as a lacy white appearance on the tongue and/or cheeks; a less common but more painful form produces red and white ulcerated lesions), and Pemphigus vulgaris (i.e., red, bleeding tissues resulting from trauma but heal without scarring). Untreated lesions can develop into large, infected regions that require immediate medical attention: recurrent aphthous stomatitis (canker sores; that is, well-circumscribed lesions that develop under the tongue, inside the lips and cheeks, and most commonly heal within 7 to 10 days). Dental professionals diagnose oral mucosal diseases, but nurses need to be aware of any abnormal findings and report them immediately.

Nurses also need to assess patients for their functional ability and manual dexterity to provide oral hygiene. Nurses need to observe older adults providing their oral hygiene to ensure that it is effective. The primary focus for nurses is to maintain older adults' function so that they may participate in their own daily care. Once older adults provide their oral hygiene, nurses must follow-up as appropriate to complete the oral hygiene.

Assessment Tools

The Oral Health Assessment Tool (OHAT) is an eight-category screening tool that can be used with cognitively intact or impaired older adults. The OHAT provides an organized, efficient method for nurses to document their oral assessment. The eight categories (i.e., lips, tongue, gums and tissues, saliva, natural teeth, dentures, oral cleanliness, and dental pain) are scored from 0 (healthy) to 2 (unhealthy). Total scores range from 0 to 16; the higher the score, the poorer the older adult's oral health (Chalmers, King, Spencer, Wright, & Carter, 2005 [Level III]). The OHAT may be implemented in any health care setting. (See the Resources for access to this tool.)

Intervention and Care Strategies

The "gold standard" for providing oral hygiene is the toothbrush. Toothbrushes should have soft nylon bristles (Fischman, 1997 [Level V]). It is the mechanical action of the toothbrush that is important for plaque removal, and research has shown that the manual toothbrush remains the primary method of maintaining good oral hygiene. If older adults have any decrease in their function or manual dexterity, the nursing staff needs to assess their ability to provide effective oral hygiene and provide assistance as needed. Foam swabs are available in numerous facilities to provide oral hygiene. Research has shown that foam swabs cannot remove plaque as well as toothbrushes (Pearson & Hutton, 2002 [Level II]). Foam swabs may be used for cleaning the oral mucous of an edentulous older adult.

Lemon glycerin swabs/swabsticks are drying to the oral mucosa and cause erosion of the tooth enamel. Combined with decreased salivary flow and an increased rate of xerostomia in older adults, use of potentates the corrosive effect of lemon-glycerin swabs (Meurman et al., 1996 [Level II]). Lemon glycerin swabs/swabsticks are detrimental to the older adult and are never to be used.

Commercial mouth rinses that contain alcohol are very trying to the oral mucosa. If an older adult is using a commercial mouth rinse with alcohol, a half commercial mouthwash/half water mixture is recommended. Toothpaste with fluoride is currently recommended by the American Dental Association (ADA) to reduce cavities and can also help reduce periodontal disease (Fischman, 1997 [Level V]).

The use of chlorhexidine in postoperative cardiac patients has been supported by scientific research for several years. It has also been shown to be effective against gram-positive bugs associated with dental caries and against fungal organisms, and it is currently recommended only for debilitated patients at risk for oral fungal infections, dental decay, and gingivitis (J. A. Ship, personal communication, February 26, 2007). The use of chlorhexidine in geriatric patients is determined by the dentist. There are some side effects of chlorhexidine (i.e., bitter taste; change in the taste of food; mouth irritation; and staining of teeth, mouth, fillings, and dentures) that may have negative outcomes for older adults. A good oral assessment by nurses on each shift is essential for geriatric patients on chlorhexidine and monitoring of their nutritional intake.

Education of the nursing staff is imperative. Two of the major barriers cited by nursing staff are (1) inadequate knowledge of how to assess and provide care, and (2) lack of appropriate supplies. Implementation of evidence-based protocols combined with educational training sessions have been shown to have a positive impact on oral care being provided and on the oral health status of older adults (Chalmers & Pearson, 2005 [Level III]; Coleman & Watson, 2006 [Level IV]; Fitch, Munro, Glass, & Pelligrini, 1999 [Level V]; Frenkel, Harvey, & Newcombe, 2001 [Level II]; Isaksson, Paulsson, Fridlund, & Nederferos, 2000 [Level III]; Nicol et al., 2005 [Level V]; Stiefel, Damron, Sowers, & Velez, 2000 [Level V]). Staff needs to be instructed on oral hygiene and the proper care of different appliances. Dentures should be brushed before placing them in a denture cup. Dentures should be removed at night; however, some elders prefer to keep their dentures in continuously. It therefore becomes even more important for nurses to perform an assessment of the oral mucosa. In the acute care and long term care settings, older adults may not have dental adhesive and, therefore, there is a high risk for food particles to get caught underneath their dentures. It is important for staff to remember to take the dentures out after each meal, rinse them and the patient's mouth, and place the dentures back in. Complete denture care should be given morning and night and as needed.

Patients on gastrostomy tubes require more frequent mouth care. Although no research studies were found specifically related to oral hygiene/oral health and patients with gastrostomy tubes, anecdotally it has been reported that patients with gastrostomy tubes tend to have an increased buildup of mucus that forms on the tongue. This causes a coating on the tongue that, if not frequently cleared off, can build up and lead to poor oral health and even respiratory distress. Therefore, it is recommended that more frequent mouth care be given to patients with gastrostomy tubes. There is no research focused on the frequency at which the care should be done; however, anecdotally, it is been found that providing oral hygiene to these patients a minimum of every 4 hours or twice in an 8-hour shift appears to prevent this buildup of mucus on the tongue.

Education of nursing staff, older adults, and families is imperative. Nurses need to be educated in oral assessment and nursing assistants need to be educated in observation of the oral cavity and what to report to nurses. Both nurses and nursing assistants need to be educated in the proper techniques for providing oral hygiene and caring for oral appliances. Patients and families need to be educated in the importance of good oral health and hygiene dispel the oral-health myths that exist about oral health and aging in general.

Education focused on the importance of good oral health and hygiene in older adults, the myths about oral health and aging, evidence-based practice protocols, implementing these protocols, and the appropriate products for providing oral hygiene to patients and residents must be provided to administrators. Without the proper supplies, it is impossible for nursing staff to provide the oral hygiene care that older adults need and to properly implement evidence-based protocols for oral health and hygiene.

Case Study and Discussion

Mrs. Smith, an 84-year-old female with a history of Alzheimer's type dementia, was admitted for recent decreased oral intake and percutaneous endoscopic gastrostomy (PEG) placement (a feeding tube placed into the stomach through the abdominal wall). Mrs. Smith was alert and oriented to herself, pleasant, cooperative with care, and able to follow simple directions. She lived at home with her family and received care from a home health aide. The initial oral assessment, done on day 2 of admission, found upper dentures and lower natural teeth, both covered with food particles. The oral mucosa was noted to be dry. The upper dentures were difficult to remove and caused pain to Mrs. Smith. The upper denture was being "kept in place" by a collection of old food that was found upon removal. The oral mucosa under the upper denture was covered with sores and ulcers and was bleeding, infected, and very painful. The health team was notified, a dental consultation was called, and an oral hygiene plan of care was implemented. Mrs. Smith's diet was changed to pureed foods while her oral mucosa was healing and the PEG placement was put on hold. Upon inquiry, it was learned from the family that their long-time aide had moved away and the new aide had been with them only a few months. It was during this time that they noticed the decline in Mrs. Smith's nutritional intake. The family chose to hire a new aide, and both the family and the new aide were educated on proper oral hygiene for Mrs. Smith. Once Mrs. Smith's oral mucosa had healed, the upper denture was replaced and she was returned to her regular diet. Mrs. Smith's oral intake returned to baseline and a PEG was no longer required.

This case study illustrates how poor oral care often goes undetected, the importance of good oral care, the need for physical assessment by nurses, and the need for staff and family education. This patient was being admitted for an invasive procedure secondary to poor oral health caused by poor oral care. Although the family was involved in Mrs. Smith's care (she had no contractures or skin breakdown), her lack of oral care had gone unnoticed by them. The admitting nurse documented that the patient had dentures on the admission form but did not do a physical oral assessment. The nurse caring for the patient on day 2 had attended an oral health seminar and included the physical oral assessment in her morning rounds. She also followed up with the nursing assistants to ensure that oral care had been provided to the patient after each meal. The implementation of an oral hygiene plan of care and the education of nursing staff, family, and home care staff ensured that Mrs. Smith received the oral care required for her oral mucosa to heal and her nutritional status to return to baseline, and prevented the unnecessary placement of a PEG.

Summary

As previously stated, many of the oral-health problems in the elderly could be avoided with routine preventive care, but many older adults believe in the myth that a decline in their oral health is a normal part of aging (Andersson, Hallberg, & Renvert, 2003 [Level IV]; Meurman & Hamalainen, 2006 [Level V]; Peltola, Vehkalahti, & Wuolijoka-Saaristo, 2004 [Level IV]; Reed, Broder, Jenkins, Spivack, & Janal, 2006 [Level IV]). To dispel this myth and improve the oral health of older adults, it is imperative that health care professionals provide continuing education to patients and families, advocate for oral health prevention, and provide oral care to older adults in all settings. Well-developed, evidence-based oral-care protocols and educational training sessions have been shown to have a positive impact on the oral-health status of older patients (Fitch et al., 1999 [Level V]; Isakasson et al., 2000 [Level III]; Stiefel et al., 2000 [Level V], see Box 17.1).

Acknowledgment

Jonathan A. Ship, DMD, Professor, Department of Oral & Maxillofacial Pathology, Radiology and Medicine; Director, Bluestone Center for Clinical Research, New York University College of Dentistry; Professor, Department of Medicine, New York University School of Medicine.

Resources

Assessment Tools

Chalmers, J. M., King, P. L., Spencer, A. J., Wright, F. A. C., & Carter, K. D. (2005). The oral health assessment tool: validity and reliability. *Australian Dental Journal, 50*(3), 191–199. Evidence Level III.

Evidence-Based Protocols

Oral Health Care in Aging www.ConsultGeriRN.org

Johnson, V., Chalmers, J., & Titler, M. (2002). *Evidence-based protocol: Oral hygiene for functionally dependent and cognitively impaired older adults.* Iowa: University of Iowa Gerontological Nursing Interventions Research Center. www.nursing.uiowa.edu/centers/gnirc/protocols.htm

Related Professional Organizations

Academy of General Dentistry www.agd.org

American Dental Association www.ada.org

American Geriatrics Society www.americangeriatrics.org

The University of Iowa Gerontological Nursing Interventions Research Center www.nursing.uiowa.edu/centers/gnirc/disseminatecore.htm

Government Information Agencies

National Institutes on Aging www.niapiblications.org

National Oral Health Information Clearinghouse www.health.gov/NHICscripts/ entry.cfm?HRCode=HR2457

National Institute of Dental and Craniofacial Research www.nidcr.nih.gov

National Center for Chronic Disease Prevention and Health Promotion www.cdc. gov/nccdphp/bb_oralhealth/index.htm

Centers for Disease Control www.cdc.gov/oralhealth/index.htm

Agency for Healthcare Research and Quality (AHRQ) www.ahrq.gov/browse/ dental.htm

Regulatory/Authoritative Sites

National Institute of Dental and Craniofacial Research www.nidcr.nih.gov

American Dental Association www.ada.org

The University of Iowa Gerontological Nursing Interventions Research Center www.nursing.uiowa.edu/centers/gnirc/disseminatecore.htm

Oral Health in America: A Report of the Surgeon General www2.nidcr.nih.gov/ sgr/sgrohweb/home.htm

Continuing Education Opportunities

CE284b Let's talk teeth: Dental health in older adults www.nursingspectrum.com www.ConsultGeriRN.org

Patient and Family Resources

American Dental Association www.ada.org

National Institute of Dental and Craniofacial Research www.nidcr.nih.gov

U.S. National Library of Medicine/National Institutes of Health www.nlm.nih. gov/medlineplus/dentalhealth.html

Box 17.1

Nursing Standard of Practice Protocol: Providing Oral Health Care to Older Adults

This standard of care protocol is based on evidence in multicomponent oral health care studies (Chalmers & Pearson, 2005 [Level IV]); Coleman & Watson, 2006 [Level IV]; Fitch, Munro, Glass, & Pelligrini, 1999 [Level V]; Frenkel, Harvey, & Newcombe, 2001 [Level II]; Isaksson, Paulsson, Fridlund, & Nederferos, 2001 [Level III]; Nicol et al., 2005 [Level V]; Stiefel, Damron, Sowers, & Velez, 2000 [Level V]).

I. OVERVIEW

The promotion of oral health through good oral hygiene is an essential of nursing care. The RN or designee provides regular oral care for functionally dependent and cognitively impaired older adults.

II. BACKGROUND

(Coleman, 2002 [Level III]; Taylor, Loesche, & Terpenning, 2000 [Level IV]; Imsand, Janssens, Auckenthaler, Mojon, & Budtz-Jorgensen, 2002 [Level V]; Terpenning et al., 2001 [Level IV]; Yoneyama et al., 2002 [Level II]; Abe, Ishara, & Okuda, 2001 [Level IV]; Mojon, 2002 [Level V]; Scannapieco, 1999 [Level V]; Fowler, 2001 [Level V])

A. Oral hygiene is directly linked with systemic infections, cardiac disease, CVA, acute MI, glucose control in diabetes, nutritional intake, comfort, ability to speak, and a patient's self-esteem and overall well-being.

B. Statistics (Ship, 2004, 2005; Ship & Ghezzi, 2005; Ship, Phelan, & Kerr, 2003)
1. More than one-half of the elderly dentate population has new or recurrent dental caries.
2. More than two-thirds of the older dentate population has evidence of gingivitis.
3. More than three-quarters of the older dentate population has experienced some form of periodontal attachment loss.

C. Definitions
1. *Oral*: refers to the mouth (natural teeth, gingival and supporting tissues, hard and soft palate, mucosal lining of the mouth and throat, tongue, salivary glands, chewing muscles, upper and lower jaw, lips)
2. *Oral cavity*: includes cheeks, hard and soft palate
3. *Oral hygiene*: the prevention of plaque-related disease, the destruction of plaque through the mechanical action of toothbrushing and flossing or use of other oral hygiene aides

4. *Edentulous*: natural teeth removed

III. PATIENT ASSESSMENT

(Chalmers, King, Spencer, Wright, & Carter, 2005 [Level III])

A. An RN conducts an oral assessment/evaluation on admission and every shift.
   1. A nurse assesses the condition of:
   2. The oral cavity (lips, oral mucosa, and tongue): The oral cavity should be pink, moist, and intact.
   3. The presence or absence of natural teeth and/or dentures: Natural teeth should be intact and dentures (partial or full) should fit comfortably and not be moving when the older adult is speaking.
   4. Ability to function with or without natural teeth and/or dentures.
   5. The patient's ability to speak, chew, and swallow.
   6. Any abnormal findings, such as dryness, swelling, sores, ulcers, bleeding, white patches, broken or decayed teeth, halitosis, ill-fitting dentures, difficulty swallowing, signs of aspiration, and pain are documented by the nurse and the health care team is informed.
B. Assessment Tool: The Oral Health Assessment Tool (OHAT). See the Resources for information about this tool.

IV. NURSING CARE STRATEGIES

(Fischman, 1997 [Level V]; Meurman et al., 1996 [Level II]; Pearson & Hutton, 2002 [Level II])

A. Oral Hygiene Plan of Care: Dependent Mouth Care of the Edentulous Patient
   1. Oral care is provided during morning care, evening care, and PRN.
   2. Wash hands and don gloves.
   3. Remove dentures by pulling the lower plate down and lift forward and out. Pull the upper plate up and forward to dislodge and remove it. Place dentures in emesis basin and proceed to the sink.
   4. Brush dentures with toothbrush/toothpaste using up and down motion.
   5. Clean the grooved area, which fits against the gum with the toothbrush. Rinse with cool water.
   6. Brush the patient's tongue.
   7. Reinsert dentures.
   8. Apply lip moisturizer.
B. Dependent Mouth Care: Patient with Teeth or Partial Dentures
   1. Oral care is provided during morning care, evening care, and PRN.
   2. Wash hands and don gloves.
   3. Place soft toothbrush at an angle against the gum line. Gently brush teeth in an up and down motion with short strokes using the toothbrush.
   4. Brush the patient's tongue.

5. Apply lip moisturizer.
For partial dentures, follow procedure for full denture cleaning and insertion.
C. Assisted/Supervised Care
   1. Oral care is provided during morning care, evening care, and PRN.
   2. Assess what a patient can do and provide assistance as needed.
   3. Set up necessary items.

V. EVALUATION OF EXPECTED OUTCOMES

A. Patient
   1. Will receive oral hygiene a minimum of once every 8 hours while in the acute care, long term care, or home setting.
   2. With gastrostomy tubes and is not unresponsive, will receive mouth care a minimum of every 4 hours while awake.
   3. With gastrostomy tubes and is unresponsive, will receive mouth care a minimum of every 4 hours.
   4. Patients and families will be referred to dental services for follow-up treatment.
   5. Patients and families will be educated on the importance of good oral hygiene and follow-up dental services.
B. Professional Caregiver/RN will:
   1. Conduct an assessment/evaluation of the oral cavity on admission and every shift.
   2. Notify the physician and dentist of any abnormalities present in the oral cavity.
   3. Assess what each a patient can do independently.
   4. Observe aspiration precautions while providing care.
   5. Provide oral care and dental care education to patients and families.
C. Institution
   1. Will provide access to dental services as appropriate.
   2. Will provide ongoing education to health care providers.
   3. Will provide a yearly oral health and dental care in-service to health care providers.

VI. OTHER CLINICAL GUIDELINES

A. Oral Health Care in Aging www.ConsultGeriRN.org
B. Johnson, V., Chalmers, J., & Titler, M. (2002). *Evidence-based protocol: Oral hygiene for functionally dependent and cognitively impaired older adults.* Iowa: University of Iowa Gerontological Nursing Interventions Research Center. www.nursing.uiowa.edu/centers/gnirc/protocols.htm

References

Abe, S., Ishihara, K., & Okuda, K. (2001). Prevalence of potential respiratory pathogens in the mouths of elderly patients and effects of professional oral care. *Archives of Gerontology and Geriatrics, 32*(1), 45–55. Evidence Level IV: Nonexperimental Study.

Al-Shammari, K. F., Al-Khabbaz, A. K., Al-Ansari, J. M., Neiva, R., & Wang, H. L. (2005). Risk indicators for tooth loss due to periodontal disease. *Journal of Periodontology, 76*(11), 1910–1918. Evidence Level IV: Nonexperimental Study.

Andersson, P., Hallberg, I. R., & Renvert, S. (2003). Comparison of oral health status on admission and at discharge in a group of geriatric rehabilitation patients. *Oral Health Prevention Dentistry, 1*(3), 221–228. Evidence Level IV: Nonexperimental Study.

Chalmers, J. M., King, P. L., Spencer, A. J., Wright, F. A. C., & Carter, K. D. (2005). The oral health assessment tool: Validity and reliability. *Australian Dental Journal, 50*(3), 191–199. Evidence Level III: Quasi-experimental Study.

Chalmers, J. M., & Pearson, A. (2005). A systemic review of oral health assessment by nurses and carers for residents with dementia in residential care facilities. *Special Care Dentistry, 25*(5), 227–233. Evidence Level III: Quasi-experimental Study.

Cianco, S. G. (2004). Medications' impact on oral health. *The Journal of the American Dental Association, 135*(10), 1440–1448. Evidence Level V: Literature Review.

Coleman, P. (2002). Improving oral health care for the frail elderly: A review of widespread problems and best practices. *Geriatric Nursing, 23*(4), 189–199. Evidence Level III: Quasi-experimental Study.

Coleman, P., & Watson, N. W. (2006). Oral care provided by certified nursing assistants in nursing homes. *Journal of the American Geriatrics Association, 54*(1), 138–143. Evidence Level IV: Nonexperimental Study.

Fischman, S. L. (1997). The history of oral hygiene products: How far have we come in 6,000 years? *Periodontology, 15*, 7–14. Evidence Level V: Literature Review.

Fitch, J., Munro, C., Glass, C., & Pelligrini, J. (1999). Oral care in the adult intensive care unit. *American Journal of Critical Care, 8*(5), 314–318. Evidence Level V: Program Evaluation.

Fowler, E. B. (2001). Peridontal disease and its association with systemic disease. *Military Medicine, 166*(1), 85–89. Evidence Level V: Literature Review.

Frenkel, H., Harvey, I., & Newcombe, R. G. (2001). Improving oral health in institutionalized elderly people by educating caregivers: A randomized controlled trial. *Community Dentistry and Oral Epidemiology, 29*, 289–297. Evidence Level II: RCT.

Imsand, M., Janssens, J. P., Auckenthaler, R., Mojon, P., & Budtz-Jorgensen, E. (2002). Bronchopneumonia and oral health in hospitalized older patients: A pilot study. *Gerodontology, 19*(2), 66–72. Evidence Level V: Review.

Isaksson, D., Paulsson, G., Fridlund, B., & Nederferos, T. (2000). Evaluation of an oral health education program for nursing personnel in special housing facilities for the elderly, Part II. *Special Care Dentistry, 20*(3), 173–180. Evidence Level III: Quasi-experimental Study.

Meurman, J. H., & Hamalainen, P. (2006). Oral health and morbidity: Implications of oral infections on the elderly. *Gerodontology, 23*(1), 3–16. Evidence Level V: Literature Review.

Meurmam, J. H., Sorvari, R., Peltari, A., Rytomaa, I., Franssila, S., & Kroon, L. (1996). Hospital mouth-cleaning aids may cause dental erosion. *Special Care in Dentistry, 16*(6), 247–250. Evidence Level II: Experimental Study.

Mojon, P. (2002). Oral health and respiratory infection. *Journal of the Canadian Dental Association, 68*(6), 340–345. Evidence Level V: Literature Review.

Nicol, R., Sweeney, M. P., McHugh, S., & Bagg, J. (2005). Effectiveness of health care worker training on oral health of elderly residents of nursing homes. *Community Dentistry and Oral Epidemiology, 33*, 115–124. Evidence Level V: Program Evaluation.

Pearson, L. S., & Hutton, J. L. (2002). A controlled trial to compare the ability of foam swabs and toothbrushes to remove dental plaque. *Journal of Advanced Nursing, 39*(5), 480–489. Evidence Level II: RCT.

Peltola, O., Vehkalahti, M. M., & Wuolijoki-Saaristo, K. (2004). Oral health and treatment needs of the long-term hospitalized elderly. *Gerodontology, 21*(2), 93–99. Evidence Level IV: Nonexperimental Study.

Reed, R., Broder, H. L., Jenkins, G., Spivack, E., & Janal, M. N. (2006). Oral health promotion among older persons and their care providers in a nursing home facility. *Gerodontology*, *23*(2), 73–78. Evidence Level IV: Nonexperimental Study.

Scannapieco, F. A. (1999). Role of bacteria in respiratory infection. *Journal of Periodontology*, *70*(7), 793–802. Evidence Level V: Literature Review.

Shimazaki, Y., Soh, I., Koga, T., Miyazaki, H., & Takehara, T. (2003). Risk factor for tooth loss in the institutionalized elderly: A six-year cohort study. *Community Dental Health, 20*(2), 123–127. Evidence Level IV: Nonexperimental Study.

Ship, J. A. (2002). Improving oral health in older people. *Journal of the American Geriatrics Society, 50*, 1454–1455. Evidence Level V: Literature Review/Care Report.

Ship, J. A. (2004). Mouth and dental disorders. In M. H. Beers, T. V. Jones, M. Berkwits, J. L. Kaplan, & R. Porter (Eds.), *The Merck manual of health and aging* (1st ed., pp. 495–506), Whitehouse Station, NJ: Merck & Co.

Ship, J. A. (2005). The oral cavity. In W. R. Hazzard, J. P. Blass, J. B. Halter, J. G. Ouslander, & M. E. Tinetti (Eds.), *Principles of geriatric medicine and gerontology* (5th ed.). New York: McGraw-Hill.

Ship, J. A., & Chavez, E. M. (2000). Management of systemic disease and chronic impairments in older adults: Oral health considerations. *General Dentistry, 48*(5), 555–565. Evidence Level V: Literature Review/Care Report.

Ship, J. A., & Ghezzi, E. M. (2005). Oral manifestations of systemic disease. In C. W. Cummings, P. W. Flint, & L. A. Harker, et al. (Eds.), *Cummings: Otolaryngology head and neck surgery* (4th ed., pp. 1493–1510). Philadelphia: Elsevier Mosby.

Ship, J. A., Phelan, J. A., & Kerr, A. R. (2003). Biology and pathology of the oral mucosa. In I. M. Freedberg, A. Z. Eisen, K. Wolff, K. F. Austen, L. A. Goldsmith, & S. I. Katz. (Eds.), *Fitzpatrick's dermatology in general medicine* (6th ed., pp. 1077–1090). New York: McGraw-Hill.

Simons, D., Brailsfords, S., Kidd, E. A. M., & Beighton, D. (2001). Relationship between oral hygiene practices and oral status in dentate elderly people living in residential homes. *Community Dentistry and Oral Epidemiology, 29*(6), 464–470. Evidence Level IV: Nonexperimental Study.

Simons, D., Kidd, E. A. M., & Beighton, D. (1999). Oral health of elderly occupants in residential homes. *Lancet, 353*, 1761. Evidence Level III: Quasi-experimental Study.

Stiefel, K., Damron, S., Sowers, N., & Velez, L. (2000). Improving oral hygiene for the seriously ill patient: Implementing research-based practice. *MedSurg Nursing, 9*(1), 40–46. Evidence Level V: Program Evaluation.

Taylor, G. W., Loesche, W. J., & Terpenning, M. S. (2000). Impact of oral diseases on systemic health in the elderly: Diabetes mellitus and aspiration pneumonia. *Journal of Public Health Dentistry, 60*(4), 313–320. Evidence Level IV: Nonexperimental Study.

Terpenning, M. S., Taylor, G. W., Lopatin, D. E., Kerr, C. K., Dominguez, L., & Loesche, W. J. (2001). Aspiration pneumonia: Dental and oral risk factors in an older veteran population. *Journal of the American Geriatrics Society, 49*(5), 557–563. Evidence Level IV: Nonexperimental Study.

Yoneyama, T., Yoshida, M., Ohrui, T., Mukaiyama, H., Okamoto, H., & Hoshiba, K., et al. (2002). Oral care reduces pneumonia in older patients in nursing homes. *Journal of the American Geriatrics Society, 50*(3), 430–433. Evidence Level II: Individual Experimental Study.

Preventing Pressure Ulcers and Skin Tears

18

Elizabeth A. Ayello
R. Gary Sibbald

Educational Objectives

On completion of this chapter, the reader should be able to:

1. complete a pressure ulcer risk assessment

2. assess risk factors associated with pressure ulcer development

3. interpret the meaning of an individual's risk assessment score

4. develop a comprehensive, holistic plan to prevent pressure ulcers in individuals at risk

5. identify elders at risk for skin tears

6. classify skin tears and develop a plan to prevent and treat skin tears

The skin is the largest external organ so preserving its integrity is an important aspect of nursing care. Florence Nightingale (1859) identified a link between skin injury (specifically, pressure ulcers) and nursing. Performing a risk assessment and implementing a consistent prevention protocol may prevent some types of skin injuries, including pressure ulcers or skin tears. Although pressure ulcers and skin tears may look similar, they are different types of skin injury: skin tears are acute traumatic wounds whereas pressure ulcers are chronic wounds. It is important, therefore, to assess the wound and to determine the correct etiology so that the proper individualized treatment plan can be implemented.

For a description of Evidence Levels cited in this chapter, see chapter 1, Developing and Evaluating Clinical Practice Guidelines, page 4.

Pressure Ulcers

Pressure ulcers are a significant health care problem worldwide. In February 2007, the National Pressure Ulcer Advisory Panel (NPUAP) revised the classic 1989 pressure ulcer definition (NPUAP, 1989) to be as follows: "A pressure ulcer is a localized injury to the skin and/or underlying tissue usually over a bony prominence, as a result of pressure, or pressure in combination with shear and/or friction. A number of contributing or confounding factors are also associated with pressure ulcers; the significance of these factors is yet to be elucidated (Black et al., 2007 [Level IV]; NPUAP, 2007 [Level IV]). Most pressure ulcers are found on the sacrum, with heels being the second most common site (Cuddigan, Ayello, & Sussman, 2001 [Level I]). In hospice patients, in addition to sacrum and heels, elbows were a common site for ulcers; most ulcers occurred within 2 weeks of death (Hanson et al., 1991 [Level IV]). Following an extensive review of the data, the NPUAP concluded that the prevalence of pressure ulcers in acute care in the United States ranged from 10% to 18%, with the best current estimate of prevalence being 15% (Cuddigan et al., 2001 [Level I]). The pressure ulcer prevalence in long term care ranged from 2.3% to 28%, whereas in home care it was 0% to 29% (Cuddigan et al., 2001 [Level I]). Incidence, or the number of new cases that develop in the particular agency during a specified period, ranged from 0.4% to 38% in acute care, with 7% being the best average (Cuddigan et al., 2001 [Level I]). A study of 20 hospitals of patients waiting for surgery determined a higher incidence of pressure ulcers for longer surgery waiting times or time in an intensive care unit (Baumgarten et al., 2003 [Level IV]). The less time patients waited to go to the operating room (OR) for repair of hip fracture resulted in fewer pressure ulcers (Hommel, Ulander, & Thorngren, 2003 [Level IV]). Length of time on the OR table also increased risk for pressure ulcers in hip-fracture patients (Houwing et al., 2004 [Level IV]). In one study of 84 surgical patients, most pressure ulcers occurred within the first 3 days post-op (Karadag & Gumuskaya, 2006 [Level IV]).

In long term care (LTC), the incidence ranged from 2.2% to 23.9%, whereas in home care it ranged from 0% to 17% (Cuddigan et al., 2001 [Level I]). In a retrospective study of more than 2,400 residents in LTC, pressure ulcers were more likely to develop in residents who were female, older, cognitively impaired, and immobile (Horn et al., 2002 [Level III]). Conversely, Horn & colleagues (2004 [Level III]) found that residents with nutritional intervention, antidepressant use, use of disposable briefs for more than 14 days, care by registered nurse of at least 0.25 hour per day (or at least 2 hours per day by a nurse's aide), or in facilities with an LPN turnover rate of less than 25% were less likely to develop pressure ulcers. A lower incidence of admission with a pressure ulcer to LTC was associated with White individuals; a higher incidence was associated with being chair or bed-bound, underweight, or in the presence of fecal incontinence (Baumgarten et al., 2003 [Level IV]).

Pressure ulcers are associated with complications including cellulitis, osteomyelitis, sepsis, increased length of stay, and financial and emotional costs (Agency for Health Care Policy and Research [AHCPR], now Agency for Healthcare Research and Quality [AHRQ], 1992 [Level I]). The Wound, Ostomy and Continence Nurses Society [WOCN] has since updated the guideline (2003 [Level I]) after a review of the literature. These ulcers occur from a combination of intensity and duration of pressure, as well as from tissue tolerance (Bergstrom, Braden, Laguzza, & Holman, 1987 [Level III]; Braden & Bergstrom, 1987 [Level II]; Braden & Bergstrom, 1989 [Level III]). Immobility as seen in bed- or chair-bound patients and those unable to change positions, undernourishment or malnutrition, incontinence, friable skin, impaired cognitive ability, and decreased ability to respond to one's environment are some of the important identified risk factors for pressure ulcers (Braden, 1998). Berlowitz and colleagues (2001 [Level IV]) found 17 characteristics of residents in LTC that were associated with pressure ulcer development, including dependence in mobility and transferring, diabetes mellitus, urinary incontinence, lower body mass index (BMI), and end-stage disease. No one single factor puts a patient at risk for pressure ulcer skin breakdown. A home care study identified increased risk of pressure ulcer development with being in bed with limited activity, dependence for putting on clothes, assistance for transfers, and urinary incontinence as predictors of stage 1 pressure ulcer occurrence (Bergquist, 2003 [Level IV]). For stage 2 or higher levels, there were other predictors, including oxygen use and the presence of a bone fracture.

Recent regulatory and government initiatives continuously support the importance of pressure ulcer prevention. An objective in Healthy People 2010 mandates the reduction of pressure ulcer incidence rates (Health Care Financing Administration [HCFA], 2000). The Centers for Medicare and Medicaid Services (CMS) released revised guidance for surveyors for Federal Regulation Tag F-314 regarding prevention of pressure ulcers in LTC in 2004. The federal regulation to prevent pressure ulcers from occurring or from existing ulcers becoming worse did not change, but the interpretation for surveyors did change. A 40-page document is provided for surveyors, but its content is based on a comprehensive review of the literature (CMS, 2004 [Level V]) and it does provide recommendations and direction for clinicians to prevent and treat pressure ulcers. Data from the Healthcare Cost and Utilization Project (HCUP) statistical review reveals that during the period 1993–2003, pressure ulcers increased in hospitalized patients by 63% even though the number of hospitalizations only increased by 11% (Russo & Elixhauser, 2006 [Level IV]). In the state of New Jersey, stage 3 or 4 pressure ulcers are now reportable in acute care (New Jersey Department of Health and Senior Services, 2004). Pressure ulcers are one of the 12 targeted areas to reduce harm to hospitalized patients in the United States as part of the Institute for Healthcare Improvement "5 Million Lives Saved Campaign" launched in December 2006 (Institute for Healthcare Improvement [IHI], 2006 [Level V]). Thus, at the beginning of the 21st century, appropriate risk assessment and preventative care take on even more important meaning. Nurses will find the NPUAP competencies for registered nurses on pressure ulcer prevention helpful in guiding their professional practice (Table 18.1).

Risk Assessment

When to Do an Assessment

Assessing relative risk is the first step of any individual patient or health care system plan for pressure ulcer prevention. Some pressure ulcer clinical

18.1 National Pressure Ulcer Advisory Panel

Purpose:
To prepare registered nurses with the minimum competencies for pressure ulcer prevention.

Competencies:
1 Identify etiologic factors contributing to pressure ulcer occurrence.
2 Identify risk factors for pressure ulcer development.
3 Recognize the presence of factors affecting tissue tolerance.
4 Conduct risk assessment using a valid and reliable tool.
5 Conduct a thorough skin assessment considering the individual's uniqueness.
6 Develop and implement an individualized program of skin care.
7 Demonstrate proper positioning to decrease pressure ulcer occurrence.
8 Select and use support surfaces as indicated by risk status.
9 Use nutritional interventions as appropriate to prevent incident pressure ulcers.
10 Accurately document results of risk assessment, skin assessment, and prevention strategies.
11 Apply critical-thinking skills to clinical decision making regarding the impact of changes in the individual's condition on pressure ulcer risk.
12 Make referrals to other health care professionals based on client assessment.

©Copyright 2001: National Pressure Ulcer Advisory Panel, used with permission.

Source: National Pressure Ulcer Advisory Panel. (2001). Pressure ulcer prevention: A competency-based curriculum. Retrieved April 21, 2007, from www.npuap.org/prevwrr.pdf

guidelines recommend that patients be assessed for pressure ulcer development on admission to a facility, on discharge, whenever the patient's condition changes, and then reassessed periodically (AHCPR, 1992; WOCN, 2003 [both Level I]). Although some clinicians have suggested reassessment intervals of every 48 hours in acute care (Ayello & Braden, 2001, 2002 [both Level V]), the IHI recommends daily pressure ulcer risk assessment (IHI, 2006 [Level V]). In LTC, research has shown that most pressure ulcers occur soon after admission (Bergstrom & Braden, 1992 [Level III]); as a result, it is recommended that LTC patients be reassessed weekly for the first 4 weeks, then at least monthly to quarterly or whenever the patient's condition changes. The best interval to do pressure ulcer risk assessment in home care has yet to be determined. In home care, reassessment for pressure ulcer risk may occur as often as at each nursing visit (Ayello & Braden, 2001, 2002 [both Level V]). Bergquist and Frantz (2001 [Level IV]) found that in 1,711 home care patients, risk assessment should be done on admission, weekly for the first 4 weeks, and then every other week. Research by Bergstrom and Braden (1992 [Level III]) found no difference in risk assessment scores performed at different times of day in the acute-care and LTC setting. Risk assessment can be done on either the day or evening shift, depending on which works best for the facility.

Pressure Ulcer Risk Assessment Tools

The AHRQ Panel Guidelines (AHCPR, 1992 [Level V]) recommend that an assessment for pressure ulcer risk be done using a valid and reliable assessment tool. Although there are several risk assessment scales available, research supports only the reliability and validity of the Braden (Pancorbo-Hidalgo, Garcia-Fernandez, Lopez-Medina, & Alvarez-Nieto, 2006 [Level I]) and Norton Scales (Norton, McLaren, & Exton-Smith, 1962); therefore, they are the only scales mentioned in the 1992 AHRQ prevention guidelines. A recent study of 429 patients in acute care found the modified Braden scale to be a better predictor than the Norton Scale (Kwong et al., 2005 [Level IV]). Although there are some concerns about methodology, one study found the Gosnell Scale to have better predictive validity than the Braden, Norton, and Waterlow to which it was compared (Jalali & Rezaie, 2005 [Level IV]).

The Braden Scale was created in 1987 as part of a research study (Bergstrom et al., 1987 [Level III]) and is the most widely used in the United States. Each of its six factors assesses the etiologic factors in pressure ulcer development. Sensory perception, mobility, and activity address clinical situations that predispose the patient to intense and prolonged pressure. Moisture, nutrition, and friction/shear address factors that alter tissue tolerance for pressure. Each of the six categories is ranked with a numerical score, with 1 representing the lowest possible subscore with the greatest risk. The sum of the six subscores is the final Braden score, which can range from 6 to 23. Braden Scale scores are as follows: 1 = highly impaired, 3–4 = moderate to low impairment, total points possible = 23, risk-predicting score = 16 or less.

A low Braden Scale score indicates that a patient is at risk for pressure ulcers. The increased risk score for the development of a pressure sore on the Braden Scale was originally determined to be 16 (Bergstrom et al., 1987 [Level III]). Further research in older adults (Bergstrom & Braden, 1992 [Level III]) and in people with darkly pigmented skin (Lyder et al., 1998, 1999 [both Level IV]) indicates that a risk score of 18 should be used in patients from these populations. The prevention protocols should be initiated for patients whose Braden Scale score is at or below the risk score. Bergquist (2001 [Level IV]) found that whereas the Braden Scale subscores of friction/shear, limited mobility, and moisture were most predictive of pressure ulcer occurrence in 1,684 home care patients, the summative score was most strongly related to the development of pressure ulcers. Interesting research by Chan, Tan, Lee, & Lee (2005 [Level IV]) also found that the total Braden Score was the only significant predictor of pressure ulcers in hospitalized patients.

However, in direct contrast, it is not just about the total score as far as regulatory agencies are concerned. CMS recommends that prevention protocols be implemented for low scores in *any* of the subscales in the Braden Scale (CMS, 2004 [Level V]). The use of prevention protocols has shown a 60% drop in pressure ulcer incidence as well as a decrease in severity of ulcers and cost of care (Braden & Bergstrom, 1989 [Level III]). Unfortunately, in another study, the use of an AHRQ prevention protocol demonstrated that the decrease in pressure ulcer incidence and the increase in length of time before a pressure ulcer developed was not sustained over time (Xakellis, Frantz, Lewis, & Harvey, 2001 [Level IV]). Frantz and Baranoski (2001 [Level V]) summarized studies from 1990–2000 assessing the effectiveness of pressure ulcer prevention in various settings. The prevention programs included risk assessment, pressure-reduction interventions, and staff education. Pressure ulcer incidence declined in all studies regardless of setting. A decrease in incidence in the four LTC studies ranged from 3.5% to 24%, which was more variable than the range in the five acute-care studies of 11% to 16%. A process for implementing prevention guidelines using a systems approach was suggested by Bryant and Rolstead (2001 [Level V]). Aurigemma (2005 [Level III]) found a lower incidence of pressure ulcers (3%) for hospitalized LTC residents who participated in a monitored order system and prevention program as compared to 34% in those who did not participate in the program.

Does Race Make a Difference?

When it comes to severity of pressure ulcers, race may make a difference. Ayello and Lyder (2001 [Level V]) analyzed and summarized the existing data about pressure ulcers across the skin-pigmentation spectrum. Lyder (1991, 1996 [both Level IV]) pioneered research about incidence rates and stage I pressure ulcers in Blacks and Latinos. One study by Bergstrom and Braden (2002 [Level IV]) found no difference in risk between Blacks and Whites in a multisite study of the predictive validity of the Braden Scale in nursing homes. Blacks have the lowest incidence (19%) of superficial tissue damage classified as stage I pressure ulcers, and Whites have the highest at 46% (Barczak, Barnett, Childs, & Bosley, 1997 [Level IV]). The more severe tissue injury seen in stages II–IV pressure ulcers is higher in persons with darkly pigmented skin (Barczak et al., 1997; Meehan, 1990, 1994 [all Level IV]). Three national surveys showed that Blacks had 39% (Barczak et al., 1997 [Level IV]), 16% (Meehan, 1990 [Level IV]); and 41% (Meehan, 1994 [Level IV]) higher incidence of stage II pressure ulcers. Subsequent studies by Lyder and colleagues (1998, 1999 [both Level IV]) continue to support a higher incidence of pressure ulcers in persons with darkly pigmented skin. Baumgarten et al. (2004 [Level IV]) found a significantly high incidence of pressure ulcers for Black residents compared to White residents in nursing homes. Therefore, early identification of stage I pressure ulcers in this population is critical to identify early damage prior to skin breakdown.

The clinician assessment of Black skin may lack the sensitivity and specificity by clinicians assessing patients with darkly pigmented skin and may contribute to the increased severity and incidence of higher stage pressure ulcers (Barczak et al., 1997; Henderson et al., 1997; Lyder et al., 1998, 1999 [all Level IV]). Inadequate detection of stage I pressure ulcers in persons with darkly pigmented skin may be because clinicians erroneously believe that dark skin tolerates pressure better than light skin (Bergstrom, Braden, Kemp, Champagne, & Ruby, 1996) or that only color changes (see Table 18.2 on NPUAP stage I definitions) indicate an ulcer (Barczak et al., 1997 [Level IV]; Bennett, 1995 [Level V]; Henderson et al., 1997 [Level IV]; Lyder, 1996 [Level IV]; Lyder et al., 1998, 1999 [both Level IV]). Bennett (1995, p. 35 [Level V]) defined darkly pigmented skin as "the obvious color of intact dark skin which remains unchanged when pressure is applied over a bony prominence." In 1998, the NPUAP approved a

18.2   2007 NPUAP Pressure Ulcer Staging System

Pressure Ulcer Definition

A pressure ulcer is a localized injury to the skin and/or underlying tissue usually over a bony prominence, as a result of pressure, or pressure in combination with shear and/or friction. *A number of contributing or confounding factors are also associated with pressure ulcers; the significance of these factors is yet to be elucidated.*

Pressure Ulcer Stages

Suspected deep-tissue injury

Purple or maroon localized areas of discolored intact skin or a blood-filled blister due to damage of underlying soft tissue from pressure and/or shear. The area may be preceded by tissue that is painful, firm, mushy, boggy, warmer, or cooler as compared to adjacent tissue.

Further description

Deep-tissue injury may be difficult to detect in individuals with dark skin tones. Evolution may include a thin blister over a dark wound bed. The wound may further evolve and become covered by thin eschar. Evolution may be rapid, exposing additional layers of tissue even with optimal treatment.

Stage I:

Intact skin with non-blanchable redness of a localized area usually over a bony prominence. Darkly pigmented skin may not have visible blanching: its color may differ from the surrounding area.

Further description:

The area may be painful, firm, soft, warmer, or cooler as compared to adjacent tissue. Stage I may be difficult to detect in individuals with dark skin tones. May indicate "at risk" persons (a heralding sign of risk)

Stage II:

Partial thickness loss of dermis presenting as a shallow open ulcer with a red-pink wound bed, without slough. May also present as an intact or open/ruptured serum-filled blister.

Further description:

Presents as a shiny or dry shallow ulcer without slough or bruising.* This stage should not be used to describe skin tears, tape burns, perineal dermatitis, maceration, or excoriation.

*Bruising indicated suspected deep-tissue injury.

18.2   2007 NPUAP Pressure Ulcer Staging System

Stage III:

Full thickness tissue loss. Subcutaneous fat may be visible but bone, tendon, or muscle is *not* exposed. Slough may be present but does not obscure the depth of tissue loss. *May* include undermining and tunneling.

Further description:

The depth of a stage III pressure ulcer varies by anatomical location. The bridge of the nose, ear, occiput, and malleolus do not have subcutaneous tissue and stage III ulcers can be shallow. In contrast, areas of significant adiposity can develop extremely deep stage III pressure ulcers. Bone/tendon is not visible or directly palpable.

Stage IV:

Full thickness tissue loss with exposed bone, tendon, or muscle. Slough or eschar may be present on some parts of the wound bed. *Often* include undermining and tunneling.

Further description:

The depth of a stage IV pressure ulcer varies by anatomical location. The bridge of the nose, ear, occiput, and malleolus do not have subcutaneous tissue and these ulcers can be shallow. Stage IV ulcers can extend into muscle and/or supporting structures (e.g., fascia, tendon, or joint capsule) making osteomyelitis possible. Exposed bone/tendon is visible or directly palpable.

Unstageable:

Full thickness tissue loss in which the base of the ulcer is covered by slough (yellow, tan, gray, green, or brown) and/or eschar (tan, brown, or black) in the wound bed.

Further description:

Until enough slough and/or eschar is removed to expose the base of the wound, the true depth and, therefore, stage cannot be determined. Stable (dry, adherent, intact without erythema or fluctuance) eschar on the heels serves as "the body's natural (biological) cover" and should not be removed.

See NPUAP Web site www.npuap.org; Black et al., 2007

revised definition of a stage I pressure ulcer to include assessment variables other than color—specifically, skin temperature, skin consistency, and sensation (NPUAP, 1998 [Level V]).

Research has begun to validate these assessment characteristics in the stage I definition. Lyder and colleagues (2001 [Level III]) reported a higher diagnostic accuracy rate of 78% using the revised definition compared with 58% using the original definition. Sprigle, Linden, McKenna, Davis, and Riordan (2001 [Level IV]) found changes in skin temperature, in particular, that warmth, then coolness, accompanied most stage I pressure ulcers.

Clinicians should pay careful attention to a variety of factors when assessing a client with darkly pigmented skin for stage I pressure ulcers. Differences in skin over bony prominences (e.g., the sacrum and the heels) as compared with surrounding skin may be indicators of a stage I pressure ulcer. The skin should be assessed for alterations in pain or local sensation. Also, a change of skin color should be noted by being familiar with the range of skin pigmentation that is normal for a particular patient (Bennett, 1995 [Level V]; Henderson et al., 1997 [Level IV]). The correct lighting source is important to accurately perform the skin assessment; where possible, natural or halogen light should be used when performing the assessment (Bennett, 1995 [Level V]). Fluorescent light should be avoided because it casts a bluish hue to the skin (Bennett, 1995 [Level V]). Clinicians may find the application of the limited studies and expert opinion helpful in the early detection of skin injury as seen in stage I pressure ulcer clients across the skin- pigment continuum.

Interventions Aimed at Prevention

Determining a patient's risk for developing a pressure ulcer is only the first step in providing best practice care. Once risk is identified, implementing a consistent protocol to prevent the development of a pressure ulcer is essential. A nursing standard of practice protocol for pressure ulcer prevention is presented to facilitate proactive interventions to prevent pressure ulcers (Box 18.1). A change in attitude of health care professionals may be required to get them to act on prevention modalities (Buss, Halfens, Abu-Saad, & Kok, 2004 [Level III]). Several clinical guidelines on preventing and treating pressure ulcers exist. Most are based on the AHRQ (now AHCPR) Panel for Prediction and Preventions (1992 [Level V]; Bergstrom & the AHCPR Treatment of Pressure Ulcers Guideline Panel, 1994 [Level 1]) guidelines, with WOCN (2003 [Level I]) guidelines being the most recently evidenced updated nursing guidelines. Components of a pressure ulcer prevention protocol should minimally include interventions targeting skin care, pressure redistribution, repositioning, and nutrition.

Skin Care

Skin that is too dry or too wet has been associated with pressure ulcers. Frantz, Xakellis, Harvey, & Lewis (2003 [Level IV]) found that pressure ulcer rates were decreased when appropriate interventions were implemented to treat incontinence in residents in a nursing home. Although there is limited research, dry skin is believed to predispose ulcer formation (Allman, Goode, Patrick, Burst & Bartolucci, 1995 [Level IV]). One quasi-experimental study demonstrated a reduction in incidence of stages I and II pressure ulcers through a combination of using body wash and skin-protectant products along with proper education of the staff (Thompson, Langemo, Anderson, Hanson, & Hunter, 2005 [Level III]). After implementation of an early prevention protocol for skin prevention in two nursing homes, stage I and stage II pressure ulcer incidence decreased from 19.9% to 8.1% (Hunter et al., 2003 [Level III]). In Australia, where real medical sheepskin is available, one study that had some questionable methodology found that patients randomly assigned to the real sheepskin mattress overlay during their hospital stay had a 9.6% incidence risk of pressure ulcers compared to the control group that had 16.6% (Jolley et al., 2004 [Level II]).

Pressure Redistribution

Because immobility is a risk factor in the development of pressure ulcers in hospitalized patients (Lindgren, Unosson, Fredrikson, & Ek, 2004 [Level VI]), efforts must be made to address pressure. Although turning and repositioning patients is a key intervention to redistribute the pressure and prevent pressure ulcers, the best frequency for turning and repositioning, as well as which support surface to use, remains a challenge (De Floor, De Bacquer & Grypdonck, 2005 [Level III]; Norton, McLaren & Exton-Smith, 1975 [Level IV]; Young, 2004 [Level IV]). Redistributing pressure is a key component of preventing pressure ulcers. Hampton and Collins (2005 [Level II]) found a reduction in pressure ulcers when visco-elastic mattresses or cushions were used for residents in a nursing home. When compared to alternating pressure overlays, alternating pressure mattresses reduced length of stay for hospitalized patients, thereby decreasing costs, as well as the added benefit of delaying the time to when a pressure ulcer appeared (Iglesias et al., 2006 [Level II]; Nixon et al., 2006 [Level II]). The incidence of heel pressure ulcers has been decreased when the appropriate heel-suspending device has been used to relieve pressure (Gilcreast et al., 2005 [Level II]). Attention to pressure redistribution also needs to be brought into the OR.

Nutrition

There is lack of consensus about the best way to assess nutritional impairment. Cavalcanti-Cordeiro and colleagues (2005 [Level IV]) found that decreased concentrations of ascorbic acid and alpha-tocopherol were significantly decreased in patients with pressure ulcers or infection. In a randomized double-blind study on the effect of a daily supplement with protein, arginine, zinc, and antioxidants versus a water-based placebo supplement in patients with hip fractures, the incidence of stage II pressure ulcers showed a 9% difference between the nutritionally supplemented group and the placebo group (Houwing, Rozendaal, Wouters-Wessling, Beulens, & Buskens, 2003 [Level II]). The Cochrane Database review of the role of nutrition in pressure ulcer prevention and treatment concluded that due to the lack of high-quality trials, no firm conclusions of the effect of the provision of enteral or parenteral nutrition could be determined (Langer,

Schloemer, Knerr, Kuss, & Behrens, 2003 [Level I]). When and how patients should be nutritionally supplemented to prevent pressure ulcers remains unclear (Haalboom, 2003 [Level II]; Reddy, Gill, & Rochon, 2006 [Level I]; Stratton et al., 2005 [Level I]); at times the literature is contradictory.

Skin Tears

Skin tears are traumatic wounds caused by shear and friction (O'Regan, 2002 [Level V]). This skin injury occurs when the epidermis is separated from the dermis (Malone, Rozario, Gavinski, & Goodwin, 1991 [Level IV]). Because aging skin has a thinner epidermis, a flatter dermal–epidermal junction, and decreased dermal collagen, older persons are more prone to skin injury from mechanical trauma (Baranoski, 2000 [Level V]; Payne & Martin, 1993 [Level IV]; White, Karam, & Cowell, 1994 [Level IV]). Therefore, skin tears are common in older adults, with more than 1.5 million occurring annually in institutionalized adults in the United States (Thomas, Goode, LaMaster, Tennyson, & Parnell, 1999 [Level III]). Skin tears are frequently located at areas of age-related purpura (Malone et al., 1991 [Level IV]; White et al., 1994 [Level IV]).

Assessment of Skin Tears

The following areas should be assessed for skin tears: shins, face, dorsal aspect of hands, and plantar aspect of the foot (Malone et al., 1991 [Level IV]). In addition to elders, others with thinning skin who are at risk for skin tears are patients on long-term steroid therapy, women with decreased hormone levels, people with peripheral vascular disease or neuropathy (i.e., the decreased sensation making them more susceptible to injury), and those with inadequate nutritional intake (O'Regan, 2002 [Level V]).

The three-group risk assessment tool, developed during a research study by White and colleagues (1994 [Level IV]), may be employed to assess for risk of skin tears. Within the tool, there are three groups delineated by level of risk: groups I, II, and III. Group I refers to a positive history of skin tears within the last 90 days or skin tears that are already present. A positive score in this group requires that the patient be put on a skin tear prevention protocol. Group II requires four of the next six criteria to identify an increased risk-related items: (1) decision-making skills are either impaired or slightly impaired, or extensive assistance/total dependence for activities of daily living (ADLs) is noted; (2) wheelchair assistance needed; (3) loss of balance; (4) bed or chair confined; (5) unsteady gait; and (6) bruises. If a patient has a score of four or more items in Group II, then implement a skin tear prevention protocol. Group III includes the following 14 items, requiring any 5 for an increased risk: (1) physically abusive; (2) resists ADL care; (3) agitation; (4) hearing impaired; (5) decreased tactile stimulation; (6) wheels self; (7) manually/mechanically lifted; (8) contractures of arms, legs, shoulders, and/or hands; (9) hemiplegia/hemiparesis; (10) trunk, partial, or total inability to balance or turn body; (11) pitting edema of legs; (12) open lesions on extremities; (13) three or four discrete senile purpura lesions on extremities; and (14) dry, scaly skin. An increased risk has also been identified in individuals with a combination of three items in group II and three items in group III. Positive responses to five or more items in group III or three items in both groups II and III should also trigger the implementation of a skin tear prevention protocol.

Several authors have suggested protocols to prevent skin tears (Baranoski, 2000 [Level V]; Mason, 1997 [Level IV]; O'Regan, 2002 [Level V]; White et al., 1994 [Level IV]). Some nursing home research supports the value of skin ulcer care protocols to reduce the incidence of skin tears (Bank, 2005 [Level IV]; Birch & Coggins, 2003 [Level IV]; Hanson, Anderson, Thompson, & Langemo, 2005 [Level III]). After changing to a no-rinse, one-step bed product from bathing with soap and water, skin tears declined from 23.5% to 3.5% in one nursing home (Birch & Coggins, 2003 [Level IV]). Hanson and colleagues (2005 [Level III]) also found that skin tears could be reduced in two different nursing homes when staff were educated in appropriate skin cleaning and protection strategies. Using longer-lasting moisturizer-lotion sleeves to protect the arms and padded side rails yielded a reduction in the monthly average of skin tears from 18 to 11 in another nursing home study (Bank, 2005 [Level IV]). A protocol of guidelines is presented for high risk patients with skin tears (Table 18.2).

Interventions for Skin Tears

If a skin tear does occur, it is important to correctly identify it and begin an appropriate plan of care. The Payne and Martin (1993 [Level IV]) classification system may be used to describe skin tears. The three categories are as follows:

- Category I: a skin tear without tissue loss
- Category II: a skin tear with partial tissue loss
- Category III: a skin tear with complete tissue loss, where the epidermal flap is absent

The usual healing time for skin tears is 3 to 10 days (Krasner, 1991 [Level VI]). Although skin tears are prevalent in the elderly, there is no consistent approach to managing these skin injuries (Baranoski, 2000 [Level V]; O'Regan, 2002 [Level V]). Research is just beginning to provide evidence as to which dressing is best to use for skin tears. One study (Edwards, Gaskill, & Nash, 1998 [Level III]) compared the use of four different types of dressings in treating skin tears in a nursing home: three occlusive (i.e., transparent film, hydrocolloid, and polyurethane foam) and one nonocclusive dressing of steri-strips covered by a nonadhesive cellulose-polyester material. The nonocclusive dressing facilitated healing at a faster rate than the occlusive dressings. Another study by Thomas and colleagues (1999 [Level III]) studied older-adult skin tears in three nursing homes and determined that a higher rate of complete healing occurred with foam dressings compared to transparent films.

Goals of care for skin tears include retaining the skin flap, if present; providing a moist, nonadherent dressing; and protecting the site from further injury (O'Regan, 2002 [Level V]). A consensus protocol for treating skin tears based on suggested plans of care has been developed by several authors (Baranoski, 2000 [Level V]; Edwards et al., 1998 [Level III]); O'Regan, 2002 [Level V]) and is in Table 18.2.

Case Study 1 and Discussion

Randy Gonnagetawound, age 70, has diabetes mellitus with several micro- and macro-vascular complications. He was admitted to the hospital after a right-sided cerebral vascular accident. Past history includes retinal hemorrhages, a previous myocardial infarction, peripheral vascular disease, and a neuro-ischemic foot ulcer (healed after a left femoral-popliteal bypass, intravenous antibiotics, and plantar pressure redistribution with deep-toed shoes and orthotics). He is incontinent of feces and urine and responds by nodding to verbal commands. The left arm and leg are paralyzed. He has a gag reflex but cannot swallow. His Braden score is 10.

Current Data

Physical exam: There is an area of persistent erythema with bruising on the left buttock along with a number of superficial nonpalpable purpuric lesions on the arms and legs.

Physical Assessment and Pertinent Admission History

General: Responds to verbal questioning, but he cannot move his left side. In the past 3 days he has been increasingly fatigued, completely bedridden. He can change position only with movement of the right side.

Vital signs: Temperature = 39.2°C
Respiration: 10 per minute and regular
Pulse: 88 and irregular
Blood pressure: 162/94
Weight: 195 pounds
Height: 5 feet, 9 inches

Abdominal: Intake has been limited to half a bowl of cereal twice a day and a piece of toast and tea for lunch for the past 3 days. Last bowel movement was 3 days ago; + bowel sounds.

Cardiovascular: Irregular heart beat, No S_3S_4 at apex, +1 pedal edema, faintly palpable pedal pulses; capillary refill prolonged at 8 seconds

Respiratory: Crackles over right lower lobe, coughing periodically, nonproductive of mucous

Renal: Episodes of urinary incontinence for the past 3 days prior to admission

Integumentary: Skin is warm, dry, translucent; tenting noted

Laboratory data: Hg 10, HCT 28, RBC: 3.2, WBC: 11,000 shift to the left. Albumin 3.0 g/dL, K: 3.1, BUN: 32 mg/100 mL, glucose and/or HbA1c not available

Medical Orders

$D_5{}^1/_2NS$ with 10 mEq KCL at 100 cc/h
Colace 100 mg PO tid
Pulse oximetry monitoring continuously
Metamucil 1 package QD
Bedrest
Multivitamin 1 tablet QD
Daily weights
Soft diet as tolerated

Mr. Gonnagetawound is a prime candidate for developing a pressure ulcer. His low numerical score on the Braden Scale (10) puts him at high risk. Immediate strategies to prevent the occurrence of an ulcer are needed. Immobility is a leading risk factor for pressure ulcer development, so a major part of his plan of care needs to first be directed to get him moving as much as possible. A physiotherapy consult is needed to evaluate and recommend a plan of progressive exercise and activity. The plan should be to get him out of bed and moving within the constraints of his limitations from the stroke, as well as being in the chair rather than the bed. When in the chair, he needs to be sitting on a gel cushion. He will need to be repositioned every hour when in the chair. A group II, alternating low-air-loss mattress needs to be placed on his bed. For the limited time when he is in bed, he needs to be turned and positioned. His skin should be assessed every shift to evaluate signs for early skin injury.

A consult to a speech therapist is essential. A swallowing study is warranted to determine his ability to safely take an oral diet. A nutritional consult with a dietician will address his needs for appropriate calories, protein, and vitamins and minerals. A toileting regimen needs to be implemented to address the fecal and urinary incontinence. A discussion with the prescribing health care provider can explore whether he should continue on the colace and Metamucil. His skin needs cleansing after each episode of incontinence. Use of a no-rinse bathing system is preferred rather than soap and water. This vulnerable skin needs protection by using one of the many skin barriers available on the market.

Both Mr. Gonnagetawound and his family need instruction as to why it is so important to get him moving and why nutrition, skin care, turning, and positioning are so critical to his skin health.

Considering his general health, low hemoglobin, possibility of sepsis, and increased capillary refill must be also be monitored and addressed. It would be beneficial to know the HbA1C to determine blood sugar control and prevent long-term complications.

Case Study 2 and Discussion

Mrs. Keri Sight, 88-year-old, presents with a diagnosis of senile dementia of the Alzheimer's type with impaired communication skills. She has a history of congestive heart failure and osteoporosis. She spends most of the day in a wheelchair and needs two-person assistance for ambulation. Her skin is thin and dry, resembling an onion; each arm and leg has a purpura area. She is 15 pounds below her ideal body weight and has difficulty swallowing. Laboratory values are total protein 5.5 g/dL, albumin 2.6 g/dL, and BUN 28. She is verbally aggressive to the staff on whom she depends for assistance for ADLs.

Assessment of Mrs. Sight on admission to the LTC facility needs to be done. Because she has four of the criteria from group II of the Skin Tear Risk Assessment Tool developed by White and colleagues (1994 [Level IV]) (i.e., impaired decision-making skills due to senile dementia, dependence for ADLs, wheelchair/bed confined, unsteady gait), she is at risk for developing skin tears. Other factors that would put her at risk are her thin, dry skin with four purpura present and poor nutritional status. Her dependence on staff for ADLs and assistance coupled with her dementia predispose her to skin injury during bathing and other ADLs.

A skin tear prevention protocol needs to be immediately implemented for Mrs. Sight. To achieve a safe environment for her, the staff must know how to approach her with her dementia. To address her nutrition and hydration risk factors, a dietary consultation should be performed. Her ability to safely swallow needs to be evaluated by a speech therapist. After the swallowing evaluation, a plan to encourage frequent fluids and assist with eating should be implemented. To protect Mrs. Sight's skin from additional injury, avoid using hot water to bathe her and instead use one of the nonrinse soapless bathing products. Her family can be asked to bring in a soft fleece jogging suit for her to wear. The purpura areas on her arms and legs should be covered with stockinette or some other soft, nonadherent dressing or product to further protect these areas. Her bedrails and the arms and legs of her wheelchair should be padded. Staff should use the palm of their hands and a turn sheet when repositioning Mrs. Sight in bed. Lotion can be applied twice a day to her dry skin. Daily assessment of her skin including the five minimal characteristics proposed by CMS should be done (CMS, 2004 [Level V]).

Summary

Skin is the largest organ, so pay attention to it. Although the research into prevention strategies is limited, there is support for doing the appropriate risk assessment for these two types of skin injuries, assessing the skin for breakdown, protecting the skin by using appropriate bathing techniques and products to minimize the effects of friction and shear on the skin, and paying attention to nutritional status. In the case of pressure ulcers, redistributing the pressure by turning and repositioning and appropriate use of support surfaces are also critical. Immediate initiation of prevention protocols after risk identification is key.

By doing so, skin integrity problems such as tears and pressure ulcers can be prevented and treated.

Resources

Tools

Ayello, E. A. (Updated 2007). Try this: Predicting pressure ulcer risk, Issue #5 (PDF). Access at the The Hartford Institute for Geriatric Nursing, College of Nursing, New York University Web site.
http://www.ConsultGeriRN.org/publications/trythis/issue05.pdf

Braden, B., & Bergstrom, N. (1988). *Braden Scale for predicting pressure ulcer risk.*
http://www.bradenscale.com/braden.PDF

Authoritative Sites

Agency for Health Research and Quality (AHRQ, formerly AHCPR) USDHHS supported Clinical Guidelines: Pressure Ulcers. Retrieved May 5, 2007, at www.guideline.gov

National Pressure Ulcer Advisory Panel (NPUAP)
Pressure ulcer prevention and treatment, research, and policy information.
http://npuap.org/

Wound, Ostomy, and Continence Nursing Society (WOCN)
Guidelines, position statements, best practices, and much more.
http://www.wocn.org/

Other Related Professional Organizations

European Pressure Ulcer Advisory Panel (EPUAP)
http://www.epuap.org/

World Council of Enterostomal Therapists (WCET)
http://www.wcetn.org/

Wound Healing Society (WHS)
http://www.woundheal.org/

American Professional Wound Care Association (APWCA)
http://www.apwca.org/

World Union of Wound Healing Societies (WUWHS)
http://www.wuwhs.org/

These data retrieved May 4, 2007.

Box 18.1

Nursing Standard of Practice Protocol: Pressure Ulcer Prevention

I. GOALS

   A. Prevention of pressure ulcers (PU)
   B. Early recognition of PU development/skin changes

II. BACKGROUND AND STATEMENT OF PROBLEM

A. Prevalence: 15% (Cuddigan et al., 2001 [Level I])
   1. Acute-care range: 10% to 18%
   2. Long term care range: 2.3% to 28%
   3. Home care range: 0% to 29%
B. Incidence: 7%
   1. acute-care range: 0.4% to 38%
   2. long term care range: 2.2% to 23.9%
   3. home care range: 0% to 17%
C. Healthy People 2010 Objective: Reduce the proportion of nursing home residents with a current diagnosis of pressure ulcers.
D. A sentinel event in long term care (HCFA, 2000)
E. Etiology and/or epidemiology
   1. Risk factors (immobility, under or malnutrition, incontinence, friable skin, impaired cognitive ability)
   2. Higher incidence stage II and higher in persons with darkly pigmented skin

III. PARAMETERS OF ASSESSMENT

A. Assess for intrinsic and extrinsic risk factors
B. Braden Scale risk score
   1. 18 or below for elderly and persons with darkly pigmented skin
   2. 16 or below for other adults

IV. NURSING CARE STRATEGIES AND INTERVENTIONS

A. Risk assessment documentation
   1. On admission to a facility
   2. Reassessment intervals whenever the client's condition changes and based on patient care setting:
      a. acute care: every 48 hours
      b. long term care: weekly for first 4 weeks, then monthly/quarterly
      c. home care: every nursing visit
   3. Use a reliable and standardized tool for doing a risk assessment, such as the Braden Scale (available at http://www.bradenscale.com/braden.PDF).
   4. Document risk assessment scores and implement prevention protocols based on cut score.
B. General Care Issues and Interventions
   1. Culturally sensitive early assessment for stage I pressure ulcers in clients with darkly pigmented skin.
      a. Use a halogen light to look for skin color changes—may be purple hues
      b. Compare skin over bony prominences to surrounding skin—may be boggy or stiff, warm or cooler

2. AHCPR (1992) prevention recommendations:
   a. Assess skin daily.
   b. Clean skin at time of soiling; avoid hot water and irritating cleaning agents.
   c. Use moisturizers on dry skin.
   d. Do not massage bony prominences.
   e. Protect skin of incontinent clients from exposure to moisture.
   f. Use lubricants, protective dressings, and proper lifting techniques to avoid skin injury from friction/shear during transferring and turning of clients.
   g. Turn and position bed-bound clients every 2 hours if consistent with overall care goals.
   h. Use a written schedule for turning and repositioning clients.
   i. Use pillows or other devices to keep bony prominences from direct contact with each other.
   j. Raise heels of bed-bound clients off the bed; do not use donut-type devices (Gilcrest, Warren, & Yoder, 2005 [Level II]).
   k. Use a 30-degree lateral side lying position; do not place clients directly on their trochanter.
   l. Keep head of the bed at lowest height possible.
   m. Use lifting devices (trapeze, bed linen) to move clients rather than dragging them in bed during transfers and position changes.
   n. Use pressure-reducing devices (static air, alternating air, gel or water mattresses) (Iglesias et al., 2006 [Level II]; Hampton & Collins, 2005 [Level II]).
   o. Reposition chair- or wheelchair-bound clients every hour. In addition, if client is capable, have him or her do small weight shifts every 15 minutes.
   p. Use a pressure-reducing device (not a donut) for chair-bound clients.
3. Other care issues and interventions
   a. Keep the patient as active as possible; encourage mobilization.
   b. Do not massage reddened bony prominences.
   c. Avoid positioning the patient directly on his or her trochanter.
   d. Avoid using donut-shaped devices.
   e. Avoid drying out the patient's skin; use lotion after bathing.
   f. Avoid hot water and soaps that are drying when bathing elderly. Use body wash and skin protectant (Hunter et al., 2003 [Level III]).
   g. Teach patient, caregivers, and staff the prevention protocols.
   h. Manage moisture:
      i. Manage moisture by determining the cause; use absorbent pad that wicks moisture.
      ii. Offer a bedpan or urinal in conjunction with turning schedules.

i. Manage nutrition:
   Consult a dietitian, and correct nutritional deficiencies in-crease
   i. protein and calorie intake and A, C, or E vitamin supple-ments as needed (Houwing et al., 2003 [Level II]; CMS, 2004 [Level V]).
   ii. Offer a glass of water with turning schedules to keep patient hydrated.
j. Manage friction and shear:
   i. Elevate the head of the bed no more than 30 degrees.
   ii. Have the patient use a trapeze to lift self up in bed.
   iii. Staff should use a lift sheet or mechanical lifting device to move patient.
   iv. Protect high risk areas such as elbows, heels, sacrum, and back of head from friction injury.
C. Interventions Linked to Braden Risk Scores (Adapted from Ayello & Braden, 2001)
   Prevention protocols linked to Braden risk scores are as follows:
   1. At risk: score of 15–18
      a. Frequent turning; consider q 2 h schedule; use a written schedule.
      b. Maximize patient's mobility.
      c. Protect patient's heels.
      d. Use a pressure-reducing support surface if patient is bed- or chair-bound.
   2. Moderate risk: score of 13–14
      a. Same as above, but provide foam wedges for 30-degree lateral position.
   3. High risk: score of 10–12
      a. Same as above, but add the following.
         i. Increase the turning frequency.
         ii. Do small shifts of position.
   4. Very high risk: score of 9 or below
      a. Same as above, but use a pressure-relieving surface.
      b. Manage moisture, nutrition, and friction/shear.

V. EVALUATION AND EXPECTED OUTCOMES

A. Patient
   1. Skin will remain intact.
   2. Pressure ulcer will heal.
B. Provider/Nurse
   1. Nurses will accurately perform PU risk assessment using stan-dardized tool.
   2. Nurses will implement PU prevention protocols for clients inter-preted as at risk for PU.

   3. Nurses will perform a skin assessment for early detection of pressure ulcers.
C. Institution
   1. Reduction in development of new pressure ulcers.
   2. Increased number of risk assessments performed.
   3. Cost-effective prevention protocols developed.

VI. FOLLOW-UP MONITORING OF CONDITION

A. Monitor effectiveness of prevention interventions.
B. Monitor healing of any existing pressure ulcers.

Box 18.2

Nursing Standard of Practice Protocol: Skin Tear Prevention

I. GOALS

A. Prevent skin tears in elderly clients.
B. Identify clients at risk for skin tears (White et al., 1994 [Level IV]).
C. Foster healing of skin tears by
   1. Retaining skin flap
   2. Providing a moist, nonadherent dressing (Edwards et al., 1998 [Level III]; Thomas et al., 1999 [Level III])
   3. Protecting the site from further injury

II. BACKGROUND AND STATEMENT OF PROBLEM

A. Traumatic wounds from mechanical injury of skin.
B. Need to clearly differentiate etiology of skin tears from pressure ulcers.
C. Common in the elderly, especially over areas of age-related purpura.

III. PARAMETERS OF ASSESSMENT

A. Use the three-group risk assessment tool (White et al., 1994 [Level IV]) to assess for skin tear risk.
B. Use the Payne and Martin (1993 [Level IV]) classification system to assess clients for skin tear risk.
   1. Category I: a skin tear without tissue loss
   2. Category II: a skin tear with partial tissue loss

3. Category III: a skin tear with complete tissue loss, where the epidermal flap is absent

IV. NURSING CARE STRATEGIES AND INTERVENTIONS

(Baranoski, 2000 [Level V])
A. Preventing Skin Tears
   1. Provide a safe environment:
      a. Do a risk assessment of elderly patients on admission.
      b. Implement prevention protocol for patients identified as at risk for skin tears.
      c. Have patients wear long sleeves or pants to protect their extremities (Bank, 2005 [Level IV]).
      d. Have adequate light to reduce the risk of bumping into furniture or equipment.
      e. Provide a safe area for wandering.
   2. Educate staff or family caregivers in the correct way of handling patients to prevent skin tears. Maintain nutrition and hydration:
      a. Offer fluids between meals.
      b. Use lotion, especially on dry skin on arms and legs, twice daily (Hanson et al., 2005 [Level III]).
      c. Obtain a dietary consultation.
   3. Protect from self-injury or injury during routine care:
      a. Use a lift sheet to move and turn patients.
      b. Use transfer techniques that prevent friction or shear.
      c. Pad bedrails, wheelchair arms, and leg supports (Bank, 2005 [Level IV]).
      d. Support dangling arms and legs with pillows or blankets.
      e. Use nonadherent dressings on frail skin.
         i. Apply petroleum-based ointment, steri-strips, or a moist nonadherent wound dressing such as hydrogel dressing with gauze as a secondary dressing. Telfa type dressings are also used.
         ii. If you must use tape, be sure it is made of paper, and remove it gently. Also, you can apply the tape to hydrocolloid strips placed strategically around the wound rather than taping directly onto fragile surrounding skin around the skin tear.
      f. Use gauze wraps, stockinettes, flexible netting, or other wraps to secure dressings rather than tape.
      g. Use no-rinse soapless bathing products (Birch & Coggins, 2003 [Level IV]; Mason, 1997 [Level IV]).
      h. Keep skin from becoming dry, apply moisturizer (Hanson et al., 2005 [Level III]; Bank, 2005 [Level IV]).
B. Treating Skin Tears (Baranoski & Ayello, 2004 [Level V])
   1. Gently clean the skin tear with normal saline.
   2. Let the area air dry or pat dry carefully.

3. Approximate the skin tear flap.
4. Use caution if using film dressings because skin damage can occur when removing dressings.
5. Consider putting an arrow to indicate the direction of the skin tear on the dressing to minimize any further skin injury during dressing removal.
   a. Skin sealants, petroleum-based products, and other water-resistant product such as protective barrier ointments or liquid barriers may be used to protect the surrounding skin from wound drainage or dressing/tape removal trauma.
   b. Always assess the size of the skin tear; consider doing a wound tracing.
   c. Document assessment and treatment findings.

V. EVALUATION AND EXPECTED OUTCOMES

A. No skin tears will occur in at-risk clients.
B. Skin tears that do occur will heal.

VI. FOLLOW-UP MONITORING OF CONDITION

A. Continue to reassess for any new skin tears in older adults.

References

Agency for Health Care Policy and Research (AHCPR, now AHRQ) (1992, May). Panel for the prediction and prevention of pressure ulcers in adults. In *Pressure ulcers in adults: Prediction and prevention.* (Clinical Practice Guideline No. 3; AHCPR Pub. No. 92-0047). Rockville, MD: Publisher. Evidence Level V: Literature Review.

Allman, R. M., Goode, P. S., Patrick, M. M., Burst, N., & Bartolucci, A. A. (1995). Pressure ulcer risk factors among hospitalized patients with activity limitations. *Journal of the American Medical Association, 273,* 865–870. Evidence Level IV: Nonexperimental Study.

Aurigemma, R. (2005). The effectiveness of the senior order systems assessment and prevention program. *Long Term Care Interface, 6*(5), 26–30. Evidence Level III: Quasi-experimental Study.

Ayello, E. A., & Braden, B. (2001). Why is pressure ulcer risk so important? *Nursing, 31*(11), 74–79. Evidence Level V: Review.

Ayello, E. A., & Braden, B. (2002). How and why to do pressure ulcer risk assessment. *Advances in Skin and Wound Care, 15*(3), 125–131. Evidence Level V: Review.

Ayello, E. A., & Lyder, C. H. (2001). Pressure ulcers in persons of color: Race and ethnicity. In J. Cuddigan, E. A. Ayello, & C. Sussman (Eds.), *Pressure ulcers in America: Prevalence, incidence, and implications for the future* (pp. 153–162). Reston, VA: National Pressure Ulcer Advisory Panel. Evidence Level V: Review.

Bank, D. (2005). Decreasing the incidence of skin tears in a nursing and rehabilitation center. *Advances in Skin and Wound Care, 18,* 74–75. Evidence Level IV: Nonexperimental Study.

Baranoski, S. (2000). Skin tears: The enemy of frail skin. *Advances in Skin and Wound Care, 13*(3), 123–126. Evidence Level V: Review.

Baranoski, S., & Ayello, E. A. (2004). *Wound care essentials: Practice principles* (pp. 54–58). Springhouse, PA: Lippincott, Williams, & Wilkins. Evidence Level V: Review.

Barczak, C. A., Barnett, R. I., Childs, E. J., & Bosley, L. M. (1997). Fourth national pressure ulcer prevalence survey. *Advanced Wound Care, 10*(4), 18–26. Evidence Level IV: Nonexperimental Study.

Baumgarten, M., Margolis, D., Berlin, J. A., Strom, B. L., Garino, J., Kagan, S. H., et al. (2003). Risk factors for pressure ulcers among elderly hip-fracture patients. *Wound repair and regeneration, 11*(2), 96–103. Evidence Level IV: Nonexperimental Study.

Baumgarten, M., Margolis, D., van Doorn, C., Gruber-Baldini, A. L., Hebel, J. R., Zimmerman, S., et al. (2004). Black/White differences in pressure ulcer incidence in nursing home residents. *Journal of the American Geriatrics Society, 52*(8), 1293–1298. Evidence Level IV: Nonexperimental Study.

Bennett, M. A. (1995). Report of the task force on the implications for darkly pigmented intact skin in the prediction and prevention of pressure ulcers. *Advances in Wound Care, 8*(6), 34–35. Evidence Level V: Review.

Bergquist, S. (2001). Subscales, subscales, or summative score: Evaluating the contribution of Braden Scale items for predicting pressure ulcer risk in older adults receiving home health care. *Journal of Wound, Ostomy, and Continence Nursing, 28*(6), 279–289. Evidence Level IV: Nonexperimental Study.

Bergquist, S. (2003). Pressure ulcer predication in older adults receiving home health care: Implications for use with the OASIS. *Advances in Skin & Wound Care, 16*(3), 132–139. Evidence Level IV: Nonexperimental Study.

Bergquist, S., & Frantz, R. (2001). Braden Scale: Validity in community-based older adults receiving home care. *Applied Nursing Research 14*(1), 36–43. Evidence Level IV: Nonexperimental Study.

Bergstrom, N., & the AHCPR Treatment of Pressure Ulcers Guideline Panel (1994). *Treatment of pressure ulcers* (Clinical Practice Guideline No. 15; AHCPR Pub. No. 95-0652). Rockville, MD: U.S. Department of Health and Human Services, Public Health Service, and Agency for Health Care Policy and Research. Evidence Level I: Systematic Review.

Bergstrom, N., & Braden, B. J. (1992). A prospective study of pressure sore risk among institutionalized elderly. *Journal of the American Geriatrics Society, 40*, 747–758. Evidence Level III: Quasi-experimental Study.

Bergstrom, N., & Braden, B. J. (2002). Brief report: Predictive validity of the Braden Scale among Black and White subjects. *Nursing Research, 51*(6), 398–403. Evidence Level IV: Nonexperimental Study.

Bergstrom, N., Braden, B. J., Kemp, M., Champagne, M., & Ruby, E. (1996). Multi-site study of incidence of pressure ulcers and the relationship between risk level, demographic characteristics, diagnoses, and prescription of preventive interventions. *Journal of the American Geriatrics Society, 44*(1), 22–30.

Bergstrom, N., Braden, B. J., Laguzza, A., & Holman, V. (1987). The Braden Scale for predicting pressure sore risk. *Nursing Research, 36*, 205–210. Evidence Level III: Quasi-experimental Study.

Berlowitz, D. R., Brandeis, G. H., Morris, J. H., Ash, A. S., Anderson, J. J., Kader, B., et al. (2001). Deriving a risk-adjustment model for pressure ulcers development using the minimum data set. *Journal of the American Geriatrics Society, 49*(7), 866–871. Evidence Level IV: Nonexperimental Study.

Birch, S., & Coggins, T. (2003). Non-rinse, one-step bed bath: The effects on the occurrence of skin tears in a long term care setting. *Ostomy/Wound Management, 49*, 64–67. Evidence Level IV: Nonexperimental Study.

Black, J., Baharestani, M. M., Cuddigan, J., Dorner, B., Edsberg, L., Langemo, D., et al. (2007). National Pressure Ulcer Advisory Panel's updated pressure ulcer staging system. *Advances in Skin and Wound Care, 20*(5), 269–274. Evidence Level IV: Nonexperimental Study.

Braden, B. J. (1998). The relationship between stress and pressure sore formation. *Ostomy Wound Management, 44* (Suppl. 3A), 265–265.

Braden, B. J., & Bergstrom, N. (1987). A conceptual schema for the study of the etiology of pressure sores. *Rehabilitation Nursing, 12*(1), 8–16. Evidence Level II: Single Experimental Study.

Braden, B. J., & Bergstrom, N. (1989). Clinical utility of the Braden Scale for predicting pressure sore risk. *Decubitus, 2*(3), 44–51. Evidence Level III: Quasi-experimental Study.

Bryant, R. A., & Rolstead, B. S. (2001). Utilizing a systems approach to implement pressure ulcer prediction and prevention. *Ostomy/Wound Management, 47*(9), 26–36. Evidence Level V: Review.

Buss, I. C., Halfens, R. J., Abu-Saad, H. H., & Kok, G. (2004). Pressure ulcer prevention in nursing homes: Views and beliefs of enrolled nurses and other health care workers. *Journal of Clinical Nursing, 13*(6), 668–676. Evidence Level III: Quasi-experimental Study.

Cavalcanti-Cordeiro, M. B., Antonelli, E. J., Ferreira da Cunha, D., Jordao, A. A. J., Rodrigues, V. J., & Vannucchi, H. (2005). Oxidative stress and acute-phase response in patients with pressure sores. *Nutrition 21*(9), 901–907. Evidence Level IV: Nonexperimental Study.

Centers for Medicare and Medicaid Services (CMS) (2004). *Guidance for surveyors in long term care.* Tag F 314. Pressure ulcers. Retrieved December 30, 2006, from http://www.cms. hhs.gov/manuals/downloads/som107ap_pp_guidelines_ltcf.pdf. Evidence Level V: Literature Review.

Chan, R. Y., Tan, S. L., Lee, C. K., & Lee, J. Y. (2005). Prevalence, incidence and predictors of pressure ulcers in a tertiary hospital in Singapore. *Journal of Wound Care, 14*(8), 383–384, 396–398. Evidence Level IV: Nonexperimental Study.

Cuddigan, J., Ayello, E. A., & Sussman, C. (Eds.) (2001). *Pressure ulcers in America: Prevalence, incidence, and implications for the future.* Reston, VA: National Pressure Ulcer Advisory Panel. Evidence Level I: Systematic Review/Meta-Analysis.

De Floor, T., De Bacquer, D., & Grypdonck M. (2005). The effect of various combinations of turning and pressure-reducing devices on the incidence of pressure ulcers. *International Journal of Nursing Studies, 42*(1), 37–46. Evidence Level III: Quasi-experimental Study.

Edwards, H., Gaskill, D., & Nash, R. (1998). Treating skin tears in nursing home residents: A pilot study comparing four types of dressings. *International Journal of Nursing Practice, 4,* 25–32. Evidence Level III: Quasi-experimental Study.

Frantz, R. A., & Baranoski, S. (2001). Pressure ulcer prevention programs in various settings: What works? What doesn't? In J. Cuddigan, E. A. Ayello, & C. Sussman. (Eds.), *Pressure ulcers in America: Prevalence, incidence, and implications for the future* (pp. 119–123). Reston, VA: National Pressure Ulcer Advisory Panel. Evidence Level V: Review.

Frantz, R. A., Xakellis, G. C., Harvey, P. C., & Lewis, A. R. (2003). Implementing an incontinence management protocol in long term care: Clinical outcomes and costs. *Journal of Gerontological Nursing, 29*(8), 46–53. Evidence Level IV: Nonexperimental Study.

Gilcreast, D. M., Warren, J. B., Yoder, L. H., Clark, J. J., Wilson, J. A., & Mays, M. Z. (2005). Research comparing three heel ulcer-prevention devices. *Journal of Wound, Ostomy, and Continence Nursing, 32*(2), 112–120. Evidence Level II: Single Experimental Study.

Haalboom, J. R. (2003). A randomized, double-blind assessment of the effect of nutritional supplementation on the prevention of pressure ulcers in hip-fracture patients. *Clinical Nutrition, 22*(4), 401–405. Evidence Level II: RCT.

Hampton, S., & Collins, F. (2005). Reducing pressure ulcer incidence in a long-term setting. *British Journal of Nursing, 14*(15), S6–S12. Evidence Level II: RCT.

Hanson, D. H., Anderson, J., Thompson, P., & Langemo, D. (2005). Skin tears in long term care: Effectiveness on skin care protocols on prevalence. *Advances in Skin and Wound Care, 18,* 74. Evidence Level III: Quasi-experimental Study.

Hanson, D., Langemo, D. K., Olson, B., Hunter, S., Sauvage, T. R., Burd, C., et al. (1991). The prevalence and incidence of pressure ulcers in the hospice setting: Analysis of two methodologies. *American Journal of Hospice Palliative Care, 8*(5), 18–22. Evidence Level IV: Nonexperimental Study.

Health Care Financing Administration (HCFA) (2000, June). *Investigative protocol, guidance to surveyors: Long term care facilities* (Rev. 274). Washington, DC: U.S. Department of Health and Human Services.

Henderson, C. T., Ayello, E. A., Sussman, C., Leiby, D. M., Bennett, M. A., Dungog, E. F., et al. (1997). Draft definition of stage I pressure ulcers: Inclusion of persons with darkly pigmented skin. *Advances in Wound Care, 10*(5), 16–19. Evidence Level IV: Nonexperimental Study.

Hommel, A., Ulander, K., & Thorngren, K. (2003). Improvements in pain relief, handling time and pressure ulcers through internal audits of hip-fracture patients. *Scandinavian Journal of Caring Sciences, 17*(1), 78–83. Evidence Level IV: Nonexperimental Study.

Horn, S. D., Bender, S. A., Bergstrom, N., Cook, A. S., Ferguson, M. L., Rimmasch, H. L., et al. (2002). Description of the national pressure ulcer long term care study. *Journal of the American Geriatrics Society*, *50*(11), 1816–1825. Evidence Level III: Quasi-experimental Study.

Horn, S. D., Bender, S. A., Ferguson, M. L., Smout, R. J., Bergstrom, N., Taler, G., et al. (2004). The national pressure ulcer long term care study: Pressure ulcer development in long term care residents. *Journal of the American Geriatrics Society*, *2*(3), 359–367. Evidence Level III: Quasi-experimental Study.

Houwing, R. H., Rozendaal, M., Wouters-Wesseling, W., Beulens, J. W., & Buskens, E. (2003). A randomised, double-bind assessment of the effect of nutritional supplementation on the prevention of pressure ulcers in hip-fracture patients. *Clinical Nutrition*, *22*(4), 401–405. Evidence Level II: RCT.

Houwing, R., Rozendaal, M., Wouters-Wessling, W., Buskens, E., Keller, P., & Haalboom, J. (2004). Pressure ulcer risk in hip-fracture patients. *Acta Orthopaedica Scandinavica*, *75*(4), 390–393. Evidence Level IV: Nonexperimental Study.

Hunter, S., Anderson, J., Hanson, D., Thompson, O., Langemo, D., & Klug, M. G. (2003). Clinical trial of a prevention treatment protocol for skin breakdown in two nursing homes. *Journal of Wound, Ostomy, and Continence Nurses Society (WOCN)*, *30*(5), 250–258. Evidence Level III: Quasi-experimental Study.

Iglesias, D., Nixon, J., Cranny, G., Nelson, E. A., Hawkins, K., Phillips, A., et al. (2006). Pressure relieving support surfaces (PRESSURE) Trial: Cost-effectiveness analysis. *British Medical Journal*, *332*(7555), 1416. Evidence Level II: Single Experimental Study.

Institute for Healthcare Improvement (IHI) (2006). 5 Million Lives Saved Campaign: Pressure Ulcers. Retrieved December 31, 2006, from http://www.ihi.org/IHI/Programs/Campaign/ Evidence Level V: Review.

Jalali, R., & Rezaie, M. (2005). Predicting pressure ulcer risk: Comparing the predictive validity of 4 scales. *Advances in Skin & Wound Care*, *18*(2), 92–97. Evidence Level IV: Nonexperimental Study.

Jolley, D. J., Wright, R., McGowan, S., Hickey, M. B., Campbell, D. A., Sinclair, R. D., et al. (2004). Preventing pressure ulcers with the Australian medical sheepskin: An open-label randomized controlled trial. *The Medical Journal of Australia*, *180*(7), 324–327. Evidence Level II: Single Experimental Study.

Karadag, M., & Gumuskaya, N. (2006). The incidence of pressure ulcers in surgical patients: A sample hospital in Turkey. *Journal of Clinical Nursing*, *15*(4), 413–421. Evidence IV: Nonexperimental Study.

Krasner, D. (1991). An approach to treating skin tears. *Ostomy/Wound Management*, *32*, 56–58. Evidence Level VI: Expert Opinion.

Kwong, E., Pamg, S., Wong, T., Ho, J., Shaoling, X., & Lijun, T. (2005). Predicting pressure ulcer risk with the modified Braden, Braden, and Norton scales in acute-care hospitals in mainland China. *Applied Nursing Research*, *18*(2), 122–128. Evidence Level IV: Nonexperimental Study.

Langer, G., Schloemer, G., Knerr, A., Kuss, O., & Behrens, J. (2003). Nutritional interventions for preventing and treating pressure ulcers. *Cochrane Database of Systematic Reviews*. Evidence Level I: Systematic Review.

Lindgren, M., Unosson, M., Fredrikson, M., & Ek, A. (2004). Immobility: A major risk factor for development of pressure ulcers among adult hospitalized patients: A prospective study. *Scandinavian Journal of Caring Sciences*, *18*(1), 57–64. Evidence Level VI: Expert Opinion.

Lyder, C. H. (1991). Conceptualization of the stage I pressure ulcer. *Journal of Enterostomal Therapy Nursing*, *18*(5), 162–165. Evidence Level IV: Nonexperimental Study.

Lyder, C. H. (1996). Examining the inclusion of ethnic minorities in pressure ulcer prediction studies. *Journal of Wound Ostomy and Continence Nursing*, *23*(5), 257–260. Evidence Level IV: Nonexperimental Study.

Lyder, C. H., Preston, J., Grady, J., Scinto, J., Allman, R., Bergstrom, N., et al. (2001). Quality of care for hospitalized Medicare patients at risk for pressure ulcers. *Archives of Internal Medicine*, *161*, 1549–1554. Evidence Level III: Quasi-experimental Study.

Lyder, C. H., Yu, C., Emerling, J., Mangat, R., Stevenson, D., Empleo-Frazier, O., et al. (1999). The Braden Scale for pressure ulcer risk: Evaluating the predictive validity in Black and Latino/Hispanic elders. *Applied Nursing Research*, *12*(2), 60–68. Evidence Level IV: Nonexperimental Study.

Lyder, C. H., Yu, C., Stevenson, D., Mangat, R., Empleo-Frazier, O., Emerling, J., et al. (1998). Validating the Braden Scale for the prediction of pressure ulcer risk in Blacks and Latino/Hispanic elders: A pilot study. *Ostomy/Wound Management, 44* (Suppl. 3A), 42S–50S. Evidence Level IV: Nonexperimental Study.

Malone, M. L., Rozario, N., Gavinski, M., & Goodwin, J. (1991). The epidemiology of skin tears in the institutionalized elderly. *Journal of the American Geriatrics Society, 39,* 591–595. Evidence Level IV: Nonexperimental Study.

Mason, S. R. (1997). Type of soap and the incidence of skin tears among residents of a long term care facility. *Ostomy/Wound Management, 43*(8), 26–30. Evidence Level IV: Nonexperimental Study.

Meehan, M. (1990). Multisite pressure ulcer prevalence survey. *Decubitus, 3*(4), 14–17. Evidence Level IV: Nonexperimental Study.

Meehan, M. (1994). National pressure ulcer prevalence survey. *Advances in Wound Care, 7*(3), 27–30, 34. Evidence Level IV: Nonexperimental Study.

National Pressure Ulcer Advisory Panel (NPUAP) (1989). Pressure ulcers prevalence, cost, and risk assessment: Consensus development conference statement. Retrieved February 18, 2007, from www.npuap.org. *Decubitus, 2*(2), 24–28.

National Pressure Ulcer Advisory Panel (1998). NPUAP statement on reverse staging of pressure ulcers. Retrieved June 22, 2002, from http://www.npuap.org. Evidence Level V: Review.

National Pressure Ulcer Advisory Panel (2001). Pressure ulcer prevention: A competency-based curriculum. Retrieved February 18, 2007, from www.npuap.org/prercurr.pdf.

National Pressure Ulcer Advisory Panel (2007). Updated Staging. Retreived May 14, 2007, from www.npuap.org/pr2.htm. Evidence Level IV: Nonexperimental Study.

New Jersey Department of Health and Senior Services (NJDHSS) (December 2004). Mandatory patient safety reporting requirements for general hospitals. Patient safety reporting initiative. Health Care Quality Assessment, New Jersey Department of Health and Senior Services, December 6, 2004. Retrieved June 5, 2007, from http://www.state.nj.us/health/ps/documents/irr.pdf.

Nightingale, F. (1859). *Notes on nursing: What it is and what it is not.* Philadelphia: Lippincott.

Nixon, J., Cranny, G., Iglesias, C., Nelson, E. A., Hawkins, K., Phillips, A., et al. (2006). Randomised, controlled trial of alternating pressure mattresses compared with alternating pressure overlays for the prevention of pressure ulcers: PRESSURE (pressure relieving support surfaces) trial. *British Medical Journal, 332*(7555), 1413. Evidence Level II: RCT.

Norton, D., McLaren, R., & Exton-Smith, A. (1975). *An investigation of geriatric nurse problems in hospitals.* Edinburgh, UK: Churchill, Livingston. Evidence Level IV: Nonexperimental Study.

Norton, D., McLaren, R., & Exton-Smith, A. N. (1962). *An investigation of geriatric nursing problems in hospitals.* London, UK: National Corporation for the Care of Old People.

O'Regan, A. (2002). Skin tears: A review of the literature. *Journal of Wound, Ostomy, and Continence Nursing, 22*(2), 26–31. Evidence Level V: Literature Review.

Pancorbo-Hidalgo, P. L., Garcia-Fernandez, F. P., Lopez-Medina, I. M., & Alvarez-Nieto, C. (2006). Risk assessment scales for pressure ulcer prevention: A systematic review. *Journal of Advanced Nursing, 54*(1), 94–110. Evidence Level I: Meta-Analysis.

Payne, R. L., & Martin, M. C. (1993). Defining and classifying skin tears: Need for common language. *Ostomy/Wound Management, 39*(5), 16–19, 22–24, 26. Evidence Level IV: Nonexperimental Study.

Reddy, M., Gill, S. S., & Rochon, P. A. (2006). Preventing pressure ulcers: A systematic review. *Journal of the American Medical Association, 296*(8), 974–984. Level I: Systematic Review/Meta-Analysis.

Russo, C. A., & Elixhauser, A. (2006). *Hospitalizations related to pressure sores, 2003. Healthcare cost and utilization project.* Rockville, MD: Agency for Healthcare Research and Quality. Retrieved December 19, 2006, from http://www.hcup-us.ahrq.gov/reports/statbriefs/sb3.pdf. Evidence Level IV: Nonexperimental Study.

Sprigle, S., Linden, M., McKenna, D., Davis, K., & Riordan, B. (2001). Clinical skin temperature measurement to predict incipient pressure ulcers. *Advances in Skin and Wound Care, 14*(3), 133–137. Evidence Level IV: Nonexperimental Study.

Stratton, R. J., Ek, A. C., Engfer, M., Moore, Z., Rigby, P., & Wolfe, R., et al. (2005). Enteral nutritional support in prevention and treatment of pressure ulcers: A systematic review and meta-analysis. *Ageing Research Review*, *4*(3), 422–450. Evidence Level I: Systematic Review/Meta-Analysis.

Thomas, D. R., Goode, P. S., LaMaster, K., Tennyson, T., & Parnell, L. K. S. (1999). A comparison of an opaque foam dressing versus a transparent film dressing in the management of skin tears in institutionalized subjects. *Ostomy/Wound Management*, *45*(6), 22–28. Evidence Level III: Quasi-experimental Study.

Thompson, P., Langemo, D., Anderson, J., Hanson, D., & Hunter, S. (2005). Skin care protocols for pressure ulcers and incontinence in long term care: A quasi-experimental study. *Advances in Skin and Wound Care*, *18*(80), 422–429. Evidence Level III: Quasi-experimental Study.

U.S. Department of Health and Human Services (2000). *Healthy people 2010: Understanding and improving health* (2nd. ed.). Washington, DC: U.S. Government Printing Office.

White, M. W., Karam, S., & Cowell, B. (1994). Skin tears in frail elders: A practical approach to prevention. *Geriatric Nursing*, *15*(2), 95–98. Evidence Level IV: Nonexperimental Study.

Wound, Ostomy, and Continence Nurses Society (WOCN) (2003). *Guideline for prevention and management of pressure ulcers*. Number 2, WOCN Clinical Practice Guideline Series. Glenview, IL: WOCN. Evidence Level I: Systematic Review.

Xakellis, G. C., Frantz, R. A., Lewis, A., & Harvey, P. (2001). Translating pressure ulcer guidelines into practice: It's harder than it sounds. *Advances in Skin and Wound Care*, *14*(5), 249–256, 258. Evidence Level IV: Nonexperimental Study.

Young, T. (2004). The 30-degree tilt position versus the 90-degree lateral and supine positions in reducing the incidence of non-blanching erythema in a hospital inpatient population: A randomized controlled trial. *Journal of Tissue Viability*, *14*, 88–96. Evidence Level IV: Nonexperimental Study.

Age-Related Changes in Health

19

Constance M. Smith
Valerie T. Cotter

Educational Objectives

On completion of this chapter, the reader should be able to:

1. describe the structural and functional changes that occur during the normal aging process in the cardiovascular, pulmonary, renal, genitourinary, oropharyngeal, gastrointestinal, musculoskeletal, and nervous systems

2. understand the clinical significance of these age-related changes with regard to the health and disease risks of older adults

3. discuss the components of a nursing assessment for older adults in light of the manifestations of normal aging

4. with consideration of age-dependent changes, identify care strategies to promote successful aging in elders

The process of normal aging, independent of disease, is accompanied by myriad changes in body systems. As evidenced by longitudinal studies such as the Baltimore Longitudinal Study of Aging (Baltimore Longitudinal Study of Aging, 2005), modifications occur in both structure and function of organs and are most pronounced in advanced age of 85 years or older (Hall, 2002). Many of these alterations are characterized by a decline in physiological reserve so that, although baseline functionality is preserved, organ systems become progressively less capable of maintaining homeostasis in the face of stresses imposed by the environment, disease, or medical therapies (Miller, 2003). Age-related changes are strongly impacted by genetics (Wang, 2003) as well as by long-term

For a description of Evidence Levels cited in this chapter, see chapter 1, Developing and Evaluating Clinical Practice Guidelines, page 4.

lifestyle factors including physical activity, diet, alcohol consumption, and tobacco use (Taffet & Lakatta, 2003). Further, great heterogeneity occurs among
older individuals; clinical manifestations of aging can range from stability to
significant decline in function of specific organ systems (Beck, 1998).

The clinical implications of these gerontological alterations are critically important in nursing assessment and care of older adults for several reasons. First,
changes associated with normal aging must be differentiated from pathological
processes in order to develop appropriate interventions (Levelser & Shakoor,
2003). Manifestations of aging can also adversely impact the health and functionality of elders and require therapeutic strategies to correct (Matsumura &
Ambrose, 2006). Age-associated changes predispose older persons to selected
diseases (Taffet & Lakatta, 2003); therefore, nurses' understanding of these risks
can serve to develop more effective approaches to assessment and care. Finally,
aging and illness may interact reciprocally, resulting in altered presentation of
illness, response to treatment, and outcomes (Hall, 2002).

This chapter describes age-dependent changes for the cardiovascular, pulmonary, renal, genitourinary, oropharyngeal, gastrointestinal, musculoskeletal,
and nervous systems. Clinical implications of these alterations for each body system, including associated disease risks, are then discussed, followed by nursing
assessment and care strategies related to these changes, and a clinical practice
protocol, see Box 19.1.

Cardiovascular System

Cardiac reserve declines in normal aging. This alteration does not affect cardiac function at rest and resting heart rate, ejection fraction, and cardiac output remain virtually unchanged with age; however, under physiological stress
with increased cardiac demand, such as physical activity or infection, the ability of an older adult's heart to increase rate and cardiac output is compromised
(Lakatta, 2000). Such diminished functional reserve results in reduced exercise
tolerance, fatigue, shortness of breath, slow recovery from tachycardia (Watters,
2002 [Level V]), and intolerance of volume depletion (Mick & Ackerman, 2004
[Level V]). Further, because of the decreased maximal attainable heart rate with
aging, a rapid heart rate of more than 90 beats per minute in an older adult indicates significant physiological stress (Taffet & Lakatta, [Level VI] 2003).

Age-dependent changes in both the vasculature and the heart contribute
to the impairment in cardiac reserve. An increase in the wall thickness and
stiffness of the aorta and carotid arteries results in diminished vessel compliance and greater systemic vascular resistance (Tully, 2002). Elevated systolic
blood pressure with constant diastolic pressure follows, increasing the risk of
isolated systolic hypertension and widened pulse pressure (Joint National Committee [JNC], 2004). Strong arterial pulses, diminished peripheral pulses, and
increased potential for inflamed varicosities occur commonly with age. Reductions in capillary density restrict blood flow in the extremities, producing cool
skin (Mick & Ackerman, 2004 [Level V]).

As an adaptive measure to increased workload against noncompliant arteries, the left ventricle and atrium hypertrophy and become rigid. The ensuing
impairment in relaxation of the left ventricle during diastole places greater dependence on atrial contractions to achieve left ventricular filling (Lakatta, 2000).

In addition, sympathetic response in the heart is blunted due to diminished β-adrenergic sensitivity, resulting in decreased myocardial contractility (Tully, 2002).

Additional age-related changes include sclerosis of atrial and mitral valves, which impairs their tight closure and increases the risk of dysfunction. The ensuing leaky heart valves may result in aortic regurgitation or mitral stenosis, presenting on exam as heart murmurs (Santinga, 2003). Loss of pacemaker and conduction cells contributes to changes in the resting electrocardiogram of older adults (Saksena & Reddy, 2003). Isolated premature atrial and ventricular complexes are common arrhythmias and the risk of atrial fibrillation is increased (Hebbar & Hueston, 2002a, 2002b). Due to atrial contractions in diastole, S_4 frequently develops as an extra heart sound (Schretzman & Strumpf, 2002).

Baroreceptor function, which regulates blood pressure, is impaired with age, particularly with change in position. Postural hypotension with orthostatic symptoms may follow (Mukai & Lipsitz, 2002), especially after prolonged bedrest, dehydration, or cardiovascular drug use, and can cause dizziness and potential for falls (Kenny, 2003 [Level V]).

Cardiac assessment of an older adult includes performing an electrocardiogram (ECG) (Saksena & Reddy, 2003 [Level V]) and monitoring heart rate (40 to 100 bpm within normal limits), rhythm (noting whether it is regular or irregular) (Docherty, 2002 [Level I]), heart sounds (S_1, S_2, or extra heart sounds S_3 in heart disease or S_4 as a common finding), and murmurs (noting location where loudest). The apical impulse is displaced laterally. In palpation of the carotid arteries, asymmetric volumes and decreased pulsations may indicate aortic stenosis and impaired left cardiac output, respectively. Auscultation of bruit potentially suggests occlusive arterial disease. Peripheral pulses should be assessed bilaterally at a minimum of one pulse point in each extremity. Assessment may reveal asymmetry in pulse volume, suggesting insufficiency in arterial circulation (Seidel, Ball, Dains, & Benedict, 2003 [Level VI]). Examine lower extremities for varicose veins and note dilation or swelling (Bickley, 2003 [Level VI]). Evaluate for dyspnea with exertion and exercise intolerance (Mahler, Fierro-Carrion, & Baird, 2003 [Level V]).

Blood pressure should be measured at least twice (Kestel, 2005 [Level V]) on an older adult and performed in a comfortably seated position with back supported and feet flat on the floor. The B/P should then be repeated after 5 minutes of rest. Measurements in both supine and standing positions evaluate postural hypotension (Kenny, 2003 [Level V]) and should be performed on all older adults.

Nursing-care strategies include referrals for older adults who have irregularities of heart rhythm and decreased or asymmetric peripheral pulses. The risk of postural hypotension emphasizes the need for safety precautions (Kenny, 2003 [Level V]) to prevent falls. These include avoiding prolonged recumbency or motionless standing and encouraging the older adult to rise slowly from lying or sitting positions and wait 1 to 2 minutes after a position change to stand or transfer. Overt signs of hypotension such as a change in sensorium or mental status, dizziness, or orthostasis should be monitored and fall-prevention strategies should be instituted. Sufficient fluid intake is advised to ensure adequate hydration and prevent hypovolemia for optimal cardiac functioning (Docherty, 2002 [Level I]; Watters, 2002 [Level V]).

Older adults should be encouraged to adopt lifestyle practices for cardiovascular fitness with the aim of a healthy body weight (i.e., BMI 18.5 to 24.9 kg/m^2) (Lewington, Clarke, Qizilbash, Peto, & Collins, 2002; Lichtenstein et al., 2006 [both Level I]) and normal blood pressure (JNC, 2004 [Level I]). These practices involve a healthful diet (Knoops et al., 2004 [Level II]; Sacks et al., 2001 [Level II]), physical activity appropriate for age and health status (Fogelholm & Kukkonen-Harjula, 2000; Netz, Wu, Becker, & Tenenbaum, 2005 [both Level I]), and elimination of the use of and exposure to tobacco products (Barnoya & Glantz, 2005; U.S. Department of Health and Human Services [USDHHS], 2004b [both Level I]).

Pulmonary System

Respiratory function slowly and progressively deteriorates with age. This decline in ventilatory capacity seldom affects breathing during rest or customary limited physical activity in healthy older adults (Zeleznik, 2003 [Level V]); however, with greater-than-usual exertional demands, pulmonary reserve against hypoxia is readily exhausted and dyspnea occurs (Seidel et al., 2003 [Level VI]).

Several age-dependent anatomic and physiologic changes combine to impair the functional reserve of the pulmonary system. Respiratory muscle strength and endurance deteriorate to restrict maximal ventilatory capacity (Kelley, 2002 [Level V]). Secondary to calcification of rib-cage cartilage, the chest wall becomes rigid (Schretzman & Strumpf, 2002 [Level VI]), limiting thoracic compliance. Loss of elastic fibers reduces recoil of small airways that can collapse and cause air-trapping, particularly in dependent portions of the lung. Decreases in alveolar surface area, vascularization, and surfactant production adversely affect gaseous exchange (Zeleznik, 2003 [Level V]).

Additional clinical consequences of aging include an increased anteroposterior chest diameter due to skeletal changes (Seidel et al., 2003 [Level VI]). An elevated respiratory rate of 12 to 24 breaths per minute accompanies reduced tidal volume for rapid, shallow breathing. Limited diaphragmatic excursion and chest/lung expansion can result in less effective inspiration and expiration (Mick & Ackerman, 2004 [Level V]). Due to decreased cough reflex effectiveness and deep-breathing capacity, mucus and foreign matter clearance is restricted, predisposing to aspiration, infection, and bronchospasm (Watters, 2002 [Level V]). Further elevating the risk of infection is a decline in ciliary and macrophage activities and drying of the mucosal membranes with more difficult mucous excretion (Kelley, 2002 [Level V]). With the loss of elastic recoil comes the potential for atelectasis. Due to reduced respiratory-center sensitivity, ventilatory responses to hypoxia and hypercapnia are blunted (Imperato & Sanchez, 2006), putting an elder at risk for development of respiratory distress with illness or administration of narcotics (Zeleznik, 2003 [Level V]).

The modifications in ventilatory capacity with age are reflected in changes in pulmonary-function tests measuring lung volumes, flow rates, diffusing capacity, and gas exchange. Whereas total lung capacity remains constant, vital capacity is reduced and residual volume is increased. Reductions in all measures of expiratory flow (i.e., FEV$_1$, FVC, FEV$_1$/FVC, PEFR) quantify a decline in useful air movement (Imperato & Sanchez, 2006). Due to impaired alveolar function, diffusing capacity (DLCO) declines as does arterial oxygen tension (PaO_2), indicating impaired oxygen exchange; however, arterial pH and carbon dioxide tension ($PaCO_2$) remain constant (Enright, 2003). Reductions in arterial oxygen saturation and cardiac output restrict the amount of oxygen available for use by tissues, particularly in the supine position, although arterial blood gas seldom limits exercise in healthy subjects (Zeleznik, 2003).

Respiratory assessment includes determination of breathing rate, rhythm, regularity, volume (hyper/hypoventilation), depth (shallow, deep) (Docherty, 2002 [Level I]), and effort (dyspnea) (Mahler et al., 2003 [Level V]). Auscultation of breath sounds throughout the lung fields may reveal decreased air exchange at the lung bases (Mick & Ackerman, 2004 [Level V]). Thorax and symmetry of chest expansion should be inspected. A history of respiratory disease (tuberculosis, asthma), tobacco use (expressed as pack years), and extended exposure to environmental irritants through work or avocation is contributory (Seidel et al., 2003 [Level VII]).

Subjective assessment of cough includes questions on quality (productive/nonproductive), sputum characteristics (note hemoptysis; purulence indicating possible infection), and frequency (during eating or drinking, suggesting dysphagia and aspiration) (Smith & Connolly, 2003 [Level V]). Evaluation for pneumococcal pneumonia includes monitoring for typical symptoms such as productive cough, fever, and dyspnea as well as insidious, atypical symptoms including tachypnea, lethargy (Bartlett et al., 2000 [Level I]), weakness, falls, decline in functional status, or increased/new-onset confusion with absent high fever and elevated white blood cell count. Decreased appetite and dehydration may be the only initial symptoms in an older adult (Kelley, 2002 [Level V]).

Secretions and decreased breathing rate during sedation can reduce ventilation and oxygenation (Watters, 2002 [Level V]). Oxygen saturation can be followed through arterial blood gases and pulse oximetry (Zeleznik, 2003 [Level V]) and breathing rate (greater than 24 bpm), accessory muscle use, and skin color (cyanosis, pallor) should also be monitored (Docherty, 2002 [Level I]). The inability to expectorate secretions, dyspnea, and decreased SaO2 levels suggests the need for suctioning to clear airways (Smith & Connolly, 2003 [Level V]). Optimal positioning to facilitate respiration should be regularly monitored with use of upright positions (Fowler's or orthopneic position) recommended (Docherty, 2002 [Level I]; Watters, 2002 [Level V]). Pain assessment may be necessary to allow ambulation and deep breathing (Mick & Ackerman, 2004 [Level V]).

Nursing-care strategies useful in facilitating respiration and maintaining patent airways in older adults include positioning to allow maximum chest expansion through the use of semi- or high-Fowler's or orthopneic position (Docherty, 2002 [Level I]). Additionally, frequent repositioning in bed or encouraging ambulation, if mobility permits, is advised (Watters, 2002 [Level V]).

Hydration is maintained through fluid intake (six to eight 8-ounce glasses per day) and air humidification, which prevent desiccation of mucous membranes and loosen secretions to facilitate expectoration (Suhayda & Walton, 2002 [Level V]). Suctioning may be necessary to clear airways of secretions (Smith & Connolly, 2003 [Level V]) while oxygen should be provided as needed (Docherty, 2002 [Level I]). Incentive spirometry, with use of sustained maximal inspiration devices (SMIs), can improve pulmonary ventilation, mainly inhalation, as well as loosen respiratory secretions, particularly in older adults who are unable to ambulate or declining in function (Dunn, 2004 [Level V]).

Medications for respiratory problems include bronchodilators (β_2 agonists, xanthines), which reduce bronchospasm, open congested airways, and facilitate ventilation (National Heart, Lung, and Blood Institute, 1996 [Level I]). Analgesics may be necessary for ambulation and deep breathing (Mick & Ackerman, 2004 [Level V]).

Deep-breathing exercises, such as abdominal (diaphragmatic) and pursed-lip breathing, in addition to controlled and huff coughing, can further facilitate respiratory function. Techniques for healthy breathing, including sitting and standing erect, nose breathing (Dunn, 2004 [Level V]), and regular exercise (Netz et al., 2005 [Level I]) should be promoted. For individuals older than 65, immunization is recommended against pneumococcal infections every 5 years (Centers for Disease Control and Prevention [CDC], 1997 [Level I]) and against influenza annually (CDC, 2000 [Level I]). Education on eliminating the use of and exposure to tobacco products should be emphasized (Barnoya & Glantz, 2005 [Level I]; USDHHS, 2004b [Level I]).

Renal and Genitourinary Systems

In normal aging, the mass of the kidney declines with a loss of functional glomeruli and tubules in addition to a reduction in blood flow. Concomitantly, changes occur in the activity of the regulatory hormones, vasopressin (antidiuretic hormone), atrial natriuretic hormone, and renin-angiotensin-aldosterone system (Miller, 2003 [Level V]). These alterations combine to result in diminished glomerular filtration rate (GFR), with a 10% decrement per decade starting at age 30, as well as impaired electrolyte and water management (Beck, 1998 [Level V]).

Despite these changes, older adults maintain the ability to regulate fluid balance under baseline conditions; however, with age, the renal system is more limited in its capacity to respond to externally imposed stresses. This reduced functional reserve increases vulnerability to disturbances in fluid homeostasis as well as to renal complications and failure (Miller, 2003 [Level V]), particularly from fluid/electrolyte overload and deficit, medications, or illness (Wiggins, 2003 [Level VI]).

The decline in functional nephrons emphasizes the risk from nephrotoxic agents including NSAIDs, β-lactam antibiotics, and radiocontrast dyes (Bailey & Sands, 2003 [Level VI]). Reduced GFR impairs an older adult's ability to excrete renally cleared medications such as aminoglycoside antibiotics (e.g., gentamycin) and digoxin, increasing the risk of adverse drug reactions. Dosages should be based on GFR estimated by the Cockcroft-Gault equation for creatinine clearance rather than by serum creatinine concentration (Beyth & Shorr, 2002 [Level V]). Values of serum creatinine remain unchanged despite an age-associated decline in GFR because of the parallel decrease in both elders' skeletal muscle mass, which produces creatinine, and GFR for creatinine elimination. Thus, serum-creatinine levels overestimate GFR to result in potential drug overdose (Beck, 1998 [Level V]).

Increased risk of electrolyte imbalances can result from an age-dependent impairment in the excretion of excessive sodium loads, particularly in heart failure and with NSAID use, leading to intravascular volume overload. Clinical indicators include weight gain (>2%); intake>output; edema; change in mental status; tachycardia; bounding pulse; pulmonary congestion with dyspnea, rales, SOB (Beck, 1998 [Level V]); increased B/P and CVP; and distended neck/peripheral veins (Kozier, Erb, Berman, & Burke, 2000 [Level VI]).

Conversely, sodium wasting, or excess sodium excretion when maximal sodium conservation is needed, can occur with diarrhea. Hypovolemia and dehydration may ensue (Stern, 2006 [Level V]), manifesting as acute change in mental status (possible initial symptom), weight loss (>2%), decreased tissue turgor, dry oral mucosa, tachycardia, decreased B/P, postural hypotension, flat neck veins, poor capillary refill, oliguria (<30 mL/h), increased hematocrit and specific gravity of urine, BUN:plasma creatinine ratio >20:1, and serum osmolality >300 mOsm/kg (Mentes, 2006 [Level V]).

Impaired potassium excretion puts an elder at risk for hyperkalemia, particularly in heart failure and with use of potassium supplements, potassium-sparing diuretics, NSAIDs, and ACE inhibitors (Mick & Ackerman, 2004 [Level V]). Clinical indicators include diarrhea, change in mental status, cardiac dysrhythmias or arrest, muscle weakness and areflexia, paresthesias and numbness in extremities, ECG abnormalities, and serum potassium >5.0 mEq/L (Beck, 1998 [Level V]; Kozier et al., 2000 [Level VI]).

Limited acid excretion capability can cause metabolic acidosis during acute illness in an older adult (Beck, 1998 [Level V]). This condition presents as Kussmaul's respirations, change in mental status, nausea, vomiting, arterial blood pH<7.35, serum bicarbonate <22 mEq/L, and $PaCO_2$<38 mm Hg with respiratory compensation (Kozier et al., 2000 [Level VI]).

Causes of abnormal water metabolism with age include diminution in maximal urinary concentrating ability, which, in concert with blunted thirst sensation and total body water, can result in hypertonic dehydration and hypernatremia (Mentes, 2006 [Level V]). Often associated with insensible fluid loss from fever (Miller, 2003 [Level V]), hypernatremia presents with thirst; dry oral mucosa; dry, furrowed tongue; postural hypotension; weakness; lethargy; serum sodium >150 mEq/L; and serum osmolality >290 mOsm/kg. Disorientation, seizures, and coma occur in severe hypernatremia (Suhayda & Walton, 2002 [Level V]).

Impaired excretion of a water load, exacerbated by ACE inhibitors, thiazide diuretics (Miller, 2003), and SSRIs (Mentes, 2006 [Level V]), predisposes an elder to water intoxication and hyponatremia (Beck, 1998 [Level V]). Clinical indicators involve lethargy, nausea, muscle weakness and cramps, serum sodium <135 mEq/L, and serum osmolality <290 mOsm/kg. Confusion, coma, and seizures are seen in severe hyponatremia (Suhayda & Walton, 2002 [Level V]).

Changes in the lower urinary tract with age include reduced bladder elasticity and innervation, which contribute to decreases in urine flow rate, voided volume, and bladder capacity, as well as increases in postvoid residual and involuntary bladder contractions (Kevorkian, 2004). A delayed or decreased perception of the signal from the bladder to void translates into urinary urgency (Bradway & Yetman, 2002 [Level V]). Increased nocturnal urine flow, which results from altered regulatory hormone production, impaired ability to concentrate urine, and bladder-muscle instability, can lead to nocturnal polyuria

(Miller, 2003 [Level V]). In older men, benign prostatic hyperplasia (BPH) can result in urinary urgency, hesitancy, and frequency. All these changes combine to increase the risk of urinary incontinence in an older adult, whereas increased risk of falls accompanies urgency and nocturia. Changes in the physiology of the urinary tract also contribute to development of bacteriuria, with potential for urinary tract infection (UTI) (Stern, 2006 [Level V]).

Renal assessment includes monitoring for renal function, based on creatinine clearance, particularly in acute and chronic illness (Beck, 1998 [Level V]). The choice, dose, need, and alternatives for nephrotoxic and renally excreted agents should be considered (Beyth & Shorr, 2002 [Level V]).

Dehydration, volume overload, and electrolyte status are assessed first by screening for risk of fluid/electrolyte imbalances based on an older adult's age, medical and nutritional history, medications, cognitive and functional abilities, psychosocial status, and bowel and bladder patterns. Data on fluid intake and output, daily weights, and vital signs, including orthostatic blood pressure measurements, are needed. Heart rate is a less reliable indicator for dehydration in older adults due to the effects of medications and heart disease (Suhayda & Walton, 2002 [Level V]).

Physical assessment for fluid/electrolyte status focuses on skin for edema and turgor. Note that turgor in older adults is a less reliable indicator for dehydration due to poor skin elasticity, and assessment over the sternum or inner thigh is recommended. Additional assessment involves the oral mucosa for dryness as well as cardiovascular, respiratory, and neurologic systems. Acute changes in mental status, reasoning, memory, or attention may be initial symptoms of dehydration (Suhayda & Walton, 2002 [Level V]). Pertinent laboratory tests include serum electrolytes, serum osmolality, CBC, urine pH and specific gravity, BUN, hematocrit (Mentes, 2006 [Level V]), and arterial blood gases (Beck, 1998 [Level V]).

Regarding the lower urinary tract, evaluations of urinary incontinence, UTI, and nocturnal polyuria using a 72-hour voiding diary are recommended. UTI in older adults may present with classical symptoms of dysuria, flank or suprapubic discomfort, hematuria, and urinary frequency and urgency, or atypical symptoms of new-onset/worsening incontinence, anorexia, confusion, nocturia, or enuresis. A voiding history and rectal exam are required to diagnose BPH (Bradway & Yetman, 2002 [Level V]). Fall risk should be addressed when nocturnal or urgent voiding is present (see chapter 9, *Preventing Falls in Acute Care*).

Ongoing care involves monitoring for renal function by creatinine clearance calculation and for levels of nephrotoxic and renally cleared drugs (Beyth & Shorr, 2002 [Level V]). Maintenance of fluid/electrolyte balance is paramount (Beck, 1998 [Level V]). To prevent dehydration, older adults weighing between 50 and 80 kg are advised to have a minimum fluid intake of 1,500 to 2,500 ml/day (unless contraindicated by medical condition) (Suhayda & Walton, 2002 [Level V]) from both fluids and food sources including fruits, vegetables, soups, and gelatin with avoidance of high salt and caffeine. Education on appropriate food choices and encouragement to follow recommendations should be provided (Mentes, 2006 [Level V]). Simmons and colleagues (2001 [Level II]) found that verbal prompting and complying with beverage preferences increased fluid intake among nursing-home residents.

Referrals to specialists in incontinence and urology should be provided for management of voiding problems. Incontinence care and exercise can improve performance, including reduced incontinence, of nursing-home residents, as demonstrated by Schnelle and colleagues (2002 [Level II]). Behavioral interventions recommended for nocturnal polyuria include limited fluid intake in the evening, avoidance of caffeine and alcohol, and prompted voiding schedule (Miller, 2003 [Level V]). Institution of safety precautions and fall-prevention strategies are needed in nocturnal or urgent voiding (see chapter 9, *Preventing Falls in Acute Care*).

Oropharyngeal and Gastrointestinal Systems

Age-specific alterations in the oral cavity can adversely affect an older adult's nutritional status. Deterioration in the strength of muscles of mastication as well as potential for tooth loss and xerostomia due to dehydration or medications may reduce food intake (Jensen, McGee, & Binkley, 2001). Contributing to poor appetite are an altered taste perception and a diminished sense of smell (Ritchie, 2002) (see chapter 17, *Oral Health Care)*.

Changes in the esophagus with age include delayed emptying in addition to decreases in upper and lower esophageal sphincter pressures, sphincter relaxation, and peristaltic contractions. Although these alterations rarely impair esophageal function and swallowing sufficiently to cause dysphagia or aspiration in normal aging, such conditions can develop in conjunction with disease or medication side effects in older adults (Achem & DeVault, 2005; Shaker & Staff, 2001 [Level V]). Diminished gastric motility with delayed emptying contributes to altered oral drug passage time and absorption in the stomach; elevated risk of gastroesophageal reflux disease (GERD) (Hall, 2003); and decreased postprandial hunger, leading to diminished food intake and possible malnutrition (Blechman & Gelb, 1999). Reduced mucin secretion impairs the protective function of the gastric mucosal barrier and increases the incidence of NSAID-induced gastric ulcerations (Hila & Castell, 2003). Although the motility and most absorptive functions of the small intestine are preserved with age, absorption of vitamin B_{12}, folic acid, and carbohydrates declines (Holt, 2001). In addition, malabsorption of calcium and vitamin D contributes to the risk of osteoporosis. Supplementation with calcium and vitamins D and B_{12} is now recommended for older adults (Institute of Medicine, 1997; USDHHS, 2005).

Age-dependent weakening of the large intestine wall predisposes older adults to diverticulosis and may lead to diverticulitis (Hall, 2003). Because motility of the colon appears to be preserved with age, increased self-reports of constipation in older adults may be attributed instead to altered dietary intake, medications, inactivity, or illness (Jensen et al., 2001). Diminished rectal elasticity, internal anal sphincter thickening, and impaired sensation to defecate contribute to the risk of fecal incontinence in elders (Tariq, 2004 [Level V]), although this condition is primarily found in combination with previous bowel surgery or disease and not in normal aging (Schiller, 2001).

Pancreatic exocrine output of digestive enzymes is preserved to allow normal digestive capacity with aging. An age-related decrease in gallbladder function increases the risk of gallstone formation (Ross & Forsmark, 2001). Although liver size and blood flow decline with age, reserve capacity maintains adequate hepatic function and values of liver-function tests remain stable; however, the liver is more susceptible to damage by stressors including alcohol and tobacco. Associated with changes in the hepatic and intestinal cytochrome P450 system (Hall, 2003), clearance of a range of medications, including many benzodiazepines, declines to result in increased potential for dose-dependent adverse reactions to these drugs (Regev & Schiff, 2001).

Decreased immune response of the gastrointestinal tract with age contributes to a high risk for infectious and inflammatory diseases of this system (Blechman & Gelb, 1999). Further, impaired enteric neuronal function may blunt an older adult's reaction to inflammation and infection and result in atypical presentation with symptoms such as confusion and fatigue rather than the typical rigidity of peritonitis (Hall, 2002 [Level V]).

In the gastrointestinal evaluation, the abdomen and bowel sounds are assessed. Liver size as well as reports of pain, anorexia, nausea, vomiting, and altered bowel habits should be noted (Edwards, 2002 [Level V]). Assessment of the oral cavity includes dentition and chewing capacity (see chapter 17, *Oral Health Care*).

Weight is monitored with calculation of body mass index (BMI) and compared to recommended values (Lichtenstein et al., 2006 [Level I]). Deficiencies in diet can be identified through comparisons of dietary intake, using a 24- to 72-hour food intake record, with nutritional guidelines (Roberts & Dallal, 2005 [Level I]; USDHHS, 2000, 2005 [both Level I]). In addition, laboratory values of serum albumin, prealbumin, and transferrin are useful nutritional indicators. Low albumin concentration can also affect efficacy and potential for toxicity of selected drugs, including digoxin and warfarin (Beyth & Shorr, 2002 [Level V]). Several instruments for screening the nutritional status, eating habits, and appetite of elders are available (McGee & Jensen, 2000 [Level V]) (see the Resources and chapter 15, *Nutrition*).

Signs of dysphagia such as coughing or choking with solid or liquid food intake should be reported for further evaluation (Shaker & Staff, 2001 [Level V]). If aspiration from dysphagia is suspected, the lungs must be assessed for the presence of infection, typically indicated by uni- or bilateral basilar crackles in the lungs, dyspnea, tachypnea, and cough (Seidel et al., 2003 [Level VI]). A decline in function or change in mental status may signal atypical presentation of respiratory infection from aspiration (Kelley, 2002 [Level V]). Evaluation of GERD is based on typical presenting symptoms of heartburn (pyrosis) and acid regurgitation and atypical symptoms in older adults of dysphagia, chest pain, hoarseness, vomiting, chronic cough, or recurrent aspiration pneumonia (Edwards, 2002 [Level V]).

To assess constipation or fecal incontinence, a careful history with a 2-week bowel log noting laxative use is needed (Tariq, 2004 [Level V]). Fecal impaction is assessed by digital examination of the rectum as a hardened mass of feces, which can be palpated. The impaction may also be palpated through the abdomen (Kozier et al., 2000 [Level VI]).

For continuing care, referrals should be provided to a registered dietician for poor food intake, unhealthy BMI (healthy BMI: 18.5–24.9 kg/m^2; overweight: 25–29.9kg/m^2; obesity: $\geq$30kg/m^2) (Lichtenstein et al., 2006 [Level I]), and unintentional weight loss of ≥10% in 6 months (Hark, Bowman, & Bellini, 1999 [Level VI]); to a dentist for dentition and problems of the oral cavity; and to a speech pathologist for dysphagia. Drug levels and liver-function tests are monitored if drugs are metabolized hepatically (Beyth & Shorr, 2002 [Level V]). Education on lifestyle modifications and over-the-counter medications is valuable in treatment of GERD (Edwards, 2002 [Level V]). Explanation of normal bowel frequency, the importance of diet and exercise, and recommended types of laxatives addresses constipation problems (Harari, 2003 [Level V]). Mobility should be encouraged to prevent constipation and prophylactic laxatives should be provided if constipating medications such as opiates are prescribed (Stern, 2006 [Level V]). Community-based food and nutrition programs (Krassie & Roberts, 2001 [Level V]) and education on healthful diets utilizing the food pyramid for elders may be useful in improving dietary intake (JNC, 2004 [Level I]; USDHHS, 2000, 2005 [both Level I]) (see chapter 15, *Nutrition*). Screening for colorectal cancer is effective in reducing mortality from colorectal cancer and should be encouraged (Takahashi, Okhravi, Lim, & Kasten, 2004 [Level V]; U.S. Preventive Services Task Force [USPSTF], 2002 [Level I]).

Musculoskeletal System

Musculoskeletal tissues undergo age-associated changes that can negatively impact function in older adults (Levelser & Shakoor, 2003). In sarcopenia, or the loss of muscle mass and strength, a decline in the size, number, and quality of skeletal muscle fibers occurs with aging. Lean body mass is replaced by fat and fibrous tissue (Levelser & Delbono, 2003) so that by age 75, only 15% of the total body mass is muscle compared to 30% in a young, healthy adult (Matsumura & Ambrose, 2006). These alterations result in diminished contractile muscle force with increased weakness and fatigue plus poor exercise tolerance (Fried & Walston, 2003). Age-specific physiological alterations contributing to sarcopenia include reductions in muscle innervation, insulin activity, and sex-steroid (i.e., estrogen, testosterone) and growth-hormone levels. Additionally, individual factors such as weight loss, protein deficiency, and physical inactivity can accelerate development of this condition to progress to a clinically significant problem. Sarcopenia has been documented to adversely affect function in older adults by increasing the risk of disability, falls, unstable gait, and need for assistive devices. Physical activity, particularly strength training, and adequate intake of energy and protein can prevent or reverse sarcopenia (Roubenoff & Hughes, 2000).

Age-dependent bone loss occurs in both sexes and at all sites in the skeleton. Whereas bone mass peaks between ages 30 and 35 (USDHHS, 2004a), density decreases thereafter at a rate of 0.5% per year. This decrement, due to reduced osteoblast activity in the deposition of new bone, is accompanied by deterioration in bone architecture and strength. Further, for 5 to 7 years following menopause during estrogen decline, bone loss in women accelerates to a 3% to 5% annual rate (Simon, 2005). This loss, resulting from osteoclast activation with elevated bone breakdown or resorption, occurs mainly in cancellous or trabecular bone such as the vertebral body and may develop into Type I osteoporosis in women ages 51 to 75 who risk vertebral fractures. Following this postmenopausal period, bone loss slows again in women and involves cortical bone in the long bones of the extremities (Dempster, 2003). With aging, both women and men may develop Type II osteoporosis and are susceptible to hip fractures and kyphosis from vertebral compression fractures in later life (Prestwood & Duque, 2003).

An age-associated decline in the strength of ligaments and tendons, which are integral to normal joint function, predisposes to increased ligament and tendon injury, more limited joint range of motion, and reduced joint stability, leading to osteoarthritis (Levelser & Shakoor, 2003). Degeneration of intervertebral discs, due to dehydration and poor nutrient influx, elevates the risk of spinal osteoarthritis, spondylosis, and stenosis with aging (Levelser & Delbono, 2003).

Gerontological changes in articular cartilage, which covers the bone endings in joints to allow smooth movement, involve increased dehydration, stiffening, crystal formation, calcification, and roughening of the cartilage surface. Although these alterations have a minor effect on joint function under baseline conditions, the aging joint is less capable of withstanding mechanical stress such as caused by obesity or excess physical activity and is also more susceptible to disease including osteoarthritis (Levelser & Delbono, 2003).

Age-dependent changes in stature include dorsal kyphosis, reduction in height, flexion of the hips and knees, and a backward tilt of the head to compensate for the thoracic curvature (Seidel et al., 2003 [Level VI]). A shorter stride, reduced velocity, and broader base of support with feet more widely spaced characterize modifications in gait with age (Sudarsky, 2001).

The musculoskeletal assessment includes inspection of posture, gait, balance, symmetry of body parts, and alignment of extremities. Kyphosis, bony enlargements, or other abnormalities should be noted. Palpate bones, joints, and surrounding muscles. Evaluate muscle strength on a scale of 0/5, symmetry, and signs of atrophy of major upper and lower extremity muscle groups. Assess active and passive range of motion for major joints and report pain, limitation of range of motion (ROM), and joint laxity. Joint stabilization and slow movements in ROM examinations are advised to prevent injury (Seidel et al., 2003 [Level VI]). Functionality, mobility, fine and gross motor skills, balance (Robbins, Waked, & Krouglicof, 1998 [Level II]), and fall risk (Baum, Capezuti, & Driscoll, 2002 [Level V]) should be assessed (see chapter 3, *Assessment of Function*, and chapter 9, *Preventing Falls in Acute Care*).

For continuing care, referrals to physical or occupational therapy may be needed. Increased physical activity, including exercises for ROM (Netz et al., 2005 [Level I]) and muscle strengthening and power (Fielding et al., 2002 [Level II]) are recommended to maintain maximal function. Several interventions have been evaluated to promote such behavior in elders and involve health education, goal setting, and self-monitoring (Conn, Minor, Burks, Rantz, & Pomeroy, 2003; Conn, Valentine, & Cooper, 2002 [both Level I]). Pain medication should be provided if needed to enhance functionality (see chapter 10, *Pain Management*). Strategies to prevent falls (Carter, Kannus, & Kahn, 2001 [Level I]; see chapter 9, *Preventing Falls in Acute Care*) and avoid physical restraints (see chapter 22, *Physical Restraints and Side Rails in Acute and Critical Care Settings: Legal, Ethical and Practice Issues*) are appropriate.

To prevent and treat osteoporosis, adequate daily intake of calcium (i.e., 1,200 mg for women aged 50 and older) and vitamin D (400 IU for women aged 50 to 70 and 600 IU for women aged 71 and older) (USDHHS, 2004a [Level I]), physical exercise, and smoking cessation are recommended (USDHHS, 2004b [Level I]; USPSTF, 1996 [Level I]). In addition, routine bone-mineral density screening for osteoporosis is advised for women 65 years and older as well as women 60 to 64 years at increased risk of osteoporotic fractures (USPSTF, 2002 [Level I]).

Nervous System and Cognition

Gerontological alterations in the nervous system can affect function and cognition in elders. Changes include a reduced number of cerebral (Seidel et al., 2003 [Level VI]) and peripheral neurons (Hall, 2002 [Level V]), modifications in dendrites and glial support cells in the brain, and loss and remodeling of synapses. Decreased levels of neurotransmitters, particularly dopamine, as well as deficits in systems that relay signals between neurons and regulate neuronal plasticity, also occur with aging (Mattson, 2003 [Level V]).

Combined, these neurological changes contribute to impairments in general muscle strength; deep-tendon reflexes; sensation of touch, pain, and vibration; and nerve conduction velocity (Hall, 2002 [Level V]), which result in slowed coordinated movements and increased response time to stimuli (Matsumura & Ambrose, 2006). These clinical consequences, although relatively mild in normal aging, cause an overall slowing of motor skills with potential deficits in balance, gait, coordination, reaction time, and agility (Pakkar & Cummings, 2003 [Level VI]). Such decline in function can adversely affect an elder's daily activities, notably ambulation and driving, and predispose to falls and injury (Craft, Cholerton, & Reger, 2003 [Level V]).

Neurological changes, along with thinning of the skin, compromise thermoregulation in older adults, resulting in decreased sensitivity to ambient temperature as well as impaired heat conservation, production, and dissipation with predisposition to hypothermia and hyperthermia (Abrass, 2003). In addition, febrile responses to infection may be blunted, particularly in the very old, frail, or malnourished elder (Watters, 2002 [Level V]).

With age, the speed of cognitive processing slows (Bashore & Ridderinkhof, 2002 [Level I]) and some degree of cognitive decline is common (Park, O'Connell, & Thomson, 2003 [Level I]) but not universal in the elder population (Stewart, 2004). Older adults demonstrate significant heterogeneity in cognitive performance, which may be positively impacted by education, good health, and physical activity (Christensen, 2001; Colcombe & Kramer, 2003 [Level I]).

Specific cognitive abilities exhibit differing levels of stability or decline with age. For example, crystallized intelligence, or the information and skills acquired from experience, remains largely intact, whereas fluid intelligence, or creative reasoning and problem-solving, declines (Christensen, 2001). Sustained attention is unaffected by aging, although divided attention, or the ability to concentrate on multiple tasks concurrently, appears to deteriorate. The mild decline in executive function, which includes the capability of directing behavior, making appropriate decisions, completing multistep tasks, and solving complex problems, usually has minimal impact on an older adult's ability to manage daily activities. Although language abilities and comprehension appear stable, spontaneous word finding may deteriorate and is often a complaint of older adults (Craft et al., 2003). Remote memory, or recalling events in the distant past, and procedural memory, or remembering ways to perform tasks, remain intact, but declarative memory, or learning new information, is slowed (Bopp & Verhaeghen, 2005). However, despite some deficits, memory functions are adequate for normal life in successful aging (Henry, MacLeod, Phillips, & Crawford, 2004 [Level I]).

Changes in the nervous system increase the risk of sleep disorders (Floyd, 2002 [Level I]) and delirium in older adults, especially in acute care (see chapter 7, *Delirium: Prevention, Early Recognition, and Treatment*). In addition, age-specific alterations predispose neurons to degeneration, contributing to Alzheimer's disease (Charter & Alekoumbides, 2004), Parkinson's disease, and Huntington's disease, although neurotropic factors, including insulin-like growth factor (Arwert, Deijen, & Drent, 2005), can counteract such neurodegeneration (Mattson, 2003 [Level V]).

Assessment, with periodic reassessment, of baseline functional status (see chapter 3, *Assessment of Function*) should include evaluation of fall risk, gait, and balance (see chapter 9, *Preventing Falls in Acute Care*) as well as basic, instrumental, and advanced ADLs. During acute illness, functional status and symptoms of delirium (see chapter 7, *Delirium: Prevention, Early Recognition, and Treatment*) should be monitored. Evaluation of baseline cognition with periodic reassessment (see chapter 4, *Assessing Cognitive Function*) and sleep disorders (Floyd, 2002 [Level I]) is warranted. The impact of physical and cognitive changes of aging on an older adult's level of safety and attentiveness in daily tasks, such as driving, should be determined (Bashore & Rudderinkhof, 2002 [Level I]; Craft et al., 2003 [Level V]; Henry et al., 2004 [Level I]; Park et al., 2003 [Level I]). Temperature indicating hypothermia (<35°C) or hyperthermia (>40.6°C) must be closely watched (Abrass, 2003 [Level V]), whereas symptoms of infection may present atypically with the absence of fever. Common symptoms to be monitored (Watters, 2002 [Level V]) include fatigue (Hall, 2002 [Level V]), decline in function, increased/new-onset confusion, and decreased appetite (Kelley, 2002 [Level V]).

For care of an older adult, fall-prevention strategies should be implemented (see chapter 9, *Preventing Falls in Acute Care*). If delirium is identified, nursing interventions for its treatment are needed (see chapter 7, *Delirium: Prevention, Early Recognition, and Treatment*). Particularly during surgery, procedures such as the use of warmed intravenous fluids and humidified gases should be instituted to maintain normal temperatures and prevent hypothermia in the older patient (Watters, 2002 [Level V]). Several lifestyle modifications are recommended to improve cognitive function and include regular physical exercise, particularly aerobic fitness training for executive function (Colcombe & Kramer, 2003 [Level I]), intellectual stimulation (Mattson, 2003 [Level V]), and a healthful diet (JNC, 2004 [Level I]; USDHHS, 2000 [Level I]). Reaction time training and safe driving courses can serve to improve safety in the older adult (Craft et al., 2003 [Level V]). Behavioral interventions for sleep disorders may be warranted (Irwin, Cole, & Nicassio, 2006 [Level I]).

Case Study and Discussion

Ms. M. is an 89-year-old woman presenting with productive cough, dyspnea, fatigue, and increased confusion during the past week. Her vital signs are pulse, 96 bpm; temperature, 98.6°F; respirations, 31 bpm; and B/P 110/55. A chest radiograph shows multilobe infiltrates with a diagnosis of pneumonia. How severe is her pneumonia?

Ms. M.'s symptoms of a respiratory rate of greater than 30 bpm, multilobe infiltrates on a chest radiograph, and diastolic blood pressure of less than 60 mm Hg characterize her pneumonia as severe (Bartlett et al., 2000) and she is likely to require admission to an intensive care unit. However, several age-related changes affect her symptoms of pneumonia. Pneumonia may present in an older adult with typical symptoms of productive cough, fever, and dyspnea or with more insidious, atypical symptoms of tachypnea, lethargy (Bartlett et al., 2000), weakness, falls, decline in functional status, or increased/new-onset confusion. Decreased appetite and dehydration may be the only initial symptoms (Kelley, 2002 [Level V]).

Because of reduced sympathetic innervation of the heart with age, the heart rate of an older adult does not increase in response to stress comparable to that of a younger individual (Taffet & Lakatta, 2003 [Level VI]). Thus, 96 bpm in an 89-year-old person is tachycardic and indicates a severe stress reaction. Further, because of a blunted febrile response to infection particularly in a very old, frail, or malnourished adult (Watters, 2002 [Level V]), a fever or elevated WBC count may not be a presenting symptom/sign even with severe infection.

Conclusion

Changes that occur with age strongly impact the health and functionality of older adults. Thus, recognition of and attention to these alterations are critically important in nursing assessment and care. Armed with knowledge of age-related changes and utilizing the clinical protocol described in this chapter, nurses can play a vital role in improving geriatric standards of practice. Designing interventions that consider gerontological changes, educating patients and family caregivers on these alterations, and sharing information with professional colleagues all serve to ensure optimal care of older adults.

Resources

Agency for Healthcare Research and Quality, AHRQ, part of the U.S. Department of Health and Human Services, provides evidence-based clinical practice guidelines including U.S. Preventive Services Task Force recommendations. Http://www.ahrq.gov

Administration on Aging The Administration on Aging, an agency in the U.S. Department of Health and Human Services, develops comprehensive systems of long-term care for older adults in the community. Web-based information for professionals is available. http://www.aoa.gov

National Institute on Aging Part of the U.S. National Institutes of Health, the NIA maintains a Web site with information on aging research as well as links to other government Web sites on aging. http://www.nia.nih.gov

Health and Age Foundation HAF is an independent nonprofit organization providing Web-based information on health care for older adults for the general public and health care professionals. http://www.healthandage.org

American Federation of Aging Research The Web site of AFAR, a nonprofit organization that supports research on aging, contains information on the biology of aging and approaches for successful aging. http://www.afar.org

Alliance for Aging Research The Web site of this nonprofit organization that supports aging research has a searchable database on information pertaining to aging. http://www.agingresearch.org

Smith-Kettlewell Eye Research Institute This nonprofit institute conducted a longitudinal study of vision in older adults. http://www.ski.org

CRONOS The goal of the CRONOS (Cross-cultural Research on the Nutrition of Older Subjects) project is to develop protocols to study the interaction of nutrition and aging. Gross, R., Solomons, N. W., Barba, C. V., de Groot, L., & Lin Khor, G. (September 1997). *Food and Nutrition Bulletin 18*(3). Tokyo: United Nations University Press. Retrieved on February 13, 2007, from http://www.unu.edu/unupress/food/V183e/begin.htm

National Council on Aging (NCOA) This nonprofit organization with a national network of more than 14,000 organizations and leaders from senior centers, area agencies on aging, adult day service centers, faith-based service organizations, senior housing facilities, employment services, consumer groups, and leaders from academia, business, and labor has information to help older people remain healthy and independent, find jobs, increase access to benefits programs, and discover meaningful ways to continue contributing to society. http://www.ncoa.org/index.cfm

The National Gerontological Nursing Association (NGNA) This national nursing organization is dedicated to the clinical care of older adults across diverse care settings. http://www.ngna.org/all.php

The National Conference of Gerontological Nurse Practitioners (NCGNP) NCGNP represents nearly 3,500 certified GNPs in the country and a multitude of family and adult NPs in geriatric practice. NCGNP has become the organization of choice for NPs who want to pursue continuing education in geriatric care and who seek peer support from experienced clinicians. The Web site has information on regulatory and practice issues, continuing education, and links to other sites. http://www.ncgnp.org/

The American Geriatrics Society (AGS) This is a not-for-profit organization of 7,000 health professionals devoted to improving the health, independence, and quality of life of all older people. The Society provides leadership to health care professionals, policy makers, and the public by implementing and advocating for programs in patient care, research, professional and public education, and public policy. Information on clinical practice guidelines for older adult care is available at the Web site. http://www.americangeriatrics.org/

Box 19.1

Nursing Standard of Practice Protocol: Age-Related Changes in Health

I. GOAL: To identify anatomical and physiological changes, which are attributed to the normal aging process.

II. OVERVIEW: Age-associated changes are most pronounced in advanced age of 85 years or older, may alter the older person's response to illness, show great variability among individuals, are often impacted by genetic and long-term lifestyle factors, and commonly involve a decline in functional reserve with reduced response to stressors.

III. STATEMENT OF PROBLEM: Gerontological changes are important in nursing assessment and care because they can adversely affect health and functionality and require therapeutic strategies; must be differentiated from pathological processes to allow development of appropriate interventions; predispose to disease, thus emphasizing the need for risk evaluation of the older adult; and can interact reciprocally with illness, resulting in altered disease presentation, response to treatment, and outcomes.

IV. AGE-ASSOCIATED CARDIOVASCULAR CHANGES

    A. Definition:
       Isolated systolic hypertension: systolic BP >140 mm Hg and diastolic BP <90 mm Hg.
    B. Etiology
       1. Arterial wall thickening and stiffening, decreased compliance.
       2. Left ventricular and atrial hypertrophy.
       3. Sclerosis of atrial and mitral valves.
       4. Strong arterial pulses, diminished peripheral pulses, cool extremities.
    C. Implications
       1. Decreased cardiac reserve.
          a. At rest: No change in heart rate, cardiac output.
          b. Under physiological stress and exercise: Decreased maximal heart rate and cardiac output, resulting in fatigue, SOB, slow recovery from tachycardia.
          c. Risk of isolated systolic hypertension; inflamed varicosities.
          d. Risk of arrhythmias, postural and diuretic-induced hypotension. May cause syncope.

V. PARAMETERS OF CARDIOVASCULAR ASSESSMENT

    A. Cardiac assessment: ECG; heart rate, rhythm, murmurs, heart sounds (S_4 common, S_3 in disease) (Seidel et al., 2003 [Level VI]).

B. Assess BP (lying, sitting, standing) and pulse pressure (Kenney, 2003 [Level V]).

C. Palpate carotid artery & peripheral pulses for symmetry (Seidel et al., 2003 [Level VI]).

VI. AGE-ASSOCIATED CHANGES IN THE PULMONARY SYSTEM

A. Etiology
  1. Decreased respiratory muscle strength; stiffer chest wall with reduced compliance.
  2. Diminished ciliary & macrophage activity, drier mucus membranes. Decreased cough reflex.
  3. Decreased response to hypoxia and hypercapnia.
B. Implications
  1. Reduced pulmonary functional reserve.
     a. At rest: No change.
     b. With exertion: Dyspnea, decreased exercise tolerance.
  2. Decreased respiratory excursion and chest/lung expansion with less effective exhalation. Respiratory rate 12 to 24 bpm.
  3. Decreased cough and mucus/foreign matter clearance.
  4. Increased risk of infection and bronchospasm with airway obstruction.

VII. PARAMETERS OF PULMONARY ASSESSMENT

A. Assess respiration rate, rhythm, regularity, volume, depth (Docherty, 2002 [Level I]), exercise capacity (Mahler et al., 2003 [Level V]). Ascultate breath sounds throughout lung fields (Mick & Ackerman, 2004 [Level V]).

B. Inspect thorax appearance, symmetry of chest expansion. Obtain smoking history (Seidel et al., 2003 [Level VI]).

C. Monitor secretions, breathing rate during sedation, positioning (Docherty, 2002 [Level I]; Watters, 2002 [Level V]), arterial blood gases, pulse oximetry (Zeleznik, 2003 [Level V]).

D. Assess cough, need for suctioning (Smith & Connolly, 2003 [Level V]).

VIII. NURSING-CARE STRATEGIES

A. Maintain patent airways through upright positioning/repositioning (Docherty, 2002 [Level I]), suctioning (Smith & Connolly, 2003 [Level V]), bronchodilators (National Heart, Lung, and Blood Institute, 1996 [Level I]).

B. Provide oxygen as needed (Docherty, 2002 [Level I]).

C. Incentive spirometry as indicated, particularly if immobile or declining in function (Dunn, 2004 [Level V]).

D. Maintain hydration and mobility (Watters, 2002 [Level V]).

E. Education on cough enhancement (Dunn, 2004 [Level V]), smoking cessation (USDHHS, 2004b [Level I]).

IX. AGE-ASSOCIATED CHANGES IN THE RENAL AND GENITOURINARY SYSTEMS

A. Definitions:
Cockcroft-Gault Equation: Calculation of creatinine clearance in older adults:
For Men

$$\text{Creatinine clearance (mL/min)} = \frac{(140 - \text{age in years}) \times (\text{body weight in kg})}{72 \times (\text{serum creatinine, mg/dL})}$$

For women, the calculated value is multiplied by 85% (0.85).

B. Etiology
1. Decreases in kidney mass, blood flow, glomerular filtration rate (10% decrement/decade after age 30). Decreased drug clearance.
2. Reduced bladder elasticity, muscle tone, capacity.
3. Increased postvoid residual, nocturnal urine production.
4. In males, prostate enlargement with risk of benign prostatic hyperplasia (BPH).

C. Implications
1. Reduced renal functional reserve; risk of renal complications in illness.
2. Risk of nephrotoxic injury and adverse reactions from drugs.
3. Risk of volume overload (in heart failure), dehydration, hyponatremia (with thiazide diuretics), hypernatremia (associated with fever), hyperkalemia (with potassium-sparing diuretics). Reduced excretion of acid load.
4. Increased risk of urinary urgency, incontinence (not a normal finding), UTI, nocturnal polyuria. Potential for falls.

X. PARAMETERS OF RENAL AND GENITOURINARY ASSESSMENT

A. Assess renal function (creatinine clearance) (Beck, 1998 [Level V]).
B. Assess choice/need/dose of nephrotoxic agents and renally cleared drugs (Beyth & Shorr, 2002 [Level V]) (see chapter 12, *Reducing Adverse Drug Events*).
C. Assess for fluid/electrolyte and acid/base imbalances (Suhayda & Walton, 2002 [Level V]).
D. Evaluate nocturnal polyuria (Miller, 2003 [Level V]), urinary incontinence, BPH. Assess UTI symptoms (Bradway & Yetman, 2002 [Level V]).
E. Assess fall risk if nocturnal or urgent voiding (see chapter 9, *Preventing Falls in Acute Care*)

XI. NURSING-CARE STRATEGIES

A. Monitor nephrotoxic and renally cleared drug levels (Beyth & Shorr, 2002 [Level V]).

B. Maintain fluid/electrolyte balance. Minimum 1,500–2,500 mL/day from fluids and foods for 50 to 80 kg adults to prevent dehydration (Suhayda & Walton, 2002 [Level V]).
C. For nocturnal polyuria: limit fluids in evening, avoid caffeine, use prompted voiding schedule (Miller, 2003 [Level V]).
D. Fall prevention for nocturnal or urgent voiding (see chapter 9, *Preventing Falls in Acute Care*).

XII. AGE-ASSOCIATED CHANGES IN THE OROPHARYNGEAL AND GASTROINTESTINAL SYSTEMS

A. Definition:
   BMI: Healthy: 18.5–24.9 kg/m^2; overweight: 25–29.9 kg/m^2; obesity: $\geq$30 kg/m^2.
B. Etiology
   1. Decreases in strength of muscles of mastication, taste, and thirst perception.
   2. Decreased gastric motility with delayed emptying. Atrophy of protective mucosa.
   3. Malabsorption of carbohydrates, vitamins B$_{12}$ and D, folic acid, calcium.
   4. Impaired sensation to defecate.
   5. Reduced hepatic reserve. Decreased metabolism of drugs.
C. Implications
   1. Risk of chewing impairment, fluid/electrolyte imbalances, poor nutrition.
   2. Gastric changes: altered drug absorption, increased risk of gastroesophageal reflux disease (GERD), maldigestion, NSAID-induced ulcers.
   3. Constipation not a normal finding. Risk of fecal incontinence with disease (not in healthy aging).
   4. Stable liver function tests. Risk of adverse drug reactions.

XIII. PARAMETERS OF OROPHARYNGEAL AND GASTROINTESTINAL ASSESSMENT

A. Assess abdomen, bowel sounds (Edwards, 2002 [Level V]).
B. Assess oral cavity (see chapter 17, *Oral Health Care*); chewing and swallowing capacity, dysphagia (coughing, choking with food/fluid intake) (Shaker & Staff, 2001 [Level V]). If aspiration, assess lungs (rales) for infection and typical/atypical symptoms (Bartlett et al., 2000 [Level I]; Kelley, 2002 [Level V]).
C. Monitor weight, calculate BMI, compare to standards (Lichtenstein et al., 2006 [Level I]). Determine dietary intake, compare to nutritional guidelines (USDHHS, 2005 [Level I]) (see chapter 15, *Nutrition*).

D. Assess for GERD (Edwards, 2002 [Level V]); constipation and fecal incontinence; fecal impaction by digital examination of rectum or palpation of abdomen (Tariq, 2004 [Level V]).

XIV. NURSING-CARE STRATEGIES

A. Monitor drug levels and liver function tests if on medications metabolized by liver. Assess nutritional indicators (McGee & Jensen, 2000 [Level V]).
B. Educate on lifestyle modifications and OTC medications for GERD (Edwards, 2002 [Level V]).
C. Educate on normal bowel frequency, diet, exercise, recommended laxatives. Encourage mobility, provide laxatives if on constipating medications (Harari, 2003 [Level V]).
D. Encourage participation in community-based nutrition programs (Krassie & Roberts, 2001 [Level V]); educate on healthful diets (US-DHHS, 2000, 2005 [both Level I]).

XV. AGE-ASSOCIATED CHANGES IN THE MUSCULOSKELETAL SYSTEM

A. Definition:
    Sarcopenia: Decline in muscle mass and strength associated with aging.
B. Etiology
    1. Sarcopenia with increased weakness and poor exercise tolerance.
    2. Lean body mass replaced by fat with redistribution of fat.
    3. Bone loss in women and men after peak mass at 30 to 35 years.
    4. Decreased ligament and tendon strength. Intervertebral disc degeneration. Articular cartilage erosion. Changes in stature with kyphosis, height reduction.
C. Implications
    1. Sarcopenia: increased risk of disability, falls, unstable gait.
    2. Risk of osteopenia and osteoporosis.
    3. Limited ROM, joint instability, risk of osteoarthritis.

XVI. NURSING-CARE STRATEGIES

A. Encourage physical activity through health education and goal setting (Conn et al., 2003 [Level I]; Conn et al., 2002 [Level I]) to maintain function (Fielding et al., 2002 [Level II]; Netz et al., 2005 [Level I]).
B. Pain medication to enhance functionality (see chapter 10, *Pain Management*). Implement strategies to prevent falls (Carter et al., 2001 [Level I]) (see chapter 9, *Preventing Falls in Acute Care*, and chapter 22, *Physical Restraints and Side Rails in Acute and Critical Care Settings: Legal, Ethical, and Practice Issues*).

C. Prevent osteoporosis by adequate daily intake of calcium and vitamin D (USDHHS, 2004a [Level I]), physical exercise, smoking cessation (USDHHS, 2004b [Level I]; USPSTF, 1996 [Level I]). Advise routine bone-mineral density screening (USPSTF, 2002 [Level I]).

XVII. AGE-ASSOCIATED CHANGES IN THE NERVOUS SYSTEM AND COGNITION

A. Etiology
1. Decrease in neurons and neurotransmitters.
2. Modifications in cerebral dendrites, glial support cells, synapses.
3. Compromised thermoregulation.
B. Implications
1. Impairments in general muscle strength; deep-tendon reflexes; nerve conduction velocity. Slowed motor skills and potential deficits in balance and coordination.
2. Decreased temperature sensitivity. Blunted febrile response to infection.
3. Slowed speed of cognitive processing. Some cognitive decline is common but not universal. Most memory functions adequate for normal life.
4. Increased risk of sleep disorders, delirium, neurodegenerative diseases.

XVIII. PARAMETERS OF NERVOUS SYSTEM AND COGNITION ASSESSMENTS

A. Assess, with periodic reassessment, baseline functional status (Craft et al., 2003 [Level V]) (see chapter 3, *Assessment of Function*, and chapter 9, *Preventing Falls in Acute Care*). During acute illness, monitor functional status and delirium (see chapter 7, *Delirium: Prevention, Early Recognition, and Treatment*).
B. Evaluate, with periodic reassessment, baseline cognition (see chapter 4, *Assessing Cognitive Function*) and sleep disorders (Floyd, 2002 [Level I]) (see chapter 20; *Excessive Sleepiness*).
C. Assess impact of age-related changes on level of safety and attentiveness in daily tasks (e.g., driving) (Henry et al., 2004 [Level I]; Park et al., 2003 [Level I]).
D. Assess temperature during illness or surgery (Abrass, 2003 [Level V]). Monitor atypical symptoms of infection, absent fever.

XIX. NURSING-CARE STRATEGIES

A. Institute fall preventions strategies (see chapter 9, *Preventing Falls in Acute Care*).

B. To maintain cognitive function, encourage lifestyle practices of regular physical exercise (Colcombe & Kramer, 2003 [Level I]), intellectual stimulation (Mattson, 2003 [Level V]), and healthful diet (Joint National Committee, 2004 [Level I]).

C. Recommend reaction time training and safe driving courses to improve safety (Craft et al., 2003 [Level V]).

D. Recommend behavioral interventions for sleep disorders (Irwin et al., 2006 [Level I]).

XX. EVALUATION AND EXPECTED OUTCOMES (FOR ALL SYSTEMS)

A. Older adult will experience successful aging through appropriate lifestyle practices and health care.

B. Health care provider will:
  1. Identify normative changes in aging and differentiate these from pathological processes.
  2. Develop interventions to correct for adverse effects associated with aging.

C. Institution will:
  1. Develop programs to promote successful aging.

D. Will provide staff education on age-related changes in health.

XXI. FOLLOW-UP MONITORING OF CONDITION

A. Continue to reassess effectiveness of interventions.

B. Incorporate continuous quality improvement criteria into existing programs.

References

Abrass, I. (2003). Disorders of temperature regulation. In W. R. Hazzard, J. P. Blass, J. B. Halter, J. G. Ouslander, & M. E. Tinetti (Eds.), *Principles of geriatric medicine and gerontology* (pp.1587–1591). NY: McGraw-Hill. Evidence Level V: Literature Review.

Achem, S. R., & DeVault, K. R. (2005). Dysphagia in aging. *Journal of Clinical Gastroenterology, 39*, 357–371.

Arwert, L. I., Deijen, J. B., & Drent, M. L. (2005). The relation between insulin-like growth factor I levels and cognition in healthy elderly: A meta-analysis. *Growth Hormone & IGF Research, 15*(6), 416–422.

Bailey, J. L., & Sands, J. M. (2003). Renal disease. In W. R. Hazzard, J. P. Blass, J. B. Halter, J. G. Ouslander, & M. E. Tinetti (Eds.), *Principles of geriatric medicine and gerontology* (pp. 551–568). NY: McGraw-Hill. Evidence Level VI: Expert Opinion.

Baltimore Longitudinal Study of Aging (2005). Retrieved October 5, 2006, from http://www.grc.nia.nih.gov/branches/blsa/blsa.htm.

Barnoya, J., & Glantz, S. A. (2005). Cardiovascular effects of secondhand smoke: Nearly as large as smoking. *Circulation, 111*, 2684–2698. Evidence Level I: Systematic Review.

Bartlett, J. G., Dowell, S. F., Mandell, L. A., File, T. M., Musher, D. M., & Fine, M. J. (2000). Practice guidelines for the management of community-acquired pneumonia in adults. *Clinical Infectious Diseases, 31*, 347–382. Evidence Level I: Systematic Review.

Bashore, T. R., & Ridderinkhof, K. R. (2002). Older age, traumatic brain injury, and cognitive slowing: Some convergent and divergent findings. *Psychological Bulletin, 128*(1), 151–198. Evidence Level I: Meta-analysis.

Baum, T., Capezuti, E., & Driscoll, G. (2002). Falls. In V. T. Cotter & N. E. Strumpf (Eds.), *Advanced practice nursing with older adults: Clinical guidelines* (pp. 245–269). NY: McGraw-Hill. Evidence Level V: Literature Review.

Beck, L. H. (1998). Changes in renal function with aging. *Clinics in Geriatric Medicine, 14,* 199–209. Evidence Level V: Literature Review.

Beyth, R. J., & Shorr, R. I. (2002). Principles of drug therapy in older patients: Rational drug prescribing. *Clinics in Geriatric Medicine, 18,* 577–592. Evidence Level V: Literature Review.

Bickley, L. S. (2003). *Bates' guide to physical examination and history taking.* Philadelphia: Lippincott, Williams & Wilkins. Evidence Level VI: Expert Opinion.

Blechman, M. B., & Gelb, A. M. (1999). Aging and gastrointestinal physiology. *Clinics in Geriatric Medicine, 15,* 429–438.

Bopp, K. L., & Verhaeghen, P. (2005). Aging and verbal memory span: A meta-analysis. *Journals of Gerontology Series B-Psychological Sciences & Social Sciences, 60*(5), P223–P233.

Bradway, C. W., & Yetman, G. (2002). Genitourinary problems. In V. T. Cotter & N. E. Strumpf (Eds.), *Advanced practice nursing with older adults: Clinical guidelines* (pp. 83–102). NY: McGraw-Hill. Evidence Level V: Literature Review.

Carter, N. D., Kannus, P., & Khan, K. M. (2001). Exercise in the prevention of falls in older people: A systematic literature review examining the rationale and the evidence. *Sports Medicine, 31*(6), 427–438. Evidence Level I: Systematic Review.

Centers for Disease Control and Prevention (1997). Prevention and control of pneumococcal disease: Recommendations of the Advisory Committee on Immunization Practices (ACIP). *MMWR Morbidity Mortality Weekly Report 46*(RR-8), 1–24. Evidence Level I: Systematic Review.

Centers for Disease Control and Prevention (2000). Prevention and control of influenza: Recommendations of the Advisory Committee on Immunization Practices (ACIP), *MMWR Morbidity Mortality Weekly Report 49*(RR-3), 1–38. Evidence Level I: Systematic Review.

Charter, R. A., & Alekoumbides, A. (2004). Evidence for aging as the cause of Alzheimer's disease. *Psychological Reports, 95*(3, Part 1), 935–945.

Christensen, H. (2001). What cognitive changes can be expected with normal ageing? *Australian and New Zealand Journal of Psychiatry, 35,* 768–775.

Colcombe, S., & Kramer, A. F. (2003). Fitness effects on the cognitive function of older adults: A meta-analytic study. *Psychological Science, 14*(2), 125–130. Evidence Level I: Meta-analysis.

Conn, V. S., Minor, M. A., Burks, K. J., Rantz, M. J., & Pomeroy, S. H. (2003). Integrative review of physical activity intervention research with aging adults. *Journal of the American Geriatrics Society, 51*(8), 1159–1168. Evidence Level I: Systematic Review.

Conn, V. S., Valentine, J. C., & Cooper, H. M. (2002). Interventions to increase physical activity among aging adults: A meta-analysis. *Annals of Behavioral Medicine, 24*(3), 190–200. Evidence Level I: Meta-analysis.

Craft, S., Cholerton, B., & Reger, M. (2003). Aging and cognition: What is normal? In W. R. Hazzard, J. P. Blass, J. B. Halter, J. G. Ouslander, & M. E. Tinetti (Eds.), *Principles of geriatric medicine and gerontology* (pp. 1355–1372). NY: McGraw-Hill. Evidence Level V: Literature Review.

Dempster, D. W. (2003). The pathophysiology of bone loss. *Clinics in Geriatric Medicine, 19,* 259–270.

Docherty, B. (2002). Cardiorespiratory physical assessment for the acutely ill: 1. *British Journal of Nursing, 11*(11), 750–758. Evidence Level I: Systematic Review.

Dunn, D. (2004). Preventing perioperative complications in an older adult. *Nursing2004, 34,* 36–41. Evidence Level V: Literature Review.

Edwards, W. F. (2002). Gastrointestinal problems. In V. T. Cotter & N. E. Strumpf (Eds.), *Advanced practice nursing with older adults: Clinical guidelines* (pp. 201–216). NY: McGraw-Hill. Evidence Level V: Literature Review.

Enright, P. L. (2003). Aging of the respiratory system. In W. R. Hazzard, J. P. Blass, J. B. Halter, J. G. Ouslander, & M. E. Tinetti (Eds.), *Principles of geriatric medicine and gerontology* (pp. 511–515). NY: McGraw-Hill.

Fielding, R. A., LeBrasseur, N. K., Cuoco, A., Bean, J., Mizer, K., & Singh, M. A. F. (2002). High-velocity resistance training increases skeletal muscle peak power in older women. *Journal of the American Geriatrics Society, 50*(4), 655–662. Evidence Level II: Single Experimental Study.

Floyd, J. A. (2002). Sleep and aging. *Nursing Clinics of North America, 37*(4), 719–731. Evidence Level I: Systematic Review.

Fogelholm, M., & Kukkonen-Harjula, K. (2000). Does physical activity prevent weight gain: A systematic review. *Obesity Reviews, 1*, 95–111. Evidence Level I: Systematic Review.

Fried, L. P., & Walston, J. (2003). Frailty and failure to thrive. In W. R. Hazzard, J. P. Blass, J. B. Halter, J. G. Ouslander, & M. E. Tinetti (Eds.), *Principles of geriatric medicine and gerontology* (pp. 1487–1502). NY: McGraw-Hill.

Hall, K. E. (2002). Aging and neural control of the GI tract. II. Neural control of the aging gut: Can an old dog learn new tricks? *American Journal of Physiology Gastrointestinal and Liver Physiology, 283*, G827–G832. Evidence Level V: Literature Review.

Hall, K. E. (2003). Effect of aging on gastrointestinal function. In W. R. Hazzard, J. P. Blass, J. B. Halter, J. G. Ouslander, & M. E. Tinetti (Eds.), *Principles of geriatric medicine and gerontology* (pp. 593–600). NY: McGraw-Hill.

Harari, D. (2003). Constipation in older people. In W. R. Hazzard, J. P. Blass, J. B. Halter, J. G. Ouslander, & M. E. Tinetti (Eds.), *Principles of geriatric medicine and gerontology* (pp. 655–670). NY: McGraw-Hill. Evidence Level V: Literature Review.

Hark, L., Bowman, M., & Bellini, L. (1999). Nutrition assessment in medical practice. In G. Morrison & L. Hark (Eds.), *Medical nutrition & disease* (pp. 3–20). Malden, MA: Blackwell Science, Inc. Evidence Level VI: Expert Opinion.

Hebbar, A. K., & Hueston, W. J. (2002a). Management of common arrhythmias: Part I. Supraventricular arrhythmias. *American Family Physician, 65*, 2479–2486.

Hebbar, A. K., & Hueston, W. J. (2002b). Management of common arrhythmias: Part II. Ventricular arrhythmias and arrhythmias in special populations. *American Family Physician, 65*, 2491–2496.

Henry, J. D., MacLeod, M. S., Phillips, L. H., & Crawford, J. R. (2004). A meta-analytic review of prospective memory and aging. *Psychology and Aging, 19*(1), 27–39. Evidence Level I: Meta-analysis.

Hila, A., & Castell, D. O. (2003). Upper gastrointestinal disorders. In W. R. Hazzard, J. P. Blass, J. B. Halter, J. G. Ouslander, & M. E. Tinetti (Eds.), *Principles of geriatric medicine and gerontology* (pp. 613–640). NY: McGraw-Hill.

Holt, P. R. (2001). Diarrhea and malabsorption in the elderly. *Gastroenterology Clinics of North America, 30*, 427–444.

Imperato, J., & Sanchez, L. D. (2006). Pulmonary emergencies in the elderly. *Emergency Medicine Clinics of North America, 24*, 317–338.

Institute of Medicine (IOM) (1997). *Dietary reference intakes for calcium, phosphorus, magnesium, vitamin D, and fluoride.* Washington, DC: National Academy Press.

Irwin, M. R., Cole, J. C., & Nicassio, P. M. (2006). Comparative meta-analysis of behavioral interventions for insomnia and their efficacy in middle-aged adults and in older adults 55+ years of age. *Health Psychology, 25*(1), 3–14. Evidence Level I: Meta-analysis.

Jensen, G. L., McGee, M., & Binkley, J. (2001). Nutrition in the elderly. *Gastroenterology Clinics of North America, 30*, 313–334.

Joint National Committee (2004). Seventh report of the Joint National Committee on prevention, detection, evaluation, and treatment of high blood pressure. Retrieved August 31, 2006, from http://www.nhlbi.nih.gov/guidelines/hypertension/jnc7full.htm. Evidence Level I: Systematic Review.

Kelley, M. F. (2002). Respiratory problems in older adults. In V. T. Cotter & N. E. Strumpf (Eds.), *Advanced practice nursing with older adults: Clinical guidelines* (pp. 67–82). NY: McGraw-Hill. Evidence Level V: Literature Review.

Kenny, R. A. (2003). Syncope. In W. R. Hazzard, J. P. Blass, J. B. Halter, J. G. Ouslander, & M. E. Tinetti (Eds.), *Principles of geriatric medicine and gerontology* (pp. 1553–1562). NY: McGraw-Hill. Evidence Level V: Literature Review.

Kestel, F. (2005, December 12). The best BP. *Advance for Nurses*, 33–34. Evidence Level V: Care Report.

Kevorkian, R. (2004). Physiology of incontinence. *Clinics in Geriatric Medicine, 20*, 409–425.

Knoops, K. T., de Groot, L. C., Kromhout, D., Perrin, A. E., Moreiras-Varela, O., Menotti, A., et al. (2004). Mediterranean diet, lifestyle factors, and 10-year mortality in elderly European men and women: The HALE project. *JAMA, 292*, 1433–1439. Evidence Level II: Single Experimental Study.

Kozier, B., Erb, G., Berman, A. J., & Burke, K. (2000). *Fundamentals of nursing*. Upper Saddle River, NJ: Prentice-Hall, Inc. Evidence Level VI: Expert Opinion.

Krassie, J., & Roberts, D. C. (2001). The independent older Australian: Implications for food and nutrition recommendations. *Journal of Nutrition, Health & Aging, 5*(1), 11–16. Evidence Level V: Program Evaluation.

Lakatta, E. G. (2000). Cardiovascular aging in health. *Clinics in Geriatric Medicine, 16*, 419–443.

Levelser, R. F., & Delbono, O. (2003). Aging of the muscles and joints. In W. R. Hazzard, J. P. Blass, J. B. Halter, J. G. Ouslander, & M. E. Tinetti (Eds.), *Principles of geriatric medicine and gerontology* (pp. 905–918). NY: McGraw-Hill.

Levelser, R. F., & Shakoor, N. (2003). Aging or osteoarthritis: Which is the problem? *Rheumatic Disease Clinics of North America, 29*, 653–673.

Lewington, S., Clarke, R., Qizilbash, N., Peto, R., & Collins, R. (2002). Prospective Studies Collaboration. Age-specific relevance of usual blood pressure to vascular mortality: A meta-analysis of individual data for 1 million adults in 61 prospective studies. *Lancet, 360*, 1903–1913. Evidence Level I: Meta-analysis.

Lichtenstein, A. H., Appel, L. J., Brands, M., Carnethon, M., Daniels, S., Franch, H. A., et al. (2006). Diet and lifestyle recommendations, revision 2006. A scientific statement from the American Heart Association Nutrition Committee. *Circulation, 114*, 82–96. Evidence Level I: Systematic Review.

Mahler, D. A., Fierro-Carrion, G., & Baird, J. C. (2003). Evaluation of dyspnea in the elderly. *Clinics in Geriatric Medicine, 19*, 19–33. Evidence Level V: Literature Review.

Matsumura, B. A., & Ambrose, A. F. (2006). Balance in the elderly. *Clinics in Geriatric Medicine, 22*, 395–412.

Mattson, M. (2003). Cellular and neurochemical aspects of the aging human brain. In W. R. Hazzard, J. P. Blass, J. B. Halter, J. G. Ouslander, & M. E. Tinetti (Eds.), *Principles of geriatric medicine and gerontology* (pp. 1341–1354). NY: McGraw-Hill. Evidence Level V: Literature Review.

McGee, M., & Jensen, G. L. (2000). Nutrition in the elderly. *Journal of Clinical Gastroenterology, 30*, 372–380. Evidence Level V: Literature Review.

Mentes, J. (2006). Oral hydration on older adults: Greater awareness is needed in preventing, recognizing, and treating dehydration. *American Journal of Nursing, 106*, 40–49. Evidence Level V: Literature Review.

Mick, D. J., & Ackerman, M. H. (2004). Critical care nursing for older adults: Pathophysiological and functional considerations. *Nursing Clinics of North America, 39*, 473–493. Evidence Level V: Literature Review.

Miller, M. (2003). Disorders of fluid balance. In W. R. Hazzard, J. P. Blass, J. B. Halter, J. G. Ouslander, & M. E. Tinetti (Eds.), *Principles of geriatric medicine and gerontology* (pp. 581–592). NY: McGraw-Hill. Evidence Level V: Literature Review.

Mukai, S., & Lipsitz, L. A. (2002). Orthostatic hypotension. *Clinics in Geriatric Medicine, 18*, 253–268.

National Heart, Lung, & Blood Institute (1996). *National Asthma Education and Prevention Program Working Group Report: Considerations for diagnosing and managing asthma in the elderly*. Bethesda, MD: National Institutes of Health. Evidence Level I: Systematic Review.

Netz, Y., Wu, M. J., Becker, B. J., & Tenenbaum, G. (2005). Physical activity and psychological well-being in advanced age: A meta-analysis of intervention studies. *Psychology & Aging, 20*(2), 272–284. Evidence Level I: Meta-analysis.

Pakkar, A., & Cummings, J. L. (2003). Mental status and neurologic examination in the elderly. In W. R. Hazzard, J. P. Blass, J. B. Halter, J. G. Ouslander, & M. E. Tinetti (Eds.), *Principles of geriatric medicine and gerontology* (pp. 111–119). NY: McGraw-Hill. Evidence Level VI: Expert Opinion.

Park, H. L., O'Connell, J. E., & Thomson, R. G. (2003). A systematic review of cognitive decline in the general elderly population. *International Journal of Geriatric Psychiatry, 18*(12), 1121–1134. Evidence Level I: Meta-analysis.

Prestwood, K. M., & Duque, G. (2003). Osteoporosis. In W. R. Hazzard, J. P. Blass, J. B. Halter, J. G. Ouslander, & M. E. Tinetti (Eds.), *Principles of geriatric medicine and gerontology* (pp. 973–986). NY: McGraw-Hill.

Regev, A., & Schiff, E. R. (2001). Liver disease in the elderly. *Gastroenterology Clinics of North America, 30*, 547–563.

Ritchie, C. S. (2002). Oral health, taste, and olfaction. *Clinics in Geriatric Medicine, 18*, 709–717.

Robbins, S., Waked, E., & Krouglicof, N. (1998). Improving balance. *Journal of the American Geriatrics Society, 46*(11), 1363–1370. Evidence Level II: Single Experimental Study.

Roberts, S. B., & Dallal, G. E. (2005). Energy requirements and aging. *Public Health Nutrition, 8*(7A), 1028–1036. Evidence Level I: Meta-analysis.

Ross, S. O., & Forsmark, C. E. (2001). Pancreatic and biliary disorders in the elderly. *Gastroenterology Clinics of North America, 30*, 531–545.

Roubenoff, R., & Hughes, V. A. (2000). Sarcopenia: Current concepts. *Journal of Gerontology: Medical Sciences, 55A*, M716–M724.

Sacks, F. M., Svetkey, L. P., Vollmer, W. M., Appel, L. J., Bray, G. A., Harsha, D., et al. (2001). Effects on blood pressure of reduced dietary sodium and the Dietary Approaches to Stop Hypertension (DASH) diet. *New England Journal of Medicine, 344*, 3–10. Evidence Level II: Single Experimental Study.

Saksena, S., & Reddy, V. J. (2003). Cardiac arrhythmias in elderly people: Advances in diagnosis and management. In W. R. Hazzard, J. P. Blass, J. B. Halter, J. G. Ouslander, & M. E. Tinetti (Eds.), *Principles of geriatric medicine and gerontology* (pp. 475–490). NY: McGraw-Hill. Evidence Level V: Literature Review.

Santinga, J. (2003). Valvular heart disease. In W. R. Hazzard, J. P. Blass, J. B. Halter, J. G. Ouslander, & M. E. Tinetti (Eds.), *Principles of geriatric medicine and gerontology* (pp. 445–452). NY: McGraw-Hill.

Schiller, L. R. (2001). Constipation and fecal incontinence in the elderly. *Gastroenterology Clinics of North America, 30*, 497–515.

Schnelle, J. F., Alessi, C.A., Simmons, S. F., Al-Samarrai, N. R., Beck, J. C., & Ouslander, J. G. (2002). Translating clinical research into practice: A randomized controlled trial of exercise and incontinence care with nursing-home residents. *Journal American Geriatrics Society, 50*, 1476–1483. Evidence Level II: Single Experimental Study.

Schretzman, D., & Strumpf, N. E. (2002). Principles guiding care of older adults. In V. T. Cotter & N. E. Strumpf (Eds.), *Advanced practice nursing with older adults: Clinical guidelines* (pp. 5–25). NY: McGraw-Hill. Evidence Level VI: Expert Opinion.

Seidel, H. M., Ball, J. W., Dains, J. E., & Benedict, G. W. (2003). *Mosby's guide to physical examination*. St. Louis, MO: Mosby, Inc. Evidence Level VI: Expert Opinion.

Shaker, R., & Staff, D. (2001). Esophageal disorders in the elderly. *Gastroenterology Clinics of North America, 30*, 335–361. Evidence Level V: Literature Review.

Simmons, S. F., Alessi, C., & Schnelle, J. F. (2001). An intervention to increase fluid intake in nursing-home residents: Prompting and preference compliance. *Journal American Geriatrics Society, 49*, 926–933. Evidence Level II: Single Experimental Study.

Simon, L. S. (2005). *Osteoporosis. Clinics in Geriatric Medicine, 21*, 603–629.

Smith, H. A., & Connolly, M. J. (2003). Evaluation and treatment of dysphagia following stroke. *Topics in Geriatric Rehabilitation, 19*, 43–59. Evidence Level V: Literature Review.

Stern, M. (2006). Neurogenic bowel and bladder in the older adult. *Clinics in Geriatric Medicine, 22*, 311–330. Evidence Level V: Literature Review.

Stewart, R. (2004). Review: In older people, decline of cognitive function is more likely than improvement, but rate of change is very variable. *Evidence-Based Mental Health, 7*(3), 92.

Sudarsky, L. (2001). Gait disorders: Prevalence, morbidity, and etiology. *Advances in Neurology, 87*, 111–117.

Suhayda, R., & Walton, J. C. (2002). Preventing and managing dehydration. *Medsurg Nursing, 11*, 267–278. Evidence Level V: Literature Review.

Taffet, G. E., & Lakatta, E. G. (2003). Aging of the cardiovascular system. In W. R. Hazzard, J. P. Blass, J. B. Halter, J. G. Ouslander, & M. E. Tinetti (Eds.), *Principles of geriatric medicine and gerontology* (pp. 403–421). NY: McGraw-Hill. Evidence Level VI: Expert Opinion.

Takahashi, P. Y., Okhravi, H. R., Lim, L. S., & Kasten, M. J. (2004). Preventive health care in the elderly population: A guide for practicing physicians. *Mayo Clinic Proceedings, 79*, 416–427. Evidence Level V: Literature Review.

Tariq, S. (2004). Geriatric fecal incontinence. *Clinics in Geriatric Medicine, 20*, 571–587. Evidence Level V: Literature Review.

Tully, K. C. (2002). Cardiovascular disease in older adults. In V. T. Cotter & N. E. Strumpf (Eds.), *Advanced practice nursing with older adults: Clinical guidelines* (pp. 29–65). NY: McGraw-Hill.

U.S. Department of Health and Human Services (2000). Healthy People 2010. Retrieved February 12, 2007, from http://www.health.gov/healthypeople. Evidence Level I: Systematic Review.

U.S. Department of Health and Human Services (2004a). Bone health and osteoporosis: A report of the Surgeon General. Retrieved February 13, 2007, from http://www.surgeongeneral.gov/library/bonehealth. Evidence Level I: Systematic Review.

U.S. Department of Health and Human Services (2004b). The health consequences of smoking: A report of the Surgeon General. Retrieved April 13, 2007, from http://www.cdc.gov/tobacco/data`statistics/sgr/sgr`2004. Evidence Level I: Systematic Review.

U.S. Department of Health and Human Services (2005). Dietary guidelines for Americans. Retrieved April 13, 2007, from http://www.healthierus.gov/dietaryguidelines. Evidence Level I: Systematic Review.

U.S. Preventive Services Task Force (1996). Guide to clinical preventive services: Report of the U.S. Preventive Services Task Force. Baltimore, MD: Williams & Wilkins. Evidence Level I: Systematic Review.

U.S. Preventive Services Task Force (2002). Guide to clinical preventive services: Report of the U.S. Preventive Services Task Force. Retrieved January 23, 2007, from http://www.ahrq.gov/uspstfix.htm. Evidence Level I: Systematic Review.

Wang, E. (2003). Genetics of age-dependent human diseases. In W. R. Hazzard, J. P. Blass, J. B. Halter, J. G. Ouslander, & M. E. Tinetti (Eds.), *Principles of geriatric medicine and gerontology* (pp. 17–33). NY: McGraw-Hill.

Watters, J. M. (2002). Surgery in the elderly. *Canadian Journal of Surgery, 45*, 104–108. Evidence Level V: Literature Review.

Wiggins, J. (2003). Changes in renal function. In W. R. Hazzard, J. P. Blass, J. B. Halter, J. G. Ouslander, & M. E. Tinetti (Eds.), *Principles of geriatric medicine and gerontology* (pp. 543–549). NY: McGraw-Hill. Evidence Level VI: Expert Opinion.

Zeleznik, J. (2003). Normative aging of the respiratory system. *Clinics in Geriatric Medicine, 19*, 1–18. Evidence Level V: Literature Review.

Excessive Sleepiness

20

Eileen R. Chasens
Laura L. Williams
Mary Grace Umlauf

Educational Objectives

On completion of this chapter, the reader should be able to:

1. identify the signs and symptoms of excessive sleepiness and quantify them using a standardized scale
2. describe the signs, symptoms, and usual treatments for the most primary sleep disorders causing excessive sleepiness in older adults: obstructive sleep apnea, restless leg syndrome, and insomnia
3. discuss the implications of chronic illness and medications on sleep
4. plan appropriate sleep hygiene interventions for the patient with excessive sleepiness
5. provide nursing care that incorporates sleep hygiene measures and provides consistent ongoing treatment for existing sleep disorders
6. educate patients and families about sleep disorders and sleep hygiene measures

Excessive sleepiness, sometimes called excessive daytime sleepiness, is common in the elderly. Distinct from fatigue, which manifests as difficulty in sustaining a high level of performance, excessive sleepiness refers to the inability to maintain alertness, with characteristic hypersomnolence. Causes for excessive sleepiness include age-related changes in chronobiology and sleep disorders, as well as other medical and psychological disorders, medications, environmental factors, and lifestyle factors. In older adults, the most common primary sleep

For a description of Evidence Levels cited in this chapter, see chapter 1, Developing and Evaluating Clinical Practice Guidelines, page 4.

disorders are obstructive sleep apnea (OSA), restless leg syndrome, and insomnia. The extent to which changes in sleep patterns experienced by older adults are due to normal physiological alterations, pathological events, sleep disorders, or poor sleep hygiene remains unclear. The cause of excessive sleepiness may also be a chronic health condition that interferes with sleep quality or quantity. Thus, the problem of excessive sleepiness can be more complicated than a straightforward diagnosis and treatment. There are many effective treatments for sleep disorders, but the first step is to identify the cause of excessive daytime sleepiness and to quantify and aggressively treat this condition in the older adult. The primary purpose of this chapter is to provide a brief summary of sleep disorders common in older adults because many practicing nurses have no background in the science of sleep (see Box 20.1 for clinical practice protocol).

Daytime sleepiness is viewed as normal or unpreventable behavior in older adults. This misperception prevents many older adults from seeking medical attention and also reduces the likelihood that health care providers will evaluate, treat, or refer patients who present with clear symptoms of excessive sleepiness. However, this symptom should not be dismissed as an insignificant condition. Additionally, the disorder underlying the excessive sleepiness can have significant health effects. OSA, for example, is associated with cardiovascular disease and diabetes. The Sleep Heart Health Study showed that mild to moderate sleep-disordered breathing is associated with cardiovascular disease (Newman et al., 2000 [Level III]; Nieto et al., 2000 [Level III]) and reduced vitality, and severe sleep-disordered breathing is more broadly associated with poorer quality of life (Baldwin et al., 2001 [Level III]). In addition, car crashes (George, 2001 [Level III]) and falls (Brassington, King, & Bliwise, 2000 [Level III]) are some of the obvious consequences of sleepiness. Further, in acute care settings, the care of patients with excessive sleepiness become more complicated when either the underlying causes of sleepiness are not yet diagnosed or the plan of care does not reflect maintenance of ongoing treatments for excessive sleepiness.

Background

The Institute of Medicine (IOM) (Colten & Altevogt, 2006) reports that 50 million to 70 million Americans are affected by chronic disorders of sleep and wakefulness. These conditions are among the most common health problems, yet health care providers frequently overlook them. The combined effects of undiagnosed and untreated sleep disorders along with sleep deprivation constitute an unmet public health problem. For example, according to the 2002 "Sleep in America" survey (National Sleep Foundation, 2002 [Level III]), 27% of Americans categorize their sleep as fair or poor. Of the 1,010 subjects polled, 37% reported symptoms of sleepiness (i.e., 7% daily or almost daily; 9%, a few days a week; and 20%, a few days a month). However, far fewer of those surveyed had been diagnosed with the most common causes of sleepiness, such as insomnia (6%), sleep apnea (4%), or restless legs syndrome (4%), and even fewer had been treated for these conditions (4%, 2%, and 1%, respectively). The Cardiovascular Health Study documented excessive sleepiness in 20% of 4,578 subjects older than age 65 (Whitney et al., 1998 [Level III]). It is not surprising that excessive daytime sleepiness and sleep disorders are more common in patients in acute- and chronic-care settings. For example, among persons older than 65, Ancoli-Israel and colleagues (1991 [Level IV], 1987 [Level IV]) found undiagnosed OSA in 24% of those living independently, in 33% of those in acute care settings, and in 42% of older adults in nursing home settings.

Consequences of Excessive Sleepiness

The primary consequences of sleepiness are decreased alertness, delayed reaction time, and reduced cognitive performance. Decreased reaction time and lack of sustained attention can contribute to accidental and work-related injuries. For example, approximately 56,000 car crashes per year are attributed to falling asleep at the wheel (Knipling & Wang, 1994 [Level IV]). Furthermore, the effects of sleepiness can be long-lasting. Recent studies show that daytime sleepiness is significantly associated with declining cognitive function (Cohen-Zion et al., 2001 [Level III]), falls (Brassington et al., 2000 [Level III]), and cardiovascular events (Whitney et al., 1998 [Level III]). In the Cardiovascular Health Study, daytime sleepiness was the only sleep symptom associated with mortality, incident cardiovascular disease morbidity and mortality, myocardial infarction, and congestive heart failure, particularly among women (Newman et al., 2000 [Level III]). Thus, sleep loss or sleep disorders may play a part in accidental or workplace injury, cardiovascular morbidity, or cognitive impairment among older adults with excessive sleepiness.

Physiological Changes in Sleep That Accompany Aging

Normal changes in sleep that occur as part of human development should be differentiated from pathological sleep conditions that increase in prevalence with aging. Although older adults require as much sleep as younger adults, older adults may divide their sleep between nighttime slumber and daytime naps, rather than a single consolidated period at night. The endogenous circadian pacemaker located in the suprachiasmatic nucleus, along with exogenous environmental cues and a homeostatic need for sleep, mediate the normal wake and sleep pattern. With aging, the circadian pattern for sleep–wake decreases in amplitude, possibly in association with less robust changes in core body temperature (Richardson, Carskadon, & Orav, 1982). Compared with younger adults, healthy older adults have a more pronounced biphasic pattern of sleepiness during the afternoon hours (about 2 p.m. to 6 p.m.) and a phase advancement of nighttime sleepiness earlier in the evening (Roehrs, Turner, & Roth, 2000 [Level IV]).

Changes in sleep architecture associated with normal aging include an increase in transient arousals, an increase in time until sleep onset as well as stage 1 sleep, and a decrease in the quantity and amplitude of restorative slow-wave sleep (stages 3 and 4). Although older women report more sleep disturbances than older men; studies indicate that their sleep is less disturbed than that of men (Rediehs, Reis, & Creason, 1990 [Level I]).

Primary Causes of Excessive Daytime Sleepiness

Obstructive Sleep Apnea

OSA is a condition in which intermittent pharyngeal obstruction causes cessation of respiratory airflow (for at least 10 seconds) and often oxygen desaturation. This results in an arousal that restores upper-airway patency, permitting breathing and airflow to resume. According to the American Academy of Sleep Medicine Task Force (1999 [Level I]), OSA is diagnosed when these events occur at a rate of greater than five per hour of sleep and is accompanied by snoring, gasping, daytime sleepiness, and impaired daytime functioning. However, it is common for patients with severe symptoms to experience multiple arousals during the night, which severely fragmented sleep, preventing the deep sleep (stages 3 and 4) and rapid eye movement (REM) sleep necessary for healthy mental and physical functioning.

OSA is both an age-related and an age-dependent condition, with an overlap in both distributions in the 60- to 70-year-old age range (Bliwise, King, & Harris, 1994). Age-related risk factors for OSA in older adults include an increased prevalence of overweight and obesity; age-dependent risk factors with old age are increased collapsibility of the upper airway, decreased lung capacity, altered ventilatory control, decreased muscular endurance, and altered sleep architecture (Brassington et al., 2000 [Level III]).

Treatments for sleep apnea depend on the contributing pathology and patient preference and include nocturnal positive airway pressure, surgical procedures (i.e., palatoplasty to reduce airway encroachment), and other techniques designed to increase the posterior pharyngeal area, oral appliances, and weight reduction when obesity is a contributing factor. Nasal continuous positive airway pressure (CPAP) therapy is currently the "gold standard" for treating OSA and is highly effective when individually titrated to eliminate apneas and hypopneas (Morgenthaler et al., 2006 [Level I]). Older adults tolerate CPAP therapy, with patterns of compliance similar to that of middle-aged adults (Weaver & Chasens, 2007 [Level I]).

Insomnia

Insomnia can be defined as delayed sleep onset, premature waking, and/or very early arousals that result in nonrestorative sleep (Ancoli-Israel & Ayalon, 2006 [Level I]). Although it remains unclear whether insomnia is an organic, psychological, pharmacological, chronobiological or behavioral problem and is associated with cardiovascular, respiratory, gastrointestinal, renal, and musculoskeletal disorders. Insomnia can be transient or chronic, and the perception of sleep duration may not correspond to objective assessment. The frequent awakenings suggestive of insomnia may be a conditioned arousal response due to environmental (e.g., noise or extremes of temperature) or behavioral cues. Anxiety associated with emotional conflict, stress, recent loss, feeling insecure at night, or change in living arrangements can also produce insomnia (Ancoli-Israel & Ayalon, 2006 [Level I]). The general anxiety and conditioned arousal response at sleep onset associated with insomnia may prompt frequent use of hypnotic medication, a common treatment for insomnia. Although the use of hypnotics may produce temporary symptom relief, they also affect sleep architecture and consequently lead to deterioration in the quality of sleep. A cycle of dependency and abuse can occur and is a potential problem in this age group (see chapter 12, *Reducing Adverse Drug Events*).

Research has shown the negative effects of continued hypnotic use in the elderly; however, recent data suggest otherwise. Avidan et al. (2005 [Level I]) examined the effects of hypnotic use and insomnia as predictors of falls in the elderly in more than 34,000 residents of Michigan nursing homes. They found that insomnia was a predictor of falls but hypnotic use was not a significant indicator. Thus, there is an ongoing debate regarding insomnia, the use of hypnotics, and falls among nursing home residents. At this time, the general recommendation is that when hypnotics are indicated that the most short-acting drug should be selected and, optimally, used in conjunction with an appropriate behavioral intervention (Ancoli-Israel, 2000 [Level I]).

The cause and duration of insomnia should be the primary determinant of the most appropriate treatment. For example, insomnia associated with a psychological origin, such as depression or anxiety, is best treated from that perspective. If pain is affecting sleep adjustment, pain medication should be attempted first and strategies to promote sleep onset should be added to the pain-management plan. If insomnia is of recent onset, then short-term pharmacotherapy is suitable for transient symptoms. Where insomnia is "learned" and this maladaptation interferes with the initiation of sleep, behavioral interventions are most appropriate. The American Academy of Sleep Medicine has published a comprehensive review of nonpharmacologic treatments used for chronic insomnia (Morin et al., 1999 [Level I]). Their findings indicate that 70% to 80% of patients benefit from behavioral therapies and that improvement in sleep is sustained for a minimum of 6 months after treatment. The three treatments that meet the American Psychological Association criteria for empirically supported effectiveness for insomnia are stimulus control, progressive muscle relaxation, and paradoxical intention. In addition, sleep restriction, biofeedback, and multifaceted cognitive-behavior therapy meet their criteria for "probable" effectiveness.

Restless Legs Syndrome

Restless legs syndrome is a disorder characterized by an almost irresistible urge to move the limbs, usually associated with disagreeable leg sensations that are worse during inactivity and often interferes with initiating and maintaining sleep. As a secondary condition, this movement disorder can be caused by iron-deficiency anemia, uremia, neurological lesions, diabetes, Parkinson's disease, or rheumatoid arthritis, or it can be a side effect of certain drugs (e.g., tricyclic antidepressants, serotonin reuptake inhibitors, lithium, dopamine blockers, xanthines). Periodic leg movement disorder is a similar chronic condition also known as *nocturnal myoclonus*. This condition is characterized by involuntary flexion of the leg and foot that produces micro-arousals or full arousals from sleep, which fragment sleep and interfere with achieving and maintaining restorative slow-wave sleep (i.e., stages 3 and 4). Although the etiology and associated mechanism of this specific movement disorder are not well defined, these movements have been linked to metabolic, vascular, and neurologic

20.1   The Epworth Sleepiness Scale

Instructions to the patient: The following questionnaire will help you measure your general level of daytime sleepiness. It asks you to rate the likelihood that you will doze off or fall asleep during various routine daytime situations. How likely are you to doze off or fall asleep in the following situations, in contrast to just feeling tired? Even if you haven't done some of these things recently, think about how they would have affected you.

Use the following scale to choose the most appropriate number for each situation:

    0 = would never doze
    1 = slight chance of dozing
    2 = moderate chance of dozing
    3 = high chance of dozing

Situation	Circle your score for each item			
Sitting and reading	0	1	2	3
Watching television	0	1	2	3
Sitting inactive in a public place, for example, a theater or meeting	0	1	2	3
Riding as a passenger in a car for an hour without a break	0	1	2	3
Lying down to rest in the afternoon	0	1	2	3
Sitting and talking to someone	0	1	2	3
Sitting quietly after lunch (when you've had no alcohol)	0	1	2	3
In a car, while stopped in traffic	0	1	2	3

Score Results:

1–6	Getting enough sleep
7–8	Tends to be sleepy but is average
9–16	Very sleepy and should seek medical advice
≥ 17	Dangerously sleepy

Printed with permission: Johns, M. W. (1991). A new method for measuring daytime sleepiness: The Epworth Sleepiness Scale. *Sleep, 14,* 540–545.

causes. Dopaminergic drugs are the most effective agents for treating restless legs syndrome and periodic leg movement disorder. Other drugs, including opioids, benzodiazepines, anticonvulsants, adrenergics, and iron supplements, are also used to treat these disorders. However, their efficacy for long-term treatment in older adults has not been sufficiently evaluated (Ancoli-Israel & Ayalon, 2006 [Level I]; Gamaldo & Earley, 2006 [Level I]).

Secondary Causes of Excessive Daytime Sleepiness

Medical and psychiatric illness can also disturb sleep or interfere with sleep quality and quantity. For example, psychiatric illnesses such as depression or anxiety can cause insomnia. Also, painful chronic conditions, such as arthritis, reduce sleep efficiency by causing the elder to wake frequently due to the pain caused by simply changing body position during sleep. Likewise, because older adults frequently have multiple medical conditions, they are also more likely to take over-the-counter (OTC) and prescription medications to manage their symptoms. However, many medications and nonprescription drugs (e.g., pseudoephedrine, alcohol, caffeine, and nicotine) interfere with sleep. Thus, health care providers must be acutely aware of the role that illness and OTC medications may play in contributing to sleep disturbances. Both symptom management and prevention of polypharmacy are important aspects of care of older adults to protect and promote sleep in this high risk group (Ancoli-Israel, 2005 [Level I]).

Assessment of Excessive Sleepiness

Several valid and reliable measures are useful to screen for sleepiness. One of the most commonly used instruments is the Epworth Sleepiness Scale (Table 20.1) (Johns, 1991 [Level IV]), which has been widely disseminated on the Internet in recent years. The likelihood of having OSA can be determined using the Multivariable Apnea Prediction Index (Maislin et al., 1995 [Level IV]). The Functional Outcomes of Sleep Questionnaire (Weaver et al., 1997 [Level IV]) evaluates the impact of daytime sleepiness on functional status, and the Pittsburgh Sleep Quality Scale (Buysse, Reynolds, Monk, Berman, & Kupfer, 1989 [Level IV]) quantifies sleep quality over the past month (see Sleep topic at www.ConsultGeriRN.org). Because it is so readily available, many sleep clinicians use the Epworth Sleepiness Scale to track sleepiness over the previous week that may occur during common activities, such as sitting and reading, watching TV, or riding in a car. It is easy to administer and to score, and it has scoring parameters to indicate when sleepiness clearly warrants a more complete evaluation by a sleep specialist. A brief sleep history can be obtained by using the questionnaire in Table 20.2. Table 20.3 presents the criteria for grading the severity of sleepiness developed by the American Academy of Sleep Medicine Task Force (1999 [Level I]). In a sleep laboratory, quantitation of sleep parameters is done using polysomnography. Additional electrophysiological tests, such as the Multiple Sleep Latency Test, are also used to assess daytime sleepiness. Most important in the assessment of sleepiness is an evaluation of

20.2 Sleep History

Basic Sleep History Questions	Follow-Up Questions	Sleep Disorders to Consider
■ Do you have any difficulty falling asleep? ■ Are you having any difficulty sleeping until morning? ■ Are you having difficulty sleeping throughout the night? ■ Have you or anyone else ever noticed that you snore loudly or stop breathing in your sleep? ■ Do you find yourself falling asleep during the day when you don't want to?	■ What time do you usually go to bed? ■ Fall asleep? ■ What prevents you from falling asleep? ■ Review intake of alcohol, nicotine, caffeine, all medications. ■ Review of depressive symptoms; weight loss, sadness, or recent losses. ■ How often do you waken? ■ How long are you awake? ■ Do you have any pain, discomfort, or shortness of breath during the night? ■ What prevents you from falling back to sleep? ■ Are you sleepy or tired during the day? ■ Review risk factors (e.g., obesity, arthritis, poorly controlled illnesses). ■ If you laugh or get angry, do you feel weak (as if you might fall down or drop what you are holding)? ■ Do your legs kick or jump around while you sleep?	■ Shift work/sleep schedule disorders ■ Psychophysiologic insomnia ■ Restless legs syndrome ■ Psychiatric disorders ■ Substance/medications- related disorders ■ Depression ■ Insomnia ■ Medical causes of sleep disturbance ■ Obstructive sleep apnea ■ Functional impairment resulting from sleep disorder ■ Narcolepsy ■ Periodic leg movement disorders

Source: Adapted from Avidan (2005) and National Center on Sleep Disorders Research Working Group (1999).

the patient's knowledge and application of sleep-hygiene measures (Table 20.4) to complement clinical findings and as simple behavioral strategies to consolidate sleep, as well as to promote and protect sleep.

Interventions and Care Strategies

The first line of defense against excessive sleepiness is a lifestyle that promotes and ensures adequate sleep and rest. Although there is a natural drive to sleep, environment and habituation—that is, sleep hygiene—plays an important part in

20.3 Severity Criteria for Sleepiness

Mild	Episodes of unwanted sleepiness or involuntary sleep occur only during activities that require little attention, such as watching television, reading, or traveling as a passenger in a moving vehicle.
Moderate	Episodes of unwanted sleepiness or involuntary sleep occur during activities that require some attention.
	Sleepiness causes moderate impairment of social and occupational function.
	Occurs during activities such as attendance at concerts, presentations, and meetings.
Severe	Episodes of unwanted sleepiness or involuntary sleep occur when more active attention is required, such as while eating, walking, standing, driving, or even during conversations or sex.
	Sleepiness markedly impairs social and occupational function.

Source: Adapted from American Academy of Sleep Medicine Task Force, 1999.

20.4 Sleep Hygiene Measures

- Use the bed only for sleeping or sex.
- Develop consistent and rest-promoting bedtime routines.
- Maintain the same bedtime and waking time every day.
- Exposure to bright sunlight is desirable upon awakening but should be avoided just before bedtime.
- Upon awakening, get out of bed slowly, no matter what time it is, to prevent postural hypotension.
- If awakened during the night, avoid looking at the clock; frequent time checks may heighten anxiety and hinder sleep onset.
- Avoid naps entirely or limit naps to 10 to 15 minutes' duration.
- Sleep in a cool, quiet environment.
- If you cannot fall asleep after 15 or 20 minutes in bed, get up and go into another room, read, or do a quiet activity, using dim lighting, until you are sleepy again. (Avoid watching television because it emits a bright light.)
- Sleeping alone is more restful than sleeping with another person or pets. If pets or bed partners add to the problem, move to the couch for a couple of nights, and restrict pets from sharing the bed.
- Before bedtime, avoid the following:
  - caffeine and nicotine after noon
  - alcohol intake (more than 3 drinks)
  - large meals or exercise 3 to 4 hours before bedtime
  - emotional upset or emotionally charged activities

being able to obtain quality sleep. Sleep hygiene has many components and each bears review and reinforcement over time. Regardless of health status, sleep-hygiene measures are as important for older adults as they are for children, adolescents, and other adults.

It bears repeating that excessive daytime sleepiness is only the general symptom of a more specific problem. Consequently, individualized plans of care must include treatment of known sleep disorders, and nurses in acute care settings must be able to identify sleep disorders in their patients. Sleep disorders are not just bothersome, they can complicate care and pose important risks if they are not diagnosed and treated.

Case Study and Discussion

Scenario

Mrs. M. complained to her friends that her husband snores "loud enough to wake the dead" and "stops breathing for maybe 30 seconds or so," which keeps her awake at night. She relates that they "don't have sex very often," he had difficulty with "doing it," they are both too tired to be "in the mood," and she has started sleeping in another room. Her friends have urged her to have her husband report the history and symptoms to his primary-care physician.

History

Mr. M. is a 62-year-old man who is obese (height, 6'2"; weight, 260 lbs.; BMI, 33.4). He is hypertensive (sitting blood pressure, 154/98 mm Hg) and takes several medications to control his blood pressure (i.e., amlodipine, digoxin, hydrochlorothiazide, lisinopril, pravastatin, enteric-coated aspirin). He was diagnosed with Type II diabetes almost 10 years ago (HgbA1c, 8.2%) and is on metformin 1,000 mg BID and glimepiride 2 mg daily.

Symptoms

Mr. M. says, "I have no energy. I can sleep anytime and anywhere, but I am tired all the time. I went to the Diabetic Educator and learned what I need to do with exercise and diet but, usually, I am so tired I just grab some fast food and want to sit down and do nothing when I get home." He reports that he wakes unrefreshed, has morning headaches, and that his sleep is disturbed by nocturia four times per night. He also says that he has heartburn at night and his legs jerk during sleep. He says that he has loss of energy, has difficulty staying awake, has difficulty in driving long distances because of extreme sleepiness, and cannot attend church or movies without falling asleep. He also takes frequent naps, consumes more than six cups of coffee per day, and drinks one or two alcoholic beverage in the evenings before bedtime. He has a history of snoring (more than 20 years) and was a smoker until 12 years ago.

20.5	Results of Overnight Polysomnography		
Total recording time	368 min	REM sleep	0
Total sleep time	256 min	Stage 1 sleep	92%
Sleep efficiency	70%	Stage 2 sleep	8%
Lowest O_2 saturation	65%	Stages 3 & 4 sleep	0
Apnea/Hypopnea Index	56/hour of sleep	Longest apnea	39 sec

Assessment

The patient has severe daytime excessive sleepiness and symptoms of OSA. Sleep hygiene habits are poor. He self-medicates with caffeine as a daytime stimulant and uses alcohol as a hypnotic. He is obese, and obesity is a prime risk factor for both OSA and Type II diabetes. Although nocturia can result from an osmotic diuresis secondary to a blood glucose that is higher then the renal threshold of 180 mg/dL, it is also an important symptom of undiagnosed and untreated OSA. Clearly, this patient is a driving risk, even during daylight hours. Although depression can cause sleep disruption, this patient's medical history and symptoms are compelling indicators of excessive sleepiness and warrant a referral to a sleep specialist for evaluation and treatment.

Interventions

The immediate intervention was referral to a sleep specialist, who ordered an overnight polysomnography to assess for OSA (Table 20.5). Intermediate interventions include a referral to the dietician for assistance in maintaining his diabetic diet and weight loss, instruction on sleep-hygiene measures, avoidance of sedating OTC drugs (i.e., alcohol), which can exacerbate OSA symptoms, and avoidance of driving long distances, especially alone or at night, until treatment of OSA has begun. If the patient does go on to receive treatment by positive airway pressure and is compliant, he may be more successful at weight loss, which can improve hypertension and glucose control. In addition, effective treatment of OSA often improves nighttime symptoms of nocturia.

Diagnosis

Severe Obstructive Sleep Apnea.

Treatment

Due to the obstructive character of the patient's sleep-related breathing disorder, continuous positive airway pressure (CPAP) at 14 cm water pressure.

Outcome

Six months after starting CPAP: Mr. M. has lost 30 lbs and his CPAP pressures and antihypertensive medications already have been titrated downward. His blood pressure has dropped to 132/88 mm Hg, his HgbA1c has improved (7.6%), and he seldom has nocturia or takes naps. The patient reduced his caffeine intake to one or two cups of coffee per day and stopped using OTC products or alcohol as a sleeping aid. He no longer feels tired and has driven his car on several car trips without feeling sleepy. Mr. M. also states that he has started to walk with his wife for 30 minutes at least four times a week. He reports, "I did not know how tired I was until I started on this breathing machine at night. I will admit, a few nights I haven't used it. But, the next day, I always know that I made a mistake by skipping the night before."

Summary

Nurses must be able to identify, screen, and refer patients for sleep disorders. Nurses see patients sleep more than other health care providers do, and sleep disorders can affect patient outcomes on a daily basis. Sleep medicine is a relatively new specialty and many health care providers have had no background in sleep disorders. Nurses also must incorporate sleep-hygiene measures and ongoing treatment of existing sleep disorders into the plan of care for older adults to ensure adequate, restful sleep in all settings: acute care, primary care, and at home. Failing to identify, diagnose, or treat excessive sleepiness and its underlying cause(s) can adversely affect the health and longevity of older adults.

Web Resources for Nurses and Consumers

Sleep Disorders and Sleep Deprivation: An Unmet Public Health Problem

This report was issued by the Institute of Medicine in April 2006 to increase public and health-professional awareness of the personal and economic consequences of sleep disorders and sleep loss. It is a valuable resource for understanding the current status of the science of sleep and sleep research. The report outlines the impact of sleep loss in America and provides recommendations to improve the recognition and treatment of sleep disorders. This publication is available online from National Academies Press at http://www.nap.edu/catalog/11617.html.

National Institutes of Health, National Center on Sleep Disorders Research

This site includes brochures that may be downloaded or printed for distribution to patients or for the education of other health care providers.

For patients and the general public: http://www.nhlbi.nih.gov/health/public/sleep/index.htm

For health care professionals: http://www.nhlbi.nih.gov/health/prof/sleep/index.htm

Sleep Research Society

This professional organization fosters scientific investigation, professional education, and career development in sleep research and academic sleep medicine. It is an excellent resource for nurses who are interested in studying issues of sleep and circadian processes.
http://www.sleepresearchsociety.org/

Society for Research on Biological Rhythms

This is a professional group formed to promote the advancement of basic and applied research in all aspects of biological rhythms and to disseminate the important results of that research among scientists, agencies that fund research, and the general public.
http://www.srbr.org/

American Academy of Sleep Medicine (AASM)

This organization for sleep professionals is also a great source of information for the public and for practice guidelines for professionals.
http://www.aasmnet.org/

Narcolepsy Network

The primary focus of this national nonprofit, patient-support organization is to improve the lives of those with the lifelong neurological sleep disorder narcolepsy.
http://www.narcolepsynetwork.org

Restless Legs Syndrome Foundation

This organization is dedicated to improving the lives of the men, women, and children who live with this often-devastating disease. The organization's goals are to increase awareness of RLS, to improve treatments, and, through research, to find a cure.
http://www.rls.org

Basics of Sleep Guide

This Sleep Research Society publication is designed for students, sleep researchers and non-sleep professionals interested in studying sleep across the life cycle, sleep deprivation/restriction, and sleep physiology. Information about this publication and how to order it can be found on the *Sleep Research Society* Web site.
http://www.sleepresearchsociety.org/AnnouncementDetails.aspx?id=14

New Abstracts and Papers in Sleep

This free online subscription service is an excellent resource for professionals to find the most recent research on sleep disorders and their treatments on a regular basis. Services include weekly personalized e-mail alerts of new citations, author abstracts, a compilation of the current week's literature in sleep, an archive of the current year's literature in sleep, search-and-retrieval capabilities customized for sleep, computer-generated reprint request forms, and notification of topical information pertaining to particular areas of interest.

http://www.websciences.org/bibliosleep/NAPS/

Box 20.1

Nursing Standard of Practice Protocol: Excessive Sleepiness

I. GOAL: Older adults will maintain an optimal state of alertness while awake and optimal quality and quantity of sleep during their preferred sleep interval.

II. BACKGROUND

A. Definition

Excessive sleepiness: somnolence, hypersomnia, excessive daytime sleepiness, subjective sleepiness. Sleepiness is a ubiquitous phenomenon, experienced not only as a symptom in a number of medical, psychiatric, and primary sleep disorders but also as a normal physiological state by most individuals over any given 24-hour period. Pathology is inferred both when its presence becomes pervasive (as in narcolepsy) or in its absence (as in insomnia). Alternatively, sleepiness can be considered abnormal when it occurs at inappropriate times or does not occur when desired (Shen, Barbera, & Shapiro, 2006).

III. ETIOLOGY AND EPIDEMIOLOGY

A. Excessive sleepiness may be due to difficulty initiating sleep, impaired sleep maintenance, waking prematurely and not being able to return to sleep, or sleep fragmentation.

B. There are many types of sleep diagnoses; the most common disorders reported by older adults are obstructive sleep apnea, insomnia, and restless legs syndrome.

C. Many sleep disorders share excessive sleepiness as a common symptom, but this symptom is often not evaluated or treated because health care providers are uninformed about the nature of sleep disorders, the symptoms of these disorders, and the many effective treatments available for these conditions.

IV. PARAMETERS OF ASSESSMENT

A. A sleep history (see Table 20.2) should include information from both the patient and family members. People who share living and sleeping spaces can provide important information about sleep behavior that the patient may not be able to convey.

B. The Epworth Sleepiness Scale (Johns, 1991 [Level IV]; Avidan, 2005 [Level I]; National Center on Sleep Disorders Work Group, 1999 [Level VI]) (Table 20.1) is a brief instrument to screen for severity of daytime sleepiness in the community setting. It can also be found under Resources at http://www.ConsultGeriRN.org.

C. Table 20.3 outlines key points in obtaining salient information from older patients and their family members as well as gauging severity of symptoms (American Academy of Sleep Medicine Task Force, 1999 [Level I]).

D. The Pittsburgh Sleep Quality Index (Buysse et al., 1989 [Level IV]) is useful to screen for sleep problems in the home environment and to monitor changes in sleep quality. This instrument can be found under Resources at http://www.ConsultGeriRN.org.

V. NURSING CARE STRATEGIES

A. Vigilance by nursing staff in observing patients for snoring, apneas during sleep, excessive leg movements during sleep, and difficulty staying awake during normal daytime activities (Ancoli-Israel & Ayalon, 2006 [Level I]; Avidan, 2005 [Level I]).

B. Management of medical conditions, psychological disorders, and symptoms that interfere with sleep, such as depression, pain, hot flashes, anemia, or uremia (Ancoli-Israel & Ayalon, 2006 [Level I]; Avidan, 2005 [Level I]).

C. For patients with a current diagnosis of a sleep disorder, ongoing treatments such as CPAP should be documented, maintained, and reinforced through patient and family education (Avidan, 2005 [Level I]). Nursing staff should reinforce patient instruction in cleaning and maintaining positive airway pressure equipment and masks.

D. Instruction for patients and families regarding sleep-hygiene techniques to protect and promote sleep among all family members (see Table 20.4) (Avidan, 2005 [Level I]).

E. Review and, if necessary, adjustment of medications that interact with one another or whose side effects include drowsiness or sleep impairment (Ancoli-Israel & Ayalon, 2006 [Level I]).

F. Referral to a sleep specialist for moderate or severe sleepiness or a clinical profile consistent with major sleep disorders such as obstructive sleep apnea or restless legs syndrome (Avidan, 2005 [Level I]).

G. Aggressive planning, monitoring, and management of patients with obstructive sleep apnea when sedative medications or anesthesia are given (Avidan, 2005 [Level I]).

H. Ongoing assessment of adherence to prescriptions for sleep hygiene, medications, and devices to support respiration during sleep (Avidan, 2005 [Level I]).

VI. EVALUATION AND EXPECTED OUTCOMES

A. Quality Assurance Actions
   1. Provide staff education on the major causes of excessive sleepiness (i.e., obstructive sleep apnea, insomnia, restless legs syndrome).
   2. Provide staff with in-services on how to use and monitor CPAP equipment.
   3. Have individual nursing units conduct environmental surveys regarding noise level during the night hours and then develop strategies to reduce sleep disruption due to noise and care patterns.
   4. Add sleep as a parameter of the admission assessment for patients and provide written instructions for patients using CPAP at home to always bring the equipment with them to the hospital. Include sleep quality (e.g., see PSQI tool, www.ConsultGeriRN.org.)
   5. Include sleep quality (e.g., Pittsburgh Sleep Quality Index) (Buysse et al., 1989) to posthospital surveys of patient satisfaction and provide feedback for nursing staff (see www.ConsultGeriRN.org, Sleep topic).
B. Quality Outcomes: Improved quality and/or quantity of sleep during normal sleep intervals as reported by patients and staff.

VII. FOLLOW-UP MONITORING

A. Depending on the diagnosis, follow-up may include long-term reinforcement of the original interventions along with support for adhering to treatments prescribed by a sleep specialist. For example, patient compliance with CPAP therapy for OSA is critical to its efficacy and should be assessed during the first week of treatment (Weaver et al., 1997 [Level IV]). All patients benefit from positive reinforcement while trying to acclimate to nightly use of a positive airway pressure device.
B. CPAP masks may require minor adjustments or refitting to find the most comfortable fit. Most such changes are needed during the acclimation period, but patients should be encouraged to seek assistance if mask problems develop (Weaver et al., 1997 [Level IV]). In the acute care setting, respiratory-care technicians are valuable in-house resources when staff from a sleep center are not readily available.
C. During the initial treatment phase of insomnia, sleep deprivation may cause rebound sleepiness, which should subside over time. Follow-up should include ongoing assessment of napping habits and sleepiness to track treatment effectiveness (Avidan, 2005 [Level I]).
D. If obesity has been a complicating health factor, weight loss is a desirable long-term goal. With reduction in daytime sleepiness, the timing is ripe for increasing the activity level. Treatment of sleep disorders should include planning for strategic changes in lifestyle that include regular exercise, which is also consistent with cardiovascular health and long-term diabetes control (Ancoli-Israel & Ayalon, 2006 [Level I]; Avidan, 2005 [Level I]).

References

American Academy of Sleep Medicine Task Force (1999). Sleep-related breathing disorders in adults: Recommendations for syndrome definition and measurement techniques in clinical research. *Sleep*, *22*(5), 667–689. Evidence Level I: Systematic Review.

Ancoli-Israel, S. (2000). Insomnia in the elderly: A review for the primary care practitioner. *Sleep*, *23* (Suppl. 1), S23–S30; discussion S26–S28. Evidence Level I: Systematic Review.

Ancoli-Israel, S. (2005). Sleep and aging: Prevalence of disturbed sleep and treatment considerations in older adults. *Journal of Clinical Psychiatry*, *66* (Suppl. 9), 24–30. Evidence Level I: Systematic Review.

Ancoli-Israel, S., & Ayalon L. (2006). Diagnosis and treatment of sleep disorders in older adults. *American Journal of Geriatric Psychiatry*, *14*(2), 95–103. Evidence Level I: Systematic Review.

Ancoli-Israel, S., & Kripke, D. F. (1991). Prevalent sleep problems in the aged. *Biofeedback & Self Regulation*, *16*(4), 349–359. Evidence Level IV: Nonexperimental Study.

Ancoli-Israel, S., Kripke, D. F., & Mason, W. (1987). Characteristics of obstructive and central sleep apnea in the elderly: An interim report. *Biological Psychiatry*, *22*(6), 741–750. Evidence Level IV: Nonexperimental Study.

Avidan, A. Y. (2005). Sleep disorders in the older patient. *Primary Care: Clinics in Office Practice*, *32*(2), 563–586. Evidence Level I: Systematic Review.

Avidan, A. Y, Fries, B. E., James, M. L., Szafara, K. L., Wright, G. T., & Chervin, R. D. (2005). Insomnia and hypnotic use, recorded in the minimum data set, as predictors of falls and hip fractures in Michigan nursing homes. *Journal of the American Geriatric Society*, *53*(6), 955–962. Evidence Level I: Systematic Review.

Baldwin, C. M., Griffith, K. A., Nieto, F. J., O'Connor, G. T., Walsleben, J. A., & Redline, S. (2001). The association of sleep-disordered breathing and sleep symptoms with quality of life in the Sleep Heart Health Study. *Sleep*, *24*(1), 96–105. Level of Evidence III: Quasi-experimental Study.

Bliwise, D. L., King, A. C., & Harris, R. B. (1994). Habitual sleep durations and health in a 50- to 65-year-old population. *Journal of Clinical Epidemiology*, *47*(1), 35–41.

Brassington, G. S., King, A. C., & Bliwise, D. L. (2000). Sleep problems as a risk factor for falls in a sample of community-dwelling adults aged 64-99 years. *Journal of the American Geriatrics Society*, *48*(10), 1234–1240. Evidence Level III: Quasi-experimental Study.

Buysse, D. J., Reynolds, C. F., Monk, T. H., Berman, S. R., & Kupfer, D. J. (1989). The Pittsburgh Sleep Quality Index: A new instrument for psychiatric practice and research. *Psychiatry Research*, *28*(2), 193–213. Evidence Level IV: Nonexperimental Study.

Cohen-Zion, M., Stepnowsky, C., Marler, S.T., Shochat, T., Kripke, D. F., & Ancoli-Israel, S. (2001). Changes in cognitive function associated with sleep-disordered breathing in older people. *Journal of the American Geriatrics Society*, *49*(12), 1622–1627. Evidence Level III: Quasi-Experimental Study.

Colten, H. R., & Altevogt, B. M. (Eds). (2006). *Sleep disorders and sleep deprivation: An unmet public health problem*. Institute of Medicine, Committee on Sleep Medicine and Research. Washington, DC: The National Academies Press.

Gamaldo, C. E., & Earley, C. J. (2006). Restless legs syndrome: A clinical update. *Chest*, *130*(5), 1596–1604. Evidence Level I: Systematic Review.

George, C. F. (2001). Reduction in motor vehicle collisions following treatment of sleep apnea with nasal CPAP. *Thorax*, *56*(7), 508–512. Evidence Level III: Quasi-experimental Study.

Johns, M. W. (1991). A new method for measuring daytime sleepiness: The Epworth sleepiness scale. *Sleep*, *14*, 540–545.

Knipling, R. R., & Wang, J. S. (1994). *Crashes and fatalities related to driver drowsiness/fatigue*. Research Note: National Highway Traffic Safety Administration, U.S. Department of Transportation. Evidence Level IV: Nonexperimental Study.

Maislin, G., Pack, A. I., Kribbs, N. B., Smith, P. L., Schwartz, A. R., Kline, L. R., et al. (1995). A survey screen for prediction of apnea. *Sleep*, *18*(3), 158–166. Evidence Level IV: Nonexperimental Study.

Morgenthaler, T. I., Kapen, S., Lee-Chiong, T., Alessi, C., Boehlecke, B., Brown, T., et al. (2006). Practice parameters for the medical therapy of obstructive sleep apnea. *Sleep*, *29*(8), 1031–1035. Evidence Level IV: Systematic Review.

Morin, C. M., Hauri, P. J., Espie, C. A., Spielman, A. J., Buysse, D. J., & Bootzin, R. R. (1999). Nonpharmacologic treatment of chronic insomnia. *An American Academy of Sleep Medicine Review*. *Sleep*, *22*, 1134–1156. Evidence Level I: Systematic Review.

National Center on Sleep Disorders Research Working Group (1999). Recognizing problem sleepiness in your patients. *American Family Physician*, *59*(4), 937–944. Evidence Level VI: Expert Opinion.

National Sleep Foundation (2002). *Sleep in America Poll*. Washington, DC.

Newman, A. B., Spiekerman, C. F., Enright, P., Lefkowitz, D., Manolio, T., Reynolds, C. F., et al. (2000). Daytime sleepiness predicts mortality and cardiovascular disease in older adults. The Cardiovascular Health Study Research Group. *Journal of the American Geriatrics Society*, *48*(2), 115–123. Evidence Level III: Quasi-experimental Study.

Nieto, F. J., Young, T. B., Lind, B. K., Shahar, E., Samet, J. M., Redline, S., et al. (2000). Association of sleep-disordered breathing, sleep apnea, and hypertension in a large community-based study. *JAMA*, *283*(14), 1829–1836. Evidence Level III: Quasi-experimental Study.

Rediehs, M. H., Reis, J. S., & Creason, N. S. (1990). Sleep in old age: Focus on gender differences. *Sleep*, *13*, 410–424. Evidence Level I: Systematic Review.

Richardson, G. S., Carskadon, M. A., & Orav, E. J. (1982). Circadian variation of sleep tendency in elderly and young adult subjects. *Sleep*, *5*, S82–S94.

Roehrs, T., Turner, L., & Roth, T. (2000). Effects of sleep loss on waking actigraphy. *Sleep*, *23*(6), 793–797. Evidence Level IV: Nonexperimental Study.

Shen, J., Barbera, J., & Shapiro, C.M. (2006). Distinguishing sleepiness and fatigue: Focus on definition and measurement. *Sleep Medicine Reviews*, *10*(1), 63–76.

Weaver, T. E., & Chasens, E. R. (2007). Continuous Positive Airway Pressure and Sleep Apnea in Older Adults *(in press, Sleep Medicine Review)*. Evidence Level I: Systematic Review.

Weaver, T. E., Chugh, D. K., Maislin, G., Schwab, R. J., George, C. F. P., Kader, G. A., et al. (1997). Impact of obstructive sleep apnea on the conduct of daily activities. *Sleep Research*, *26*, 530. Evidence Level IV: Nonexperimental Study.

Whitney, C. W., Enright, P. L., Newman, A. B., Bonekat, W., Foley, D., & Quan, S. F. (1998). Correlates of daytime sleepiness in 4,578 elderly persons: The Cardiovascular Health Study. *Sleep*, *21*(1), 27–36. Evidence Level III: Quasi-experimental Study.

Sensory Changes

21

Pamela Z. Cacchione

Educational Objectives

At the completion of this chapter, the reader will be able to:

1. describe the normal changes of aging that affect the senses in older adults

2. identify common sensory disorders that impact the senses in older adults

3. determine how best to assess sensory status in older adults

4. identify nursing strategies to manage sensory impairment in older adults

5. recognize interprofessional team members who can assist older adults with sensory impairment

Background and Statement of Problem

Individuals interact with their environment through their senses. Vision, hearing, smell, taste, and peripheral sensation allow us to experience the world around us. As people age, they often experience changes in their sensory function (i.e., vision, hearing, smell, taste, and peripheral sensation). These sensory changes can negatively impact older adults' ability to interact with their environment, decreasing their quality of life. For example, changes in hearing can impact an older person's communication skills; changes in vision can impact the ability to take medications safely. Healthy People 2010 stresses the importance

For a description of Evidence Levels cited in this chapter, see chapter 1,
Developing and Evaluating Clinical Practice Guidelines, page 4.

of vision and hearing ability as essential to language, whether spoken, signed, or read (USDHHS, 2000 [Level VI]). Decreases in sense of smell can interfere with an older adult's ability to smell smoke in a fire or recognize spoiled food. Many adults report a decrease in taste that impacts their desire to eat. Decreased peripheral sensation sets up an individual for falls.

Understanding how to assess the senses as well as manage sensory deficits is essential to holistic nursing. A goal of Healthy People 2010 is to improve the visual and hearing health of the nation through prevention, early detection, treatment, and rehabilitation (USDHHS, 2000 [Level VI]). This chapter on sensory changes addresses common changes with the senses that occur with advancing age, as well as disease states and injuries to the senses that occur more commonly with aging. Nursing care related to the Healthy People 2010 goals regarding sensory changes are also addressed.

Normal Changes of Aging Senses

Almost all the senses change with aging, usually presenting with a slowing of function. Table 21.1 describes the changes that occur and the functional outcomes for each sense.

Vision

There are several changes that occur with vision as people age. The eyelids start to lag, the pupil takes longer to dilate and contract, and presbyopia is widespread.

Presbyopia

A loss of elasticity in the lens of the eye leads to a decrease in the eyes' ability to change the shape of the lens to focus on near objects, such as fine print, and a decrease in the ability to adapt to light (Warnat & Tabloski, 2006; Whiteside, Wallhagen, & Pettengill, 2006 [both Level VI]).

Hearing

Normal changes of aging impacting hearing include the decrease in function of the hair fibers in the ear canal that normally aid in the natural removal of cerumen and the protection of the ear canal from external elements.

Presbycusis

Presbycusis is the most common form of hearing loss in the United States (Bagai, Thavendiranathan, & Detsky, 2006 [Level I]). This high-frequency sensorineural hearing loss is a multifactorial process that varies in severity and is associated with aging (Gates & Mills, 2005 [Level V]). Presbycusis usually has a bilateral progressive onset and is due to gradual loss of hair cells and fibrous changes in the small blood vessels that supply the cochlea. Presenting symptoms are difficulty hearing high-pitched sounds such as *t, s, z, sh, and ch* (Wallhagen,

21.1   Normal Changes of Aging

Sense	Change of Aging	Functional Outcome
Vision	■ Decreased dark adaptation	■ Increased safety risk in changing environmental light
	■ Decreased upward gaze	■ Decreased field of vision
	■ Eyes become drier and produce fewer tears	■ Dry irritated eyes
	■ Cornea becomes less sensitive	■ Slow to recognize injury to the cornea
	■ Pupils decrease in size	■ Inability to adjust to glare and change in lighting conditions
	■ Visual fields become smaller	■ Safety risk for driving and maneuvering in the environment
Hearing	■ Eardrum thickens	■ Thickened eardrum decreases sound moving across the ear canal
	■ Loss of high frequency hearing acuity	■ Decreased ability to hear sounds such as *p, w, f, sh,* and women's and children's voices
	■ Decreased ability to process sounds after age 50	■ Requires more time to process and respond to auditory stimuli
	■ Increased cerumen impactions	■ Decreased hearing due to blockage of sound
Smell	■ Decreased ability to identify odors	■ Inability to identify spoiled food or smoke
	■ Impacts ability to taste	■ Limits enjoyment in eating
Taste	■ Decreased number of tastebuds	■ Decreased sensitivity to flavors
	■ Limited decrease in taste supported by studies	
	■ Less saliva production	■ Dry mouth affecting ability to swallow
Sensation	■ Decreased vibratory sense	■ Increases risk for injury
	■ Decreased two-point discrimination	■ Decreased ability to sense pressure
	■ Decreased temperature sensitivity	■ Decreased protective response to withdraw from hot objects
	■ Decreased balance	■ Risk of falls
	■ Decreased Proprioception	■ Risk of falls
	■ Changed pain sensation	■ Decreased protective mechanism

Source: Adapted from Bromley, 2000 [Level VI]; Linton, 2007 [Level V]; Murphy et al., 2002 [Level III]; Schiffman, 1997 [Level V]; Seilberling & Conley, 2004 [Level V]; Wallhagen et al., 2006 [Level VI]; Whiteside et al., 2006 [Level V].

Pettengill, & Whiteside, 2006 [Level VI]). Background noise further aggravates this hearing deficit.

Smell

Changes in smell are common as people age but are not considered a normal part of aging. Changes in the sense of smell have been found to correlate with neurological conditions such as Parkinson's disease and Alzheimer's disease (Albers, Tabert, & Devanand, 2006 [Level I]; Hummel & Nordin, 2003 [Level VI]; Wilson, Arnold, Schneider, Tang, & Bennett, 2007 [Level II]).

Taste

Common changes in taste include a decreased ability to detect the intensity of tastes, when compared to younger adults (Schiffman, 1997 [Level V]). However, changes in taste are more often related to dental concerns and medications.

Peripheral Sensation

Peripheral nerve function that controls the sense of touch declines slightly with age. Two-point discrimination and vibratory sense both decrease with age. The ability to perceive painful stimuli is preserved in aging. However, there may be a slowed reaction time for pulling away from painful stimuli with aging (Linton, 2007 [Level V]).

Epidemiology of Sensory Impairment in Older Adults

Vision

The prevalence of visual impairment increases with age and the settings in which older adults live. Older adults comprise 12.8% of the U.S. populationbut account for 30% of all visually impaired individuals (Desai, Pratt, Lentzer, & Robinson, 2001 [Level V]). Of adults older than the age of 70, 19% are visually impaired (Desai et al., 2001 [Level V]). Studies evaluating older adults in long term care settings demonstrate a prevalence rate of visual impairment of 40% to 54% (Bron & Caird, 1997 [Level VI]; Cacchione, Culp, Dyck, & Laing, 2002 [Level III]). More than 90% of older adults report that they wear eyeglasses (Campbell, Crews, Moriarty, Zack, & Blackman, 1999 [Level II]). Uncorrected refractive error was also found to be common in visually impaired older adults. Of the 8.8% of the older adults found to be visually impaired, 59% of those were impaired due to an uncorrected refractive error (Vitale, Cotch, & Sperduto, 2006 [Level III]). Leading causes of visual impairment include cataracts, macular degeneration, and glaucoma (Congdon et al., 2004 [Level III]). Cataracts, one of the leading causes of blindness, are the fifth most common chronic condition in adults older than 75 (NAAS, 1999 [Level II]). The definition of visual impairment varies by different groups and by country (AHRQ, 2004 [Level VI]). The United States defines low vision as best corrected visual acuity:

- Normal vision: visual acuity of 20/20 or better
- Mild vision impairment: 20/25 to 20/50

21.2   Vision History Questions

- When was your last eye exam?
- How would you describe your eyesight?
- Any change in your eyesight?
- When did you notice this change?
- Are you experiencing any blurred vision?
- Are you having any double vision?
- Are you bothered by glare?
- Are you experiencing any eye pain?
- Are you using any eye drops for any reason?
- Any history of trauma or injury to your eyes?
- Have you had any eye surgeries?
- Do you have cataracts?
- Any family history of eye problems?

Source: Adapted from Cacchione, 2007, and Whiteside et al., 2006 [both Level VI].

- Moderate visual impairment: 20/60 to 20/160
- Severe visual impairment (legally blind): 20/200 to 20/400
- Profound vision impairment: 20/400 to 20/1000
- Near-total vision loss: less than or equal to 20/1250
- Total blindness: no light perception (AHRQ, 2004)

Low vision can also be defined based on visual-field limitations. Severe visual impairment is defined as best corrected field less than or equal to 20 degrees (i.e., legal blindness). Profound visual impairment is defined as visual field less than or equal to 10 degrees (AHRQ, 2004 [Level VI]).

Nursing Assessment of Vision

The health history is an essential part of vision assessment. Several health conditions predispose older adults to visual impairment. Diabetes is one of the leading causes of disease-related blindness related to diabetic retinopathy (Baker, 2003 [Level I]; Munoz et al., 2000 [Level II]; Tielsch, Sommer, Witt, Katz, & Royall, 1990 [Level II]). Hypertension carries with it the risk of hypertensive retinopathy. Ascertaining a thorough baseline health history with yearly reviews and updates is essential in maintaining visual health. Health questions related to visual health are detailed in Table 21.2 (Cacchione, 2007; Whiteside, Wallhagen & Pettengill, 2006 [both Level VI]).

Examination of the Eye

The external structures can cause decreased vision if the lids lag due to laxity of the skin of the upper eyelid. Lid lag can interfere with visual acuity and fields and may require surgery. Cataracts in severe cases can be visible with the naked eye and appear as a whitish-gray pupil instead of black. Cloudiness of the whole cornea of the eye is indicative of a corneal problem, not a cataract. If the person has had cataract surgery, the lens implant may be visible on close inspection.

Fundus Exam. Using an ophthalmoscope, a nurse can visualize the red reflex and, with experience and practice, the fundus of the eye. This is often difficult with small pupils. Darkening the room may help to dilate the pupils. Optometrists and ophthalmologists dilate the pupils to allow for a better view of the fundus. Cataracts will appear as dark shadows in the anterior portion of the lens in front of the retina.

Vision Testing. Vision testing should be completed before the eyes are dilated and completed with both uncorrected and corrected (i.e., with glasses) vision.

Distance Vision. The "gold standard" in eye charts, the Snellen Chart, is one of the most commonly used to assess distance vision. Visual acuity is tested at 20 feet. The individual is asked to read the letters on the chart until they miss more than two on a line of acuity. Acuity equals the line above the line with more than two errors. Acuity measures range from 20/10 to 20/800 on the Snellen Chart.

ETDRS. The Early Treatment of Diabetic Retinopathy Study (ETDRS) (Ferris, Kassoff, Bresnick, & Bailey, 1982 [Level III]) eye chart is also used frequently and can be used at a distance of 4 meters. At this distance, the greatest visual acuity measured is 20/200—the equivalent of legal blindness.

Pin-Hole Test. With best vision with or without glasses, a card with a small pin hole in the center is placed in front of the eye, and the vision is tested at the last line that the individual is able to read. If individuals can read farther down the chart with the pin hole, their vision may be improved with better refraction of their eyeglasses or, if they do not have glasses, with eyeglasses.

Near Vision. Near vision is important for health literacy, especially in regard to reading food or medication labels. There are several ways to assess near vision. Two commonly used tools are the Rosenbaum Pocket Eye Screener and the Lighthouse for the Blind Near Vision Screener. The Rosenbaum Pocket Eye Screener, a non-copyrighted tool based on the Snellen test, can be useful in assessing near vision in acute- and primary-care settings. It is true to scale when compared with the Snellen Chart at the 20/200, 20/400, and 20/800 acuity levels. However, the other levels are slightly too large, causing an overestimation of visual acuity (Horton & Jones, 1997 [Level VI]).

Light House for the Blind Near Vision Screener (Light House for the Blind): This handheld vision screener has a cord that can be used at 40 and 20 centimeters to measure the proper distance for testing near vision. This near-vision screener mimics the ETDRS eye chart in a smaller version but is not pocket size. It does not, however, have the questions about matching scale of the ETDRS distance acuity level. For research purposes, it has the added feature of the cord for measuring a consistent distance.

Contrast Sensitivity. Contrast sensitivity is often compromised by aging and diseases or conditions of the eye. Decreases in contrast sensitivity occur with cataracts, glaucoma, and retinopathies (Mantyjarvi & Laitinen, 2001; Wilensky & Hawkins, 2001 [both Level III]). Contrast sensitivity provides information on how well an individual may perform in real-life conditions. Decline in contrast sensitivity impacts the ability to distinguish when one step ends and another begins, identify light switches on the wall, read materials not printed in high contrast font, and identify the buttons on the remote control. Intact contrast sensitivity is important for day-to-day functioning within the environment.

The Pelli–Robson Contrast Sensitivity Chart (Pelli, Robson, & Wilkins, 1988 [Level III]) is read at the 1- or 3-meter distance. All letters are presented at the 20/200 acuity level but in decreasing shades of black to gray. The Pelli–Robson Contrast Sensitivity Chart is widely used in practice and works well for older adults who are experienced in recognizing letters (Hirvela, Koskela, & Laatikainen, 1995 [Level III]; Morse & Rosenthal, 1997 [Level VI]).

The Vistech Contrast Sensitivity Test, another contrast sensitivity measure, has four patches of gray circles with lines in different directions (Kennedy & Dunlap, 1990 [Level II]). The person being examined points to the direction the lines within the circle are pointed (Morse & Rosenthal, 1997 [Level VI]).

Visual Fields. Fields of vision refers to the area of peripheral vision visible when an individual is focusing straight ahead (Cassin, 2001 [Level IV]). The vision in visual fields can be affected by many eye conditions, as well as neurological disorders that inhibit eye movement or affect the blood supply to the optic nerve. Intact visual fields are important to function safely in the environment. In assessing visual fields by confrontation, a gross clinical measure of visual fields, the examiner faces the patient and determines if the patient can identify the examiner's moving fingers as they are moving into their field of view (Seidel, Dains, Ball, & Benedict, 2003 [Level IV]). Although subjective and dependent on the examiner having normal fields of vision, the confrontation test is useful in quickly identifying large losses in visual fields.

The Humphrey Visual Field Test is completed by an ophthalmologist and assesses visual fields using a static type of perimetry (Gianutsos & Suchoff, 1997 [Level VI]). This measure provides a more reliable measure of functional visual fields. The Goldman VI4e kinetic perimetry visual field testing, on the other hand, assesses kinetic type of functional visual fields (Gillmore, 2002 [Level VI]). Kinetic perimetry entails the introduction of a moving stimulus moving from a nonvisible area toward the fixed point of view. The Goldman perimeter visual field testing is difficult to standardize because it is operator-dependent (Gillmore, 2002 [Level VI]); therefore, automated methods are more widely used. The location of the visual field deficit may clue the examiner as to the type of eye condition. For example, unilateral visual field deficits may be related to a cerebral vascular accident, glaucoma affects the peripheral fields, and macular degeneration has associated central field of vision loss.

Conditions of the Eye

Diseases That Alter Vision Seen More Frequently as People Age

Cataracts. Clouding of the crystalline lens that presents as a painless, progressive loss of vision can be unilateral or bilateral (NIA, 2005 [Level VI]). Cataracts can be hereditary, injury-related, or related to medications. The management of cataracts includes early identification and monitoring followed by surgical extraction and lens implantation once vision is affected.

Macular Degeneration. The development of drusen deposits in the retinal pigmented epithelium is the leading cause of central vision loss and legal blindness in older adults. Macular degeneration is more common in fair-haired, blue-eyed individuals. Other risk factors include smoking and excessive sunlight exposure. There are wet and dry forms of macular degeneration. The wet form is more easily treated than the dry form. Newer treatments of expensive injectable medications are available to slow the progression of dry macular degeneration.

Glaucoma. Glaucoma is a progressive, serious form of eye disease. Primary Open Angle Glaucoma is the most common form (Linton, 2007 [Level V]). Increased intraocular pressure causes atrophy and cupping of the optic nerve head, leading to visual field deficits that can progress to blindness. Vision changes include loss of peripheral vision, intolerance to glare, decreased perception of contrast, and decreased ability to adapt to the dark.

Diabetic Retinopathy. This results from end-organ damage from diabetes causing retinopathy and spotty vision. Risk can be reduced by strict blood-sugar control. Almost 6% of diabetics aged 65 to 74 develop diabetic retinopathy (NEI, 2004 [Level VI]). Diabetic retinopathy that starts as nonproliferative and progresses to proliferative should be treated with laser photocoagulation.

Hypertensive Retinopathy. This is caused by end-organ damage from poorly controlled hypertension causing background and eventual proliferative retinopathy. Hypertensive retinopathy is usually treated with laser photocoagulation and strict blood pressure control.

Temporal Arteritis. This is an autoimmune disorder that causes inflammation of the temporal artery, also known as giant cell arteritis. It presents as malaise, scalp tenderness, unilateral temporal headache, jaw claudication, and sudden vision loss (usually unilateral). This vision loss is a medical emergency but is potentially reversible if identified immediately. If symptoms develop, an individual should see an ophthalmologist or go immediately to the emergency room.

Detached Retina. This is a condition that can occur in patients with cataracts or recent cataract surgery, trauma, or spontaneously. A detached retina presents as a curtain coming down across a patient's line of vision. An individual experiencing this should see an ophthalmologist or immediately go to the emergency room. Table 21.3 lists the implications of vision changes on an older adult's function.

Nursing-Care Strategies

Vision

Nurses should obtain a past medical history to avoid disruption in the management of chronic eye conditions, assuring continuation of ongoing regimens

21.3	Implications of Vision Changes in Older Adults

Impact on Safety
Inability to read medication labels
Difficulty navigating stairs or curbs
Difficulty driving
Difficulty crossing streets

Impact on Quality of Life
Reduces ability to remain independent
Difficulty or unable to read
Falls

such as eye drops for glaucoma. Without the continuation of an individual's eye drops, eye pressures could precipitously increase causing an acute exacerbation of the glaucoma, potentially dramatically limiting vision. If an acute change in an individual's vision occurs, the primary-care provider should be notified immediately. Depending on the signs and symptoms present, the individual may need to see an ophthalmologist or go to the emergency room to receive treatment to restore the vision or limit the deterioration.

Lighting is important in an individual's environment. Too little light can limit vision. Too much light, depending on an individual's eye condition such as cataracts, may cause eye pain and glare. It is important to ascertain whether an individual is sensitive to light. If so, indirect light and night lights may be helpful to provide a safe environment. The majority of older adults benefit from improved lighting. To avoid glare, directing incandescent lamps directly on a task, such as sewing or reading, often improves visual acuity and is well tolerated. Glare occurs when a light shines directly into the eye or reflects off a shiny surface. Low-vision specialists recommend trying different positions and wattage of lighting to find what works best for each individual (Community Services for the Blind and Partially Sighted, 2004 [Level VI]).

Encourage the use of the person's eyeglasses. Older adults' eyeglasses should be labeled with their name so they can be reconnected to their owner if they are set down and left behind. Even with eyeglasses, magnification may be helpful. Have family provide lighted magnification if needed (large lighted magnifiers are available at low-vision centers).

Contrast sensitivity is a problem with several eye conditions, including cataracts, glaucoma, and macular degeneration. Adding contrast to the fixtures in the home if light switches blend into the wall or faucets blend into the sink can create a safer and more functional environment.

Nurses should encourage an annual dilated-eye examination with either an optometrist or an ophthalmologist. This is crucial in people who have a diagnosis of diabetes or hypertension. Nurses are members of the interprofessional team responsible for preventing unnecessary disability. Therefore, nurses should ensure that there is a mechanism in place to trigger these visits on an annual basis.

Hearing Impairment

Hearing impairment is the third leading chronic condition affecting adults older than 75 (NAAS, 1999 [Level I]). More than 50% of adults older than 75 are hearing impaired. For older adults in nursing homes, the estimates run as high as 90% (Lewis-Culinan & Janken, 1990 [Level II]; Newman, 1990 [Level III]). Hearing loss is greater in men than women (NIDCD, 2007 [Level VI]). The American Academy of Audiology defines hearing loss based on decibels or loudness and the Hertz or the pitch of sound. Normal speech is in the 0 to 25 dB level and mild hearing loss is defined as hearing in the 25- to 40-dB level. Hearing between 40 and 70 dBs is considered moderate hearing loss; severe hearing loss is between 70 and 90 dBs. Greater than 90 dBs is considered profound hearing loss (Mehr, 2007 [Level IV]). Aging impairs hearing of the sounds in the higher frequencies or pitch, which are often more difficult to hear.

Assessment of Hearing

It is easy to determine when older adults are hard of hearing just from having a conversation with them. The older adult may lean closer in an attempt to hear better, turn their head to their "good ear," or cup their hand behind their ear. Older adults may have to ask for things to be repeated, and often have trouble hearing their grandchildren's or other's high-pitched voices. Older adults often complain that people are mumbling. Any or all of these signs may be present. Regardless of whether any of these signs are present, all older adults should have their hearing screened annually at their primary-care visit (Bagai et al., 2006 [Level I]). Methods of screening are described herein.

Hearing Handicap for the Elderly-Screen

The Hearing Handicap for the Elderly- Screen (HHIE-S) (Ventry & Weinstein, 1983 [Level III]) is a 10-item scale to determine how hearing impacts an older adult's daily life and to assist in identifying who might benefit from a hearing aid and an audiologic referral. The scale takes approximately 5 minutes to complete and is targeted for community-dwelling older adults. This scale is available online through the Hartford Institute for Geriatric Nursing *Try This Best Practices in Care for Older Adults* (Demers, 2001 [Level V]) (access at www.ConsultGeriRN.org). The HHIE-S has reported excellent sensitivity and specificity for severe hearing loss, but the sensitivity and specificity decreases as the level of hearing impairment lessens (Sindhusake et al., 2001 [Level II]).

Whisper Test

The whisper test involves covering or rubbing one ear canal and, from a distance of 2 feet, whispering a three-syllable word on an exhale that the patient either correctly or incorrectly repeats back. An incorrect response triggers a repeat attempt to see if the older adult can identify a different three-syllable word. The consistency of the level of the whispered word makes this test difficult to compare among examiners. However, despite this difficulty, it has been found to be a valid and reliable test to screen for hearing loss (Pirozzo, Papinczak, & Glasziou, 2003 [Level I]).

Finger-Rubbing Test

The finger-rubbing test is less dependent on volume of the whispered three-syllable word. It entails having the examiner rub the thumb and first two fingers together, starting at 2 inches from the patient's ear, and then slowly moving the fingers away from the ear. The patient reports when they can no longer hear the fingers rubbing together on each side. The sensitivity and specificity has been reported as 80% and 49%, respectively, at 6 to 8 in, and 90% sensitivity and 85% specificity at 3 inches (Patterson, 1994 [Level V]).

Handheld Audioscope

The handheld audioscope is a device developed to specifically screen for hearing impairment. It has a test tone that is presented at the 60-dB level. The decibel levels that may be tested include the 20-, 25-, and 40-dB levels at the 500-, 1,000-, 2,000-, and 4,000-Hz levels. The audioscope has an otoscope that allows for the visualization of the tympanic membrane or cerumen impactions, which can result in conductive hearing loss present in up to 30% of older adults (Lewis-Culinan & Janken, 1990 [Level II]). Testing using the audioscope should be performed in a quiet setting and may not be as useful in the long term care environment with high noise levels.

Pure Tone Audiometry

This is the "gold standard" of hearing testing, particularly if completed in a soundproof booth with 92% sensitivity and 94% specificity in detecting sensorineural hearing loss (Frank & Petersen, 1987 [Level II]). Pure tone audiometry allows for testing of a wide range of decibels and Hertz levels, or loudness and pitch or frequencies, allowing for testing at the 5- to 120-dB level and 250 to 4,000 Hz. Portable pure tone audiometers with noise-reduction earphones are available and can be used in the community, outpatient, and long term care settings when access to an audiologist is limited. The wide range of tones allows for a better understanding of an individual's functional hearing. Pure tone audiometry by an audiologist is the next step after screening identifies a hearing deficit (Yueh, Shapiro, MacLean, & Shekelle, 2003 [Level I]).

Tuning Fork Tests

Two tuning fork tests have been used in hearing screenings, although a recent systematic review discouraged their use because they were found to be unreliable with limited accuracy (Bagai et al., 2006 [Level I]). The tuning fork should be either 256 or 512 Hz (Wallhagen, et al., 2006 [Level VI]). The Rinne Test is meant to differentiate whether an older adult hears better by bone or air conduction and can help determine if an individual had sensorineural or conductive hearing loss. The Weber Test is used to help identify unilateral hearing loss.

Hearing Changes Common in Older Adults

Conductive hearing loss involves the outer and/or middle ear including the ear canal, tympanic membrane, and bones in the outer and middle ear (Marcincuk & Roland, 2002 [Level VI]). Causes of conductive hearing impairment include cerumen impactions or foreign bodies, ruptured eardrum, otitis media, and otosclerosis (Wallhagen et al., 2006 [Level VI]).

Sensorineural hearing loss, the most common form of hearing loss in older adults (Linton, 2007 [Level V]), involves damage to the inner ear, the cochlea, or the fibers of the eighth cranial nerve. Causes of sensorineural hearing loss include hereditary causes, viral or bacterial infections, trauma, tumors, noise exposure, cardiovascular conditions, ototoxic drugs, and Meniere's disease (Wallhagen et al., 2006 [Level VI]).

Central auditory processing disorder is an uncommon disorder that includes an inability to process incoming signals and is often found in stroke patients and older adults with neurological conditions such as Alzheimer's dementia and Parkinson's disease (Pekkonen et al., 1999 [Level II]). The person's hearing is intact but the ability to process the sound is impaired.

Tinnitis, which is otherwise known as ringing in the ear, is of two types: subjective and objective. Subjective tinnitus is a condition in which there is perceived sound in the absence of acoustic stimulus (Ahmad & Seidman, 2004 [Level VI]; Lockwood, Salvi, & Burkard, 2002 [Level V]). Objective tinnitus is considered rare and presents as ringing in the ear that is audible by the individual and others. It is thought to have a vascular or neurological condition or Eustachian-tube dysfunction (Crummer & Hassan, 2004 [Level VI]). Subjective ringing in the ears may fluctuate and can be due to damage to the hair receptors of the cochlear nerve and age-related changes in the organs of hearing and balance. Patients with tinnitis should be referred to an ear, nose, and throat (ENT) specialist.

Meniere's disease is characterized by fluctuating hearing loss, dizziness, vertigo, tinnitus, and a sensation of pressure in the affected ear (NIDCD, 2001 [Level VI]). Unfortunately, the fluctuating hearing loss can become permanent hearing loss over time. Possible causes of Meniere's disease include hypothyroidism, diabetes, and neurosyphillis.

Implications of Hearing Changes

Older adults who have hearing impairment experience a decreased quality of communication, social isolation, low self-esteem, and generally lower quality of life. Decreased hearing impacts an individual's word recognition, decreasing the ability to communicate. This in turn can lead to significant safety issues. For example, if patient education about medication administration is provided only verbally, key information can be misheard and misinterpreted. Difficulty understanding the spoken word can lead to fatigue and speech paucity of friends and loved ones.

Speech paucity is described as decreased attempts to have meaningful conversations due to the difficulty in getting the message through to a hearing-impaired loved one. Speech paucity (Wallhagen, 2006 [Level VI]) leads to social isolation of the hearing impaired because only the necessary information is transferred and no everyday social information is shared (Wallhagen,

Strawbridge, Shema, & Kaplan, 2004 [Level III]). This can lead to depression and low self-esteem in a hearing-impaired individual and the partner. Other factors that lead to social isolation in hearing-impaired older adults include the inability to hear the telephone or the doorbell ringing or knocking at the door.

Ideally, an older adult who develops hearing loss will see an audiologist and obtain unilateral or bilateral hearing aids to improve the ability to communicate with the people around them. Unfortunately, the stigma, cost, and delay in pursuing hearing aids are barriers to their success. Hearing aids should be pursued early in the course of hearing impairment. For example, hearing aids can be very helpful when hearing is impaired to the point that background noise interferes with understanding the spoken word. Success in using hearing aids at this level of hearing improves the chance that older adults will continue with hearing aids. Once older adults become used to the silence, it is difficult to adapt to the increased ambient noise heard with hearing aids. Often, older adults require extensive coaching from an audiologist to get through the transition phase of wearing hearing aids. Technology has improved to the point of analog hearing aids that can be finely tuned to the individual's needs (Wallhagen et al., 2006 [Level VI]). In one intervention group of older adults fitted with hearing aids, 98% experienced benefit and their caregivers perceived significant benefit as well (Tolson, Swan, & Knussen, 2002 [Level II]). University settings are often the most cost-effective locations to pursue hearing aids. The cost of hearing aids is an important factor because most insurance plans, including Medicare, do not cover hearing aids.

Cochlear implants are another technological advancement that has demonstrated positive outcomes in older adults in the areas of speech recognition. A cochlear implant works by bypassing the damaged parts of the ear and stimulating the auditory nerve. These impulses are sent to the brain through the auditory nerve and the brain recognizes them as sound (NIDCD, 2006 [Level VI]). Severe hearing impairment must be present unilaterally or bilaterally before this surgical intervention will be considered. Cochlear implants were found in one study to improve word recognition and health-related quality of life (Francis, Chee, Yeagle, Cheng, & Niparko, 2002 [Level III]). Despite these improvements, relatively few adults have received this new technology. According to the U.S. Food and Drug Administration, nearly 22,000 adults have received cochlear implants (NIDCD, 2006 [Level VI]). Technological advances will continue to improve the options for hearing-impaired older adults.

Smell and Taste

Smell and taste are two senses that are difficult to separate because they overlap, particularly when food is involved. Both these senses depend on *chemosensation*, the ability of the nose, mouth, and throat to identify tastes and smells based on chemical reactions that occur when odors or tastes are present in the environment (AAO-HNS, 2007 [Level VI]). The sense of smell and ability to identify odors decrease due to normal changes in aging. Up to 50% of octogenarians have smell disorders (Murphy et al., 2002 [Level III]). This can be problematic for safety reasons. An inability to smell smoke, for instance, could put an older adult at risk. Studies have also linked the loss of smell to Alzheimer's dementia and

Parkinson's disease (Mesholam, Moberg, Mahr, & Doty, 1998 [Level I]; Muller, Reichmann, Livermore, & Hummel, 2002 [Level II]).

Changes in Smell and Taste Common to Older Adults

There are four medical terms used when describing olfactory disorders: (1) *hyposmia* is the reduction of the sense of smell; (2) *parosmia* is the distortion in the sense of smelling the presence of an odor; (3) *anosmia* is no sense of smell; and (4) *phantosmia* is the perception of an odor when no odor source is present (Hummel & Nordin, 2003 [Level VI]). Olfactory disorders impact quality of life in older adults. Common complaints from people with olfactory disorders include difficulty with cooking, decreased appetite, eating spoiled food, too little perception of body odor, and inability to detect gas leaks or smoke (Miwa, et al., 2001 [Level II]; Temmel, Quint, Schickinger-Fischer, & Hummel, 2005 [Level III]).

Because of the impact on quality of life, it is important to take a complete history and physical with older adults, asking questions regarding the olfactory system. A thorough cranial nerve exam and head and neck examination should be included. If an olfactory disorder is identified, the individual should be referred to an otorhinolaryngologist (ENT) (Hummel & Nordin, 2005 [Level VI]).

Most changes in taste are thought to occur due to an oral condition, xerostomia (i.e., dry mouth), decreased sense of smell, medications, diseases, and tobacco use (Seiberling & Conley, 2004 [Level V]). Dysgeusias, or taste disorders, may resolve spontaneously. However, due to the poor outcomes for older adults with taste disorders, referral for treatment is indicated either to an otolaryngologist, neurologist, or subspecialist at a smell and taste center (Bromley, 2000 [Level VI]).

As with olfactory disorders, disorders of taste are often identified on history, not by physical exam. There are few tests to assess for taste disorders. Therefore, the history is essential. Substance abuse including tobacco, alcohol, and cocaine should be reviewed. The individual's dietary habits should be reviewed. Questions regarding recent dental work or procedures should also be asked. Ascertaining whether an individual has a history of gastric reflux could surface manageable conditions impacting taste. A thorough review of medications is fundamental in the evaluation of a taste disorder (Bromley, 2000 [Level V]).

Diseases That Alter Taste Seen More Frequently as People Age

Burning Mouth Syndrome

This is a sensation that the tongue is tingling or burning. There may be several contributing factors: Vitamin B deficiencies, local trauma, gastrointestinal disorders causing reflux, allergies, salivary dysfunction, and diabetes.

Xerostomia

Dry mouth is common with many medications used to treat disorders common to older adults, including anticholinergic medications, antidepressants, antihistamines, ACE-inhibitors, lipid-lowering agents, antiparkinsonian medications, and anticonvulsants to name a few (Bromley, 2000 [Level VI]; Seiberling & Conley, 2004 [Level V]).

Implications of Taste and Smell Changes

Inability to smell limits some of the pleasures of everyday life. The smell of a spring rain, a Christmas tree, flowers, or coffee brewing may not be detectable. Taste is diminished due to inability to smell. Of significant concern in older adults who have smell and taste disorders is malnutrition. Appetite is detrimentally affected due to inability to smell and taste the food. Inability to smell is a safety hazard due to the inability to smell smoke in a fire or a gas leak. Decreased sense of taste may also result in inability to recognize spoiled food, resulting in nausea, vomiting, or infectious diarrhea.

Peripheral Sensation

Peripheral neuropathy is one of the most common neurological disorders encountered in a general medical practice, with estimates of 2% to 7% of all patients having symptoms of neuropathy (Smith & Singleton, 2004 [Level II]). An assessment of 894 participants in the Women's Health and Aging Study indicated that 58% of women showed evidence of neuropathy by age 65 (Resnick, Vinik, Heimovitz, Brancati, & Guralnik, 2001 [Level II]).

Changes in peripheral sensation common to older adults

Diseases that alter peripheral sensation are seen more frequently as people age and include peripheral neuropathy, diabetic neuropathy, phantom limb pain, and acute sensory loss.

Peripheral neuropathy. This is nerve pain in the distal extremities related to nerve damage from circulatory problems or vitamin deficiencies. Common vitamin deficiencies that impact peripheral nerves include B_6, B_{12}, and folate.

Diabetic neuropathy. This is end-organ damage to the peripheral nerves from microvascular changes that occur with diabetes. It often leads to loss of sensation in the feet of diabetics, contributing to undetected trauma to the extremities and subsequent refractory infections due to poor vascular supply to the extremity. It is extremely important to teach diabetics and patients with peripheral neuropathy to provide special care to their feet.

Phantom-limb pain. This is the experience of pain that can range from dull ache to crushing pain where an amputated limb once was. The sensory cortex of the brain has influence in this mechanism. This pain is often chronic and requires special interventions to control and manage it, including electronic prosthetics, analgesics, and psychosocial support.

Acute sensory loss. Acute sensory loss may be due to a stroke, acute nerve entrapment in the spine, or compartment syndrome due to trauma to a limb. It presents with acute onset of numbness, tingling, or lack of sensation and function in the affected extremity.

Implications of Peripheral Sensation Changes

The inability to recognize position sense, pressure, or ascertain where the feet are on the floor can lead to falls, burns, lacerations, calluses, and pressure ulcers. Intact peripheral sensation is essential for keeping safe in the environment.

Nursing Assessment and Care Strategies of Peripheral Sensation

Nurses should take appropriate health histories to ascertain the presence of decreased sensations in limbs. Physical exams should always include a thorough inspection of an individual's feet (Hellman, 2002 [Level VI]). Diabetics and people known to have peripheral neuropathy should have a thorough neurological exam including vibratory sense with a tuning fork over bony prominences and Semmes-Weinstein monofilament testing of the feet and proprioception (Boike & Hall, 2002 [Level VI]).

Semmes-Weinstein Monofilament Test

This inexpensive and simple procedure is used to screen for decreased sensation in several plantar sites on the foot. The monofilament is placed against the sole of the foot in eight different areas. The individual is asked to report any sensations (Boike & Hall, 2002 [Level VI]). The Semmes-Weinstein nylon monofilament 5.04 gauge buckles at a pressure of 10 grams. Loss of sensation at this level of pressure indicates a risk for ulcer development. Identification of this risk is important for improving the vigilance of foot care (Armstrong & Lavery, 1998 [Level VI]).

Vibratory Sense

This is assessed by using a 128-Hz vibrating tuning fork on lower extremity bony prominences and asking individuals if they feel any vibration (Boike & Hall, 2002 [Level VI]). Older adults should be able to feel the vibration.

Proprioception

This is the ability for an individual to determine where they are in space. To assess for deficits in proprioception in the feet that may set up an older adult for falls and local trauma, ask the individual to close his or her eyes. Then hold the large toe on the sides and move the foot up or down. Ask the individual to identify which direction the toe was moved. Inability to correctly identify the direction is an indication of decreased proprioception.

Individualized Sensory Enhancement of the Elderly (I-SEE)

The Individualized Sensory Enhancement of the Elderly (I-SEE) program was developed to tailor nursing interventions to the type and level of sensory impairment experienced by older adults (Cacchione, 2007 [Level VI]). Originally developed to address hearing and visually impaired older adults, the I-SEE can logically be extended to address sensory impairment in smell, taste, and peripheral sensation. There are three levels to the I-SEE program: nursing assessments, nursing actions, and nursing referrals.

Case Study and Discussion

Mr. Sweets is a 75-year-old African American male living by himself in the community. He lives in a senior apartment building where he receives housekeeping services and can participate in a meal plan. He arrives on the Ace Unit in your hospital with a diagnosis of hyperglycemia and a urinary tract infection. He also has a history of hypertension, hyperlipidemia, and osteoarthritis of the left hip. He is widowed and has three children: two live in the area, the other lives out of state. His medications include Amaryl 6 mg, which was recently increased from 4 mg; Zocor, 40 mg p.o. daily; Lisinopril, 20 mg daily; HCTZ, 25 mg daily; and Tylenol ES 1,000 mg, three times a day for his hip discomfort. He is a retired aeronautical engineer.

In the admission assessment, you determine that he remembers receiving verbal instructions to cut his diabetic pills in half. Therefore, since that appointment, he has only been taking 2 mg of Amaryl rather than 6 mg. His primary-care provider had instructed him to take $1\frac{1}{2}$ tabs of his Amaryl, not just a $\frac{1}{2}$ tab. You are not sure if it was just a misunderstanding or if Mr. Sweets has difficulty hearing. You are also concerned that his vision may be a problem as well due to his 5-year history of known diabetes.

After you complete your history taking, you gather your supplies to complete your physical exam, including an audioscope, Lighthouse for the Blind near-vision screener, three plastic bags—one each of coffee, baby powder, and peppermint candies—tuning fork, and a Semmes-Weinstein Monofilament Test. The audioscope reveals that Mr. Sweets' ear canals are completely occluded with cerumen and he can only hear the test tone that is delivered at the 60-dB level. On the near-vision screener, he scored 20/125 in both eyes with his dirty glasses. Unfortunately, because his blood sugar is and has been elevated, it is unclear how much of the decreased vision is related to that and how much to possible diabetic retinopathy. Mr. Sweets was able to correctly identify each scent in the plastic bags. When you examine his feet, you identify that he has significant sensation loss on the bottom of his feet. He has intact vibratory sense in the ankle but it is decreased in both toes. His feet are free of any calluses, deformities, or open wounds. He does have some thickened toenails.

These assessments impact the care plan for Mr. Sweets. His sensory deficits most likely precipitated his hospital admission. Written instructions may have helped prevent this, but his near vision may have interfered with the understanding of the written directions as well. He should have written instructions in large font, ideally in 24-point font. Due to the bilateral cerumen impactions, he will need cerumen-softening drops started and the cerumen removed with a cerumen spoon after a few days. If this is not successful, he may need to be seen by an otolaryngologist (ENT) to have the wax removed. If his hearing is still impaired after the cerumen is removed, Mr. Sweets should see an audiologist.

If his vision does not improve with blood-sugar control, he should be seen by an ophthalmologist to determine any treatments for his diabetic retinopathy. He also should see an ophthalmologist if he has not been to one in a year. He would qualify for low-vision services if his acuity remained at 20/125. He also would benefit from increased contrast, which older adults with diabetic retinopathy often need. This can be achieved by adding red or white to light fixtures, remote controls, and other electrical devices that are usually solid colors with limited contrast. A low-vision specialist could help to make his home environment more safe and user-friendly.

Mr. Sweets should be evaluated by a diabetic foot nurse to have his nails trimmed and to learn more about foot care. He will need to learn how to complete daily foot inspections as well as assistance in learning what type of footwear is appropriate for his feet. His hip may cause him some difficulty in reaching his feet. It will be important for him to use mirrors and palpation to assist him in his self-care. A diabetic nurse educator can assist him with further information on the management of the disease and empower him to ask more questions and clarify when information does not appear compatible with his symptoms.

Mr. Sweets was discharged from the hospital after 4 days. His Amaryl was increased to 6 mg; he is afebrile and discharged on oral antibiotics for his urinary tract infection. He had his ears cleaned during those 4 days so his hearing improved to where he can hear at the 40-dB level. He has an appointment with an audiologist as well as with an ophthalmologist. Follow-up appointments have also been made with the endocrinologist, diabetic nurse educator, and diabetic foot nurse on the same visit. These appointments were written out on a 4-x -6-inch index card with a black marker that he could read with his glasses.

Sensory impairment is an interprofessional health care problem. Good communication among disciplines is essential in maintaining Mr. Sweets's functional status and ability to stay in the community. Nurses are best prepared to help Mr. Sweets navigate and coordinate visits to the other disciplines. Screening completed by nurses either in the community, acute care, or long term care settings can identify problems that have often been passed off by an older adult as just getting older.

Related Professional Organizations and Informational Web Sites

Administration on Aging
http://www.aoa.gov/prof/notes/notes_low_vision.asp
American Speech-Language-Hearing Association
www.asha.org
Assisted Listening Devices: Summary of available assisted listening devices
www.entcolumbia.org/acd.htm
Cochlear Implants: General information including video on cochlear implants
www.fda.gov/cdrh/cochlear

Hear Now: 1(800) 648-HEAR (4327)

Will accept donated hearing aids to refit for the under-served

Lighting Research Center: Consumer, Builders, and Health Professional infor-mation on lighting

www.lrc.rpi.edu/programs/lightHealth/AARP/index.asp

The Lighthouse for the Blind: Consumer and health professional information on visual impairment and dual impairment

www.lighthouse.org

National Institute on Aging Information Center

www.nia.nih.gov

National Institute on Deafness and Other Communication Disorders. Contains information for health care providers and consumers

www.nidcd.nih.gov

The National Eye Institute: Contains health information for consumers and health professionals. Also has images of eye diseases and eye charts.

www.nei.nih.gov

Talking Tapes: Access to talking books for visually impaired elders

www.talkingtapes.org

Patient and Family Resources

Aging in the Know: Your gateway to health and aging resources on the Web. Created by the American Geriatrics Society Foundation for Health in Aging (FHA)

www.healthinaging.org/agingintheknow/

League for Hard of Hearing

www.lhh.org/

Prentis Care Networks Project. Care Networks for Formal and Informal Care-givers of Older Adults

http://caregiving.case.edu

Box 21.1

Nursing Standard of Practice Protocol: Nursing Sensory Assessments

I. HISTORY

    A. Ask questions about changes in hearing, vision, and senses of smell and taste, as well as any numbness and tingling in extremities.

    B. Review medications that may be exacerbating the sensory prob-lem, such as anticholinergic medications, antibiotics, aminoglyco-sides, and high-dose aspirin.

    C. Determine if symptoms occurred suddenly or gradually.

    D. Clarify if symptoms are unilateral or bilateral.

    E. Inquire whether the individual has had any prior treatment for sen-sory conditions.

F. Ascertain if sensory conditions interfere with daily function.

G. Ask about the ability to drive. Driving can be affected by vision, hearing, and the peripheral nervous system.

H. Determine interest in receiving treatment for these conditions.

For each positive symptom reported, gather more information by asking about the character, associated symptoms, radiation, location, intensity, and duration, as well as what makes it better; which medications the individual has tried for these symptoms; and what makes it worse. These questions can be easily remembered by using the acronym CAR LID BMW. These questions provide a better understanding of the individual's concerns.

II. PHYSICAL EXAM FOR ALL SYSTEMS

A. Inspect the external structures of the eyes and ears, and examine the ear canal for cerumen using an otoscope.

B. Check visual acuity with a near-vision screener, distance-acuity measure, and contrast sensitivity.

C. Perform a whisper test to assess rough hearing, If available in your setting, use a handheld audioscope to assess up to a 40-dB hearing. If a greater range of hearing testing is needed, use a portable audiometer with noise-reduction earphones. A referral to an audiology professional may be indicated.

D. Assess the nares and determine if they are patent using the otoscope.

E. Inspect the mouth and tongue for any obvious lesions or deviations from normal.

F. Perform a neurosensory exam of the extremities including a monofilament test. Complete a monofilament test on all diabetics. This test quantifies the level of sensory impairment in the feet of diabetic patients.

G. Assess vibratory sense of the extremities with a tuning fork and proprioception.

III. NURSING ACTIONS

A. Vision

1. Avoid disruption in the management of chronic eye conditions by obtaining past history and assuring continuation of ongoing regimens, such as eye drops for glaucoma.

2. Notify the primary-care provider of any acute change in vision.

3. Encourage the use of good lighting in patient rooms. Avoid glare whenever possible.

4. Encourage the use of the patient's eyeglasses. Have family provide lighted magnification if needed (i.e., large magnifiers with a light attached available at low-vision centers).

5. Add contrast to the fixtures and electronics in the room if light switches blend into the wall or faucets blend into the sink. Other

       low-contrast items in the environment include remote controls, television sets, and radios.

    6. Encourage annual eye exams with either an optometrist or an ophthalmologist.

    7. Schedule an annual dilated-eye exam for patients with diabetes and hypertension by an ophthalmologist.

B. Hearing

    1. Assess for cerumen impactions. Request cerumen-softening drops followed by cerumen removal or ENT consultation.

    2. Get the person's attention and face them before speaking to assist the individual with lip reading, a common compensatory mechanism for older adults.

    3. Have at least one pocket amplifier on the nursing unit to use with hearing-impaired individuals.

    4. Do not shout at people with hearing impairments; rather, use a lower tone of your voice.

    5. Provide written instructions (use a large black marker if the person is also visually impaired).

    6. Ensure appropriate care for hearing aids: remove batteries at night; use the brush provided to gently clean the tubes to reduce wax accumulation.

    7. Before sending bed linens or clothing to the laundry, make sure the hearing aid is in the patient's ear or in the designated location (e.g., bedside table or medication cart).

    8. Notify the primary-care provider of any sudden change in hearing.

    9. Referral to an audiologist and/or ENT as indicated.

C. Taste and Smell

    1. Take seriously all complaints of inability or decreased ability to smell or taste. Do not pass them off to medications or poor dentition.

    2. Notify primary-care provider of an abrupt change in taste or smell.

    3. Schedule an ENT referral for evaluation for a sudden change in smell or taste.

    4. Patient teaching should focus on safety issues regarding odors of gas and spoiled food.

    5. Educate seniors about carbon-monoxide detectors in their home and to evaluate food with methods other than the sense of smell and taste.

D. Peripheral Sensation

    1. Individuals should be taught to examine their feet daily as well as look inside their shoes before putting them on each day.

    2. Individuals should be instructed to inform their primary provider of any lesions, calluses, or red areas.

    3. Extremities should be clean and thoroughly dry before applying lotion.

4. Encourage individuals to bring in footwear for evaluation by the advanced practice nurse if they have concerns about safety. Most medical-supply companies carry diabetic healing shoes that have wide toe boxes and Velcro straps, which can be purchased for less than $50.
5. Refer diabetics to facilities with a Certified Diabetes Educator and foot-care specialist.
6. Implement fall precautions and initiate referral to physical therapy for all diabetics with peripheral neuropathy.
7. Refer all older adults with decreased sensation or circulation to a podiatrist or foot-care specialist for ongoing foot care.

IV. EXPECTED OUTCOMES

A. Baseline visual acuity and hearing acuity for all older patients will be performed prior to discharge from the hospital and upon admission to home care or a nursing home.
B. Fall precautions should be in place for all older patients with sensory impairments.
C. Older adults should avoid falls and injuries to extremities if they have decreased sensation of the lower extremities.
D. Accidental exposure to toxins either in the air or food due to decreased sense of smell or taste should be avoided.

V. FOLLOW-UP MONITORING

A. Annual vision assessment: Medicaid in most states will pay for a new pair of eyeglasses every 2 years.
B. When vision is worse than 20/125, individuals should be referred to a low-vision specialist to provide training in the use of visual assistive devices.
C. Given that hearing can change significantly over time, an audiological evaluation for hearing-impaired older adults every 2 years is important. Some states pay through Medicaid for one hearing aid under limited conditions. Hearing aids have been shown to be better accepted if older adults receive them when they start having difficulty with word finding with background noise. Encouragement is needed to improve the consistent use of a hearing aid. Audiologists can help train older adults and their families in the use of hearing aids if necessary.
D. When abrupt changes in smell or taste are reported, a referral to a dentist or ENT is indicated.
E. Long-term adjustments must be made in the home when smell and taste are affected. First, food should be dated and discarded after 48 hours to avoid accidentally eating spoiled food.
F. When xerostomia (i.e., severe dry mouth) is found, a referral to a dentist is indicated.

G. Older adults with decreased peripheral sensation should be followed regularly by a podiatrist or foot-care specialist.

VI. INTERPROFESSIONAL CARE OF SENSORY CHANGES

Care of the aging senses is an interdisciplinary endeavor. Nurses, who frequently have the most contact with patients, can take the lead in assessing and screening older adults for decreased sensory function. Once these deficits are identified, it is important to take the appropriate steps and identify the resources available to older adults. Occupational therapists, low-vision specialists, audiologists, nutritionists, otolaryngologists, and neurologists are just some of the professionals who may be part of the team caring for sensory-impaired older adults. Good communication among disciplines is essential to help older adults benefit from each specialist.

References

Ahmad, N., & Seidman, M. (2004). Tinnitus in the older adult. *Drugs and Aging, 21*(5), 297–305. Evidence Level VI: Expert Opinion.

AHRQ (2004). Technology Assessment: Vision rehabilitation for elderly individuals with low vision or blindness. Rockville, MD: Agency for Healthcare Research and Quality. Evidence Level VI: Expert Opinion.

Albers, M. W., Tabert, M. H. M., & Devanand, D. P. (2006). Olfactory dysfunction as a predictor of neurodegenerative disease. *Current Neurology & Neuroscience Reports, 6*(5), 379–386. Evidence Level I: Systematic Review.

American Academy of Otolaryngology–Head and Neck Surgery (AAO–HNS) (2007). Smell and Taste. Accessed March 15, 2007, at http://www.entet/org/healthinfo/topics/smell_taste.cfm. Evidence Level: VI: Expert Opinion.

Armstrong, D. G., & Lavery, L. A. (1998). Diabetic foot ulcers: Prevention, diagnosis, and classification. *American Family Physician, 57*, 1325–1332, 1337–1338. Evidence Level VI: Expert Opinion.

Bagai, A., Thavendiranathan, P., & Detsky, A. S. (2006). The rational clinical examination: Does this patient have hearing impairment? *Journal of the American Medical Association, 295*(4), 416–428, 448. Evidence Level I: Systematic Review.

Baker, R. S. (2003). Diabetic retinopathy in African Americans: Vision impairment, prevalence, incidence, and risk factors. *International Ophthalmology Clinics, 43*(4), 105–122. Evidence Level I: Systematic Review.

Boike, A. M., & Hall, J. O. (2002). A practical guide for examining and treating the diabetic foot. *Cleveland Clinic Journal of Medicine, 69*, 342–348. Evidence Level VI: Expert Opinion.

Bromley, S. M. (2000). Smell and taste disorders: A primary care approach. *American Family Physician, 61*, 427–436, 438. Evidence Level VI: Expert Opinion.

Bron, A. J., & Caird, R. I. (1997). Conference report: Loss of vision in the ageing eye. *Age and Ageing, 26*, 159–162. Evidence Level VI: Expert Opinion.

Cacchione, P. Z. (2007). Nursing care of older adults with age-related vision loss. In S. Crocker-Houde (Ed.), *Vision loss in older adults* (pp. 131–148). New York: Springer Publishing Company. Evidence Level VI: Expert Opinion.

Cacchione, P. Z., Culp, K., Dyck, M, & Laing, J. (2002). Risk for acute confusions in sensory-impaired rural LTC elders. *Clinical Nursing Research, 12*, 145–158. Evidence Level III: Quasi-experimental study.

Campbell, V., Crews, H., Moriarty, D., Zack, M., & Blackman, D. (1999). Surveillance for sensory impairment, activity limitation and health-related quality of life among older adults: United States, 1993–1997. *MMR Surveillance Summaries, 48* (SS08), 131–156. Evidence Level II: Individual Experimental Study.

Cassin, B. (2001). *Dictionary of eye terminology*. Gainesville, FL: Triad Publishing. Retrieved November 20, 2006, from www.eyeglossary.net. Evidence Level IV: Nonexperimental Study.

Community Services for the Blind and Partially Sighted (2004). Enhancing low vision: Lighting. http://csps.com/publicinfo/lighting.pdf. Accessed on April 20, 2007. Evidence Level VI: Expert Opinion.

Congdon, N., Vingerlin, J. R., Klein, B. E., West, S., Friedman, D. S., Kempen, J., et al. (2004). Causes and prevalence of visual impairment among adults in the United States. *Archives of Ophthalmology, 122*, 477–485. Evidence Level III: Quasi-experimental Study.

Crummer, R. W., & Hassan, G. A. (2004). Diagnostic approach to tinnitus. *American Family Physician, 64*, 120–126, 127–128. Evidence Level VI: Expert Opinion.

Demers, K. (2001). Hearing screening. *Try this: Best practices in nursing care for older adults*. Hartford Institute for Geriatric Nursing, 12. Evidence Level V: Review.

Desai, M., Pratt, L. A., Lentzer, H., & Robinson, K. N. (2001). Trends in vision and hearing among older Americans. *Aging Trends* (2), 1–8. Evidence Level V: Review.

Ferris, F., Kassoff, A., Bresnick, G. H., & Bailey, I. (1982). New visual acuity charts for clinical research. *American Journal of Ophthalmology, 94*, 91–96. Evidence Level III: Quasi-experimental Study.

Francis, H. W., Chee, N., Yeagle, J., Cheng, A., & Niparko, J. (2002). Impact of cochlear implants on the functional health status of older adults. *Laryngoscope, 112*(8 Pt 1), 1482–1488. Evidence Level III: Quasi-experimental Study.

Frank T., & Petersen, D. R. (1987). Accuracy of a 40 dB HL audioscope and audiometer screening for adults. *Ear and Hearing, 8*, 180–183. Evidence Level II: Individual Experimental Study.

Gates, G. A., & Mills, J. H. (2005). Presbycusis. *Lancet, 366*, 1111–1120. Evidence Level V: Review.

Gianutsos, R., & Suchoff, I. B. (1997). Visual fields after brain injury: Management issues for the occupational therapist. In M. Scheiman (Ed.), *Understanding and managing vision deficits: A guide for occupational therapists* (pp. 333–358). Thorogare, NJ: SLACK. Evidence Level VI: Expert Opinion.

Gillmore, G. (2002). Modules 12: Visual Field Testing. Glaucoma I, Continuing Education Module. Retrieved April 20, 2007, from www.eyetec.net/group3/M12Start.htm. Evidence Level VI: Expert Opinion.

Hellman, C. (2002). Nurse practitioner management of the patient with diabetic foot ulcers. *Clinical Excellence for Nurse Practitioners, 5*(5), 11–15. Evidence Level VI: Expert Opinion.

Hirvela, H., Koskela, P., & Laatikainen, L. (1995). Visual acuity in a population aged 70 years or older: Prevalence and causes of visual impairment. *ACTA Ophtalmologica Scandinavia, 73*, 99–104. Evidence Level III: Quasi-experimental Study.

Horton, J. C., & Jones, M. R. (1997). Warning on inaccurate Rosenbaum Cards for testing near vision. *Survey of Ophthalmology, 42*(2), 169–174. Evidence Level VI: Expert Opinion.

Hummel, T., & Nordin, S. (2003). Quality of life in olfactory dysfunction: A White Paper. *Sense of Smell Institute*. Retrieved January 19, 2005, from http://www.senseofsmell.org/feature/whitepaper/whitepaper_print.html. Evidence Level VI: Expert Opinion.

Kennedy, R. S., & Dunlap, W. P. (1990). Assessment of the Vistech contrast sensitivity test for repeated-measures applications. *Optometry & Vision Science, 67*, 248–251. Evidence Level II: Single Experimental Study.

Lewis-Culinan, C., & Janken, J. (1990). Effect of cerumen removal on hearing ability in geriatric patients. *Journal of Advanced Nursing, 15*, 594–600. Evidence Level II: Individual Experimental Study.

Linton, A. D. (2007). Age-related changes in the special senses. In A. D. Linton & H. W. Lach (Eds.), *Matteson & McConnell's gerontological nursing, concepts and practice* (3rd ed., pp. 600–630). St. Louis, MO: Saunders, Elsevier. Evidence Level V: Review.

Lockwood, A. H., Salvi, R. J., & Burkard, R. F. (2002). Tinnitis. *New England Journal of Medicine, 347*(12), 904–910. Evidence Level V: Review.

Mantyjarvi, M., & Laitinen, T. (2001). Normal values for the Pelli-Robson contrast sensitivity test. *Journal of Cataract Refraction Surgery, 27*(2), 261–266. Evidence Level III: Quasi-experimental Study.

Marcincuk, M. C., & Roland, P. S. (2002). Geriatric hearing loss: Understanding the causes and providing appropriate treatment. *Geriatrics, 57*(4), 44. Evidence Level VI: Expert Opinion.

Mehr, AS. (2007). Understanding your audiogram. American Association of Audiology. http://audiology.org/aboutaudiology/consumered/guides/audiogram.htm?PF=1 (accessed January 31, 2007). Evidence Level IV: Nonexperimental Study.

Mesholam, R. I., Mober, P. J., Mahr, R. N., & Doty, R. L. (1998). Olfaction in neurodegenerative disease: A meta-analysis of olfactory functioning in Alzheimer's and Parkinson's diseases. *Archives of Neurology, 55*(1), 84–90. Evidence Level I: Systematic Review.

Miwa, T., Furukawa, M., Tsukatani, T., Costanzo, R. M., DiNardo, L. J., & Reiter, E. R. (2001). Impact of olfactory impairment on quality of life and disability. *Archives of Otolaryngology—Head and Neck Surgery, 127*, 497–503. Evidence Level II: Single Experimental Study.

Morse, A. R., & Rosenthal, B. P. (1997). Vision and vision assessment. In J. A. Teresi, M. P. Lawton, D. Holmes, & M. Ory (Eds.), *Measurement in elderly chronic care populations*. Evidence Level VI: Expert Opinion.

Muller, A., Reichmann, H., Livermore, A., & Hummel, T. (2002). Olfactory function in idiopathic Parkinson's disease (IPD): Results from cross-sectional studies in IPD patients and long-term follow-up of de-novo IPD patients. *Journal of Neural Transmission, 109*, 805–811. Evidence Level II: Single Experimental Study.

Munoz, B., West, S. K., Rubin, G. S., Schein, O. D., Quigley, H. A., Bressler, S. B., et al. (2000). Causes of blindness and visual impairment in a population of older Americans: The Salisbury Eye Evaluation Study. *Archives of Ophthalmology, 118*, 819–825. Evidence Level II: Individual Experimental Study.

Murphy, C., Schubert, C. R., Cruickshanks, K. J., Klein, B. E., Klein, R., & Nondahl, D. M. (2002). Prevalence of olfactory impairment in older adults. *Journal of the American Medical Association, 288*, 2307–2312. Evidence Level III: Quasi-experimental Study.

National Academy on an Aging Society (NAAS) (1999). *Chronic Conditions: A challenge for the 21st century*, Number 1. www.agingsociety.org. Evidence Level II: Individual Experimental Study.

National Academy on an Aging Society (NAAS) (1999). *Hearing loss: A growing problem that affects quality of life*, Number 2. www.agingsociety.org. Evidence Level I: Systematic Review.

National Eye Institute (NEI) (2004). Age-related eye diseases study – results: background. Retrieved February 20, 2007, from http://www.nei.nih.gov/amd/background.asp. Evidence Level VI: Expert Opinion.

National Eye Institute (2004). Statistics and data: Prevalence of blindness data. Retrieved March 1, 2007, from http://www.nei.nih.gov/eyedata/pbd_tables.asp. Evidence Level VI: Expert Opinion.

National Institute on Deafness and Other Communication Disorders (NIDCD) (2007). *Statistics about hearing disorders, ear infections, and deafness*. Retrieved April 22, 2007, from http://www.nidcd.nih.gov/health/statistics/hearing.asp. Evidence Level VI: Expert Opinion

National Institute on Deafness and Other Communication Disorders (NIDCD) (2006). Cochlear Implants. Retrieved April 22, 2007, from http://www.nidcd.nih.gov/health/hearing/coch.asp. Evidence Level VI: Expert Opinion.

National Institute on Deafness and Other Communication Disorders (NIDCD) (2001). Meniere's Disease. http://www.nidcd.nih.gov/health/balance/meniere.asp. Retrieved April 21, 2007. Evidence Level VI: Expert Opinion.

Newman, D. (1990). Assessment of hearing loss in elderly people: The feasibility of a nurse-administered screening test. *Journal of Advanced Nursing, 15*, 400–409. Evidence Level III: Quasi-experimental Study.

Patterson, C. (1994). Prevention of hearing impairment and disability in the elderly. In *Canadian task force on periodic health examination: Canadian guide to clinical prevention health care* (pp. 954–963). Canada: Ottowa Health. Evidence Level V: Review.

Pekkonen, E., Jaaskelainen, I. P., Hietanen, M., Huotilainen, M., Naatanen, R., Ilmoniemi, R. J., et al. (1999). Impaired preconscious auditory processing and cognitive functions in Alzheimer's disease. *Clinical Neurophysiology, 110*, 1942–1947. Evidence Level II: Individual Experimental Study.

Pelli, D. G., Robson, J. G., & Wilkins, A. J. (1988). The design of a new letter chart for measuring contrast sensitivity. *Clinical Vision Science, 2*, 187–199. Evidence Level III: Quasi-Experimental Study.

Pirozzo, S., Papinczak, T., & Glasziou, P. (2003). Whispered voice test for screening for hearing impairment in adults and children: Systematic review. *British Medical Journal, 327*(7421), 967. Evidence Level I: Systematic Review.

Resnick, H. E., Vinik, A. I., Heimovitz, H. K., Brancati, F. L., & Guralnik, J. M. (2001). Age 85+ years accelerates large-fiber peripheral nerve dysfunction and diabetes contributes even in the oldest-old: The Women's Health and Aging Study. *Journals of Gerontology Series*

A-Biological Sciences & Medical Sciences, 56, M25–M31. Evidence Level II: Longitudinal Study.

Schiffman, S. S. (1997). Taste and smell losses in normal aging and disease. *Journal of the American Medical Association, 278*(16),1357–1362. Evidence Level V: Review.

Seiberling, K. A., & Conley, D. G. (2004). Aging and olfactory and taste function. *Otolaryngologic Clinics of North America, 37,* 1209–1228. Evidence Level V: Review.

Seidel, H. M., Dains, J. E., Ball, J. W., & Benedict, G. W. (2003). *Mosby's guide to physical examination* (pp. 278–312). St. Louis, MO: Mosby. Evidence Level VI: Nonexperimental Study.

Sindhusake, D., Mitchell, P., Smith, W., Golding, M., Newell, P., Hartley, D., et al. (2001). Validation of self-reported hearing loss: The Blue Mountains Hearing Study. *International Journal of Epidemiology, 30,* 1371–1378. Evidence Level II: Individual Experimental Study.

Smith, A. G., & Singleton, J. R. (2004). The diagnostic yield of a standardized approach to idiopathic sensory-predominant neuropathy. *Archives of Internal Medicine, 164,* 1021–1025. Evidence Level III: Quasi-experimental study.

Temmel, A. F., Quint, C., Schickinger-Fischer, B., & Hummel (2005). Taste function in xerostomia before and after treatment with saliva substitute containing carboxymethylcellulose. *Journal of Otolaryngology, 34*(20),116–120. Evidence Level III: Quasi-experimental study.

Tielsch, J. M., Sommer, A., Witt, K., Katz, J., & Royall, R. M. (1990). Blindness and visual impairment in an American urban population: The Baltimore Eye Survey. *Archives of Ophthalmology, 108*(2), 286–290. Evidence Level II: Individual Experimental Study.

Tolson, D., Swan, I., & Knussen, C. (2002). Adult/elderly care nursing: Hearing disability: A source of distress for older people and carers. *British Journal of Nursing, 11*(15), 1021–1025. Evidence Level II: Single Experimental Study.

U.S. Department of Health and Human Services (USDHHS) (2000). Healthy People 2010: With understanding and improving health and objectives for improving health. Washington, DC: Government Printing Office. Evidence Level VI: Expert Opinion.

Ventry, I. M., & Weinstein, B. E. (1983). Identification of elderly people with hearing problems. *American Speech and Hearing Association, 25*(7), 37–42. Evidence Level III: Quasi-experimental Study.

Vitale, S., Cotch, M. F., & Sperduto, R. D. (2006). Prevalence of visual impairment in the United States. *Journal of the American Medical Association, 295,* 2158–2163. Evidence Level III: Quasi-experimental Study.

Yueh, B., Shapiro, N., MacLean, C. H., & Shekelle, P. G. (2003). Scientific review and clinical applications: Screening and management of adult hearing loss in primary care: Scientific review. *Journal of the American Medical Association, 289*(15), 1976–1985. Evidence Level I: Systematic Review.

Wallhagen, M. I. (2006). Personal communication at the Geronotological Society of America Meeting, Dallas, TX. Evidence Level VI: Expert Opinion.

Wallhagen, M. I., Pettengill, E., & Whiteside, M. (2006). Sensory impairment in older adults: Part 1, Hearing Loss. *American Journal of Nursing, 106*(11), 52–61. Evidence Level VI: Expert Opinion.

Wallhagen, M. I., Strawbridge, W. J., Shema, S. J., & Kaplan, G. A. (2004). Impact of self-assessed hearing loss on a spouse: A longitudinal analysis of couples. *Journal of Gerontology. Series B: Psychological Sciences and Social Sciences, 59*(B), S190–S196. Evidence Level III: Quasi-experimental Study.

Warnat, B. M., & Tabloski, P. (2006). Sensation: Hearing, vision, taste, touch, and smell. In Tabloski, P. (Ed.), *Gerontological nursing* (pp. 384–420). Upper Saddle River, NJ: Pearson Education, Inc. Evidence Level VI: Expert Opinion.

Whiteside, M., Wallhagen, M. I., & Pettengill, E. (2006). Sensory impairment in older adults: Part 2, Vision Loss. *American Journal of Nursing, 106*(11), 52–61. Evidence Level VI: Expert Opinion.

Wilensky, J. R., & Hawkins, A. (2001). Comparison of contrast sensitivity, visual acuity, and Humphrey visual field testing in patients with glaucoma. *Training in American Ophthalmological Society, 99,* 213–218. Evidence Level III: Quasi-experimental Study.

Wilson, R. S., Arnold, S. E., Schneider, J. A., Tang, Y., & Bennett, D. A. (2007). The relationship between cerebral Alzheimer's disease pathology and odor identification in old age. *Journal of Neurology, Neurosurgery & Psychiatry, 78*(1), 30–35. Evidence Level II: Individual Experimental Study.

Physical Restraints and Side Rails in Acute and Critical Care Settings: Legal, Ethical, and Practice Issues

22

Lorraine C. Mion
Barbara L. Halliday
Satinderpal
K. Sandhu

Introduction

The Centers for Medicare and Medicaid Services (CMS; formerly Health Care Finance Administration [HCFA]) defines physical restraint as "**any** *(emphasis added)* manual method, physical or mechanical device, material, or equipment that immobilizes or reduces the ability of the patient to move his or her arms, legs, body or head freely" (Federal Register, 2006). Examples of these are wrist or leg restraints, hand mitts, Geri-chairs, and, in certain situations, full side rails and reclining chairs. Despite the federal regulations placed on hospitals since 1999, the use of physical restraints for the management of patients in

For a description of Evidence Levels cited in this chapter, see chapter 1,
Developing and Evaluating Clinical Practice Guidelines, page 4.

503

acute nonpsychiatric settings remains a controversial and challenging practice. Typically, health care professionals utilize physical restraints and/or side rails to protect the patient or others. However, the use of physical restraints or side rails for the involuntary immobilization of a patient may not only be an infringement of the patient's rights but can also result in patient harm, including soft-tissue injury, fractures, delirium, and even death (Bower, McCullough, & Timmons, 2003; Evans, Wood, & Lambert, 2003; Miles, 1993 [both Level V]).

The standards from the Joint Commission on Accreditation of Healthcare Organizations (JCAHO) and regulations from CMS have raised concerns among hospital professionals about the feasibility and safety of reducing or eliminating use of physical restraints and side rails in hospitals. The almost nonexistent use of physical restraint in the United Kingdom in comparable settings provides evidence that this can be achieved (O'Keeffe, Jack, & Lye, 1996 [Level IV]; Williams & Finch, 1997 [Level VI]). This chapter focuses on the issues of physical restraint in acute, nonpsychiatric hospital settings with particular attention to the frail elderly, decisions to use physical restraint, legal and ethical issues, administrative responsibilities, and approaches to eliminating or minimizing physical restraints on acute- and critical care units.

Legal Issues

Regulations and Accrediting Standards

In 1992, the U.S. Food and Drug Administration (FDA) issued a Medical Alert on the potential hazards of restraint devices (FDA, 1992). Any harm that arises from the use of a restraining device, which now includes bedside rails, must be reported to the FDA. The hospital standards promulgated by the JCAHO in the early 1990s began to address the use of physical restraints. Over the ensuing years, the standards have become increasingly prescriptive as well as more difficult for acute care settings to meet.

In 1999, HCFA established an interim rule for hospitals, Conditions of Participation, regulating the use of physical restraints in all settings that accepted Medicare or Medicaid participants (HCFA, 1999). In December 2006, a final rule finalized the Patients' Rights Condition of Participation (Federal Register, 2006). These conditions establish the minimum protections of patients' rights and safety and may be superseded by state regulations or accrediting agencies. In brief, use of physical restraint should be used as a last resort; only used when less restrictive mechanisms have been determined to be ineffective; the use of restraint must be in accordance with a written modification to the patient's plan of care; used in accordance with the order of a physician or licensed independent practitioner; must never be written as a PRN order; each order must be renewed every 24 hours for reasons of violent or self-destructive behavior; each order for restraint use for nonviolent reasons must be renewed according to hospital policy; and restraint must be discontinued at the earliest possible time.

Risks of Liability

A major obstacle in reducing clinicians' use of physical restraint or side rails is the fear of liability if restraints are not used. Case law has been mixed on use of physical restraints in hospitals. Hospitals have been found liable both for the use of physical restraints and for not using physical restraints (Kapp, 1994, 1999 [both Level VI]). However, the changing standards of care will lead to a different legal standard of care than that of the 1980s or 1990s. Although hospitals have a clear duty to protect patients from harm, they do not have a duty to restrain patients. Indeed, as the practice in hospitals becomes one of reduced restraints due to changing legal and accrediting standards, it will become easier for hospitals to justify non-use of restraints in instances of patient injury where use of nonrestraint interventions were clearly demonstrated (Kapp, 1999 [Level VI]). However, it will also become harder for a hospital to justify its use of restraints in instances of patient harm (Kapp, 1999 [Level VI]).

Professional Standards of Care

Several organizations have established guidelines for the use of physical restraints, including the American Geriatrics Society and The American Psychiatric Association. As early as 1994, a set of voluntary standards on physical restraints was developed for hospital nurses by the Nurses Improving Care of the Hospitalized Elderly Project, sponsored by The John A. Hartford Foundation (Mion & Strumpf, 1994 [Level V]). Subsequently, the National Quality Forum has designated physical restraint use in hospitals and nursing facilities as a patient-centered outcome for nursing-sensitive care. Last, as part of the condition for participation as a Magnet facility, hospitals must examine use of physical restraint in relation to nursing-skill mix and hours.

These guidelines have become the standard for customary practice and are used as an appropriate legal standard that defines the parameters of liability. Furthermore, these guidelines in combination with JCAHO and CMS requirements are used to establish hospital-based policies and procedures, quality of performance activity, and utilization of these criteria.

Prevalence and Rationale of Staff

Extent of Use

These standards and guidelines have led to an overall decrease in physical-restraint use in acute care and a change in practice patterns (Minnick, Mion, Johnson, Catrambone, & Leipzig, 2007; Minnick, Mion, Leipzig, Lamb, & Palmer, 1998; Whitman, Davidson, Sereika, & Rudy, 2001 [all Level IV]). In the 1980s, a number of single-site studies examined the prevalence of physical restraint on general adult units. The overall prevalence of physical restraint use on general floors ranged from 6% to 13% with higher rates (18% to 22%) among elderly patients (Mion, Minnick, Palmer, Kapp, & Lamb, 1996 [Level V]).

In the late 1990s, overall hospital restraint prevalence decreased but varied as much as threefold with rates ranging from 39 restraint-days/1,000 patient-days to 82 restraint-days/1,000 patient-days (Minnick et al., 1998 [Level IV]; Whitman et al., 2001 [Level IV]). For the first time, restraint use was examined in critical care units and was noted to be as high as 500 restraint-days/1,000 patient-days. Intensive care unit (ICU) rates varied markedly, between units in the same hospital setting as well as matched units between hospitals (Minnick et al., 1998 [Level IV]; Whitman et al., 2001 [Level IV]). During 1998–1999, a longitudinal study was conducted at two acute care settings involving six ICUs and seven non-ICUs (Mion et al., 2001 [Level III]). ICU rates were much higher than non-ICU rates (i.e., up to 482 restraint-days/1,000 patient-days versus 0.1 restraint days/1,000 patient-days). The variation in ICUs within the same hospital and by type of ICU again was present. For example, neurological ICUs had rates greater than surgical ICUs.

A national prevalence study involving 434 units in 40 acute care hospitals selected at random from five geographic areas was completed in 2005 (Minnick et al., 2007 [Level IV]). Findings from this study revealed overall hospital prevalence of 50 restraint-days/1,000 patient-days but with a 10-fold variation among hospitals from a rate of 9 to 94 restraint-days/1,000 patient-days. The majority of use was accounted for in ICUs. The pattern of differences by type of unit was again present (e.g., medical versus surgical and adult versus pediatric). However, even when controlling by type of unit, a more than 10-fold variation existed among similar settings. For example, overall prevalence among the 41 general ICUs was 202.6 restraint-days/1,000 patient-days, with a range of 9 to 351/1,000 patient-days. An examination of staffing ratios and nursing-skill mix failed to demonstrate an association with physical-restraint rates. Further analyses revealed that variation in practice persisted even when controlling for size of hospital, academic/nonacademic status, geographic region, and type of hospital (i.e., nonprofit, profit, and government). Clearly, there are patient populations associated with clinicians' decisions to use physical restraint but, more important, there are major practice differences *even when controlling for patient population.*

Rationale for Use

In the 1980s, hospital nurses cited fall prevention as the primary reason for restraint use (56% to 77%) (Mion, Frengley, Jakovcic, & Marino, 1989 [Level III]; Robbins, Boyko, Lane, Cooper, & Jahnigen, 1987 [Level IV]; Strumpf & Evans, 1988 [Level IV]). Although fall risk is still a concern, today's hospital nurses cite prevention of patient initiated therapy disruption as the primary reason for restraint use (reported for 75% of restraint-days) (Minnick et al., 2007 [Level IV]). It is somewhat disconcerting that nurses still tend to use the term *confusion* as a reason for use of physical restraints. In this study, it was cited in 25.4% of the restraint-days, and in 8.25% of the restraint-days it was the sole reason for use. Prevention of falls was identified in only 17.6% of the restraint-days. Other less commonly voiced reasons included management of agitation or violent behavior, wandering, and positioning. Most nurses cite patient-care issues for the rationale to use physical restraint. However, a small proportion of nurses have cited insufficient staffing for restrained patients (Evans & Fitzgerald, 2002 [Level IV]; Matthiesen, Lamb, McCann, Hollinger-Smith, & Walton, 1996 [Level IV]; Minnick et al., 1998 [Level IV]; Minnick et al., 2007 [Level IV]; Scherer, Janelli, Wu, & Kuhn, 1993 [Level V]; Schott-Baer, Lusis, & Beauregard, 1995 [Level V]).

There have been many studies of the perceptions of caregiving staff about their attitudes and beliefs regarding physical restraint. In the 1980s, clinicians rarely questioned the use of physical restraints, instead assuming that this widespread practice was necessary as well as appropriate (Frengley, 1996 [Level VI]; Strumpf & Evans, 1988 [Level IV]). Early studies on attitudes toward restraints, mostly conducted at single sites with small sample sizes, found that 75% to 82% of nursing staff were "comfortable" using restraints and up to 78% believed that restraints prevented injury (Houston & Lach, 1990 [Level V]; Neary, Kanski, Janelli, Scherer, & North, 1991 [Level IV]; Scherer, 1991 [Level VI]). In the late 1990s, well after JCAHO had begun more restrictive standards, a study of 799 nurses and physicians at three teaching hospitals found that only 46% felt a patient suffered loss of dignity when placed in restraints, 17% felt guilty using restraints, and 16% felt embarrassment when family entered the room of a restrained patient (Lamb, Minnick, Mion, Palmer, & Leipzig, 1999 [Level IV]). Most of the respondents believed that the benefits of restraints outweighed the risks.

With more than 5 years of federal regulations restricting their use, one wonders to what extent any of the attitudes or knowledge has changed among acute care personnel. Given the variation in actual use of restraint, it appears that the decision to use physical restraint continues to be one based on individual judgment and beliefs rather than on scientifically validated guidelines or protocols.

Ethical Issues in the Use of Physical Restraint

The use of physical restraints has been examined from an ethical perspective (Moss & La Puma, 1991 [Level VI]; Robinson, 1995; Schafer, 1985; Slomka, Agich, Stagno, & Smith, 1998 [all Level VI]). The primary ethical dilemma resulting from physical restraint is the clinician's value or emphasis of beneficence versus the patient's autonomy. The presence of a physical restraint, by its very nature, is applied against a patient's wishes and inevitably compromises the individual's dignity and diminishes respect for the person. Beneficence requires that at least no harm should arise from the use of physical restraint and that, optimally, a good outcome would result from use. The lack of beneficial results from the use of physical restraints has been well documented in many health care settings. Little is known, however, of the risk-to-benefit ratio of use or non-use of physical restraint in patients who are critically ill (Maccioli et al., 2003 [Level VI]).

The discussion of physical restraints from an ethical viewpoint must also incorporate the socioculture and political contexts. For example, clinicians have reported on low to nonexistent use of physical restraint in the United Kingdom, stemming perhaps from a legal mandate existing since the 1800s prohibiting their use. It has been suggested that in the United States, the domination of risk in geriatric assessment (e.g., prevent harm, prevent falls) shapes much of clinicians' understanding of old age (Kaufmann, 1994 [Level VI]). If one's primary focus is on the likelihood of patient risk resulting in harm, one is less likely to see self-esteem or dignity as the more important value or model to guide clinical decisions (Slomka, et al. 1998 [Level VI]). Interestingly, Slomka and associates (1998 [Level VI]) point out the contradictory nature of the frequent use of physical restraint in the United States—that is, a society that places a high value on autonomy yet is so willing to violate that autonomy in the interest of perceived patient benefit. This contradiction may stem from the youth-oriented culture that places low value on aging.

The discussion of ethics in clinical practice must also acknowledge the realities of reduced resources and escalating costs (Slomka et al., 1998 [Level VI];

Minnick et al., 2007 [Level IV]). Decisions and protocols about use of physical restraints and methods to reduce and/or eliminate restraints will be impacted by cost-containment efforts. There is a shortage of registered nurses and a need to change our models of care delivery to account for this change, at a time of sicker patients (Johnson, Billingsley, & Costa, 2006 [Level VI]). Given this scenario, clinicians and administrators alike may be reluctant to minimize or eliminate restraints. If alternatives to physical restraints in acute care settings can be shown to contribute to quality outcomes (e.g., patient safety, patient dignity/satisfaction) *and* within existing cost-containment efforts, then there is an increased likelihood of successfully implementing and maintaining practice guidelines. There is a chance, however, that if restraint-reduction efforts are seen as too expensive (e.g., use of "sitters"), then the emphasis on cost-constraint may trump other considerations (Slomka, et al., 1998 [Level VI]).

Administrative Responsibilities

Changing established practices and philosophies of care can be a daunting task. Although education and training are important, the single most important factor in affecting a major shift in the present paradigm of care to one that is restraint-free care is the commitment by administrators and key clinical leaders (Mion et al., 2001 [Level III]; Williams & Finch, 1997 [Level VI]). Indeed, the huge variation seen in the rates among 40 hospitals that cannot be explained by size of hospital, type of hospital, or geographic location lends support to this observation. The administrators, including nurse managers, set the tone for the practice on the unit. Clinical staff, especially the frontline care providers, must feel supported during the transition period. Reducing health care providers' reliance on physical restraint in managing confused or agitated patients, especially in the critical care units, is a major shift that leaves many staff uneasy. The goal set and supported by administration of a restraint-free (or restraint-minimal) environment would establish the presence of a physical restraint as an outlier that requires a full analysis as for any sentinel event. The outcome of such analyses may well lead to the recognition of system problems and organizational arrangements that can be improved, which, in turn, lead to even fewer restraints in use.

Settings of Care

The studies of the prevalence of the use of physical restraints for nonpsychiatric purposes in hospitals have shown that there is great discrepancy between general medical and surgical units and intensive-care units in terms of the extent and rationale. Therefore, the use of physical restraints and approaches to possible alternatives can be considered separately for general hospital units and critical care units.

General Medical–Surgical Units

Rates of physical restraint use on general medical and surgical units have declined in the past 20 years (Frengley & Mion, 1986 [Level IV]; Minnick et al., 2007 [Level IV]). Although the rate of use has declined, the evidence of wide variation among these units exists; the range was 3 to 123 restraint-days/1,000 patient-days on 70 medical units and 0 to 65 restraint-days/1,000 patient-days on 50 surgical units (Minnick et al., 2007 [Level IV]). It is apparent that there are units that demonstrate best practices but also that further efforts are needed to diminish this practice as a national standard. Otherwise, significant numbers of patients will continue to be restrained.

Many hospitals provide care for acutely ill, frail elderly in settings that are not designed environmentally for the care of such older people (Mion, 1992 [Level VI]; Palmer, Landefeld, Kresevic, & Kowal, 1994 [Level VI]). Environmental structure can either facilitate or inhibit monitoring and surveillance, noise control, appropriate lighting, socialization, cognition, and function (Inouye & Charpentier, 1996 [Level IV]; Palmer et al., 1994 [Level VI]). Studies in long term care settings have demonstrated that the use of environmental strategies can enhance function among those suffering from dementia; similar strategies need to be considered in acute care settings.

In addition to environmental strategies, organizational factors, such as systems to determine staffing numbers and mix, models of care delivery, and transmission or communication of the plan of care among multiple disciplines and departments, are gaining increased recognition in the patient-safety movement (Leape & Berwick, 2005 [Level VI]). Many health care providers lack the knowledge, skills, and sensitivity in providing appropriate care to older adults. The JCAHO standard to ensure age-specific education and training is a step in the right direction, but further efforts are required.

No single approach to eliminating physical restraints on general medical–surgical units can be successful. Studies in a variety of settings have shown that the use of advanced practice nurses, comprehensive interdisciplinary approaches to enhance cognitive and physical function, staff education, organizational strategies, and environmental interventions can eliminate or reduce physical restraints in a cost-effective manner while promoting other patient outcomes, such as reduced fall rates (Amato, Salter, & Mion, 2006 [Level V]; Landefeld et al., 1995 [Level II]; Mion et al., 2001 [Level III]).

Critical Care Units

The practice of physical restraints is now predominantly within ICUs to maintain needed life-sustaining therapies or life-maintaining therapies (Minnick et al., 2007 [Level IV]). Strategies that have been used with success in long term care settings, rehabilitation settings, and general hospital units are not as successful in critical care environments (Mion et al., 2001 [Level III]). The severity of illness of patients; the intensity and delivery of care; the pace of activity; and the consequences of interruptions, delays, or disruptions of therapeutic devices differ significantly among non-ICUs and ICUs. The thought of delirious patients dislodging external ventricular drains with subsequent brain damage, pulling out central lines with threat of hemorrhage, or self-extubation from mechanical ventilation with subsequent respiratory arrest is one that heavily influences critical care nurses' decisions to use physical restraints (Frengley & Mion, 1998 [Level V]; Happ, 2000 [Level V]).

Efforts to limit physical-restraint use in the ICU are hampered by lack of information regarding the extent of therapy disruption in these units or the resulting immediate and subsequent harm to patients (Maccioli et al.,

2003 [Level VI]). A number of studies, mostly single-site, have examined self-extubation from mechanical ventilation (Betbese, Perez, Bak, Rialp, & Mancebo, 1998 [Level IV]; Boulain, 1998 [Level IV]; Carrion et al., 2000 [Level IV]; Chevron et al., 1998 [Level IV]; Chiang, Lee, Lee, & Wei, 1996 [Level V]; Christie, Dethelf-sen, & Cane, 1996 [Level IV]; Fraser, Riker, Prato, & Wilkins, 2001 [Level IV]; Frezza, Carleton, & Valenziano, 2000 [Level III]; Kapadia, Bajan, & Raje, 2000 [Level IV]; Moons, Sels, De Becker, De Geest, & Ferdinande, 2004 [Level IV]). Rates have ranged from 0.3% to 14.3%, with higher rates in medical ICUs. Re-intubation after self-extubation ranged from 11% to 76%. **Importantly, 33% to 91% of those who self-extubated did so while physically restrained.** As part of the national prevalence study described earlier, the authors also examined the prevalence of patient-initiated device removal, patient contexts, patient risk-adjusted factors, and consequences (Mion, Minnick, Leipzig, Catrambone, & Johnson, n.d. [Level V]). In 49 ICUs in 39 hospitals, data was collected on 49,470 patient-days. Patients removed 1,623 devices on 1,097 occasions, for an overall rate of 22.1 episodes/1,000 patient-days. Similar to results on physical-restraint prevalence, wide variation in rates were noted: from 0 to 102.1 episodes/1,000 patient-days. Approximately one-half the episodes occurred on the day shift, and 44% were in physical restraint at the time of the episode. Patient harm occurred in 250 (23%), mostly minor in nature. In 10 (0.9%) episodes, patients incurred major harm. No deaths occurred. The authors examined rates of rein-sertion and found that these varied by type of device. Devices that are easily applied, such as monitor leads or oxygen masks, had much higher reinsertion rates than devices that are more complex and difficult to insert (e.g., endotra-cheal tubes or surgical drains). It may be that devices are utilized too long, which could contribute to prolonged use of physical restraint. In turn, physical restraint may contribute to agitation and delirium (Inouye & Charpentier, 1996 [Level IV]). Additional hospital resources (e.g., x-rays, laboratory tests) were utilized in slightly more than half the episodes; Fraser and associates (2001 [Level IV]) commented on the potential costliness of this problem.

Information gathered on staffing levels and mix showed little variation among these ICUs; hence, there was no association between staffing ratios and therapy disruptions. Of the three studies on self-extubation that examined rela-tionship to staffing levels, two also showed no association (Boulain, 1998 [Level IV]; Chevron et al., 1998 [Level IV]; Marcin et al., 2005 [Level IV]). The propor-tion of unit days were collected involving use of physical restraint and found *no* association between a unit's restraint rate and rate of therapy disruption, a finding similar to some other studies (Kapadia, Bajan, & Raje, 2000 [Level IV]; Mion et al., 2001 [Level III]) but not others (Carrion et al., 2000 [Level IV]; Frezza, Carleton, & Valenziano, 2000 [Level III]; Tominaga, Rudzwick, Scannell, & Waxman, 1995 [Level III]).

Finally, the pattern of sedation and analgesia in these units was unclear and 30% of the patients had received no analgesia or sedation in the 24 hours prior to the episode. Others have reported on inconsistent sedation and anal-gesia practices in ICUs (Bair, Bobek, Hoffman-Hogg, Mion, & Arroliga, 2000 [Level IV]; Egerod, Christensen, & Johansen, 2006 [Level IV]; Mehta et al., 2006 [Level IV]; Siegel, 2003 [Level VI]; Weinhart, Chlan, & Gross, 2001 [Level IV]). In an earlier cohort study, the authors examined ICU patient outcomes after implementing sedation and analgesia guidelines and found that those cared for with the guidelines had less self-extubations and use of physical restraints (Bair et al., 2000 [Level IV]). Examining appropriate strategies for sedation and analgesia in critically ill patients may well result in improved clinical outcomes while providing care in a more humane fashion.

Attention to the environment of the ICU is as important as any other setting. Indeed, the environment can affect more strongly persons whose personal competence is low and who are unable to exert control over the environment. Inouye and Charpentier (1996 [Level IV]) exquisitely demonstrated the inverse relationship of the individual's level of vulnerability with that of environmental or process insults on subsequent development of delirium among hospitalized older adults. Environmental features such as noise, light, and unit design have been shown to be associated with agitation, anxiety, and disorientation of ICU patients (Williams, 1988 [Level VI]).

Lack of communication with ICU patients by care providers has been documented and results in distress, anxiety, and confusion (Fontaine, 1994 [Level V]). Attention to the physical environment; use of communication techniques with seemingly noncommunicative patients; encouragement of collaborative practice among ICU disciplines; and nonpharmacologic approaches to relieve patient distress, anxiety, and agitation have been suggested but largely untested (Maccioli et al., 2003 [Level VI]). Nevertheless, a multi-prong approach to optimize physical and cognitive function, address onset as well as management of delirium, and appropriate and adequate pain control are likely to affect nurses' and physicians' reliance on physical restraint.

Alternatives to Physical Restraints

This book has provided the reader with a number of protocols addressing care issues such as falls, delirium, sleep, nutrition, medications, and function. The reader is encouraged to review these protocols closely. Implementing best practices aimed at these areas will in itself reduce the use of physical restraints. A brief overview of an approach the authors have found to be successful is presented herein.

The two major reasons for using physical restraints—to prevent therapy disruption and falls—require comprehensive yet targeted approaches. The act of self-terminating therapy among hospitalized, acutely ill older adults is most likely a manifestation of delirium and less likely a desire to enact a clinical decision, as with advanced directives. Both falls and delirium are well-known syndromes with significant morbidity and mortality among older adults. Both are complex syndromes with multiple underlying etiologies that require a combination of individual-, environmental-, and organizational-specific strategies (Tinetti, Inouye, Gill, & Doucette, 1995 [Level VI]).

Inouye and colleagues (1999 [Level II]) demonstrated an approach to preventing delirium in a randomized controlled trial. However, most strategies are based on nonrandomized trials and/or clinical experience. Given the complexity of falls and delirium, it is unlikely that any single intervention would suffice as an alternative to physical restraint. Rather, attention to the environment and organization of the unit, as described in the two previous sections, combined with patient-specific approaches provides the most successful approach to this issue (Mion et al., 2001 [Level III]; Amato et al., 2006 [Level V]). Tables 22.1 and 22.2

22.1   Interventions to Reduce Fall Risk

Patient-Centered Interventions	Organizational Interventions	Environmental Interventions
Supervised, progressive ambulation	Examine pattern of falls on unit (e.g., time of day, day of week)	Keep bed in low, locked position
PT/OT consultation: weakened or unsteady gait, trunk weakness, upper arm weakness	Examine unit factors that can contribute to falls that can be ameliorated (e.g., report in back room versus walking rounds to improve surveillance)	Safety features such as grab bars, call bells, and bed alarms are in good working order
Provide physical aids, hearing, vision, walking	Restructure staff routines to increase number of available staff throughout day	Ensure that bedside tables and dressers are in easy reach
Modify clothing: skid-proof slippers, slipper-socks; robes no longer than ankle length	Set and maintain toilet schedules	Clear pathways of hazards
Bedside commode if impaired or weakened gait	Install electronic alarms for wanderers	Bolster cushions to assist with posture, maintain seat in chair
Postural hypotension: behavioral recommendations such as ankle pumps, hand clenching, reviewing medications, elevating head of bed	Provide bed/chair alarms*	Adequate lighting, especially bathroom at night
	Moving patient closer to nurse station	Furniture to facilitate seating: reclining chairs†, extended arm rests, high back
	Increased checks on high risk patients	

*Note that alarms do not necessarily prevent a patient from attempting to arise from bed or chair or leave a unit. They are primarily to be used to ensure more timely notification to staff that patients are attempting unsupervised transfers or ambulation.

† For those with poor trunk balance and who slide out of chairs; in other instances, could be viewed as a restraint.

Although there is no strong evidence to support each of these interventions, they have been used in multicomponent interventions studies that have demonstrated reduced fall risk (Oliver et al., 2007 [Level I]).

Determining Underlying Cause for Agitation/Cognitive Impairment	Device Removal
Immediate Assessment If abrupt change in perception, attention, or level of consciousness: – Assess for life-threatening physiologic impairments: respiratory, neurologic, fever/sepsis, hypo/hyperglycemia, alcohol/substance withdrawal, fluid and electrolyte imbalance. – Notify physician of change in mental status & compromised physiologic status	*Disruption of Any Device* – Determine if medically possible to discontinue device; try alternative mode of therapy – For mild-to-moderate cognitive impairment, explain device and allow patient to feel under nurse's guidance
Differential assessment (Interdisciplinary) – Obtain baseline or pre-morbid cognitive function from family caregivers – Establish whether the patient has history of dementia or depression – Review medications to identify drug–drug interactions, adverse effects – Review current laboratory values	*Attempted or actual disruption: ventilator* – Determine underlying cause of behavior for appropriate medical and/or pharmacologic approach – More secure anchoring Start with less restrictive means: mitts, elbow extenders
Treatment (Interdisciplinary) – Treat underlying disorder(s) – Judicious, low dose use of medication if warranted for agitation – Communication techniques: low voice, simple commands, reorientation – Frequent reassurance and orientation – Surveillance/observation: Determine whether family member(s) willing to stay with patient; move patient closer to nurses' station; perform safety checks more frequently; redeploy staff to provide one-on-one observation if other measures ineffective.	*Attempted or actual disruption: Nasogastric tube* – If for feeding purposes, consult with nutritionist, speech or occupational therapist for swallow evaluation – Consider gastrotomy tube for feeding as appropriate if other measures ineffective – Anchoring of tube, either by taping techniques or commercial tube holder – If restraints needed, start with least restrictive restraints: mitts, elbow extenders
	Attempted or actual disruption: IV lines – Commercial tube holder for anchoring – Long-sleeved robes, commercial sleeves for arms – Consider Hep-Lock and cover with gauze – Taping, securement of IV line under gown, sleeves – Keep IV bag out of visual field – Consider alternative therapy: oral fluids, drugs *Attempted or actual disruption: Bladder catheter* – Proper securement, anchoring to leg; commercial tube holders available

Although there is no strong evidence to support each interventions, they have been used in a multicomponent quality improvement study that demonstrated reduced rates of therapy disruption (Mion, Fogel, Sandhu, et al., 2001 [Level III]).

display selected interventions aimed at reducing the likelihood of falls and the attenuation of delirium and subsequent disruption of therapy.

Falls are well-known, serious events in hospitalized older patients. The goal is to minimize the risk or probability of falling without compromising an older individual's mobility and functional independence. Using a systematic or standardized approach, the nurse and physician assess the patient for intrinsic (personal), extrinsic (environment), and situational (activity) factors. The evaluation need not be complex or time-consuming, and several fall risk assessment guidelines are available. For instance, a nurse can do a simple evaluation of gait and balance by simply observing a person's ability to transfer in and out of bed or chair and the ability to walk to and from the bathroom. A nurse can quickly note any difficulty with steadiness, ability to stand up independently without using a rocking motion or use of upper extremities, ability to sit down without "plopping" onto the surface of the chair, and the ability to walk steadily to the bathroom without holding onto objects or the wall. At this time, notation can be made of lightheadedness or dizziness, presence of orthostatic hypotension, and use of sedating medications.

Extrinsic factors include clothing and footwear. Shoes or slippers should be nonskid, but rubber-soled foot wear is not recommended. Furniture design, such as beds at a proper height and chairs with extended armrests for easier leverage, can facilitate mobility. Reclining chairs are helpful for those with poor trunk control and who slide out of chairs with a 90-degree seating angle. On the other hand, reclining chairs could be a type of restraint if used for patients with general deconditioning or weakened states who subsequently struggle to rise out of the chair. Although beds low to the floor assist with preventing fall injury, they may actually contribute to a fall in a person with weak quadriceps muscle strength; hence, the nurse must use clinical judgment of whether the intervention is to prevent a fall or prevent a fall injury; these goals do not necessarily result in similar interventions. Hospital equipment can also contribute to falls, such as legs collapsing on bedside commodes, wheelchairs tipping when a patient leans forward, or tubing from lower extremity intermittent compression devices that are left on when a patient gets up from bed.

The findings of either intrinsic or extrinsic factors should lead to targeted interventions. There are some fall-prevention strategies that one could consider as "universal"—that is, be implemented for all patients regardless of the risk level. For instance, all patients should have beds at appropriate heights for ease of exiting and entering, have call bells within reach, and have clear pathways. Depending on the type of unit, some units may elect to incorporate universal interventions that other floors would consider a targeted intervention. For example, an acute-stroke unit may elect to automatically place all patients on a toileting schedule at time of admission and reevaluate continually whether this intervention is required, whereas other units in the hospital would elect to use this as a targeted intervention only for those patients with cognitive impairment and incontinence. Table 22.1 provides a number of suggestions reported in the literature and based on clinical experience to reduce the risk of falls (see chapter 9, *Preventing Falls in Acute Care*, for greater detail).

Disruption of therapy or self-termination of devices can be dealt with by first identifying the underlying reason for a patient's attempts to terminate therapies. In many cases, a nurse will identify confusion as the underlying cause. As discussed in earlier chapters, nurses need to differentiate dementia, delirium, and delirium with dementia. A systematic approach to determine the cause of the behavior is necessary for treatment. For example, if an older adult is suffering from alcohol withdrawal, it is unlikely that interventions such as increased surveillance or pain relief will have much impact on the person's agitation and delirium. Refer to chapter 4, *Assessing Cognitive Function*, and chapter 7, *Delirium*, for further protocols to identify cognitive impairments and to prevent and manage delirium.

As the health care team works to address a patient's behavior, nonpharmacological approaches to protecting the device from self-termination can be made. First, determine whether the device is absolutely necessary. Even in the critical care environment, major therapy devices may not be reinserted once a patient pulls it out. Thus, always question whether the device is absolutely necessary or a less noxious device or approach may be used instead. For example, if a nasogastric tube is used for nutrition, request the assessment of other disciplines, such as speech or occupational therapists, to determine whether oral feeding could be introduced. If long-term enteral feeding is required, an interdisciplinary team plan with the patient and family is warranted given the known deleterious effects of tube feedings with certain conditions. A second approach is to use anchoring or camouflaging techniques to secure the device against the patient's attempts to dislodge the device and to "hide" the device from the patient. For instance, one cannot disguise or hide a nasogastric tube from the person. The tube, however, can be placed so as to not interfere with or interrupt the person's visual field. Seeing the tube dangling in front of one's eyes or pulling on one's nares is an obvious irritant. If a gastrostomy tube is determined to be appropriate in a person's plan of care, abdominal binders can aid in reducing the person's ability to pull it out. There are several commercial products available to secure various tubes, including nasogastric tubes, endotracheal tubes, intravenous lines, and indwelling bladder catheters. Although none of these devices is likely to prevent a determined person from pulling out a device, they do provide anchoring and stability of the device that are probably more secure than taping methods (Tasota, Hoffman, Zullo, & Jamison, 1987 [Level II]).

Side Rails

A discussion on physical restraints in hospitals would not be complete without mentioning side rails. Side rails, in and of themselves, are not considered a restraining device by either the JCAHO or CMS. It is a nurse's intent of their use that determines whether side rails are a restraining device or a protective device. This has led to some confusion by nurses. Full side rails to transfer patients in carts, during procedures (e.g., conscious sedation), or to protect a sedated or lethargic patient from rolling out of the bed can be considered as protective devices. A number of specialty beds, such as ICU pulmonary beds or bariatric beds, require full side rails in use. Many bed manufacturers have bed controls and call systems embedded in the side rail frames, resulting in patients requesting that the side rails be kept raised for ease of control. Hospital patients have also been observed to request partial to full side rails to be raised because of the narrowness of the beds or to facilitate movement (e.g., transfers, repositioning).

Full side rails to keep patients in bed who *desire* to leave bed are restraints. It does not matter the cognitive level of the person. If a severely demented patient wishes to leave the bed, full side rails are considered a restraint, even if a nurse believes the side rails are for "patient safety." Side rails have been shown to increase fall injuries because patients either try to squeeze through rails or climb over the foot of the bed; they are never a recommended strategy for fall prevention. Moreover, the FDA has received reports of more than 400 deaths as a direct result of side-rail entrapment from a variety of health care settings, including hospitals (FDA, 2006). The reader is referred to Capezuti and Braun (2001 [Level V]) for an excellent review of the legal and medical aspects of side rail use.

Conclusion

The pattern and rationale for physical-restraint use has changed over the past 2 decades. Focusing on assessment and prevention of delirium and falls will likely minimize their use. Further work is needed in the ICU settings for best strategies to identify delirium, prevent delirium, and manage delirium that would include nonpharmacological as well as pharmacological approaches. To avoid the use of physical restraints, practical and cost-effective strategies need to be devised and tested. This would best be done in an interdisciplinary patient-centered fashion.

References

Amato, S., Salter, J. P., & Mion, L. C. (2006). Physical restraint reduction in the acute rehabilitation setting: A quality improvement study. *Rehabilitation Nursing, 31,* 235–241. Evidence Level III: Review. Quasiexperimental Study.

Bair, N., Bobek, M. B., Hoffman-Hogg, L., Mion, L. C., & Arroliga, A. (2000). Introduction of sedation guidelines in an intensive care unit: Physician and nurse adherence. *Critical Care Medicine, 28,* 707–713. Evidence Level IV: Nonexperimental Study.

Betbese, A. J., Perez, M., Bak, E., Rialp, G., & Mancebo, J. (1998). A prospective study of unplanned endotracheal extubation in intensive care unit patients. *Critical Care Medicine, 26,* 1180–1186. Evidence Level IV: Nonexperimental Study.

Boulain, T. (1998). Unplanned extubations in the adult intensive care unit: A prospective multicenter study. *American Journal of Respiratory and Critical Care Medicine, 157,* 1131–1137. Evidence Level IV: Nonexperimental Study.

Bower, F., McCullough, C., & Timmons, M. (2003). A synthesis of what we know about the use of physical restraints and seclusion with patients in psychiatric and acute care settings: 2003 update. *Online Journal of Knowledge Synthesis in Nursing, 10*(1), document number 1.

Capezuti, E. A., & Braun, J. A. (2001). Medico-legal aspects of hospital side rail use. *Ethics, Law, and Aging Review, 7,* 25–57. Evidence Level V: Review.

Carrion, M. I., Ayuso, D., Marcos, M., Robles, M. P., de la Cal, M. A., Alia, I., et al. (2000). Accidental removal of endotracheal and nasogastric tubes and intravascular catheters. *Critical Care Medicine, 28,* 63–66. Evidence Level IV: Nonexperimental Study.

Chevron, V., Menard, J. F., Richard, J. C., Girault, C., Leroy, J., & Bonmarchand, G. (1998). Unplanned extubations: Risk factors of development and predictive criteria for re-intubation. *Critical Care Medicine, 26,* 1049–1053. Evidence Level IV: Nonexperimental Study.

Chiang, A. A., Lee, K. C., Lee, J. C., & Wei, C. H. (1996). Effectiveness of a continuous quality improvement program to reduce unplanned extubations: A prospective study. *Intensive Care Medicine, 22,* 1269–1271. Evidence Level V: Review.

Christie, J. M., Dethelfsen, M., & Cane, R. D. (1996). Unplanned endotracheal extubation in the intensive care unit. *Journal of Clinical Anesthesia, 8,* 289–293. Evidence Level IV: Nonexperimental Study.

Egerod, I., Christensen, B. V., & Johansen, L. (2006). Nurses' and physicians' sedation practices in Danish ICUs in 2003: A national survey. *Intensive and Critical Care Nursing, 22,* 22–31. Evidence Level IV: Nonexperimental Study.

Evans, D., & Fitzgerald, M. (2002). Reasons for physically restraining patients and residents: A systematic review and content analysis. *International Journal of Nursing Studies, 39,* 735–743. Evidence Level IV: Nonexperimental Study.

Evans, D., Wood, J., & Lambert, L. (2003). Patient injury and physical restraint devices: A systematic review. *Journal of Advanced Nursing, 41*(3), 274–282. Evidence Level V: Review.

Federal Register (December 8, 2006). Part IV. Department of Health and Human Services, Centers for Medicare and Medicaid Services. 42 CFR Part 482 Medicare and Medicaid Programs; Hospital Conditions of Participation: Patients' Rights; Final Rule (pp. 71377–71428).

Fontaine, D. K. (1994). Nonpharmacologic management of patient distress during mechanical ventilation. *Critical Care Clinics, 10,* 695–708. Evidence Level V: Review.

Francis, J. (1989). Using restraints in the elderly because of fear of litigation. *New England Journal of Medicine, 320,* 870–871. Evidence Level VI: Expert Opinion.

Fraser, G. L., Riker, R. R., Prato, S., & Wilkins, M. L. (2001). The frequency and cost of patient-initiated device removal in the ICU. *Pharmacotherapy, 21*(1), 1–6. Evidence Level IV: Nonexperimental Study.

Frengley, J. D. (1996). The use of physical restraints and the absence of kindness. *Journal of the American Geriatrics Society, 44,* 1125–1127. Evidence Level V: Expert Opinion.

Frengley, J. D., & Mion, L. C. (1986). Incidence of physical restraints on acute general medical wards. *Journal of the American Geriatrics Society, 34,* 565–568. Evidence Level IV: Nonexperimental Study.

Frengley, J. D., & Mion, L. C. (1998). Physical restraints in the acute care setting: Issues and future direction. *Clinics in Geriatric Medicine, 14*(4), 727–743. Evidence Level V: Review.

Frezza, E. E., Carleton, G. L., & Valenziano, C. P. (2000). A quality improvement and risk management initiative for surgical ICU patients: A study of the effects of physical restraints and sedation on the incidence of self-extubation. *American Journal of Medical Quality, 15,* 221–225. Evidence Level III: Quasiexperimental Study.

Happ, M. B. (2000). Preventing treatment interference: The nurse's role in maintaining technologic devices. *Heart & Lung, 29,* 60–69. Evidence Level V: Review.

Health Care Financing Administration (HCFA) (1999, July). Medicare and Medicaid Programs, hospital conditions of participation: Patient's Rights: Interim Final Rule (42CFR Part 482). *Federal Register, 64*(127).

Houston, K., & Lach, H. (1990). Restraints: How do you score? *Geriatric Nursing, 4,* 231–232. Evidence Level V: Review.

Inouye, S. K., Bogardus, S. T., Jr., Charpentier, P. A., Leo-Summers, L., Acampora, D., Holford, T. R., et al. (1999). A multicomponent intervention to prevent delirium in hospitalized older patients. *New England Journal of Medicine, 340*(9), 669–676. Evidence Level II: Single Experimental Study.

Inouye, S. K., & Charpentier, P. A. (1996). Precipitating factors for delirium in hospitalized elderly persons: Predictive model and interrelationship with baseline vulnerability. *Journal of the American Medical Association, 275,* 852–857. Evidence Level IV: Nonexperimental Study.

Johnson, J. E., Billingsley, M. C., & Costa, L. L. (2006). Xtreme nursing and the nursing shortage. *Nursing Outlook, 54*(4), 294–299. Evidence Level VI: Expert Opinion.

Joint Commission on Accreditation of Healthcare Organizations (JCAHO) (2006). *2005 comprehensive accreditation manual for hospitals: The official handbook.* Oakbrook Terrace, IL: Author.

Kapadia, F. N., Bajan, K. B., & Raje, K. V. (2000). Airway accidents in intubated intensive care unit patients: An epidemiologic study. *Critical Care Medicine, 28,* 659–664. Evidence Level IV: Nonexperimental Study.

Kapp, M. B. (1994). Physical restraints in hospitals: Risk management's reduction role. *Journal of Healthcare Risk Management, 14*(1), 3–8. Evidence Level VI: Expert Opinion.

Kapp, M. B. (1999). Physical restraint use in acute care hospitals: Legal liability issues. *Elder's Advisor, 1*(1), 1–10. Evidence Level VI: Expert Opinion.

Kaufman, S. R. (1994). Old age, disease, and the discourse on risk: Geriatric assessment in U.S. health care. *Medical Anthropology Quarterly, 8*(4), 430–447. Evidence Level VI: Expert Opinion.

Lamb, K., Minnick, A., Mion, L. C., Palmer R., & Leipzig, R. (1999). Help the health care team release its hold on restraint. *Nursing Management, 30*(12), 19–24. Evidence Level IV: Non-experimental Study.

Landefeld, C. S., Palmer, R. M., Kresevic, D. M., Fortinsky, R. H., & Kowal, J. (1995). A randomized trial of care in a hospital medical unit especially designed to improve the functional outcomes of acutely ill older patients. *New England Journal of Medicine, 332*, 1338–1344. Evidence Level II: Single Experimental Study.

Leape, L. L., & Berwick, D. M. (2005). Five years after *To Err Is Human*: What have we learned? *Journal of the American Medical Association, 293*, 2384–2390.

Maccioli, G. A., Dorman, T., Brown, B. R., Mazuski, J. E., McLean, B. A., Kuszaj, J. M., et al. (2003). Clinical practice guidelines for the maintenance of patient physical safety in the intensive care unit: Use of restraining therapies – American College of Critical Care Medicine Task Force 2001–2002. *Critical Care Medicine, 31*(11), 2665–2676. Evidence Level VI: Expert Opinion.

MacPherson, D. S., Lofgren, R. P., Granieri, R., & Myllenbeck, S. (1990). Deciding to restrain medical patients. *Journal of the American Geriatrics Society, 38*, 516–520. Evidence Level IV: Nonexperimental Study.

Marcin, J. P., Rutan, E., Rapetti, P. M., Brown, J. P., Rahnamayi, R., & Pretzlaff, R. K. (2005). Nurse staffing and unplanned extubation in the pediatric intensive care unit. *Pediatric Critical Care Medicine, 6*, 254–257. Evidence Level IV: Nonexperimental Study.

Matthiesen, V., Lamb, K. V., McCann, J., Hollinger-Smith, L., & Walton, J. C. (1996). Hospital nurses' views about physical restraint use with older patients. *Journal of Gerontological Nursing, 22*(6), 8–16. Evidence Level IV: Nonexperimental Study.

Mehta, S., Burry, L., Fischer, S., Martinez-Motta, J. C., Hallett, D., Bowman, D., et al. (2006). Canadian survey of the use of sedatives, analgesics, and neuromuscular blocking agents in critically ill patients. *Critical Care Medicine, 34*, 374–380. Evidence Level IV: Nonexperimental Study.

Miles, S. H. (1993). Restraints and sudden death. *Journal of the American Geriatrics Society, 41*, 1013. Evidence Level V: Review.

Minnick, A. F., Mion, L. C., Johnson, M. E., Catrambone, C., & Leipzig, R. M. (2007). Prevalence and variation of physical restraint use in acute care settings in the U.S. *Journal of Nursing Scholarship, 39*(1), 30–37. Evidence Level IV: Nonexperimental Study.

Minnick, A. F., Mion, L. C., Leipzig, R., Lamb, K., & Palmer, R. M. (1998). Prevalence and patterns of physical restraint use in the acute care setting. *Journal of Nursing Administration, 28*(11), 19–24. Evidence Level IV: Nonexperimental Study.

Mion, L. C. (1992). Environmental restructuring. In G. M., Bulechek, & J. C., McCloskey (Eds.), *Nursing interventions: Treatments for nursing diagnoses* (pp. 254–264). Philadelphia: W. B. Saunders. Evidence Level VI: Expert Opinion.

Mion, L. C., Fogel, J., Sandhu, S., Palmer, R. M., Minnick, A. F., Cranston, T., et al. (2001). Outcomes following physical restraint reduction programs in two acute care hospitals. *Joint Commission Journal on Quality Improvement, 27*(11), 605–618. Evidence Level III: Quasi-experimental Study.

Mion, L. C., Frengley, J. D., Jakovcic, C. A., & Marino, J. A. (1989). A further exploration of physical restraints in hospitalized patients. *Journal of the American Geriatrics Society, 37*, 949–956. Evidence Level IV: Nonexperimental Study.

Mion, L. C., Minnick, A. F., Leipzig, R. M., Catrambone, C., & Johnson, M. E. (In Press). Patient-initiated device removal in intensive care units: A national prevalence study: Critical care medicine. Evidence Level IV: Nonexperimental Study.

Mion, L. C., Minnick, A., Palmer, R., Kapp, M. B., & Lamb, K. (1996). Physical restraint use in the hospital setting: Unresolved issues and directions for research. *Milbank Quarterly, 74*(3), 411–433. Evidence Level V: Review.

Mion, L. C., & Strumpf, N. (1994). Use of physical restraints in the hospital setting: Implications for the nurse. *Geriatric Nursing, 15*(3) 127–131. Evidence Level V: Review.

Moons, P., Sels, K., De Becker, W., De Geest, S., & Ferdinande, P. (2004). Development of risk assessment tool for deliberate self-extubation in intensive care patients. *Intensive Care Medicine, 30*, 1348–1355. Evidence Level IV: Nonexperimental Study.

Moss, R. J., & La Puma, J. (1991). The ethics of mechanical restraints. *Hastings Center Report, 21*(1), 22–25. Evidence Level VI: Expert Opinion.

Neary, M. A., Kanski, G., Janelli, J., Scherer, Y., & North, N. (1991). Restraint in the 90s. Restraints as nurses' aides see them. *Geriatric Nursing, 12*(4), 191–192. Evidence Level IV: Nonexperimental Study.

O'Keeffe, S., Jack, C. I., & Lye, M. (1996). Use of restraints and bedrails in a British hospital. *Journal of the American Geriatrics Society, 44*, 1125–1127. Evidence Level IV: Nonexperimental Study.

Oliver, D., Connelly, J. B., Victor, C. R., Shaw, F., Whitehead, A., Genc, Y., et al. (2007). Strategies to prevent falls and fractures in hospitals and care homes and effect of cognitive impairment: Systematic review and meta-analyses. *British Medical Journal, 334*(82), 82–85. Evidence Level I: Systematic Review.

Palmer, R. M., Landefeld, C. S., Kresevic, D. M., & Kowal, J. (1994). A medical unit for the acute care of the elderly. *Journal of the American Geriatrics Society, 42*, 545–552. Evidence Level VI: Expert Opinion.

Robbins, L. J., Boyko, E., Lane, J., Cooper, D., & Jahnigen, D. W. (1987). Binding the elderly: A prospective study of the use of mechanical restraints in an acute care hospital. *Journal of the American Geriatrics Society, 35*, 290–296. Evidence Level IV: Non-experimental Study.

Robinson, B. E. (1995). Death by destruction of will: Lest we forget. *Archives of Internal Medicine, 155*, 2250–2251. Evidence Level VI: Expert Opinion.

Schafer, A. (1985). Restraints and the elderly: When safety and autonomy conflict. *Canadian Medical Association Journal, 132*(11), 1257–1260. Evidence Level VI: Expert Opinion.

Scherer, Y. K. (1991). The nursing dilemma of restraints. *Journal of Gerontological Nursing, 17*(2), 14–17, 32–34. Evidence Level VI: Expert Opinion.

Scherer, Y. K., Janelli, L. M., Wu, Y. W., & Kuhn, M. M. (1993). Restrained patients: An important issue for critical care nursing. *Heart Lung, 22*(1), 77–83. Evidence Level V: Review.

Schott-Baer, D., Lusis, S., & Beauregard K. (1995). Use of restraints: Change in nurses' attitudes. *Journal of Gerontological Nursing, 21*(2), 39–44. Evidence Level IV: Non-experimental Study.

Siegel, M. D. (2003). Management of agitation in the intensive care unit. *Clinics in Chest Medicine, 24*(4), 713–725. Evidence Level VI: Expert Opinion.

Slomka, L., Agich, G. J., Stagno, S., & Smith, M. L. (1998). Physical restraint elimination in the acute care setting: Ethical considerations. *Healthcare Ethics Committee Forum, 10*(3–4), 244–262. Evidence Level VI: Expert Opinion.

Strumpf, N. E., & Evans, L. K. (1988). Physical restraint of the hospitalized elderly: Perceptions of patients and nurses. *Nursing Research, 37*(3), 132–137. Evidence Level IV: Nonexperimental Study.

Tasota, F. J., Hoffman, L. A., Zullo, T. G., & Jamison, G. (1987). Evaluation of two methods used to stabilize oral endotracheal tubes. *Heart & Lung, 16*, 140–146. Evidence Level II: Simple Experimental Study.

Tinetti, M. E., Inouye, S. K., Gill, T. M., & Doucette, J. T. (1995). Shared risk factors for falls, incontinence, and functional dependence: Unifying the approach to geriatric syndromes. *Journal of the American Medical Association, 273*, 1348–1353. Evidence Level VI: Expert Opinion.

Tominaga, G. T., Rudzwick, H., Scannell, G., & Waxman, K. (1995). Decreasing unplanned extubations in the surgical intensive care unit. *American Journal of Surgery, 170*, 586–590. Evidence Level III: Quasi-experimental Study.

U.S. Food and Drug Administration (March 9, 2006). FDA News: FDA issues guidance on hospital bed design to reduce patient entrapment. P06-36. Accessed at www.fda.gov/bbs/topics/NEWS/2006/NEW01331.html.

Weinhart, C. R., Chan, L., & Gross, C. (2001). Sedating critically ill patients: Factors affecting nurses' delivery of sedative therapy. *American Journal of Critical Care, 10*, 156–165. Evidence Level IV: Nonexperimental Study.

Whitman, G. R., Davidson, L. F., Sereika, S. M., & Rudy, E. B. (2001). Staffing and pattern of mechanical restraint use across a multiple hospital system. *Nursing Research, 50*(6), 356–362. Evidence Level IV: Nonexperimental Study.

Williams, M. A. (1988). The physical environment and patient care. Annual Review of Nursing, 6, 61–84. Evidence Level VI: Expert Opinion.

Williams, C. C., & Finch, C. E. (1997). Physical restraint: Not fit for woman, man, or beast. *Journal of the American Geriatrics Society, 45,* 773. Evidence Level VI: Expert Opinion.

Health Care Decision Making

23

Ethel L. Mitty
Linda Farber Post

Educational Objectives

On completion of this chapter, the reader should be able to:

1. define informed consent and the supporting bioethical and legal principles

2. understand the role of culture in treatment decision making

3. differentiate between competence and capacity

4. understand the process of assessment of decisional capacity

5. describe a nurse's role and responsibility as an advocate for a patient's voice in treatment decision making

Overview

Until the latter half of the 20th century, patients were told which health care interventions would benefit them and they rarely questioned the doctor's instructions. The rise of the rights movement in most areas of society promoted the idea that patients would benefit from robust participation in health care decision making affecting their health outcomes. Building on the well-established doctrine of informed consent, statutory law, and case law, all states came to

For a description of Evidence Levels cited in this chapter, see chapter 1, Developing and Evaluating Clinical Practice Guidelines, page 4.

require that patient wishes and values be central to treatment decisions. The result was a greater degree of clinician–patient collaboration in planning and implementing care decisions affecting them.

Health care is about decisions. How and whether health care and treatment are provided, limited, or modified depends on who makes the decisions and according to what standards. In this chapter, *treatment* is considered a therapeutic intervention, either a single act or a coordinated plan of care, intended to affect cure or improve the disease or injury-caused process. Similarly, diagnostic interventions are specific tests intended to assist the identification and assessment of clinical conditions that may benefit from treatment. *Care* or *caring* is considered a series of acts (including treatments, diagnostic tests, activities of daily living [ADLs], planning for discharge or future therapy, and provision of comfort measures) that defines the clinical interaction. Care is seen as a philosophy or attitude of nurturing that encompasses all aspects of the therapeutic dynamic, including both cure-oriented and palliative ministrations.

Although all health care activities require principled and thoughtful decision making, treatment and diagnostic interventions—because of their benefit-burden-risk calculus—typically require specific informed consent by or on behalf of the patient. For this reason, the determination of decision-making capacity, authority, and standards becomes a most pressing clinical issue when deciding about treatment or diagnostic interventions.

Background

Ethical Principles and Professional Obligations

Core ethical principles that underlie the health care decision process and give rise to clinician obligations include the following:

- Respect for autonomy: supporting and facilitating a capable patient's exercise of self-determination
- Beneficence: promoting a patient's best interest and well-being and protecting the patient from harm
- Nonmaleficence: avoiding actions likely to cause a patient harm
- Distributive justice: allocating fairly the benefits and burdens related to health care delivery (Beauchamp & Childress, 2001)

These principles and the professional obligations they create often give rise to conflict and tension for clinicians. For example, care providers are expected to respect patients' autonomy by honoring their decisions *and* protecting them from the harm of risky choices. Care providers are also expected to provide care to patients who need it *and* be responsible stewards of limited resources. Clinical, legal, and ethically valid decisions by or for patients invoke a careful balancing of information, principles, rights, and responsibilities in the light of medical realities, cultural factors, and, increasingly, concerns about resource allocation.

Autonomy, Capacity, and Consent

The well-settled right to determine what shall be done with one's own body has two equally important components: the right to consent to treatment and the right to refuse treatment. Grounded in the ethical principle of respect for persons, this right to bodily integrity is considered so fundamental that it is protected by the U.S. Constitution, state constitutions, and decisions of the U.S. Supreme Court (Cruzan, 1990; Rivers, 1986). All persons are considered to have the potential for autonomy, expressed in the clinical setting through informed decision making. The threshold question is whether they have the *capacity* to act autonomously.

Autonomy is widely considered to be the ethical principle most central to health care decision making because of its emphasis on self-governance and choices that reflect personal values. The heightened emphasis on self-determination is largely a Western phenomenon and not universally shared. Capable patients who are elderly, those who are easily confused or with diminished or fluctuating capacity, or from cultures that do not consider autonomy a central value may not be capable of or comfortable with pure autonomous decision making. Instead, they may involve trusted others in planning their care, thus exhibiting *assisted, supported,* or *delegated* autonomy as their preferred method of decision making. For these patients, autonomy may not be reflected in self-determined decision making about treatment but rather in expressions of values and goals of care. Thus, diminished or fluctuating capacity should be seen not as the reason to ignore the patient's voice but rather as an indicator to attend more carefully to what is being communicated. The "what" and "how" of the treatment may be a decision of others to make; the "why" in the patient's voice must be heard.

Consent and Refusal

In the clinical setting, the principle of respect for autonomy is most clearly expressed in the doctrine of informed consent and refusal (Beauchamp & Childress, 2001). Because therapeutic and diagnostic interventions typically involve a range of benefits, burdens, and risks, express consent is almost always required before they are implemented. Consent should be a process over time rather than a single event or a signed document. As an expression of autonomy, the process can be solitary or, more likely, a collaborative process that includes consultation with clinicians, family, and trusted others.

Capable patients or surrogates acting on behalf of patients without capacity are engaged in a process, which is considered to include the following elements:

- decisional capacity
- disclosure of sufficient information relevant to the decision in question
- understanding of the information provided
- voluntariness (a patient's right to make health care choices free of any undue influence) in choosing among the options, and, on the basis of these
- consent to or refusal of the intervention (Lo, 2000)

Research shows that patients may lack sufficient information to make an informed, autonomous choice (Agard, Hermeren, & Herlitz, 2001 [Level II]). Education can improve decisional capacity to give safe, informed consent, even for clinically depressed older adults (Lapid, Rumman, Pankratz, & Applebaum, 2004 [Level II]). In addition, a physician's emphasis on the distinctions about the efficacy of a treatment, as to whether it would be curative or palliative, can influence a patient's decision even more than information given about the disease or treatment options; "framing" can be persuasive (van Kleffens, van Baarsen, & van Leeuwen, 2004 [Level IV]).

Decision-Making Authority

Decisions about treatment are typically made by capable patients based on their goals and values in response to information they receive about their diagnosis, prognosis, and therapeutic options. These decisions are thus an expression of autonomy, reflecting the view that health care is not something that is *done to* patients; rather, it is a collaborative endeavor in which patients and clinicians contribute to the shared goal of recovery, rehabilitation, or palliation. Only when patients are not capable of making decisions about their treatment are others asked to choose for them, basing their decisions as much as possible on what is known of the patients' preferences or what is considered to be in their best interest. Autonomous decision making is not the same as isolated decision making, and drawing on the assistance or support of trusted others does not diminish the integrity of the process. As noted previously, even capable patients may choose to include others in the process. Voluntarily delegating decision-making authority to others is also an autonomous choice, but it is one that must be explicitly confirmed, not inferred.

The determination of decision-making authority is among the most critical tasks in the clinical setting. Capable persons have a well-settled right, grounded in law and ethics, to determine what is done to their bodies, an exercise of autonomy expressed most fully in the doctrine of informed consent and refusal. When patients lack the ability to make treatment decisions, authority to act on their behalf must be vested in others—appointed agents, family, or other surrogates. The threshold determination, then, is of the patient's decisional capacity: an assessment of an individual's ability to make decisions about health care and treatment.

Assessment

Decision-Making Capacity

Although the terms *capacity* and *competence* are often used interchangeably, in the health care setting their distinctions go beyond semantics. Competence is a *legal* presumption that an adult has the mental ability to negotiate various legal tasks, such as entering into a contract, making a will, and standing for trial (Beauchamp & Childress, 2001). Incompetence is a judicial determination that because a person lacks this ability, he or she should be prevented from doing certain things (Beauchamp & Childress, 2001). Capacity is a *clinical* determination that a person has the ability to understand, make, and take responsibility for the consequences of health care decisions (Beauchamp & Childress, 2001). Because the legal system is and should be rarely involved in medical decisions, it is customary to determine a patient's capacity for decision making, an assessment made by clinicians.

The importance of capacity determination can be appreciated in the presumption that adults have decisional capacity and, absent contrary evidence, treatment decisions defer to patient wishes. Moreover, this deference usually extends to all decisions made by individuals with capacity, including those decisions that appear risky or ill advised. Capacity assessment is important because patients who lack the ability to appreciate the implications of and accept responsibility for their choices are vulnerable to the risks of deficient decision making. Whereas honoring the decisions of a capacitated patient demonstrates respect for the person, honoring the decisions of a patient without capacity is an act of abandonment. Thus, clinicians have an obligation to ensure that capable patients have the opportunity to make treatment decisions that will be implemented and that incapacitated patients will be protected by having decisions made for them by others who act in their best interest.

Fulfilling this obligation requires that clinicians appreciate the characteristics of decision-making capacity. The elements of decisional capacity include the ability to:

- understand and process information about diagnosis, prognosis, and treatment options
- weigh the relative benefits, burdens, and risks of the care options
- apply a set of values to the analysis
- arrive at a decision that is consistent over time
- communicate the decision (Roth, Meisel, & Lidz, 1997)

Capacity assessment depends on interaction with the patient over time rather than on specific tests. There is no "gold standard" instrument or "capacimeter" that assesses decisional capacity (Kapp & Mossman, 1996). The Mini-Mental Status Examination (MMSE) estimates orientation, long- and short-term memory, and mathematical and language dexterity. It is not a test of executive function (an assessment more likely to broach reasoning and recall) and is, therefore, less helpful in gauging a patient's ability to understand the implications of a decision (Allen et al., 2003 [Level IV]). It has been suggested, however, that an MMSE score below 19 or above 23 might be able to differentiate those with capacity from those who lack capacity for decision making (Karlawish, Casarett, James, Xie, & Kim, 2005 [Level IV]). Persons with mild to moderate dementia ($n = 88$) can make or at least participate in treatment decision making, but impaired memory recall might be a barrier to demonstrating their understanding of treatment options (Moye, Karel, Azar, & Gurrera, 2004 [Level IV]). Standard assessment of appreciation of diagnostic and treatment information should focus on the patient's ability to state the importance or implications of the choice on his or her future health state. Specific neuropsychological tests (e.g., MacArthur Competence Assessment Tool, Hopemount Capacity Assessment Interview) can predict decisional capacity for those with mild-to-moderate dementia, although reasoning and appreciation might differ among those with mental illness (Gurrera, Moye, Karel, Azar, & Armesto, 2006 [Level IV]).

Among a group of respondents including geriatricians, psychologists, and ethics committees members, most agreed about the elements that have to be present to determine decisional capacity for health care decision making (Volicer & Ganzini, 2003 [Level IV]). The standard of decision making most highly valued is the ability to appreciate the consequences of a decision followed by the ability to respond "yes" or "no" to a question; the standard least supported is that the decision has to seem reasonable.

A review of the research on decision-making capacity of cognitively impaired older adults (Kim & Karlawish, 2003 [Level V]) reports that of 32 relevant studies, there is no consistent standardized definition of decisional capacity. Among the studies examined, there is sufficient evidence that safe and appropriate decision making is retained in early-stage dementia. Cognitive changes associated with the stages of Alzheimer's disease (AD) were examined in relationship to different legal thresholds of competency: capacity to make a choice (minimal legal standard [LS 1]), capacity to appreciate the consequences of a decision (moderate standard [LS 3]), and capacity to understand the medical situation and options (stringent standard [LS 5]). Receptive aphasia and severe dysnomia associated with advanced AD precluded making a simple treatment choice (LS 1). Patients with mild to moderate AD, evidenced by impaired executive function, lack the capacity to identify treatment consequences (LS 3). Multiple deficits in ability to conceptualize, verbal recall, and word memory preclude AD patients' understanding of diagnoses and treatment options (LS 5) (Marson, Chatterjee, Ingram, & Harrell, 1996 [Level IV]).

Decisional capacity is a clinical judgment that should be made by care professionals most familiar with the patient. Nursing staff are ideally situated to contribute important and necessary information. Because capacity may fluctuate, decision-making ability should be assessed over time rather than at a given moment (Mezey, Mitty, & Ramsey, 1997 [Level V]).

Clinical Importance of Decisional Capacity

Accurate and useful capacity assessment depends on the recognition that capacity is decision-specific rather than global. For example, a person with diminished capacity may be able to decide what to have for lunch or when to shower. Evidence also suggests that adults with mild-to-moderate mental retardation are able to make and provide a rationale for their treatment decisions and evaluate the risks and benefits of treatment options (Cea & Fisher, 2003 [Level IV]). Because most people have the ability to make some decisions and not others, respect for autonomy requires clinicians to identify the widest range of decisions each patient is capable of making. A note in the chart saying, "Patient lacks decision-making capacity" arbitrarily precludes the individual from making any decisions about anything when, in fact, the patient may only lack the ability to make complex treatment decisions. Far more helpful would be an entry that says, "Patient lacks the capacity to make decisions about participation in a drug study."

Likewise, decisional capacity may not be constant but may fluctuate, depending on the clinical condition, medication, and/or the time of day. It is imperative for the protection of those with mild-to-moderate dementia that their understanding and reasoning with regard to treatments and interventions is periodically assessed (Moye, Karel, Gurrera, & Azar, 2006 [Level IV]). Approaching patients for discussions and decisions when they are at their most capable (e.g., during the patient's "window of lucidity") enhances their opportunities to participate in determining their treatment and health care.

Whereas disagreement with a proposed care plan or refusal of recommended treatment does not by itself demonstrate incapacity, risky or potentially harmful decisions should be carefully scrutinized to protect vulnerable patients from the consequences of deficient decision making. Because appointing a health care proxy agent requires a lower level of capacity than that needed to make the often complex decisions the agent will make, even patients with diminished capacity may be able to select the persons they want to speak for them (Mezey, Teresi, Ramsey, Mitty, & Bobrowitz, 2002 [Level IV]).

Decision Making in the Absence of Capacity

The more difficult clinical scenario is decision making on behalf of patients who have lost or never had the capacity to make decisions for themselves. Two approaches have been developed in response to the needs of incapacitated patients: advance directives and surrogate decision making. Advance directives (see chapter 24, *Advance Directives*) include the living will (i.e., a list of interventions the patient does or does not want in specified circumstances) and the preferred directive, the health care proxy (i.e., the appointment of a health care agent with the same decision-making authority as the patient).

Because only 15% to 25% of the adult population in the United States has advance directives, the majority of health care decisions for incapacitated patients are made by surrogates. Absent explicit instructions from the patient, decisions by others are based on either substituted judgment (when the patient's wishes are known or can be inferred) or the best-interest standard (when the patient did not have or articulate treatment preferences). Substituted judgment assesses what the *patient* would choose, based on prior statements and patterns of decision making. The best-interest standard is the *surrogate's* evaluation of the proposed intervention's benefits and burdens to the patient.

A health care surrogate may be any competent adult older than 18 who, although not specifically chosen or legally appointed by a patient, assumes the responsibility for making health care decisions on behalf of a person who does not have the ability to do so. In some states, statutory or case law provides authority for surrogates to make substitute decisions. Informal surrogates are individuals, usually family or others close to the patient, who are asked by the care team to participate in making treatment decisions. Most states accord considerable latitude to surrogates, especially next of kin, in consenting to treatment. Decisions about limiting treatment are more problematic and may be significantly restricted, depending on the state in which the patient is receiving care (See Resources, American Bar Association Commission on Law & Aging, for state guidelines).

Context of Health Care Decision Making

Studies indicate that individual treatment preferences can change as a patient's health and functional status changes (Fried et al., 2006 [Level IV]) and that patients may have different treatment and comfort goals than their family care-givers and professional providers (Steinhauser et al., 2000 [Level IV]). Previously unacceptable treatment states can become more acceptable. For example, patients already experiencing pain are less likely to refuse a treatment outcome that includes being in pain than patients who are not currently experiencing moderate to severe pain (Fried et al., 2006 [Level IV]). Steinhauser and colleagues found that being able to maintain a sense of humor and knowing what to expect were more important to patients than to their family members or physician (Steinhauser et al., 2000 [Level IV]).

Illness is not only a condition but a social role (Segall, 1976). Culture defines and sanctions adoption of the sick role. Being in the sick role means being exempt from social obligations (e.g., spouse, breadwinner, parent, caregiver), seeking advice, and doing as advised. The role trajectory includes recognition that being sick is an undesirable state and should be ended as soon as possible. Culture influences member attitudes toward truth-telling or disclosure, life-sustaining treatment, and decision-making processes (Kagawa-Singer & Blackhall, 2001 [Level V]). For the patient whose decision-making ability is questionable or deteriorating, the nature of communication, amount of information provided, and boundaries of acceptable decision making may impel the surrogate to protect the individual from an inappropriate and/or risky decision. Moving away from the divisive notion that decision making is either family- or patient-centered, the challenge in situations in which the individual's decisional capacity may be wavering is to determine how much support the family (and others) can give to the patient's decision making and how much decision making must be done by others.

Just as there is the right to know one's medical information, there is also a right not to be burdened with unwanted information. Some persons—for example, some older adults and those from cultures that traditionally shield patients from knowing about their illness—may prefer to have information given to and decision making assumed by a particular family member, the family as a group, or trusted others. Although it is important to respect patient preferences and cultural traditions, a patient's waiver of the disclosure obligation must be explicitly confirmed, not presumed. Since the implementation of HIPAA, many hospitals have a form for the patient to sign designating who this decision maker will be. One approach is to ask, "When we have information about your condition and decisions will need to be made, who would you like us to talk to? Would you like to be part of those discussions? What would make you comfortable?"

Trust in professional health care providers is a critical element in health care and no less so in decision-making situations in which information is given and questions have to be answered. A national sample reported that African American patients were significantly more likely than White patients to report low trust, unrelated to age or socioeconomic status (Halbert, Armstrong, Gandy, & Shaker, 2006 [Level IV]).

Using focus-group methodology, 73 male and female adults (age range 50 to 3) provided ample evidence of diversity within and across ethnic groups with regard to end-of-life treatment preferences (Duffy, Jackson, Schim, Ronis, & Fowler, 2006 [Level IV]). Among Arab Muslims, Arab Christians, Hispanic, Black, and White participants, some were against assisted suicide, telling the patient "bad news," and artificial feeding. Between groups, some participants were opposed to nursing homes and favored extending life. Within specific groups, the men and women were sometimes on opposite sides of an issue. Treatment decision making for care at the end of life clearly needs to be adapted to an individual's culturally specific preferences.

Quality-of-Life Considerations in Decision Making

Even in the presence of diminishing or questionable capacity, a patient's notion of quality of life, as death approaches, may differ from those of their physicians or families (Kim & Karlawish, 2002 [Level V]; Rosenfeld, Wenger, & Kagawa-Singer, 2000 [Level IV]; Steinhauser et al., 2000 [Level IV]). Whereas there is almost universal acknowledgment of the desire to be comfortable (i.e., relief from pain and suffering) and to achieve a sense of completion, attitudes about the importance of clergy, of being physically touched, of using all available technology can vary (Steinhauser et al., 2000). In one study, 21 older adults (average age 83), with varying degrees of functional impairment and past experiences with treatment decision making, were more interested in the outcome of a serious medical event than with the interventions that might be used to cure them (Rosenfeld et al., 2000 [Level IV]). Participants were interested in a treatment insofar as it could restore or maintain their ability to participate in activities they valued. "Acceptable health states" in the face of advanced age were relevant discussion points rather than specific interventions. Among physicians, nurses, and family members in two nursing homes in The Netherlands, decisions about withholding artificial nutrition and hydration were more influenced by a patient's medical condition, likely trajectory of illness, and inferred quality of life than by a duly executed advance directive (The, Pasman, Onwuteaka-Philipsen, Ribbe, & van der Wal, 2002 [Level IV]).

Interventions

Assessing a patient's orientation and understanding can provide critical information about decision-making behavior in different circumstances and ability to articulate wishes about care. Reporting that a patient is "disoriented to time and place" is helpful only in establishing the context in which more specific and useful assessment of decisional capacity should take place.

Documentation needs to be specific and descriptive. The entry should describe the circumstances or interaction that led to the conclusion about a patient's ability to make decisions. Because capacity is decision-specific, it is not helpful to read, "Patient lacks capacity to make decisions." The implication is that the patient lacks the ability to make any and all decisions. More accurate and useful statements are "Patient appears to lack the capacity to make decisions about discharge. She is unable to describe how she will cook or get to the bathroom at home" or "Patient lacks the capacity to make decisions about surgery; he was unable to name the type of surgery, what the surgery is supposed to correct, or what is involved or to be expected in recovery after surgery."

Communicating needed information includes determining what the decision maker(s)—including the patient or other surrogate(s)—want to know, who should participate, determining what the patient and family understand, having the relevant medical facts available, and avoiding jargon. It can be useful to consider the participants in the decision making: Who should be present? What is their actual relationship and their decision-making relationship to the patient? Why is the information necessary and how will it be used? At what level of detail? When is the information to be provided; over what period of time? Where will the discussion take place (i.e., patient's room or other private place)? Popejoy (2005 [Level V]) commented on the importance of understanding how patients and their families make decisions, the processes and steps they go through, the congruence between their expectations, and the likely goals of treatment.

Interpreters might be the only health care staff who recognize that substitute decision makers and the physician/health care professionals have differing interpretations of illness, treatment and health; disparate views about death and dying; and use language and a decision-making framework differently. An interpreter may realize that truth-telling might not only be disrespectful and dangerous but could shorten the patient's life span, as believed in certain cultures. As such, ideally, an interpreter is more than a word-for-word translator but rather a mediator, culture broker, patient advocate, witness, educator, and participator who is interpreting fact and nuance.

Case Study and Discussion

Mr. Peters is an 85-year-old man with advanced Alzheimer's disease who has been living in a nursing home for the past 6 months. His condition has been deteriorating and, when he stopped eating several weeks ago, he was hospitalized for the insertion of a PEG tube to provide artificial nutrition and hydration. He returned to the nursing home briefly but developed uncontrolled diarrhea and apparent abdominal discomfort. Two days ago, his PEG tube fell out and he has been readmitted to the hospital for treatment of the diarrhea and possible replacement of the PEG.

Mr. Peters opens his eyes and responds to painful stimuli but does not interact and appears not to recognize family members. He is clearly incapable of participating in discussions or decisions about care and has no advance directives to provide guidance about his wishes. He does have close family, however, including his son and granddaughter, who are visiting from California, and his grandson, Jason, who has been very involved for several years in providing and making decisions about care.

A clinical ethics consultation has been convened, including Mr. Peters's family, his two attending physicians, and the house and nursing staff who have cared for him most consistently. Discussion focuses on clarifying his condition and probable clinical course, the goals of care, and his likely care preferences.

Jason describes his grandfather as very active and fiercely independent until age 78, when his dementia began. With his wife, he had raised Jason and, when she died, he continued to raise the boy alone until he left for college. When the dementia worsened several years ago, Jason arranged for his grandfather and a team of 24-hour caregivers to move into an apartment next to his. That arrangement continued until Mr. Peters required care that could best be provided in a skilled-nursing facility. All three family members agree that, given Mr. Peters's personality, values, and lifetime behavior pattern, he would not have wanted to be maintained in his current condition, especially dependent on artificial nutrition and hydration. Nevertheless, they express concern about the ethics, legality, and clinical effect of not replacing the PEG tube, and they are especially uncomfortable about whether it would be considered "starving" him to death.

According to the care team, Mr. Peters's advanced dementia is not reversible and he will continue to deteriorate mentally and physically until death. The doctors referred to the considerable literature demonstrating that, in patients with advanced dementia, artificial nutrition and hydration can cause GI distress, including nausea, bloating, gas, and diarrhea, which appears to have happened to Mr. Peters. In the opinion of the care team, continued artificial nutrition and hydration would only contribute to the patient's suffering and prolong the dying process. The doctors also explain that, far from suffering, Mr. Peters appears more comfortable since the PEG fell out and the diarrhea has stopped. They assure the family that the patient could be admitted to the nursing home's hospice unit, where he will receive comfort care, including pain and other symptom management.

The ethics analysis of this case focuses on decision making for an incapacitated patient, promoting the patient's best interest, and protecting him from harm, and forgoing life-sustaining treatment, specifically artificial nutrition and hydration, at the end of life.

Surrogate decision making on behalf of patients lacking capacity uses the following standards:

- the patient's wishes as expressed directly through discussions with others or in advance directives (i.e., health care proxy appointments or living wills)
- substituted judgment (when the patient's wishes are known or can be inferred)
- the best-interest standard (when the patient's wishes are not known or inferable) (Beauchamp & Childress, 2001)

Mr. Peters has not left any explicit instructions, but his family, knowing him very well, is able to predict with confidence what he would and would not have wanted based on his characteristic patterns of behavior and decision making. In this case, the family's substituted judgment is consistent with what was considered by the family and the care team to be in the patient's best interest, protecting him from continued artificial nutrition and hydration that would have increased his suffering without providing benefit and prolonged his dying.

One of the most difficult surrogate decisions is forgoing life-sustaining treatment and, because providing nourishment is so intimately associated with love and nurturing, forgoing artificial nutrition and hydration is especially wrenching for families and caregivers. Clinicians, ethicists, and courts have consistently agreed that artificial nutrition and hydration is a medical treatment, the benefits, burdens, and risks of which should be assessed like those of any other intervention.

How these decisions are made for Mr. Peters will depend as much on state law as on his clinical condition and his family's concern for his well-being. Capable patients and the appointed health care agents of incapacitated patients have a well-settled right to refuse any treatment, including those that are life-sustaining. Absent capacity or advance directives, the family's authority to make end-of-life decisions, including forgoing artificial nutrition and hydration, depends on the laws of the state in which the patient is treated. Many states permit family and surrogates authorized by case or statutory law to make these decisions based on substituted judgment or their assessment of the patient's best interest. Other states, such as New York and Missouri, require surrogates, even next of kin, to provide explicit evidence that the patient would have refused life-sustaining treatment, particularly artificial nutrition and hydration, in order to authorize withholding or withdrawing the interventions.

Summary

Health care decision making should be, in and of itself, a therapeutic interaction between and among the key players. Paterson and colleagues (2001) suggest a paradigm for those living with and managing their chronic illness; a model that reflects the individual's pursuit of their preferences and lifestyle, and a perspective that behaviors contrary to the prescribed medical regimen should not be construed as noncompliant (Paterson, Russell, & Thorne, 2001 [Level V]). Their view of the rational decision making exercised on a daily basis by those living with chronic illness facilitates understanding that health care decision making is grounded in personal values and context. The notion of "ownership" of one's body should apply to health care decision making even at times of crisis. Paterson and colleagues advise viewing the decision-making process as one that in all likelihood contains conflicting goals and expectations among the various parties, framing issues, social and cultural factors, and complex processes in meaning making.

In summary, every capable patient who is temporarily confused or has fluctuating decisional capacity should not be denied the opportunity to make the specific health care decisions they are capable of making. A vulnerable patient who lacks capacity, despite some social or conversational skills, needs to be protected from the potentially harmful effects of uninformed, poorly reasoned, and potentially risky health care decisions. The ethical obligations that must be assumed by health care professionals are skillfully assessing the clinical situation; the benefits, burdens, and risks of the therapeutic options; the patient's capacity to make and take responsibility for the relevant decisions; and the proxy's need for guidance and information.

Resources

American Bar Association (ABA)
321 North Clark Street
Chicago, IL 60610
312.988.5000
and/or
American Bar Association (ABA)
740 15th Street, N.W.
Washington, DC 20005-1019
202.662.1000
www.abanet.org

American Bar Association Commission on Law & Aging, Legislative Updates
See link for chart that summarizes the wide variation in how states allocate
    decisional authority in the absence of patient capacity to make health care
    decisions.
http://www.abanet.org/aging/legislativeupdates/home.shtml

American Society of Bioethics and Humanities
4700 W. Lake
Glenview, IL 60025-1485
Telephone: 847.375.4745
Fax: 877.734.9385
Email: info@asbh.org
www.asbh.org

The Hastings Center
21 Malcolm Gordon Road
Garrison, NY 10524-4125
Telephone: 845.424.4040
Fax: 845.424.4545
Email: mail@thehastingscenter.org
www.thehastingscenter.org

Box 23.1

Nursing Standard of Practice Protocol: Health Care Decision Making

I. GOALS

To ensure nurses in acute care:
A. Understand the supporting bioethical and legal principles of in-
    formed consent.
B. Are able to differentiate between competence and capacity.

C. Understand the issues and process of assessing decisional capacity.
D. Can describe the nurse's role and responsibility as an advocate for the patient's voice in health care decision making.

II. OVERVIEW

A. Capable persons (i.e., those with decisional capacity) have a well-established right, grounded in law and Western bioethics, to determine what is done to their bodies.
B. In any health care setting, the exercise of autonomy (self-determination) is seen in the process of informed consent to and refusal of treatment and/or care planning.
C. Determination of decision-making capacity is a compelling clinical issue because treatment and diagnostic interventions have the potential for significant benefit, burden, and/or risk.
D. Honoring the decisions of a capable patient demonstrates respect for the person; honoring the decisions of a patient without capacity is an act of abandonment.

III. BACKGROUND AND STATEMENT OF PROBLEM

A. Introduction
1. Core ethical principles that are the foundation of clinician obligation are:
   a. Respect for autonomy, beneficence, nonmaleficence, and distributive justice.
   b. Clinically, legally, and ethically valid decisions by or for patients requires a careful balancing of information, principles, rights, and responsibilities in light of medical realities, cultural factors, and, increasingly, concerns about resource allocation.
   c. Even capable patients, including those who are elderly, easily confused, or from cultures that do not consider autonomy a central value, as well as patients with diminished or fluctuating capacity, may not be capable of or comfortable with exercising purely autonomous decision making.
   d. Care professionals have an obligation to be alert to questionable or fluctuating capacity both in patients who refuse and those who consent to recommended treatment. Capable individuals may choose to make their own care decisions or they may voluntarily delegate decision-making authority to trusted others. Delegation of decisional authority must be explicitly confirmed, not inferred.
   e. The context of decision making can include cultural imperatives and taboos, perceptions of pain, suffering and quality of life and death, education and socioeconomic status, language barriers, and advance health care planning.

B. Definitions
1. *Consent*: the informed-consent process requires evidence of decisional capacity, disclosure of sufficient information, understanding of the information provided, voluntariness in choosing among the options, and, on those bases, consent to or refusal of the intervention.
2. *Competence*: a *legal* presumption that an adult has the mental ability to negotiate various legal tasks (e.g., entering into a contract, making a will).
3. *Incompetence*: a *judicial* determination that a person lacks the ability to negotiate legal tasks and should be prevented from doing so.
4. *Decisional capacity*: a *clinical* determination that an individual has the ability to understand and to make and take responsibility for the consequences of health decisions. Because capacity is not global but decision-specific, patients may have the ability to make some decisions but not others. Capacity may fluctuate according to factors, including clinical condition, time of day, medications, and psychological and comfort status.
C. Essential Elements
1. Decisional capacity reflects the ability to understand the facts, appreciate the implications, and assume responsibility for the consequences of a decision.
2. The elements of decisional capacity: the ability to understand and process information; weigh the relative benefits, burdens, and risks of each option; apply personal values to the analysis; arrive at a consistent decision; and communicate the decision.
3. Standards of decision making:
   a. Prior explicit articulation: decision based on the previous expression of a capable person's wishes through oral or written comments or instructions.
   b. Substituted judgment: decision by others based on the formerly capable person's wishes that are known or can be inferred from prior behaviors or decisions.
   c. Best-interest standard: decision based on what others judge to be in the best interest of an individual who never had or made known health care wishes and whose preferences cannot be inferred.

IV. ASSESSMENT OF DECISIONAL CAPACITY

A. There is no "gold standard" instrument to assess capacity.
B. Assessment should occur over a period of time, at different times of day, and with attention to the patient's comfort level.
C. The MMSE or Mini-Cog is not a test of capacity. Tests of executive function might better approximate the reasoning and recall needed to understand the implications of a decision.

D. Clinicians agree that the ability to understand the consequences of a decision is an important indicator of decisional capacity.

E. Safe and appropriate decision-making is retained in early-stage dementia (Kim & Karlawish, 2002 [Level V]) and by adults with mild to moderate mental retardation (Cea & Fisher, 2003 [Level IV]).

V. NURSING CARE STRATEGIES

A. Communicate with patient and family or other/surrogate decision makers to enhance their understanding of treatment options.

B. Be sensitive to racial, ethnic, religious, and cultural mores and traditions regarding end-of-life care planning, disclosure of information, and care decisions.

C. Be aware of conflict resolution support and systems available in the care-providing organization.

D. Observe, document, and report the patient's ability to:
1. articulate his or her needs and preferences
2. follow directions
3. make simple choices and decisions (e.g., "Do you prefer the TV on or off?" "Do you prefer orange juice or water?")
4. communicate consistent care wishes

E. Observe period(s) of confusion and lucidity; document the specific time(s) when the patient seems more or less "clear." Observation and documentation of the patient's mental state should occur during the day, evening, and at night.

F. Understanding is assessed relative to the particular decision at issue. The following probes and statements are useful in assessing the degree to which the patient has the skills necessary to make a health care decision:
- "Tell me in your own words what the physician explained to you."
- "Tell me which parts, if any, were confusing."
- "What do you feel you have to *gain* by agreeing to (the proposed intervention)?"
- "Tell me what you feel you have to *lose* by agreeing to (the proposed intervention)?"
- "Tell me what you feel you have to gain/lose by refusing (the proposed intervention)?"
- "Tell me why this decision is important (difficult, frightening, etc.) to you."

G. Select (or construct) appropriate decision aids.

H. Help the patient express what he or she understands about the clinical situation, the goals of care, the expectation of the outcomes of the diagnostic or treatment interventions.

I. Help the patient identify who should participate in diagnostic and treatment discussions and decisions.

VI. EVALUATION AND EXPECTED OUTCOME(S)

A. The number of referrals to the ethics committee or ethics consultant in situations of decision-making conflict between any of the involved parties.

B. The use of interpreters in communication of, or decision-making about, diagnostic and/or treatment interventions.

C. Plan of Care: instructions regarding frequency of observation to ascertain the patient's lucid periods, if any.

D. Documentation
1. Is the process of the capacity assessment described?
2. Is the assessment specific to the decision at issue?
3. Is the informed consent and refusal interaction described?
4. Are the specifics of the patient's degree or spheres of orientation described?
5. Is the patient's language used to describe the diagnostic or treatment intervention under consideration recorded? Is the patient's demeanor during this discussion recorded?
6. Are the patient's questions and the clinician(s) answers recorded?
7. Are appropriate mental-status descriptors used consistently?

References

Agard, A., Hermeren, G., & Herlitz, J. (2001). Patients' experiences of intervention trials on the treatment of myocardial infarction: Is it time to adjust the informed consent procedure to the patient's capacity? *Heart (British Cardiac Society), 86*(6), 632–637. Evidence Level II: Single Experimental Study, RCT.

Allen, R. S., DeLaine, S. R., Chaplin, W. F., Marson, D. C., Bourgeois, M. S., Dijkstra, K., et al. (2003). Advance care planning in nursing homes: Correlates of capacity and possession of advance directives. *The Gerontologist, 43*(3), 309–317. Evidence Level IV: Nonexperimental Study.

Beauchamp, T. L., & Childress, J. F. (2001). *Principles of biomedical ethics* (5th ed). New York: Oxford University Press.

Cea, C. D., & Fisher, C. B. (2003). Health care decision making by adults with mental retardation. *Mental Retardation, 41*(2), 78–87. Evidence Level IV: Nonexperimental Study.

Cruzan v. Director, Missouri Department of Health (1990). 497 U.S. 261.

Duffy, S. A., Jackson, F. C., Schim, S. M., Ronis, D. L., & Fowler, K. E. (2006). Racial/ethnic preferences, sex preferences, and perceived discrimination related to end-of-life care. *JAGS, 54*(1), 150–157. Evidence Level IV: Nonexperimental Study.

Fried, T. R., Byers, A. L., Gallo, W. T., VanNess, P. H., Towle, V. R., O'Leary, J. R., et al. (2006). Prospective study of health status preferences and changes in preferences over time in adults. *Archives of Internal Medicine, 166*(8), 890–895. Evidence Level IV: Nonexperimental Study.

Gurrera, R. J., Moye, J., Karel, M. J., Azar, A. R., & Armesto, J. C. (2006). Cognitive performance predicts treatment decisional abilities in mild to moderate dementia. *Neurology, 66*(9), 1367–1372. Evidence Level IV: Nonexperimental Study.

Halbert, C. H., Armstrong, K., Gandy, O. H., & Shaker, L. (2006). Racial differences in trust in health care providers. *JAMA, 166*(8), 896–901. Evidence Level IV: Nonexperimental Study.

Kagawa-Singer, M., & Blackhall, L. J. (2001). Negotiating cross-cultural issues at the end of life. *JAMA, 286*(23), 2993–3002. Evidence Level V: Case Study.

Kapp, M. B., & Mossman, D. (1996). Measuring decisional capacity: Cautions on the construction of a "capacimeter." *Psychology and Public Policy Law, 2,* 73–95.

Karlawish, J. H., Casarett, D. J., James, B. D., Xie, S. X., & Kim, S. Y. (2005). The ability of persons with Alzheimer's disease (AD) to make a decision about taking an AD treatment. *Neurology, 64*(9), 1514–1519. Evidence Level IV: Nonexperimental Study.

Kim, S. Y., & Karlawish, J. H. (2002). Current state of research on decision-making competence of cognitively impaired elderly persons. *American Journal of Geriatric Psychiatry, 11*(2), 257–258. Evidence Level V: Literature Review.

Lapid, M. I., Rumman, T. A., Pankratz, V. S., & Applebaum, P. S. (2004). Decisional capacity of depressed elderly to consent to electroconvulsive therapy. *Journal of Geriatric Psychiatry and Neurology, 17*(1), 42–46. Evidence Level II: Single Experimental Study, RCT.

Lo, B. (2000). *Resolving ethical dilemmas: A guide for clinicians* (2nd ed.). Philadelphia: Lippincott, Williams & Wilkins.

Marson, D., Chatterjee, A., Ingram, K. K., & Harrell, L. E. (1996). Toward a neurologic model of competency: Cognitive predictors of capacity to consent in Alzheimer's disease using three different legal standards. *Neurology, 46*(3), 666–672. Evidence Level IV: Nonexperimental Study.

Mezey, M. D., Mitty, E., & Ramsey, G. (1997). Assessment of decision-making capacity: Nurse's role. *Journal of Gerontological Nursing, 23*(3), 28–35. Evidence Level V: Literature Review.

Mezey, M. D., Teresi, J., Ramsey, G., Mitty, E., & Bobrowitz, T. (2002). Determining a resident's capacity to execute a health care proxy. *Voices of decision in nursing homes: Respecting residents' preferences for end-of-life care.* New York: United Hospital Fund. Evidence Level IV: Nonexperimental Study.

Moye, J., Karel, M. J., Azar, A. R., & Gurrera, R. J. (2004). Capacity to consent to treatment: Empirical comparison of three instruments in older adults with and without dementia. *Gerontologist, 44*(2), 166–175. Evidence Level IV: Nonexperimental Study.

Moye, J., Karel, M. J., Gurrera, R. J., & Azar, A. R. (2006). Neuropsychological predictors of decision-making capacity over 9 months in mild-to-moderate dementia. *Journal of General Internal Medicine, 21*(1), 78–83. Evidence Level IV: Nonexperimental Study.

Paterson, B. L., Russell, C., & Thorne, S. (2001). Critical analysis of everyday self-care decision making in chronic illness. *Journal of Advanced Nursing, 35*(3), 335–341. Evidence Level V: Literature Review.

Popejoy, L. (2005). Health-related decision making by older adults and their families: How clinicians can help. *Journal of Gerontological Nursing, 31*(9), 12–18. Evidence Level V: Literature Review.

Rivers V. Katz, 67 N.Y. 485, 495 N.E. 2d 337, 504. N.Y. S. 2d 74 (1986).

Rosenfeld, K. E., Wenger, N. S., & Kagawa-Singer, M. (2000). End-of-life decision making: A qualitative study of older individuals. *Journal General Internal Medicine, 15*(9), 620–625. Evidence Level IV: Nonexperimental Study.

Roth, L. H., Meisel, A., & Lidz, C.W. (1997). Tests of competency to consent to treatment. *American Journal of Psychiatry, 134*(3), 279–284.

Segall, A. (1976). The sick role concept: Understanding illness behavior. *Journal of Health & Social Behavior, 17,* 162–169.

Steinhauser, K. E., Christakis, N. A., Clipp, E. C., McNeilly, M., McIntyre, L., & Tulsky, J. A. (2000). Factors considered important at the end of life by patients, family, physicians and other care providers. *JAMA, 284*(19), 2476–2482. Evidence Level IV: Nonexperimental Study.

The, A. M., Pasman, R., Onwuteaka-Philipsen, B., Ribbe, M., & Van Der Wal, G. (2002). Withholding the artificial administration of fluids and food from elderly patients with dementia: Ethnographic study. *British Medical Journal (Clinical Research Ed.), 325*(7376), 1326. Evidence Level IV: Nonexperimental Study.

Van Kleffens, T., van Baarsen, B., & van Leeuwen, E. (2004). The medical practice of patient autonomy and cancer treatment refusals: A patients' and physicians' perspective. *Social Science and Medicine, 58*(11), 2325–2336. Evidence Level IV: Nonexperimental Study.

Volicer, L., & Ganzini, L. (2003). Health professionals: Views on standards for decision-making capacity regarding refusal of medical treatment in mild Alzheimer's disease. *Journal of the American Geriatrics Society, 51*(5), 1270–1274. Evidence Level IV: Nonexperimental Study.

Advance Directives

24

Ethel L. Mitty
Gloria Ramsey

Educational Objectives

On completion of this chapter, the reader should be able to:

1. explain and differentiate between a Durable Power of Attorney for Health Care and a Living Will

2. describe assessment parameters to ensure that older adults receive advance directive information

3. identify strategies to ensure good communication about advance directives among patients, families, and health care professionals

4. guide a discussion of the benefits and burdens of various treatment options to assist proxy treatment decision-making

5. describe measurable outcomes to be expected from implementation of this practice protocol

Overview

One of the most difficult situations health care professionals face is how to assist with treatment decision making for those who can no longer communicate their treatment preferences. Decision-making capacity of older adults may be diminished, fluctuating, or lapsed. Substitute decision makers rely on directions or instructions left by the patient when they had capacity to express and communicate their treatment preferences and goals of care. The justification

For a description of Evidence Levels cited in this chapter, see chapter 1,
Developing and Evaluating Clinical Practice Guidelines, page 4.

Adapted from a chapter in the second edition by Gloria Ramsey and Ethel L. Mitty. (2003). Advance directives: Protecting patient's rights. In M. Mezey, T. Fulmer, & I. Abraham (Eds.), Geriatric nursing protocols for best practice (2nd ed., pp. 265–91).

for advance care planning is that a person with capacity can state their wishes, values, and treatment preferences in advance, prospectively, so that their authentic voice will be heard when their capacity has lapsed. Decision making can be especially difficult when care providers barely know the patient, have little knowledge of what treatments a patient would or would not want, or there is no one available to speak for the patient. Approximately 30% of older adults do not have a relative, friend, or guardian who can make health care decisions for them. The right to *not* complete an advance directive must also be respected. It is very important that patients are informed (and, in some cases, reassured) that neither providers nor the facility will abandon them or provide substandard care if the patient elects not to formulate an advance directive.

Background

The Patient Self Determination Act (PSDA), enacted in 1991, is the federal statutory codification of an advance planning and decision-making approach for those who are no longer able to make their own health care decisions. The PSDA requires all agencies and institutions that receive Medicare or Medicaid reimbursement to inform their clients and patients of their right to make health care decisions, including their option to complete an advance directive (AD). Predicated on the Western philosophic tradition of individual freedom and choice, self-determination as a moral right, the U.S. Supreme Court decision in the matter of Nancy Cruzan (1990) articulated the need for "clear and convincing evidence" that an incompetent patient would not want a specific treatment. Because few oral statements could meet this standard, written ADs were promulgated as constituting clear and convincing evidence.

An AD (i.e., health care proxy appointment and/or living will) is created by a capable/capacitated person to prospectively state his or her wishes and treatment preferences regarding medical care that are to be communicated and implemented in the event that the individual is unable to communicate and/or capacity has lapsed. ADs are value-neutral and can be used to request as well as refuse treatments; they provide guidance for health care professionals and families. Importantly, ADs provide immunity for health care professionals and families from civil and criminal liability when health care professionals follow the AD in good faith. State statutes generally outline the conditions under which an AD is legally valid and when it should be followed (see state statutes link in the Resources section).

Nurses need to be sensitive to the reasons why people do and do not create an AD. Approximately 25% of the general public and only slightly more than 51% of nursing home residents have an AD (Mezey, Mitty, Rappaport, & Ramsey, 1997b [Level IV]); advance planning is still not the norm for most adults (Tilden, Nelson, Dunn, Donius, & Tolle, 2000 [Level IV]). Older adults who create an AD feel that their physicians know their wishes and do not feel that the AD would be a constraint on their care. Those who do not create an AD want their families to make decisions for them and apparently fail to see the flexibility that having an AD provides (Beck, Brown, Boles, & Barrett, 2002 [Level II]). Many patients with chronic illness want pain and symptom management and supportive care rather than aggressive life-sustaining interventions (Zerzan, Stearns,

& Hanson, 2000 [Level IV]). Hospice patients who talk with their surrogates about their treatment wishes for their last week of life have a higher rate of agreement with their surrogate's understanding of their treatment wishes than patients who do not have these discussions (Engelberg, Patrick, & Curtis, 2005 [Level III]). Treatment preferences of capacitated nursing home residents are relatively stable over time and, in fact, indicate a preference for less invasive interventions as dependency increases (Berger & Majerovitz, 1998 [Level V]; Danis, Garret, Harris, & Patrick, 1994 [Level V]).

Although family surrogate decision-making is more accurate than primary physicians regarding older patients' preferences for life-sustaining treatments in hypothetical scenarios, having an AD does not improve congruence between patients' wishes and decisions made by others (Coppola, Ditto, Danks, & Smucker, 2001 [Level II]). Substitute decision makers are not necessarily making treatment choices or decisions that represent the patient's preferences (Ditto et al., 2001 [Level II]; Hines et al., 2001 [Level IV]; Mitchell, Berkowitz, Lawson, & Lipsitz, 2000 [Level IV]). The lack of concordance between a patient's stated wishes and physician orders, as found in 65% of cases in one study (Hardin & Yusufaly, 2004 [Level II]), cannot simply be viewed as a denial of a patient's rights; physicians might be relying on additional information to guide their treatment decisions. Using interview and qualitative methods with 30 pairs of patient and primary caregiver at an outpatient clinic, Rodriquez and Young (2006 [Level IV]) report that participants talk about life-sustaining treatments in terms of four goals of end-of-life care: extending life, improving quality of life, improving or maintaining a specific function, and temporary assistance. Patients feel that their professional health care providers are more interested in extending their life than with the quality of that life. In the patients' view, life-sustaining treatments were acceptable in the short term but not for an extended period. Caregivers are torn between quality of life and simply extending life. Given this body of evidence of discordance among patient wishes, surrogates' decisions, and physician orders, it can be argued that nurses have a responsibility to hear the patient's voice, to ascertain the patient's treatment wishes and goals of care, and to represent the patient when treatment decisions are made—even in the seeming absence of conflict between parties.

Types of Advance Directives

Durable Power of Attorney for Health Care

There are two types of ADs: the Durable Power of Attorney for Health Care (DPAHC) and the Living Will (LW). The DPAHC allows an individual to appoint a relative, friend, or trusted other—called a health care proxy, agent, attorney-in-fact, or surrogate—to make health care decisions if the individual loses the ability to make decisions or communicate his or her wishes. (An alternate agent should also be appointed.) A key presumption of health care proxy appointment is that the patient and proxy have discussed the patient's treatment wishes; some states require that the proxy sign the AD as an attempt to ensure that the proxy is aware of their appointment and has accepted decision-making responsibilities as the patient's voice in care planning and decision making. A proxy has the legal authority to interpret the patient's wishes on the basis of the medical circumstances of the situation and is not restricted to only deciding if life-sustaining treatment can be withdrawn or withheld. Thus, the proxy can make decisions as the need arises, and such decisions can respond directly to the situation at hand rather than being restricted only to circumstances that were thought of previously.

Thirty-one states have "family consent laws" that designate the order in which family members can make decisions for an incapacitated patient who did not appoint a proxy; a spouse is usually first, then adult children, parents, and distant relatives. The decisions of family members acting in this capacity are restricted in various ways by 41 states. This includes the requirement that the patient must be terminal or in a persistent vegetative state, comatose, and so forth. Disputes between family members who bear the same relationship to the patient (e.g., two sons) are not uncommon and often very difficult to resolve (see the section on conflict mediation). A proxy's decision legally supercedes a decision made by a family member or nonproxy concerned party. This is not to say, however, that a proxy's decision is always easy and conflict-free or that the burden is light. Whereas a living will is in effect at the end of life, the DPAHC springs into effect at any time that the patient has a temporary (or permanent) absence of decisional capacity, as might be associated with trauma, illness, or mental impairment (e.g., dementia, stroke, delirium).

Living Will

For adults who have no one to appoint as their proxy, completing a LW that outlines their wishes is preferable to not providing any information at all about care preferences. A LW is also helpful for those with a DPAHC who want to provide their proxy with some guidance about their treatment preferences and end-of-life care wishes, including artificial nutrition and hydration, ventilator support, and pain management.

A LW provides specific instructions to health care providers about particular kinds of health care treatments or interventions that an individual would or would not want in specific clinical circumstances, usually at the end of life (e.g., comfort care, all life-sustaining treatments). A LW is a prospective declaration. All but three states (i.e., New York, Massachusetts, and Michigan) have detailed statutes recognizing LWs. The usefulness of a LW is limited, however, to those clinical circumstances that were thought of before the person became incapable of making decisions. If a situation occurs that the LW does not address, providers and families may not know how to proceed and still respect the patient's wishes. Hence, it is recommended that individuals also appoint a proxy—that is, a trusted other who knows their values and wishes. When an individual completes both the LW and DPAHC, the proxy/agent might not be obligated (in some states) to follow the wishes outlined in the LW; the LW serves as a guide.

Some states have a combined directive that includes elements of the LW and the DPAHC. A section on organ donation (i.e., "anatomical gift") has been added to the AD document of some states that allows individuals to indicate if they wish to donate an organ(s). However, in New York State, for example, the proxy cannot affect this wish unless the proxy is also the identified decision maker for organ donation, a distinct statutory authority separate from a health care proxy's rights and responsibilities. Once again, this speaks to nurses knowing the relevant law regarding ADs as well as after-death decision making.

"Instructional directives" have been suggested to compensate for the deficiencies of LWs; they address specific clinical situations and interventions that are acceptable to the patient. Also known as a "Medical Directive," individuals must decide prospectively which interventions they would want in the face of four scenarios: coma with virtually no chance of recovery; coma with a small chance of recovery but restored to an impaired physical and mental state; advanced dementia and a terminal illness; advanced dementia (Emanuel & Emanuel, 1989 [Level IV]). Among the interventions are CPR, artificial hydration and nutrition, dialysis, invasive diagnostic tests, antibiotics, and blood transfusion. Nursing homes using this directive demonstrate improved patient and family satisfaction, reduced health care costs, and lower hospitalization rates (Molloy et al., 2000 [Level II]). The Medical Directive does not address a patient's desired goals of care, willingness to allow a short-term intervention, or treatment choices associated with stage of chronic illness or exacerbation.

The notion of a "research" AD has been suggested (National Bioethics Advisory Commission, 1998). The conduct of research with participants suffering from a dementing illness is daunting with regard to obtaining informed consent. A Research AD must be executed while the individual still retains decisional capacity and must contain a fairly detailed description of the person's understanding of the research intention, possible risks, benefits, and burdens. The proxy decision maker must make a determination of whether or not the person's intention to participate in research is congruent with the proposed research. A study involving patients with moderate dementia and their family proxies sought to learn whether the patients wanted to retain decision making about their participation in research in the future or allow their proxy to make the decision. Although the majority of patients granted future decision making to their proxies, it was also clear that proxies did not always want to make research participation decisions (Stocking et al., 2006 [Level IV]).

Two other AD documents that further the goals of advance care planning and that are accepted in many states are the Physician Order for Life Sustaining Treatment (POLST) and the Five Wishes document. POLST originated in Oregon in 1995 and is a state-endorsed protocol to honor an individual's wish to die in a setting of their choice without unwanted life-supporting interventions. It contains four separate categories of physician's orders that are based on patient–physician discussion about comfort measures, antibiotics, parenteral feeding, and cardiopulmonary resuscitation. Studies indicate that Oregon nursing home residents with POLST documents received more intense comfort care and fewer aggressive life-sustaining interventions, were less likely to be transferred to a hospital to die, and had more orders for narcotic analgesia at the time of death than did nursing home residents without POLSTs (Tolle, Tilden, Nelson, & Dunn, 1998 [Level IV]). The Five Wishes document combines the health care proxy, LW, values, instructional directions, and proxy designation. Open-ended statements guide individuals to express their thoughts and wishes about how they want to be physically and emotionally supported, the medical treatments they want and do not want, and the funeral arrangements and eulogy they would like. It is legally valid in all but 12 states. Values "statements" generally do not explore or express a patient's understanding of the benefits and burdens of various treatments, thereby making it difficult to act on a patient's wishes and preferences (Lo & Steinbrook, 2006 [Level V]).

Oral Advance Directive

Although the courts prefer written ADs, oral ADs are respected, especially in emergency situations, and can be persuasive in a judicial decision to withhold a life-sustaining treatment. Ten states permit a patient to orally designate a proxy in discussion with their physician rather than execute a written AD (Lo & Steinbrook, 2006 [Level V]). However, there are limitations to their applicability and they might need to be witnessed. In determining the validity of an oral AD, the court seeks information about whether the statement was made on serious or solemn occasions, consistently repeated, made by a mature person who understood the underlying issues, was consistent with the values demonstrated in other aspects of the patient's life (including the patient's religion), made before the need for the treatment decision, and specifically addressed the actual condition of the patient (Lo & Steinbrook, 2006 [Level V]). What might seem like an occasional comment made by a patient (whether in a practitioner's office or at the bedside) should be recorded for just such an occasion when "clear and convincing evidence" is required. It has been argued that oral instructions explicated during conversation with one's physician can be taken to signify the patient's genuine intent on having his or her instructions followed. This has been contrasted with statements made to family and friends that are likely to be emotion-laden and not a true reflection of the patient's wishes (Lo & Steinbrook, 2006 [Level V]).

Legal statutes stipulate that health care providers, including physicians, must heed the wishes stated in an AD; by law, a person cannot be treated without explicit permission—that is considered "battery." In most states, unless the patient has severely limited the proxy's scope, the proxy's decision has the same weight and power as the patient speaking on his or her own behalf. A proxy's power is no greater or less than the capable patient. Vague or ambiguous language in an AD (e.g., refusal of "heroic measures") deprives the proxy as well as providers of the guidance needed to honor the patient's wishes. This speaks to assisting patients and proxies in a dialogue that elicits the patient's wishes, sometimes by hypothesizing or imagining diverse illness and treatment scenarios. In such cases when, based on conscience or religion, a facility and/or physician objects to a request in an AD or a proxy's decision, the patient must be assisted with transfer to another facility and/or provider who will honor the decision/directive.

Do-Not-Resuscitate Orders

Consent to cardiopulmonary resuscitation (CPR) is presumed unless a physician writes a Do-Not-Resuscitate (DNR) order. Respecting (or not) a patient's resuscitation wishes is a frequent cause of moral distress for nurses. The SUPPORT Study (i.e., Study to Understand Prognoses and Preference for Outcomes and Risks of Treatment), a multi-hospital study involving almost 2,000 seriously ill patients, found that less than one-fourth of patients had discussed their resuscitation wishes with their physician. Among patients who had not discussed their preferences, slightly more than half were not interested in having the discussion (Hofmann et al., 1997 [Level III]). Nurses, specially trained for the study, reported that patient requests for DNR were frequently ignored; physicians were not always aware of their patient's end-of-life care wishes.

It has been suggested that CPR should not be instituted when it will not offer a medical benefit or when death is inevitable and expected (Tresch et al., 1994 [Level V]). All states have a Natural Death Act that recognizes the right of competent patients, in their written AD, to refuse life-sustaining treatments. Patients have a right to refuse CPR after they have been informed of the risks and benefits involved and may, in fact, request a DNR order. If the physician is unwilling to write a DNR order to comply with the patient's request, the physician has a duty to notify the patient or family and assist the patient to obtain another physician (Sabatino, nd). Nurses need to be aware of such situations and, as well, need to know their institution's policy and law in their state governing a DNR directive. It is important, however, that otherwise healthy elderly hospitalized patients who may benefit from CPR should not be denied this life-saving intervention.

Community-dwelling adults with a hospital-originated DNR order are likely to be resuscitated by emergency medical services (EMS), which are required to do so until the patient is at the hospital. Some states have created an acceptable community-based or certified DNR order and require the individual to have a special identifier, such as a wrist band.

Artificial Nutrition and Hydration

As health care professionals and families grapple with issues around treatments and care at the end of life, artificial nutrition and hydration continues to pose challenging ethical, legal, and cultural questions. How can you not feed or hydrate a dying person? The U.S. Supreme Court, in 1990 (before the PSDA), established that competent patients have a "constitutionally protected liberty" to refuse unwanted medical treatment. The court further established that artificial nutrition and hydration is no different than other forms of medical treatment. Many physicians and nurses are unaware that a capable patient has a legal and ethical right to discontinue artificial nutrition and hydration, and they erroneously believe that there is a legal difference between forgoing versus discontinuing artificial nutrition and hydration. The legal evidence and procedures required to forgo or discontinue artificial nutrition and hydration vary by state. Several states' statutes hold that proxies cannot make decisions about withholding unless the patient specifically directs, in the AD, that the proxy can make this decision on his or her behalf. In 20 states, the DPAHC document contains a statement and box to check, if the patient wishes, that states: "My proxy knows my wishes." Nothing has to be written regarding precisely what those wishes are. Because the LW directive in some states regards artificial nutrition and hydration as a medical treatment, whereas other states regard this intervention as a comfort measure (Gillick, 2006 [Level V]), it is important that nurses are aware of their specific state's statutes and definitions in this regard in order to accurately and appropriately inform patients, families, and proxies. Given the extensive variation between states in regulation and administration of tube feeding (Aronheim, Mulvihill, Sieger, Park, & Fries, 2001 [Level IV]), nurses need to be aware of their state law in this regard and the extent to which patients (and proxies) are correctly informed about the consequences of artificial nutrition and hydration at the end of life and the caring and comfort treatment alternatives.

Whether to institute artificial feeding and hydration or to withdraw it once started has the moral equivalence, for many people, of "killing" the patient. Decisions to withhold artificial nutrition and hydration from nursing home residents with advanced dementia are more influenced by the patient's presumed quality of life, stage of illness, and co-morbidities than by AD instructions (The, Pasman, Onwuteaka-Philipsen, Ribbe, & van der Wal, 2002 [Level IV]).

Pain Management

There is a moral as well as a professional imperative to relieve pain even in the absence of an AD. Compassionate pain relief does not require consent because it is grounded in respect for and dignity of the person (i.e., principles of autonomy and beneficence). An individual's constitutionally protected interest in pain relief was made clear in the U.S. Supreme Court ruling in Quill versus Vacco (1996). Rejecting the argument that there is a constitutionally protected right to assisted suicide, the Court reaffirmed, however, the doctrine of "double effect." This principle holds that a single act having two foreseen effects, one good and one bad, is not legally or morally wrong or prohibited if the harmful effect is not intended. For a terminally ill, incapacitated patient who lacks a directive or proxy to advocate on behalf of his or her comfort needs, it is ethically and legally appropriate to provide as much medication as necessary to relieve pain, even if the effect hastens death. For the patient with capacity, refusal of pain relief might be a value-based choice between intellectual and emotional awareness versus relief from pain.

Assessment

A primary consideration in approaching a patient about AD creation is the person's capacity to make decisions about his or her health care. "Competence" and "capacity" are not the same, yet they are frequently used synonymously and interchangeably (see chapter 23, *Health Care Decision Making*). The law presumes competency unless shown otherwise; only the court can rule that an individual is incompetent. Capacity is a clinical determination and is not determined solely by a medical or psychiatric diagnosis or test. Inability to make financial decisions or communicate verbally does not preclude the ability to communicate important information about one's treatment preferences. The determination that a patient lacks capacity is often made on the basis of a mental-status assessment test—an inappropriate measure of decisional capacity. Thus, there is a grave risk that individuals with communication disorders or those with mild dementia might not have the opportunity to appoint a health care proxy or to execute a LW.

Decisional Capacity to Create an Advance Directive

The steps in determining if a patient has sufficient decisional capacity to create an AD are similar to the basic elements of a valid consent and are based on observation of a specific set of abilities. These steps include (1) the patient appreciates and understands that he or she has the right to make a choice;(2) the patient understands the medical situation, prognosis, risks, benefits, and consequences of treatment consent (or refusal); (3) the patient can communicate the decision; and (4) the patient's decision is stable and consistent over a period of time (Roth, Meisel, & Lidz, 1977).

Not all health decisions require the same level of decision-making capacity to make a decision. Decision-making capacity is not an all-or-none, "on-off" switch. Rather, capacity should be viewed as "task-specific." An individual may be able to perform some tasks adequately, may have the ability to make some decisions, but is unable to perform all tasks or make all decisions. The notion of "decision-specific capacity" assumes that an individual has or lacks capacity for a particular decision at a particular time and under a particular set of circumstances (Meisel, 2002 [Level VI]; Mezey, Mitty, & Ramsey, 1997a [Level VI]). Most older adults have sufficient cognitive capability to make some but not all decisions. An individual might have the requisite capacity or understanding that they can choose someone to make health care decisions for them when they no longer have the capacity to make treatment choices in advance as would be required for a LW. The determination of decisional capacity becomes more exacting in relationship to the complexity and risk associated with the health care decision (Midwest Bioethics Center, 1996 [Level VI]).

The Mini-Mental Status Examination (MMSE) is a cognitive screen; it was not designed for nor is it applicable to capacity determination (Mezey, Teresi, Ramsey, Mitty, & Bobrowitz, 2002 [Level IV]). Appreciation of the consequences of an option or decision is a key component of capacity determination. Although more than three-quarters of nursing home residents (n = 68) could make a treatment choice, few understood their treatment options or the consequences of each treatment. The MMSE score explained only 6% of variance in appreciation of consequences (Allen et al., 2003 [Level IV]). There is no "gold standard" or "capacimeter" to assess capacity (Kapp & Mossman, 1996 [Level V]). It is generally agreed among bioethicists, legal scholars, and clinicians that a low level of capacity is needed to create a DPAHC and there is evidence to support this (Mezey et al., 2002 [Level IV]). As such, the informed consent necessary to ensure that the individual understands the issues relating to a proxy appointment can be simpler and less rigorous than the process required for decisions of greater risk, such as creating a LW.

Nurses can make a valuable contribution in determining decision-making capacity sufficient to create an AD. Relevant documentation about the patient includes patients' ability to express their needs, follow directions, state a preference, and exhibit stability of their choices. Objective assessment of capacity can avoid two types of mistakes: (1) mistakenly preventing persons who ought to be considered capacitated from directing the course of their treatment; and (2) failing to protect incapacitated persons from the harmful effects of their decisions.

Advance care planning is not without legal, ethical, language, communication, and cultural conundrums. Persuasive argument can be brought to set limits on the treatment preferences expressed by a formerly competent but now demented individual. It has been argued that the person with Alzheimer's disease is a different person than the one who existed prior to the profound mental changes and who stated his or her treatment preferences. The opposing position is that the now incapacitated person is the same person who expressed those treatment preferences and that any decision to disregard the wishes should be based on a judgment about the person's quality of life (as he or she is living it!) and on the benefits and burdens associated with a particular treatment decision.

Benefit–Burden Assessment

Proxy or surrogate decision makers are unlikely to know what and how a benefit–burden analysis can assist them in their decision-making responsibilities. As such, nurses can be invaluable to families and proxies simply by taking them through the steps of the analysis. A benefit–burden analysis considers the intended and unintended consequences of a particular treatment, estimates the likelihood that the intended benefit will occur, and weighs the importance of the benefit and burden to the patient. As each treatment or intervention is considered, the benefit (advantage) and burden (disadvantage, risk potential) to the patient is evaluated. The proxy can be helped to infer how the patient would evaluate the benefits and burdens based on knowledge of the patient's values, preferences, and past behavior. The nurse can ask the proxy, "If [the patient] could join this discussion, what would he say?" "Faced with similar situations in the past, how did he decide?" A survey of almost 3,429 hospitalized seriously ill older adults found that almost 75% preferred to have their family and physician make a resuscitation decision for them—not follow their previously stated wishes–should they lose decisional capacity (Puchalski et al., 2000 [Level V]). Advance care planning discussions with patients and their proxies can elucidate patients' perceptions of benefits and barriers. Higher congruence between patient and proxy regarding the patient's end-of-life care preferences was associated with a nurse-led discussion intervention compared to a patient–proxy control group. Intervention-group patients were more knowledgeable about life-sustaining treatments (LSTs), less willing to receive LSTs for a new serious medical event, and less willing to live in a state of poor health (Schwartz et al., 2002 [Level II]).

The rationale for withholding or withdrawing a treatment is to eliminate a burdensome intervention/treatment that is not producing the desired result. The motivation is not to hasten death. In those situations where the proxy has scant knowledge about the patient for whom he or she must make health care decisions (or there is no AD, proxy appointment, or person who speaks for the patient), a decision is made on what would be in the patient's best interest. Known as the "reasonable person" or "best interest" standard, the decision relies on the notion of what an average person in the patient's particular situation would consider beneficial or burdensome. Questions that could move the process along would ask, "What does [this patient] have to gain or lose as a result of this treatment?" and "In what ways will [this patient] be better or worse off as a result of this treatment—or not having this treatment?"

Cultural Perspectives on Advance Care Planning

The notion of advance care planning and written directives is not universally acceptable. In some cultures, for a closeknit family an AD is intrusive, irrelevant, and a refusal if not a legitimized denial of care. They do not view the DPAHC as the voice of the patient and a means for someone to advocate for the patient's desired care. Disinterest in creating an AD because of a present-day rather than a future orientation and an unwillingness to write, speak, or plan for one's death are pervasive cultural influences on a decision not to create an AD. As well, deference to physician decision making, the family's role in protecting the patient from the burdens of life and death decision making, and spiritual obligations or beliefs can exert a powerful influence on the decision.

Studies indicate different life-sustaining treatment preferences and decision-making contexts between racial and ethnic groups (Cox et al., 2006 [Level I]). Among four ethnic groups, Asian and Hispanic patients preferred family-centered decision-making in contrast to White and African American patients' preference for patient-directed decision-making (Kwak & Haley, 2005 [Level V]). As many have shown, White patients are more interested in and likely to discuss treatment preferences, execute a LW, refuse certain life-sustaining treatments, and appoint a health care proxy decision maker than Black or Hispanic patients (Hopp & Duffy, 2000 [Level IV]). AD completion is more concentrated among White patients with higher education and income levels than among Black and Hispanic patients at low income levels and less than a high school education (Mezey, Leitman, Mitty, Bottrell, & Ramsey, 2000b [Level IV]). In contrast, African American patients are more likely to want life-sustaining treatments to prolong life. Some Black patients believe that having an AD is a legal way to deny access to treatment and care, and they tend to distrust the health care system more than MexicanAmericans and Euro-Americans (Perkins, Geppert, Gonzales, Cortez, & Hazuda, 2002 [Level IV]). An intervention study using same-race peer mentors to discuss advance care planning with dialysis patients demonstrated a significant positive effect on Black patients but not on White patients. Positive outcomes included increased comfort in discussion and completion of ADs and improved feelings of well-being (Perry et al., 2005 [Level II]).

Cultural assimilation, as well as cultural diversity, makes even a simplistic assumption about why people do and do not create an AD extremely hazardous. When patients and health care professionals are from different ethnic backgrounds, the value systems that form the basis for AD decision making may conflict, often leading to distinct ethical and interpersonal tensions. Predictors of AD completion for multi-ethnic urban seniors include what investigators called "modifiable factors," such as an established relationship with a primary-care physician and their doctor's willingness to start the discussion, being knowledgeable about advance care planning, recognition of the family role in decision making, and prior experience with decision making about mechanical ventilation (Morrison & Meier, 2004 [Level IV]). A nurse's role in the midst of diverse cultural and religious belief systems is to approach the patient and/or the proxy with awareness, sensitivity, and competency that respect their values. These conversations occur over time; they are not interviews per se. Discussion is always patient-centered, not proxy or provider centered.

Nurses' Roles in Advance Directives

All adult patients, regardless of their gender, religion, socioeconomic status, diagnosis, or prognosis, should be approached with information about and encouraged to discuss ADs. Time and workload permitting, nurses can have a major role in checking their patients' knowledge about end-of-life treatment options and the benefits, burdens, and consequences of each option. Yet, nurses lack confidence in their knowledge and ability to assist patients to create an AD (Jezewski et al., 2005 [Level IV]). Failure to consider language barriers and hearing and visual deficits can result in the erroneous conclusion that a person lacks the capacity to execute an AD. Although surveys of the general public report positive attitudes toward ADs, few patients actually have completed one (Lynn, Schuster, & Kabcenell, 2000 [Level V]). Even patients at higher risk of becoming incapable of making decisions and who, therefore, might be more likely to need an AD are not necessarily more likely to complete a directive. Patients' understanding of their clinical and legal options about care at the end of life is limited and often mistaken. A study involving 1,000 English-speaking adult outpatients revealed that almost two-thirds did not know the difference between euthanasia and assisted suicide and did not understand treatment refusal; less than half understood treatment withdrawal (Silviera, DiPiero, Gerrity, & Feudtner, 2000 [Level IV]). Correct information/knowledge was associated with being college educated, White, and prior experience as a proxy for another.

Educating and talking with patients about ADs can make a difference in completion rates (Gutheil & Heyman, 2005 [Level II]; Patel, Sinuff, & Cook, 2004 [Level I]). Patients say that they complete ADs to ease their family's financial and emotional burden and to ease decision making. They want to discuss end-of-life care and LWs, but they expect providers to initiate these discussions. Community-dwelling older patients attending a general medical clinic were more likely to create an AD when they received AD information by mail in advance of their appointment and their physician received a reminder to discuss ADs in comparison to patients whose physicians only received a reminder to document ADs (Heiman, Bates, Fairchild, Shaykevich, & Lehmann, 2004 [Level II]). Interestingly, discussions of end-of-life care and ADs were a statistically significant predictor of satisfaction with primary-care physicians among almost 700 outpatients 50 to 75 years old (Tierney et al., 2001 [Level II]). Attitude, skills, and knowledge regarding advance care planning among medical residents caring for hospitalized older adults influenced their willingness to discuss it; as well, they had incomplete and often erroneous understanding of patients' decision-making process (Gorman, Ahern, Wiseman, & Skrobik, 2005 [Level V]).

Educating health care professionals about the virtues and methods of advance care planning can be instrumental in creating and communicating a clear and sufficiently detailed AD. Nursing home residents cared for by social workers (SWs) who were educated about ADs and given a structure for follow-up, documentation, and communication of residents' AD wishes were more likely to have their life-sustaining treatment and hospitalization preferences documented than were residents of control-group SWs who only received information about ADs (Morrison et al., 2005 [Level II]). Subsequently, control-group residents were significantly more likely than intervention-group residents to receive a treatment that was not in accordance with their stated wishes and preferences.

Nurses have a responsibility in dispelling myths and misperceptions about ADs. A pervasive myth among patients, and one influenced by a history of abuse and denial of health care, is that an AD means "Do not treat" (Sabatino, nd). Many people believe that an AD, particularly a LW, is necessary to protect one from being kept alive against their wishes, with all manner of tubes and technology. Some patients believe, erroneously, that a lawyer is needed to execute an AD and that each state has its own specific AD document that must be used. It is partially correct that absent an AD, a "surrogate decision maker," most often a family member, is the designated decision maker. This reflects custom as well as recognition of the pivotal role of the family in important decisions as well as the fact that a family member is most likely to be aware of the patient's values, wishes, and preferences. The reality in many cases is that families disagree or might be ignorant of a patient's wishes. Nurses are in a position to identify pending family conflict and act to mitigate the drastic effects of poor or delayed treatment decisions. It can also be helpful, in some circumstances, to help the patient and family/proxy think about alternative treatments and goals of care. Perhaps an intervention that is less burdensome or one that has a rapid positive result if only for the short term—for example, to satisfy a patient's wish to be present at a major personal event would be acceptable.

One way for a nurse to begin the discussion about advance care planning is by helping the patient and/or proxy explore and express what quality of life means for the patient, the importance of preservation of life, and how the patient's illness (and death) will affect others (e.g., emotionally, financially). Some patients might want to focus on the quality of their living, whereas others, the quality of their dying. Some patients might want to talk about from whom and where they will receive care at the end of life. Some may abhor their coming dependence on others; others may not like or want it but will accept it. Still others might opt for hospice care out of the home to distance their dependency on family caregivers. Patients (and proxies) might need or want to talk about what they each fear most and what will be important when dying.

Copies of the completed AD(s) should be given to the primary health care provider (physician, nurse practitioner), agency or institution, and the proxy. Wallet-size cards indicating that the person has an AD and with the name and contact information for the proxy should be carried. Nurses in virtually every kind of health care delivery setting can take the initiative to review the document with patients annually and in the event of a significant change of condition. While doing so, the nurse or other appropriate person should check whether the proxy is still alive and willing to continue to act in that capacity. If the proxy has died or is no longer willing, the nurse should discuss with the patient which person they would like to become their surrogate decision maker, follow-through that someone has been selected, and check that the new proxy is aware of the patient's wishes and preferences.

Interventions and Care Strategies

Conflict Mediation

As seen in the literature, as well as by anecdotal report, many nurses experience moral distress when patients' proxy decision makers do not appear to be honoring the patients' treatment and care wishes (Bookvar & Lachs, 1998 [Level IV]; Van Niekerk & Martin, 2002 [Level IV]). Although couched in clinical language and scenarios, there is no escaping the fact that these situations speak to patient rights and the ethical principle of respect for persons.

Differences of opinion about a patient's quality of life, goals of care, and treatment preferences should not be characterized as a "conflict" when it is not seen that way by the proxy, the patient's family, or the health care providers. A nurse's role in this kind of situation is to try to level the playing field so that all parties can voice their concerns while avoiding power struggles.

Conflict mediation can solve problems by identification of the concerned parties and determination of their needs and interests. Sometimes, the problem is not one of irrevocable conflict but rather lack of sufficient and accurate information—a communication problem (Dubler & Marcus, 1994 [Level VI]). Sensitivity to the values of all the involved parties facilitates exploration of alternatives and agreement about the best decisions for the patient. Steps in mediation and their general sequence are collection of information about the patient's medical conditions and nursing needs; discussion of the goals of care and the medical uncertainties; review of the process by which health care decisions were made in the past; and identification of any legal, ethical, cultural, or spiritual issues that exert pressure on the decision. A "principled solution" is one that reflects the fairness of the process and one that was not predetermined by the power status of any one of the parties. If this type of informal but focused deliberation is unable to arrive at resolution that reflects the patient's wishes and with which all are in accord, an ethics consultation or meeting of the institution's ethics committee may be the next step. An ethics committee should look like members of the health care team—interdisciplinary. If the institution's lawyer or risk manager is a committee member, it is essential that the potential legal risk to the institution does not dominate discussion and trump the ethical discussion relevant to the key figures.

Communication About Advance Care Planning

Under state law and JCAHO standards, patients have the right to have a qualified interpreter translate and transmit discussion between themselves and the health care professional. The interpreter may be the only person who recognizes that patients and their families have a totally different "take" than the health care team on words like "health" and "illness," on what a treatment is supposed to do, and on what dying is and what it is not. If "telling bad news" is prohibited (e.g., Navajo, Greece, Korea, Horn of Africa nations), then it will be difficult to discuss end-of-life planning. It should not be assumed that facility, family, or other interpreters are neutral and will simply "translate" words. An interpreter is communicating fact and nuance, explanation and rationale, and might influence a treatment decision by virtue of attempting a 1:1 word translation or a clumsy approximation of two distinct languages. In the presence of conflict about treatment decisions, or an unexpected decision, it may be in the patient's best interest to bring in another interpreter and repeat the exchange of information and questions.

Case Study and Discussion

Mrs. R. is an 88-year-old female, widowed for 22 years and with no next of kin, who lived alone prior to her admission to the nursing home 2 years ago, at which time she consented to a DNR order. She has severe COPD; chronic renal failure (BUN 58); dementia mild/mod (MMSE 20/30); is mildly depressed (by GDS score); and is below her IBW (-22 pounds). Mrs. R. now requires one person for all personal care; she bruises easily. Her prognosis is poor; goals of care are symptom management with comfort/palliative care. She has had multiple hospitalizations for "pneumonia"; the latest was 10 weeks ago, after which she had further weight loss and developed a grade II pressure ulcer on her right hip. She is receiving the standard meds for COPD, an anti-anxiety med, a short-acting sleeping med, and appetite stimulants. Recent discussion about her quality of life by the interdisciplinary team noted that she no longer attends parties, Sabbath candle lighting, or discussions, all of which she used to enjoy. Mrs. R. seemed unable to make health care decisions as of 6 months ago; her decisional capacity appears to fluctuate in relation to her O2 saturation.

Five years ago, Mrs. R. created a LW that stipulated "aggressive comfort care, including ventilator support." There are no verbal statements documented that might indicate Mrs. R.'s feelings about being hospitalized if she has another COPD exacerbation, which is to be expected given the trajectory of this disease.

Two days ago, Mrs. R. began to have stertorous breathing, a nonproductive cough, and episodes of diaphoresis. She appears exhausted; her solid food intake is minimal and she gets very dyspneic when taking small sips of fluid. A chest x-ray was equivocal and is to be repeated today. At present, her vital signs are T: 100.8, Pulse Ox: 82%; P and BP WNL. The nursing home has the resources to provide oxygen and IV fluids including antibiotics.

The difficulty of this case is a LW instruction, written before the disease trajectory had reached a terminal state, and that now might not be in Mrs. R.'s best interest; aggressive intervention might be more burdensome than beneficial. Whose voice will articulate the benefits and burdens of hospitalization or remaining in the nursing home for palliative/terminal care? The nurse assistants feel she should be hospitalized; their advocacy is based on 2 years of knowing her and feelings of great affection for her. The clinical professional staff argue from prognostications about the likely aggressive interventions (e.g., intubation and ventilator support) and probable multiple skin breakdowns if she is hospitalized. The standard of "substituted judgment" that a proxy uses when deciding on behalf of a patient whose wishes and preferences are known is not available to us. One could ask, "What would Mrs. R. choose if she could join the discussion?" The "best interest" standard of decision making asks what we think would promote Mrs. R.'s well-being. Can we bring her back to baseline (i.e., the status at which staff knew and loved her)? At this point, the benefit–burden assessment becomes a critical part of the discussion.

Conflict among the professional and paraprofessional staff has to be addressed. For the nurses, administering morphine to provide respiratory comfort might well hasten Mrs. R.'s death. Are we prolonging life or prolonging death? Are we treating resident or institutional anxiety? What are our learning needs? COPD is a disease with no cure; it progresses inexorably to death. What is meant by quality of life? It is a complex personal phenomenon and judgment, not a medical determination. To what extent can the facility provide a reasonable quality of life, a degree of comfort and safety that might meet Mrs. R.'s interests at this time? Life and engagement for Mrs. R. at this time will be different from the one the staff previously enjoyed with her. What are the contingencies, the "what-ifs" for the nursing home? What are the legal and ethical implications of departing from Mrs. R.'s AD? What are the risks to the nursing home in administering morphine, of the principle of double (i.e., unintended) effect?

After discussion with an ethics consultant at an interdisciplinary meeting that included the nurse assistants involved in her care, a consensus decision was made not to hospitalize Mrs. R. The decision was guided by the clinical facts, Mrs. R.'s prior wishes (for "aggressive comfort care"), education about COPD, fact-gathering, values discussion, and reflection about Mrs. R.'s condition after each hospitalization. Mechanical ventilation was likely to be more of a burden than a benefit at this point in her illness; Mrs. R. could be made comfortable with judicious use of medication and intensive nursing care. This case teaches us that advance care planning is not a static one-time event. Whether a person's wishes and preferences are stated through an AD document or verbally, they must be periodically reviewed upon a person's change of condition, lifestyle, proxy, heart, and mind. The ability to reach consensus through mediation that addressed each person's concerns but kept the discussion resident-centered was key to arriving at a medically and ethically appropriate decision that focused on the goals of care.

Conclusion

Discussions about care at the end of life should occur over time. Having such discussions shortly after hospitalization for an acute event can blur the priorities of advance care planning, focusing more on resuscitation preferences than on the long-range goals of care and treatment (Happ et al., 2002 [Level IV]). Notions of quality of life, confusion about what it looks and feels like, and how to measure this complex phenomenon influence patient, proxy, and family decisions regarding end-of-life care and interventions (O'Brien et al., 1995 [Level IV]; Suri, Egleston, Brody, & Rudberg, 1999 [Level IV]). Rather than discussing the technology of life-sustaining treatment and end-of-life care, nurses can help reorient and center the discussion on the patient's wishes and preferences. It may be wiser and more humane to discuss with patients, families, and proxies the acceptable state of health, desired functionality, and the "valued life activities" that patients want. Construing quality of life in this manner might be more meaningful and helpful.

Although hardly a justification, having an AD can be cost effective—if not for the patient, then for the health care system—and with no decrease in satisfaction with care. Patients suffering from advanced illness and approaching the end of their life were randomly assigned to a coordinated care program for advanced illness or usual care. Intervention-group patients were more satisfied with care and communication, and their surrogates reported fewer difficulties in accessing providers, in comparison to patients receiving usual care (Engelhardt et al., 2006 [Level II]). There was no difference in mortality rate; 6-month costs were lower in the intervention group. Another study demonstrated that after systematic implementation of an AD program in several nursing homes, a significant number of competent residents and families of incompetent residents created ADs in the intervention homes; satisfaction with care was no different between intervention and control homes (Molloy et al., 2000 [Level II]). There were fewer hospitalizations per resident and less resource use in the intervention homes and no difference in percentage of deaths for intervention and control homes.

An environment conducive to meaningful discussions about ADs and end-of-life care requires an appropriate time and location. An emergency admission is not an appropriate time. Distribution without discussion, commonly done in hospital admissions offices at the time of an elective admission, is not an appropriate time either. (Nursing homes tend to wait 2 weeks before discussing ADs with a new admission.) Patients may be more receptive to read about ADs if the information is part of a preadmission package or discussed as part of the discharge process when the impact of hospitalization is still fresh but the acute symptoms (and probable anxiety) are no longer present. It is unlikely that education and information about ADs will completely counteract the natural discomfort associated with discussing death and dying; this is generally as true for patients and families as it is for care providers. Awareness of the patient and family's spiritual and cultural "surround," as well as the provider's moral biases about life-sustaining treatment, gives rise to sensitive and realistic discussion. Nurses can improve care at the end of life for elderly patients by encouraging advance care planning and creation of ADs.

Bioethics Resources

American Nurses Association (ANA)
ANA Center for Ethics and Human Rights
600 Maryland Avenue, SW, Suite 100 West
Washington, DC 20024-2571
Telephone: (202) 651-7055
www.nursingworld.org

- Code for Nurses with Interpretive Statements
- Position Statements on Assisted Suicide and Active Euthanasia, Do-Not-Resuscitate, Comfort and Relief, Patient Self-Determination Act
- Selected Bibliographies on Ethical Issues Such as End-of-Life Decisions, Forgoing Artificial Nutrition and Hydration, Nursing Ethics Committees, and Assisted Suicide and Euthanasia

The American Society of Bioethics and Humanities
4700 West Lake Avenue
Glenview, IL 60025
Telephone: (847) 375-4745
www.asbh.org

■ International Journal of Nursing Ethics

Choice in Dying/Partnership for Caring, Inc.
National Office
1620 I Street NW, Suite 202
Washington, DC 20006
Telephone: (202) 296-8071
http://www.choices.org

■ Questions and Answers: Advance Directives and End-of-Life Decisions;
Medical Treatments and Your Advance Directives; Artificial Nutrition and
Hydration and End-Of-Life Decision Making; Do-Not-Resuscitate Orders
and End-of-Life Decisions
■ Video: Who's Death Is It, Anyway? (PBS special)

Hospice and Palliative Nurses Association

Medical Center East, Suite 375
211 North Whitfield Street
Pittsburgh, PA 15206-3031
Telephone: (412) 361-2470

■ Standards of Hospice Nursing
■ Symptom Management
■ Algorithms for Palliative Care

The Kennedy Institute of Ethics
P.O. Box 571212
Georgetown University
Washington, DC 20057-1212
www.georgetown.edu/research/kie/

■ Scope Note series
■ Ethics Journal (available electronically)

Last Acts
1620 I Street, NW, Suite 202
Washington, DC 20006
Telephone: (202) 296-8352
www.lastacts.org

■ Journal article summaries
■ State initiatives on EOL Care—Focus: Pain Management

- Helping employees deal with EOL issues
- Statement on diversity in EOL care

Aging With Dignity (Five Wishes AD)
P.O. Box 1661
Tallahassee, FL 32302-1661
Telephone: (888) 5WISHES (594-7437)
www.agingwithdignity.org

Physician's Orders for Life-Sustaining Treatment (POLST)
Washington State Medical Association
2033 6th Avenue, Suite 1100
Seattle, WA 98121
Telephone: (800) 552-0612
www.wsma.org/patients/polst.html

End-of-Life Nursing Education Consortium (ELNEC)
American Association of Colleges of Nursing
One Dupont Circle, NW, Suite 530.
Washington, DC 20036
Telephone: (202) 785-8320
www.aacn.nche.edu/elnec

End-of-Life Physician Education Research Center (EPERC)
Medical College of Wisconsin, MEB, Room 3235
8701 Watertown Plank Road
Milwaukee, WI 53226
Telephone: (414) 456-4353
www.eperc.mcw.edu

Box 24.1

Nursing Standard of Practice Protocol: Advance Directives Protocol

GUIDING PRINCIPALS

A. All people have the right to decide what will be done with their bodies.
B. All individuals are presumed to have decision-making capacity until deemed otherwise.
C. All patients who can participate in a conversation, either verbally or through an alternate means of communication, should be approached to discuss and record their treatment preferences and wishes.
D. Health care professionals can improve end-of-life care for elderly patients by encouraging the use of ADs.

I. BACKGROUND

A. Education about Advance Directives
1. Patients uniformly state that they want more information about ADs.
2. Patients want nurses (and doctors) to approach them about ADs.
3. Fewer than 20% of Americans have completed an AD.

B. Advance Directives
1. Allow individuals to provide directions about the kind of medical care they do or do not want if they become unable to make decisions or communicate their wishes.
2. Provide guidance for health care professionals, families, and substitute decision makers about health care decision making that reflect the person's wishes.
3. Provide immunity for health care professionals, families, and appointed proxies from civil and criminal liability when health care professionals follow the AD in good faith.

C. Two types of Advance Directives: durable power of attorney for health care (DPAHC) (also called a health care proxy) and living will (LW)
1. A *durable power of attorney* allows individuals to appoint someone, called a health care proxy, agent, or surrogate, to make health care decisions for them should they lose the ability to make decisions or communicate their wishes.
2. A *living will* provides specific instructions to health care providers about particular kinds of health care treatment an individual would or would not want to prolong life. Living wills are often used to declare a wish to refuse, limit, or withhold life-sustaining treatment.

D. Instructional or Medical Directive: Intended to compensate for the weaknesses of LWs, this kind of directive identifies specific interventions that are acceptable to a patient in specific clinical situations.

E. Oral Advance Directives (verbal directives) are allowed in some states if there is clear and convincing evidence of the patient's wishes. Clear and convincing evidence can include evidence that the patient made the statement consistently and seriously, over time; specifically addressed the actual condition of the patient; and was consistent with the values seen in other areas of the patient's life. Legal rules surrounding oral ADs vary by state.

II. ASSESSMENT PARAMETERS

A. All adult patients regardless of age (with the exception of patients with persistent vegetative state, severe dementia, or coma) should be asked if they have a LW or if they have designated a proxy.

B. All patients, regardless of age, gender, religion, socioeconomic status, diagnosis, or prognosis, should be approached to discuss ADs and advance care planning.

C. Discussions about ADs should be conducted in the patient's preferred language to enable information transfer and questions and answers.

D. Patients who have been determined to lack capacity to make other decisions may still have the capacity to designate a proxy or make some health care decisions. Decision-making capacity should be determined for each individual based on whether the patient has the ability to make the specific decision in question.

E. If a LW has been completed or proxy has been designated:
1. The document should be readily available on the patient's current chart.
2. The attending physician should know that the directive exists and has a copy.
3. The designated health care proxy should have a copy of the document.
4. The AD should be reviewed periodically by the patient, attending physician/nurse, and the proxy to determine if it reflects the patient's current wishes and preferences.

III. CARE STRATEGIES

A. Nurses should assist patients and families trying to deal with end-of-life care issues.

B. Patients may be willing to discuss their health situation and mortality with a nurse or clergyman rather than with a family member and should be supported in doing so.

C. Patients should be assisted in talking with their family/proxy about their treatment and care wishes.

D. Patients should be assessed for their ability to cope with the information provided.

E. Nurses must be mindful of and sensitive to the fact that race, culture, ethnicity, and religion can influence the health care decision-making process. The fact that patients from non-Western cultures may not subscribe to Western notions of autonomy does not mean that these patients do not want to talk about their treatment wishes or that they would not have conversations with their families about their treatment preferences.

F. Patients must be respected for their decision to not complete an AD and reassured that they will not be abandoned or receive substandard care if they do not elect to formulate an AD.

G. Nurses should be aware of the institution's mechanism for resolving conflicts between family members and the patient or proxy or between the patient/family and care providers and assist the parties in using this resource.

H. Nurses should be aware of which professional in their agency/institution is responsible for checking with the patient that copies of the AD have been given to their primary-care provider(s), to their proxy, *and* that the patient is carrying a wallet-size card with AD and contact information.

IV. EVALUATION OF EXPECTED OUTCOMES

To determine whether implementation of this protocol influenced the type as well as the number of ADs created, changes should be measurable and contribute to the facility's ongoing quality improvement program. Look at:

A. As documented in the record:
  1. whether patients are asked about advance care planning and directives
  2. whether patients do or do not have an AD
B. Of those patients with an AD, the percentage of ADs included in patient charts
C. The use of interpreters to assist staff discussion of ADs with patients for whom English is not their primary language
D. The number of ADs completed in association with admission to or receipt of services from the agency/institution
E. The number of nurse referrals to the Ethics Committee of patient or staff situations regarding ADs

References

Allen, R. S., DeLaine, S. R., Chaplin, W. F., Marson, D. C., Bourgeois, M. S., Dijkstra, K., et al. (2003). Advance care planning in nursing homes: Correlates of capacity and possession of advance directives. *The Gerontologist, 43*(3), 309–317. Evidence Level IV: Nonexperimental Study.

American Bar Association (2001). *Health care surrogate decision making legislation*. Commission on Legal Problems of the Elderly. Washington, DC.

Aronheim, J. C., Mulvihill, M., Sieger, C., Park, P., & Fries, B. E. (2001). State practice variations in the use of tube feeding for nursing home residents with severe cognitive impairment. *Journal of the American Geriatrics Society, 49*(2), 148–152. Evidence Level IV: Nonexperimental Study.

Beck, A., Brown, J., Boles, M., & Barrett, P. (2002). Completion of advance directives by older health maintenance organization members: The role of attitudes and beliefs regarding life-sustaining treatment. *Journal of the American Geriatrics Society, 50*(2), 300–306. Evidence Level II: Single Experimental Study [RCT].

Berger, J. T., & Majerovitz, D. (1998). Stability of preferences for treatment among nursing home residents. *The Gerontologist, 38,* 217–223. Evidence Level V: Case Report.

Bookvar, K. S., & Lachs, M. S. (1998). Ethical conflicts reported by certified registered rehabilitation nurses. *Rehabilitation Nursing 23*(4), 179–184. Evidence Level IV: Nonexperimental Study.

Coppola, K. M., Ditto, P. H., Danks, J. H., & Smucker, W. D. (2001). Accuracy of primary care and hospital-based physicians' predictions of elderly outpatients' treatment preferences with and without advance directives. *Archives of Internal Medicine, 161*(3), 431–440. Evidence Level II: Single Experimental Study.

Cox, C. L., Cole, E., Reynolds, T., Wandrag, M., Breckenridge, S., & Dingle, M. (2006). Implications of cultural diversity in Do Not Attempt Resuscitation (DNAR) decision making. *Journal of Multicultural Nursing & Health, 12*(1), 20–28. Evidence Level I: Systematic Review.

Cruzan v. Missouri Department of Health (1990). 497 U.S. 261, 110 SCt 2841.

Danis, M., Garret, J., Harris, R., & Patrick, D. L. (1994). Stability of choices about life-sustaining treatments. *Annals of Internal Medicine, 120*, 567–573. Evidence Level V: Program Evaluation.

Ditto, P. H., Danks, J. H., Smucker, W. D., Bookwala, J., Coppola, K. M., Dresser, R., et al. (2001). Advance directives as acts of communication: A randomized controlled trial. *Archives of Internal Medicine, 161*, 421–430. Evidence Level II: Single Experimental Study (RCT).

Dubler, N. N., & Marcus, L. J. (1994). *Mediating bioethical disputes.* New York: United Hospital Fund of New York. Evidence Level VI: Expert Opinion.

Emanuel, L. L., & Emanuel, E. J. (1989). The medical directive: A new comprehensive advance care document. *Journal of the American Medical Association, 261*(22), 3288–3293. Evidence Level IV: Nonexperimental Study.

Engelberg, R. A., Patrick, D. L., & Curtis, J. R. (2005). Correspondence between patients' preferences and surrogates' understandings for dying and death. *Journal of Pain and Symptom Management, 30*(6), 498–509. Evidence Level III: Quasi-experimental Study.

Engelhardt, J. B., McClive-Reed, K. P., Toseland, R. W., Smith, T. L., Larson, D. G., & Tobin, D. R. (2006). Effects of a program for coordinated care of advanced illness on patients, surrogates, and health care costs: A randomized trial. *American Journal of Managed Care, 12*(2), 93–100. Evidence Level II: Single Experimental Study (RCT).

Gillick, M. R. (2006). The use of advance care planning to guide decisions about artificial nutrition and hydration. *Nutrition in Clinical Practice, 21*(2), 126–133. Evidence Level V: Literature Review.

Gorman, T. E., Ahern, S. P., Wiseman, J., & Skrobik, Y. (2005). Residents' end-of-life decision making with adult hospitalized patients: A review of the literature. *Academic Medicine, 80*(7), 622–633. Evidence Level V: Literature Review.

Gutheil, I. A., & Heyman, J. C. (2005). Communication between older people and their health care agents: Results of an intervention. *Health & Social Work, 30*(2), 107–116. Evidence Level II: Single Experimental Study.

Happ, M. B., Capezuti, E., Strumpf, N. E., Wagner, L., Cunningham, S., Evans, L., et al. (2002). Advance care planning and end-of-life care for hospitalized nursing home residents. *Journal of the American Geriatrics Society, 50*(5), 829–835. Evidence Level IV: Nonexperimental Study.

Hardin, S. B., & Yusufaly, Y. A. (2004). Difficult end-of-life treatment decisions: Do other factors trump advance directives? *Archives of Internal Medicine, 164*(14), 1531–1533. Evidence Level II: Single Experimental Study.

Heiman, H., Bates, D. W., Fairchild, D., Shaykevich, S., & Lehmann, L. S. (2004). Improving completion of advance directives in the primary care setting: A randomized controlled trial. *The American Journal of Medicine, 117*(5), 318–324. Evidence Level II: Single Experimental Study (RCT).

Hines, S. C., Glover, J. J., Babrow, S., Holley, J. L., Badzek, L. A., & Moss, A. H. (2001). Improving advance care planning by accommodating family preferences. *Journal of Palliative Medicine, 4*(4), 481–489. Evidence Level IV: Nonexperimental Study.

Hofmann, J. C., Wenger, N. S., Davis, R. B., Teno, J., Connors, A. F., Jr., Desbiens, N., et al. (1997). Patient preferences for communication with physicians about end-of-life decisions. SUPPORT Investigators. Study to Understand Prognoses and Preference for Outcomes and Risks of Treatment. *Annals of Internal Medicine, 127*(1), 1–12. Evidence Level III: Quasi-experimental Study.

Hopp, F. P., & Duffy, S. A. (2000). Racial variations in end-of-life care. *Journal of the American Geriatrics Society, 48*(6), 658–663. Evidence Level IV: Nonexperimental Study.

Jezewski, M. A., Brown, J. K., Wu, Y. B., Meeker, M. A., Feng, J. Y., & Bu, X. (2005). Oncology nurses' knowledge, attitudes, and experiences regarding advance directives. *Oncology Nursing Forum, 32*(2), 319–327. Evidence Level IV: Nonexperimental Study.

Kapp, M. B., & Mossman, D. (1996). Measuring decisional capacity: Cautions on the construction of a capacimeter. *Psychology and Public Policy Law, 2*, 73–95. Evidence Level V: Literature Review.

Kwak, J., & Haley, W. E. (2005). Current research findings on end-of-life decision making among racially or ethnically diverse groups. *The Gerontologist, 45*(5), 634–641. Evidence Level V: Literature Review.

Lo, B., & Steinbrook, R. (2006). *Resuscitating Advance Directives. Archives of Internal Medicine, 164*, 1501–1506. Evidence Level V: Literature Review.

Lynn, J., Schuster, J. L., & Kabcenell, A. (2000). *Improving care for the end of life: A sourcebook for health care managers and clinicians.* New York: Oxford University Press. Evidence Level V: Literature Review.

Meisel, A. (2002). *The right to die (Vols. 1 and 2).* New York: Aspen Law & Business. Evidence Level VI: Expert Opinion.

Mezey, M., Mitty, E., Bottrell, M., Ramsey, G., & Fisher, T. (2000a). Advance directives: Older adults with dementia. *Clinics in Geriatric Medicine, 16*, 255–268. Evidence Level IV: Non-experimental Study.

Mezey, M., Mitty, E., & Ramsey, G. (1997a). Assessment of decision-making capacity: Nurse's role. *Journal of Gerontological Nursing, 23*(3), 28–35. Evidence Level VI: Expert Opinion.

Mezey, M., Mitty, E., Rappaport, M., & Ramsey, G. (1997b). Implementation of the Patient Self-Determination Act in nursing homes in New York City. *Journal of the American Geriatrics Society, 45*(1), 43–49. Evidence Level IV: Nonexperimental Study.

Mezey, M. D., Leitman, R., Mitty, E. L., Bottrell, M. M., & Ramsey, G. C. (2000b). Why hospital patients do and do not execute an advance directive. *Nursing Outlook, 48*(4), 165–171. Evidence Level IV: Nonexperimental Study.

Mezey, M., Teresi, J., Ramsey, G., Mitty, E., & Bobrowitz, T. (2002). Determining a resident's capacity to execute a health care proxy. *Voices of decision in nursing homes: Respecting residents' preferences for end-of-life care.* New York: United Hospital Fund of New York. Evidence Level IV: Nonexperimental Study.

Midwest Bioethics Center (1996). *Ethics committee consortium: Guidelines for the determination of decisional incapacity.* Kansas City: Midwest Bioethics Center. Evidence Level VI: Expert Opinion.

Mitchell, S. L., Berkowitz, R. E., Lawson, F. M., & Lipsitz, L. A. (2000). A cross-national survey of tube-feeding decisions in cognitively impaired older persons. *Journal of the American Geriatrics Society, 48*, 391–397. Evidence Level IV: Nonexperimental Study.

Molloy, D. W., Guyatt, G. H., Russo, R., Goeree, R., O'Brien, B. J., & Bedard, M. (2000). Systematic implementation of an advance directive program in nursing homes: A randomized controlled trial. *Journal of the American Medical Association, 283*(11), 1437–1444. Evidence Level II: Single Experimental Study.

Morrison, R. S., Chichin, E., Carter, J., Burack, O., Lantz, M., & Meier, D. E. (2005). The effect of a social work intervention to enhance advance care planning documentation in the nursing home. *Journal of the American Geriatrics Society, 53*(2), 290–294. Evidence Level II: Single Experimental Study (RCT).

Morrison, R. S., & Meier, D. (2004). High rates of advance care planning in New York City's elderly population. *Archives of Internal Medicine, 164*(22), 2421–2426. Evidence Level IV: Nonexperimental Study.

National Bioethics Advisory Commission (1998). *Research involving persons with mental disorders that may affect decision making capacity, Vol 1.* Rockville, MD.

O'Brien, L. A., Grisso, J. A., Maislin, G., LaPann, K., Krotki, K. P., Greco, P. J., et al. (1995). Nursing home residents' preferences for life-sustaining treatments. *Journal of the American Medical Association, 274*, 1775–1779. Evidence Level IV: Nonexperimental Study.

Patel, R. V., Sinuff, T., & Cook, D. J. (2004). Influencing advance directive completion rates in non-terminally ill patients: A systematic review. *Journal of Critical Care, 19*(1), 1–9. Evidence Level I: Systematic Review.

PSDA, Patient Self-Determination Act. Pub. L. No. 101-508 (42 U.S.C.A. 1395cc (f)(1992).

Perkins, H. S., Geppert, C. M., Gonzales, A., Cortez, J. D., & Hazuda, H. P. (2002). Cross-cultural similarities and differences in attitudes about advance care planning. *Journal of General Internal Medicine, 17*(1), 48–57. Evidence Level IV: Nonexperimental Study.

Perry, E., Swartz, J., Brown, S., Smith, D., Kelly, G., & Swartz, R. (2005). Peer mentoring: A culturally sensitive approach to end-of-life planning for long-term dialysis patients. *American Journal of Kidney Diseases, 46*(1), 111–119. Evidence Level II: Single Experimental Study.

Puchalski, C. M., Zhong, Z., Jacobs, M. M., Fox, E., Lynn, J., Harrold, J., et al. (2000). Patients who want their family and physician to make resuscitation decisions for them: Observations from SUPPORT (Study to Understand Prognoses and Preferences for Outcomes and Risks of Treatment) and HELP (Hospitalized Elderly Longitudinal Project). *Journal of the American Geriatrics Society, 48* (5 Suppl.), S84–S90. Evidence Level V: Case Report.

Quill v. Vacco, 80 F.3d 716 (2nd Cir.), 1996.

Rodriquez, K. L., & Young, A. J. (2006). Patients' and health care providers' understandings of life-sustaining treatment: Are perceptions of goals shared or divergent? *Social Science Medicine, 62*(1), 125–133. Evidence Level IV: Nonexperimental Study.

Roth, L. H., Meisel, A., & Lidz, C. W. (1977). Tests of competency to consent to treatment. *American Journal of Psychiatry, 134*(3), 279–284.

Sabatino, C. P. (nd). *10 Legal myths about advance directives*. ABA Commission on Law and Aging. Washington, DC: American Bar Association.

Schwartz, C. E., Wheeler, H. B., Hammes, B., Basque, N., Edmunds, J., Reed, G., et al. (2002). Early intervention in planning end-of-life care with ambulatory geriatric patients: Results of a pilot trial. *Archives of Internal Medicine, 162*(14), 1611–1618. Evidence Level II: Single Experimental Study (RCT).

Silviera, M. J., DiPiero, A., Gerrity, M. S., & Feudtner, C. (2000). Patients' knowledge of options at the end of life. *Journal of the American Medical Association, 284*(19), 2483–2488. Evidence Level IV: Nonexperimental Study.

Stocking, C. B., Hougham, G. W., Danner, D. D., Patterson, M. B., Whitehouse, P. J., & Sachs, G. A. (2006). Speaking of research advance directives: Planning for future research participation. *Neurology, 66*(9), 1361–1366. Evidence Level IV: Nonexperimental Study.

Suri, D. N., Egleston, B. L., Brody, J. A., & Rudberg, M. A. (1999). Nursing home resident use of care directives. *Journal of Gerontology: Series A Biological Sciences and Medical Sciences, (54A)* M225–M229. Evidence Level IV: Nonexperimental Study.

The, A. M., Pasman, R., Onwuteaka-Philipsen, B., Ribbe, M., & Van Der Wal, G. (2002). Withholding the artificial administration of fluids and food from elderly patients with dementia: Ethnographic study. *British Medical Journal, 325*(7376), 1326. Evidence Level IV: Nonexperimental Study.

Tierney, W. M., Dexter, P. R., Gramelspacher, G. P., Perkins, A. J., Zhou, X. H., & Wolinsky, F. D. (2001). The effect of discussion about advance directives on patients' satisfaction with primary care. *Journal of General Internal Medicine, 16*(1), 32–40. Evidence Level II: Single Experimental Study (RCT).

Tilden, V. P., Nelson, C. A., Dunn, P. M., Donius, M., & Tolle, S. W. (2000). Nursing's perspective on improving communication about nursing home residents' preferences for medical treatment at end of life. *Nursing Outlook, 48*(3), 109–115. Evidence Level IV: Nonexperimental Study.

Tolle, S. W., Tilden, V. P., Nelson, C. A., & Dunn, P. M. (1998). A prospective study of the efficacy of the Physician Order for Life Sustaining Treatment (1995–1997). *Journal of the American Geriatrics Society, 46*(9), 1097–1102. Evidence Level IV: Nonexperimental Study.

Tresch, D., Heudebert, G., Kutty, K., Ohlert, J., VanBeek, K., & Masi, A. (1994). Cardiopulmonary resuscitation in elderly patients hospitalized in the 1990s: A favorable outcome. *Journal of the American Geriatrics Society, 42*(2), 137–141. Evidence Level V: Review of the Literature.

Van Niekerk, B. A., & Martin, F. (2002). The impact of the nurse-physician professional relationship on nurses' experience of ethical dilemmas in effective pain management. *Journal of Professional Nursing, 18*(5), 276–288. Evidence Level IV: Nonexperimental Study.

Zerzan, J., Stearns, S., & Hanson, L. (2000). Access to palliative care and hospice in nursing homes. *Journal of the American Medical Association, 284*, 2489–2494. Evidence Level IV: Nonexperimental Study.

Comprehensive Assessment and Management of the Critically Ill

25

Michele C. Balas
Colleen M. Casey
Mary Beth Happ

Educational Objectives

On completion of this chapter, the reader will be able to:

1. identify factors that influence an older adult's ability to survive and rehabilitate from a catastrophic illness

2. list examples of an atypical presentation of illness in critically ill older adults

3. describe geriatric-specific assessment and physical examination of critically ill older adults

4. identify nursing interventions that decrease critically ill older adults' risk for adverse medical outcomes

Overview

More than half (55.8%) of all intensive care unit (ICU) days are incurred by patients older than 65 and this number is expected to increase to unprecedented levels in the next 10 years as the population ages (Angus et al., 2000 [Level IV]). Although older adults are an extremely heterogeneous group, they share some

For a description of Evidence Levels cited in this chapter, see chapter 1, Developing and Evaluating Clinical Practice Guidelines, page 4.

Adapted from the American Association of Colleges of Nursing, "Preparing nursing students to care for older adults: Enhancing gerontology in senior-level undergraduate courses" curriculum module. Assessment and Management of Older Adults with Complex Illness in the Critical Care Unit, prepared by Michele C. Balas, Colleen M. Casey, and Mary Beth Happ.

age-related characteristics and are susceptible to various geriatric syndromes and diseases that may influence ICU treatments and outcomes.

Ideally, the goals of providing nursing care to a critically ill older adult include restoring physiologic stability, preventing complications, maintaining comfort and safety, and preserving or preventing decline in pre-illness functional ability and quality of life (QOL). There is evidence, however, suggesting that many critically ill older adults are at risk for poor outcomes. A critical review of the literature found that, once hospitalized for a life-threatening illness, older adults suffer from high ICU, hospital, and long-term crude mortality rates and are at risk for deterioration in functional ability and post-discharge institutional care (Chelluri, Grenvik, & Silverman, 1995 [Level V]). Older age is also one of the factors that may lead to physician bias in refusing ICU admission (Joynt et al., 2001 [Level IV]; Mick & Ackerman, 2004 [Level VI]); the decision to withhold mechanical ventilation, surgery, or dialysis (Hamel et al., 1999 [Level III]); and an increased frequency of Do-Not-Resuscitate (DNR) orders (Hakim et al., 1996 [Level III]). Despite these findings, most critically ill older adults demonstrate resiliency, report being satisfied with their QOL post-discharge, and, if needed, would reaccept ICU care and mechanical ventilation (Chelluri et al., 1995 [Level V]; Guentner et al., 2006 [Level IV]; Kleinpell & Ferrans, 2002 [Level IV]).

Background

Chronologic age *alone* is not an acceptable or accurate predictor of poor outcomes after critical illness (Chelluri et al., 1995 [Level V]; Esteban et al., 2004 [Level IV]; Kleinpell, 2003 [Level IV]). Factors influencing an older adult's ability to survive a critical illness include severity of illness, nature and extent of co-morbidities, diagnosis, reason for/duration of mechanical ventilation, complications, length of ICU/hospital stay, preadmission nursing home residence, pulmonary artery catheterization, prehospitalization functional ability, gender, and ethnicity (Adnet et al., 2001 [Level IV]; Chelluri et al., 1995 [Level V]; Chelluri, Pinsky, Donahoe, & Grenvik, 1993 [Level IV]; Djaiani & Ridley, 1997 [Level IV]; Esteban et al., 2004 [Level IV]; Hamel et al., 1999 [Level III]; Kass, Castriotta, & Malakoff, 1992 [Level IV]; Knaus et al., 1991 [Level IV]; Mayer-Oakes, Oye, & Leake, 1991 [Level IV]; Nicolas, Le Gall, Alperovitch, Loirat, & Villers, 1987 [Level IV]; Nierman, Schechter, Cannon, & Meier, 2001 [Level IV]; Richmond, Kauder, Strumpf, & Meredith, 2002 [Level IV]; Shapira et al., 1997 [Level IV]; Wu, Rubin, & Rosen, 1990 [Level IV]). Other less well investigated variables include senescence, cognitive impairment, ageism, decreased social support, and the critical care environment (Mick & Ackerman, 2004 [Level VI]; Tullmann & Dracup, 2000 [Level VI]).

The onset of new geriatric syndromes for an older hospitalized adult, such as urinary incontinence, infection, delirium, or falls, can often be prevented with appropriate and timely ICU nursing interventions (for more information, visit www.ConsultGeriRN.org). This chapter presents strategies and rationales for comprehensive assessment of critically ill older adults to guide optimal care management.

Assessment of Problem and Nursing Care Strategies

Assessment of Baseline Health Status

Comprehensive assessment of a critically ill older adult's preadmission health status, functional and cognitive ability, and social support systems helps nurses identify risk factors that make older adults susceptible to cascade iatrogenesis (Creditor, 1993 [Level VI]), the development of life-threatening conditions, and frequently encountered geriatric syndromes.

Pre-existing Cognitive Impairment

Several anatomic and physiologic changes occur in the aged central nervous system (Table 25.1) and are not necessarily synonymous with cognitive impairment (Urden, Stacy, & Lough, 2002 [Level VI]). The additive effect of chronic illness (e.g., diabetes, hypertension, or coronary artery disease [CAD]) coupled with common aging changes and acute pathology may, however, partially explain the high rates of pre-existing cognitive impairment (31% to 42%) found in older adults admitted to medical ICUs (Pisani, Inouye, McNicoll, & Redlich, 2003 [Level IV]). Relatives or other caregivers should be asked for baseline information about memory, executive function (problem solving, planning, organization of information), and overall functional ability in daily living prior to the critical care admission (Kane, Ouslander, & Abrass, 2004 [Level VI]) (see chapter 4, *Assessing Cognitive Function*).

Developmental and Psychosocial Factors

Various living and family arrangements are evidenced in this heterogeneous age group. Although many older adults live independently or are cared for by adult children or other relatives, many elders are also caregivers themselves, caring for their aging spouses, relatives, grandchildren, and friends (Administration on Aging, 2005 [Level IV]). The lack of presence of family or a significant other threatens a nurse's ability to obtain accurate data about the person, which is often needed to make urgent, important care management decisions. The very nature of the critical illness often renders older adults physically unable to effectively communicate with the health care team.

The inability to communicate may stem from multiple factors including physiologic instability, tracheal intubation, and/or sedative and narcotic use (Happ, 2000 [Level IV]; Happ, 2001 [Level IV]). Family members are therefore a crucial source for obtaining important preadmission information such as past medical and surgical history, drug and alcohol use, nutritional status, sensory impairments, home environment, and medication use, as well as information about advance directives and decisional choices (see chapter 23, *Health Care Decision Making*, and chapter 24, *Advance Directives*).

Functional Ability

Although the majority of older adults report having at least one chronic condition, they remain relatively independent (Administration on Aging, 2005

25.1 Age-Associated Changes by Body System in the Older ICU Patient*

System	Age-Associated Changes
Respiratory	Decrease in chest-wall compliance, rib mobility, lung elasticity, ventilatory response to hypoxia and hypercapnia, strength of respiratory muscles, PaO_2 level, mucociliary clearance, total lung capacity (minimal), vital capacity, forced expiratory volume (FEV_1), peak and maximal expiratory flow rate, and maximal inspiratory and expiratory pressure Increases in: functional residual capacity, closing volume, A/A gradient, ventilation/perfusion (VQ) imbalance
Gastrointestinal	Delayed gastric emptying and thinning of smooth muscle in gastric mucosa Decrease in the number of mucus-secreting cells, mucosal prostaglandin concentrations, bicarbonate secretion, transit time of feces, pepsin and acid secretion, ability to swallow (secondary to poor mastication and decrease in the number and velocity of peristaltic contractions in esophagus), enteric nervous system neurons, and the capacity to repair gastric mucosa Increase in body fat, changes to interstitial tissue (predisposing to soft-tissue injury and increasing the time and course for mobilization of extracellular water) Decreases in calcium absorption, lean muscle mass and strength, daily energy expenditure, and intracellular water
Hepatobiliary	Decrease in the number of hepatocytes and overall weight and size of liver (compensatory increase in cell size and proliferation of bile ducts), hepatic blood flow, metabolism of and sensitivity to drugs
Genitourinary	Nephrons/glomeruli become sclerotic, functional units hypertrophy, afferent and efferent arterioles atrophy Decline in GFR, renal tubular cell function and number, renal blood flow, and creatinine clearance Ability to conserve sodium and excrete hydrogen ions falls as does ability to excrete salt and water loads, ammonia, and certain drugs Decline in the activity of the renin-angiotensin system and end organ responsiveness to antidiuretic hormone Bladder: Increase in collagen In women, alterations in estrogen cause changes in urethral sphincter In males, benign prostatic hypertrophy
Skin	Decreased subcutaneous and connective tissue, number of eccrine and sebaceous glands, vascular supply to dermis, and skin turgor

	(continued)
System	**Age-Associated Changes**
Neurologic	Decrease in size of brain, number of neurons and dendrites, length of dendrite spines, and cerebral blood flow
	Increase in liposuscins, neuritic plaques, neurofibrillary bodies, and ventricle size
	Changes in hypothalamus and neurotransmitter turnover and function
	Decline in visual acuity and depth perception (secondary to anatomic and functional changes to the auditory and vestibular apparatus) and proprioception, balance and postural control, and tactile and vibratory sensation
Cardiovascular	Decrease in number of myocytes, ventricular compliance, rate of relaxation, baroreceptor sensitivity, compliance of arteries, response of myocardium to catecholamine stimulation, resting heart rate, and heart rate with stress
	Increase in myocardial collagen content, stiffening of the outflow tract and great vessels (causing resistance to vascular emptying), ventricular hypertrophy, pulse wave velocity
	Autonomic tissue is replaced by connective tissue and fat, whereas fibrosis causes conduction abnormalities through the intranodal tracts and the Bundle of His
Immune/ Hematopoi- etic	Change in T-cell populations, products and response to stimuli; defects in B-cell function; mix of immunoglobulins change (i.e., IgM decreases, IGG and IGA increase), and decline in neutrophil function

Source: Adapted from:

Nagappan, R., & Parkin, G., 2003 [Level VI]. Geriatric critical care. *Critical Care Clinics, 19,* 253–270.

Rosenthal, R. A., & Kavic, S. M., 2004 [Level VI]. Assessment and management of the geriatric patient. *Critical Care Medicine, 32*(4 Suppl.), S92–S105.

Urden et al., 2002 [Level VI]. Gerontological Alterations and Management. In *Thelan's critical care nursing: diagnosis and management* (4th ed., pp. 199–220). St. Louis, MO: Mosby.

[Level IV]); Waldrop & Stern, 2003 [Level IV]). Ascertaining preadmission functional status is a major determinant in the recovery of critically ill older adults (Mick & Ackerman, 2004 [Level VI]; Roche, Kramer, Hester, & Welsh, 1999 [Level IV]; Tullmann & Dracup, 2000 [Level VI]). Both the Katz Index of Activities of Daily Living (Katz, Ford, Moskowitz, Jackson, & Jaffe, 1963) and the Functional Independence Measure (FIM) (Kidd et al., 1995 [Level III]) have been recommended for use with an older population (Kresevic & Mezey, 2003 [Level VI]) (see chapter 3, *Assessment of Function*).

Assessment and Interventions During ICU Stay

Although a full discussion of the physiologic changes that accompany common aging is beyond the scope of this chapter, in the following sections we provide readers with (1) an overview of the major age-related changes to organ systems;

(2) a discussion of how these changes often manifest on physical exam; (3) a discussion of atypical presentations of some common ICU diagnoses; and (4) a description of interventions that may decrease risk for untoward medical events for critically ill older adults (also see the Box 25.1). Common nursing interventions that benefit multiple organ systems are discussed only in the first section in which the intervention is introduced. These interventions include encouraging early, frequent mobilization/ambulation; obtaining timely and appropriate consults (e.g., physical, occupational, speech, respiratory, and nutritional therapy); providing proper oral hygiene and adequate pain control; securing and ensuring the proper functioning of tubes/catheters; maintaining normothermia; and reviewing and assessing medication appropriateness. The importance of these interventions and vigilance to these elements of nursing care cannot be overstated.

Respiratory System

An older ICU patient's respiratory status can become the most tenuous component of his or her recovery. Common pulmonary changes in aging include progressive decreases in the strength of respiratory muscles, lung elasticity, chest-wall compliance, PaO_2 level, ventilatory responses to hypoxia and hypercapnia, and number and efficiency of airway cilia (see Table 25.1) (Nagappan & Parkin, 2003 [Level VI]; Rosenthal & Kavic, 2004 [Level VI]; Urden et al., 2002 [Level VI]). Nurses may observe some of the skeletal changes common in aging, including possible kyphosis and an increased anteroposterior diameter of the chest (Bates, 1995 [Level VI]) and on auscultation, hear a few bibasilar crackles that clear with deep breathing and coughing (Urden et al., 2002 [Level VI]).

Common pulmonary changes in aging elevate an older adult's risk for aspiration, atelectasis, and pneumonia (Nagappan & Parkin, 2003 [Level VI]; Rosenthal & Kavic, 2004 [Level VI]; Urden et al., 2002 [Level VI]). These risks are further heightened in older adults who undergo thoracic or abdominal surgery; sustain rib fractures or chest injury; receive narcotics or sedatives; have tubes that bypass the oropharyngeal airway; or who are weak, deconditioned, dehydrated, and have poor oral hygiene (Nagappan & Parkin, 2003 [Level VI]; Rosenthal & Kavic, 2004 [Level VI]; Urden et al., 2002 [Level VI]). Pre-existing pulmonary disease and manipulations of the abdominal and thoracic cavities may lead to the unreliability of traditional values associated with central venous (CVP) and pulmonary artery occlusion (PAOP) pressures (Rosenthal & Kavic, 2004 [Level VI]). Consequently, it is important to discuss with the ICU team any unusual preexisting or acute influences on these hemodynamic parameters so that adequate trends can be monitored.

Older patients with pre-existing obstructive or restrictive lung disease who are mechanically ventilated are also at increased risk for ventilator assisted pneumonia (VAP) and delayed extubation. To minimize this complication, nurses should aggressively exercise standard VAP precautions, including keeping the head of the bed elevated to more than 30 degrees, providing frequent oral care, maintaining adequate cuff pressures, assessing the need for stress ulcer prophylaxis, turning the patient as tolerated, maintaining general hygiene practices, and advocating for weaning trials as early as possible (Kunis & Puntillo, 2003 [Level VI]).

Caring for an older adult who requires mechanical ventilation is particularly challenging. Although debate exists as to whether age influences outcome in this population, evidence suggests that chronic ventilatory dependency disproportionately affects older patients, whether as a complication of a critical illness or as a result of a chronic respiratory system limitation (Esteban et al., 2004 [Level IV]; Kleinhenz & Lewis, 2000 [Level VI]). Patients who require 4 or more days of mechanical ventilation are more likely to die in the hospital or, if they survive, to spend a considerable amount of time in an extended-care facility upon discharge, experience an increased risk for hospital readmission, suffer from continued morbidity, and experience a decreased quality of life (Chelluri et al., 2004 [Level IV]; Daly, Douglas, Kelley, O'Toole, & Montenegro, 2005 [Level II]; Douglas, Daly, Brennan, Gordon, & Uthis, 2001 [Level IV]; Douglas et al., 1997 [Level IV]; Douglas, Daly, Gordon, & Brennan, 2002 [Level IV]). In addition to advocating for weaning trials and extubation as early as possible, the health care team, including the ICU nurse, must include these potential consequences as part of a discussion of treatment options with patients and their families.

Cardiovascular System

Because so many older adults live with hypertension, peripheral vascular disease, or CAD, individual responses to treatment can dramatically differ depending on the severity of their illness and any preexisting co-morbidities. Even "disease-free" older adults may experience a decrease in their ability to respond to stressful situations due to the many changes that accompany cardiovascular aging (see Table 25.1). Upon auscultation, many healthy older adults display a fourth heart sound (S_4), an aortic systolic murmur, higher systolic blood pressure with a widening pulse pressure, and a slower resting heart rate (Bates, 1995 [Level VI]).

Cardiovascular-associated aging changes ultimately render the myocardium less compliant and responsive to catecholamine stimulation, can cause ventricular hypertrophy, and predispose the older adult to the development of arrhythmias (Nagappan & Parkin, 2003 [Level VI]; Rosenthal & Kavic, 2004 [Level VI]; Urden et al., 2002 [Level VI]). During times of stress, an older adult achieves an increase in cardiac output by increasing diastolic filling rather than increasing heart rate (Nagappan & Parkin, 2003 [Level VI]; Rosenthal & Kavic, 2004 [Level VI]; Urden et al., 2002 [Level VI]). The practical implication of this finding is that older adults often require higher filling pressures (i.e., CVPs in the 8 to 10 range, PAOPs in the 14 to 18 range) to maintain adequate stroke volume and may be especially sensitive to hypovolemia (Rosenthal & Kavic, 2004 [Level VI]). However, over-hydration of the older adult should also be avoided because it can lead to systolic failure, poor organ perfusion, and hypoxemia with subsequent diastolic dysfunction (Rosenthal & Kavic, 2004 [Level VI]). Careful monitoring of hemodynamic and fluid status is therefore essential to optimize an older patient's cardiac status.

Many conduction abnormalities (i.e., atrial arrhythmias, sick sinus syndrome, and bundle branch blocks) are common in aging. Although many of the randomized controlled trials of beta-blocker therapy are small, the weight of evidence, in aggregate, suggests that the use of preoperative beta-adrenergic blockade decreases the incidence of postoperative cardiac complications and death in patients considered high risk (Fleisher et al., 2006 [Level I]; Mangano, Layug, Wallace, & Tateo, 1996 [Level II]; Poldermans et al., 1999 [Level II]). High cardiovascular risk includes older adults with unstable coronary syndromes, decompensated heart failure, significant arrhythmias, previous myocardial infarction, and even patients with diabetes mellitus and renal insufficiency (Fleisher et al., 2006 [Level I]).

Certain drugs commonly used in the ICU setting may prove to be either not as effective (e.g., isoproterenol and dobutamine) or more effective (e.g., afterload reducers) in the older adult population (Rosenthal & Kavic, 2004 [Level VI]). Symptoms of a myocardial infarction may be blunted in older adults, requiring the need to monitor for nonspecific and atypical presentations in this patient population, including shortness of breath, acute confusion, or syncope. Finally, because older adults may have difficulty with thermoregulation, especially during a critical illness, nurses should take active measures to maintain normothermia (Rosenthal & Kavic, 2004 [Level VI]).

Neurologic System

The central and peripheral nervous system changes that accompany the aging process include decreases in both the overall size of the brain and the number of neurons, hypothalamic alterations, neurotransmitter turnover, and anatomic changes to the auditory, visual, and vestibular apparatus (see Table 25.1) (Nagappan & Parkin, 2003 [Level VI]; Rosenthal & Kavic, 2004 [Level VI]; Urden et al., 2002 [Level VI]). On physical exam, these changes are often manifested by a decreased papillary response to penlight, as well as a decrease in near and peripheral vision and loss of visual acuity to dim light (Urden et al., 2002 [Level VI]). Other alterations on physical exam findings may include evidence of muscle wasting and atrophy, presentation of a benign essential tumor, slower and less agile movement as compared to younger adults, diminished peripheral reflexes, and a decreased vibratory sense in the feet and ankles (Bates, 1995 [Level VI]).

Older adults often present to emergency departments or ICU with acute neurologic symptoms. These acute neurological changes may represent an atypical presentation of an acute illness and can be reversible (e.g., delirium), including alterations caused by infection, an imbalance of electrolytes, or drug toxicity. A thorough physical examination, with follow-up testing, must be conducted to accurately diagnose the etiology of an older adult's neurologic changes, as well as to review medications that are likely to cause delirium.

Age-related changes to the neurologic system, when coupled with acute pathology and the ICU environment, may increase a critically ill older adult's risk for cognitive dysfunction, falls, restraint use, over-sedation, alterations in body temperature, and anorexia. Most important, these changes also elevate the risk for delirium that occurs in up to 70% of older adults admitted to a medical ICU (McNicoll et al., 2003 [Level IV]; Peterson et al., 2006 [Level IV]) and is associated with increased morbidity, mortality, length of hospital stay, and poor functional outcomes (Ely et al., 2001 [Level II]). Pain, sleep deprivation, visual impairment, illness severity, prior cognitive impairment, dehydration, co-morbidities, laboratory abnormalities, multiple medications, chemical withdrawal syndromes, infections, fever, windowless units, and ICU length of stay may place a critically ill older adult at risk for delirium (Aldemir, Ozen, Kara, Sir, & Bac, 2001 [Level IV]; Dubois, Bergeron, Dumont, Dial, & Skrobik, 2001 [Level IV]; Inouye et al., 1999 [Level II]; Sveinsson, 1975; Tullmann & Dracup, 2000 [Level VI]; Wilson, 1972 [Level III]).

Achieving adequate pain control for critically ill older adults is of utmost importance, both related to and independent of its relationship to delirium; however, nurses also need to avoid over-sedation and under-treatment of pain in this population because both are associated with multiple negative outcomes, including distress, delirium, sleep disturbances, and impaired mobility (Graf & Puntillo, 2003 [Level VI]; Rosenthal & Kavic, 2004 [Level VI]). A number of tools exist to assess a critically ill patient's level of sedation and delirium status. The Richmond Agitation and Sedation Scale (RASS) (Sessler et al., 2002 [Level IV]) and the Confusion Assessment Method-ICU (CAM-ICU) (Ely et al., 2001 [Level IV]; Miller & Ely, 2006 [Level VI]) are two of the most common in the critical care setting (see the Resources section for additional information on these tools and the Protocol for interventions to reduce delirium (Box 25.1).

Gastrointestinal (GI) System

Common age-related changes to the GI system can predispose older ICU patients to complications during their ICU stay, ranging from altered presentation of illness to issues of medication effectiveness. Physiologic changes include delayed gastric emptying, alterations in the secretion of gastric enzymes and acid, loss of enteric nervous system neurons, and a decrease in the number of hepatocytes and overall weight and size of liver, all of which influence the pharmacodynamics and pharmacokinetics associated with drug dosing, metabolism, and sensitivity (see Table 25.1) (Nagappan & Parkin, 2003 [Level VI]; Rosenthal & Kavic, 2004 [Level VI]; Urden et al., 2002 [Level VI]). Older adults also experience changes in their body composition (i.e., decrease in lean body mass) and energy use that can potentiate the effect of medications on these GI system changes.

Ironically, whereas many conditions affecting the GI system are more common in older adults (e.g., constipation, under-nutrition and malnutrition, gastritis), their presence is not fully explained by the aging processes (Rosenthal & Kavic, 2004 [Level VI]). When assessing the GI function of a critically ill older adult, it is important for the nurse to realize that age may blunt the manifestations of acute abdominal disease. For example, pain may be less severe; fever less pronounced or absent; and signs of peritoneal inflammation, such as muscle guarding and rebound tenderness, may be diminished or even absent (Bates, 1995 [Level VI]). Because of changes in the secretion of gastric enzymes, the stomach wall of older adults can be more susceptible to acid injury, especially in the face of critical illness. ICU nurses must be alert for signs of gastrointestinal bleeding and be proactive in advocating for gastric ulcer prophylaxis, especially in those elders requiring mechanical ventilation.

Delayed gastric emptying may predispose older adults to abdominal distension, nausea, vomiting, aspiration, and constipation. This delayed motility is especially true in the postoperative period when many older adults are immobile and receiving narcotics. Many older adults take multiple medications, which along with age-related changes such as altered thresholds for taste and smell, a hypersensitive hypothalamic satiety center, and oropharyngeal atrophy, can inhibit their intake of solids and liquids (Rosenthal & Kavic, 2004 [Level VI]). This baseline GI functionality, in combination with their critical illness, must be proactively addressed. Nurses need to be alert for ill-fitting dentures, swallowing difficulties, silent aspiration, and the possibility of decreased saliva production (due to either salivary dysfunction or the use of drugs, such as sympathomimetics). These alterations can lead to insufficient mastication and can combine with other risk factors that put the older ICU patient at risk for aspiration. Aspiration should be considered a life-threatening situation, requiring immediate nursing intervention.

Older adults facing stress from illness, injury, or infection are also at high risk for protein-calorie malnutrition, as evidenced by low serum albumin and prealbumin levels, a decline in hepatic function, decreased muscle mass and strength, and dysfunction in those tissues with high cell turnover (Nagappan & Parkin, 2003 [Level VI]; Rosenthal & Kavic, 2004 [Level VI]). These changes lead to a breakdown in barrier function, increased susceptibility to infection, delayed wound healing, fluid shifts, deconditioning, and further impairment in absorption of essential nutrients (Rosenthal & Kavic, 2004 [Level VI]). Thus, early enteral or parental nutritional support is crucial when considering advance directives.

Reductions with age in the activity of the drugmetabolizing enzyme system and blood flow through the liver influences the liver's capacity to metabolize various drugs (Kane et al., 2004 [Level VI]; Urden et al., 2002 [Level VI]). Splanchnic blood flow is further compromised in states of shock or even mild hypotension. These changes may predispose older adults to adverse drug reactions (Urden et al., 2002 [Level VI]). For example, drugs like warfarin, which work directly on hepatocytes, may reach their therapeutic effect at lower doses (Rosenthal & Kavic, 2004 [Level VI]). Common pharmacologic agents used in the critical care setting and their common side effects often experienced by the gerontologic patient are listed in Table 25.2 (see chapter 12, *Preveating Adverse Drug Events*).

Finally, many older adults have diabetes and even those older adults without pre-existing diabetes may experience elevated blood glucose levels as a result of medications and a stress response to critical illness. Studies have shown that strict control of blood glucose using insulin drips leads to better outcomes, across ages, in terms of mortality, bloodstream infections, acute renal failure, blood transfusions needed, and polyneuropathy (van den Berghe et al., 2001 [Level II]). However, glycemic control in the older ICU patient may be more difficult because of a declining glucose tolerance associated with aging. In light of an older adult's susceptibility to iatrogenesis, strict control of the exaggerated glucose response in this population may prove especially important (Rosenthal, 2004 [Level VI]).

Genitourinary (GU) System

Preservation of the older adult's preadmission renal status is one of the goals of ICU care. Age-related renal changes to this system include declines in renal blood flow, glomerular filtration rate (GFR), and creatinine clearance, and a decreased ability to conserve sodium and excrete hydrogen ions (see Table 25.1) (Nagappan & Parkin, 2003 [Level VI]; Rosenthal & Kavic, 2004 [Level VI];

25.2 High Risk Medications Commonly Used in Older ICU Patients

Drug	Severity Rating[+]	Potential Adverse Effects
*Amiodarone (Cordarone)	High	May provoke torsades de pointes and QT interval problems. Lack of efficacy in older adults.
*Clonidine (Catapres)	Low	Orthostatic hypotension, CNS adverse effects
*Diazepam (Valium)	High	Increased sensitivity to benzodiazepines; long half-life in older patients (can be several days); prolonged sedation; increasing risk of falls/fractures; short- and intermediate-acting benzodiazepines preferred
Digoxin (Lanoxin)	Low	Decreased renal clearance may lead to increased risk of toxic effects; dose should not exceed >0.125 mg/d except when treating atrial arrhythmias
*Diphenhydramine (Benadryl)	High	Strong anticholinergic effects, confusion, over-sedation; also can cause dry mouth, urinary retention; aggravates benign prostatic hypertrophy and glaucoma; use smallest possible dose
*Ketorolac (Toradol)	High	Peptic ulceration, GI bleeding, perforation; GI effects can be asymptomatic
*Meperidine (Demerol)	High	Active metabolite accumulation may cause CNS toxicity, tremor, confusion, irritability; other narcotics preferred
*Promethazine (Phenergan)	High	Highly anticholinergic; confusion, over-sedation; also can cause dry mouth, urinary retention; aggravates benign prostatic hypertrophy and glaucoma
Propofol (Diprivan)	Unrated	Lipophilic drug; decreased clearance in older adults related to increased total body fat
Cimetidine (Tagamet) and Ranitidine (Zantac)	Low	CNS effects, confusion

*Source: Adapted from Bonk et al., 2006 [Level IV]. Potentially inappropriate medications in hospitalized senior patients. *American Journal of Health System Pharmacists, 63*(12), 1161–1165.

Fick et al., 2003. Updating the Beers criteria for potentially inappropriate medication use in older adults: Results of a U.S. consensus panel of experts. *Archives of Internal Medicine, 163* (22), 2716–2724 [Level VI].

[+]Severity Rating—Adverse effects of medications rated as high or low severity based on the probability of event occurring and significance of the outcome (Beers, 1997; Bonk et al., 2006 [Level IV]).

*Identified in Bonk et al., 2006 [Level IV] as seven most commonly prescribed Beers medications used in older hospitalized patients.

Urden et al., 2002 [Level VI]). Common age-related changes in the GU system decrease older adults' ability to excrete ammonia and drugs, diminish their capacity to regulate fluid and acid base balance, and often impair their ability to properly empty their bladder (Nagappan & Parkin, 2003 [Level VI]; Rosenthal & Kavic, 2004 [Level VI]; Urden et al., 2002 [Level VI]). The coupling of these common age-related changes with conditions commonly seen in the ICU environment such as hypovolemia, shock, sepsis, and polypharmacy render older adults at increased risk for acute renal failure, metabolic acidosis, and adverse drug events. The increased prevalence in the older population of asymptomatic bacteriuria also exacerbates an older ICU patient's infection risk related to Foley catheter use (Richards, 2003 [Level VI]).

Nurses must consider older patients' baseline cardiovascular status relative to their renal function. If an older patient was typically hypertensive prior to hospitalization, for example, this patient's renal vasculature may be accustomed to a higher than normal pressure to perfuse the kidneys. Furthermore, common indicators of dehydration, such as skin turgor, should be considered an unreliable sign in older adults, related to their loss of subcutaneous tissue (Sheehy, Perry, & Cromwell, 1999 [Level VI]). Although the Cockroft and Gault formula (see chapter 12, *Reducing Adverse Drug Events*) has been derived to estimate creatinine clearance in the healthy aged, care must be taken when applying this formula to critically ill older patients or to those patients on medications that directly affect renal function (Rosenthal & Kavic, 2004 [Level VI]). Finally, nurses should be especially cognizant of medications known to contribute to renal failure including aminoglycosides, certain antibiotics, and contrast dyes, and closely monitor laboratory results as warranted (Urden et al., 2002 [Level VI]).

Immune/Hematopoietic System

The changes that occur in the aged immune and hematological system mainly involve altered T and B cell functioning and a decrease in hematopoietic reserve (see Table 25.1) (Nagappan & Parkin, 2003 [Level VI]; Rosenthal & Kavic, 2004 [Level VI]; Urden et al., 2002 [Level VI]). The consequences of these changes include an increased susceptibility to infection, increases in auto antibodies and monoclonal immunoglobulins, and tumorigenesis (Rosenthal & Kavic, 2004 [Level VI]). These common aging changes coupled with the stress, malnutrition, and number of invasive procedures seen in the critical care environment may heighten an older adult's risk for a nosocomial infection. Furthermore, because an older adult's ability to mount a febrile response to infection diminishes with age (related to a decline in hypothalamic function), an older patient may even be septic without the warning of a fever (Urden et al., 2002 [Level VI]) and instead may exhibit only a decline in mental status. Close assessment of other nonfebrile signs of infection (i.e., restlessness, agitation, delirium, hypotension, and tachycardia) is essential and warranted.

Although recent research suggests that giving blood more liberally to patients may be associated with worse patient outcomes, these findings may not necessarily apply to the older adult population for several reasons: (1) the chronic anemia often seen in aging, (2) the exclusion of many older adults from previous clinical trials, (3) research findings that suggest higher transfusion triggers in older patients with acute myocardial infarction actually decreases mortality, and (4) the association of low hemoglobin levels with increased incidence of delirium, functional decline, and decreased mobility (Rosenthal & Kavic, 2004 [Level VI]).

Skin and Wounds

Older adults are at high risk for skin breakdown in the ICU setting due to loss of elastic, subcutaneous, and connective tissues; a decrease in sweat gland activity; and a decrease in capillary arterioles supplying the skin with age (Urden et al., 2002 [Level VI]) (see Table 25.1). On physical exam, a nurse may observe that an older adult's skin has become thin, fragile, wrinkled, loose, or transparent and is dry, flaky, rough, and often itchy. Older adults' nails lose their luster, with hair color and loss also occurring as part of aging (Bates, 1995 [Level VI]).

Because the skin changes that occur in older adults can cause difficulty with thermoregulation, can heighten the risk for skin breakdown and IV infiltrations, may delay wound healing, and can make hydration assessment difficult, nurses should make every effort to prevent heat loss, carefully monitor hydration status, and conduct thorough skin assessments (Bates, 1995; Urden et al., 2002 [both Level VI]) (see chapter 18, *Preventing Pressure Ulcers and Skin Tears*).

Case Study and Discussion

Ned Saunders is a 71-year-old man who fell off of a ladder while stringing holiday lights and suffered serious complications, including Adult Respiratory Distress Syndrome (ARDS), after laminectomy. He required a second back surgery (revision of the laminectomy) during the same hospital stay, and developed a clostridium difficile (c. difficile) infection and nutritional problems secondary to the severe diarrhea. Infection with antibiotic-resistant organisms necessitated the use of isolation protocol. Tracheostomy placement occurred on the 17th ICU day and progressive weaning trials began.

Preadmission

Mr. Saunders was a former smoker and his past medical history included mild COPD and hypertension. His medications prior to admission were Albuterol inhaler 2 puffs every 6 hours and hydrochlorothiazide 50mgs for blood pressure. He smoked a half pack per day for 30 years. A retired school teacher, Mr. Saunders was slightly overweight but active around the house and enjoyed an active social life, especially dancing with his wife at local dance halls. He was a "social drinker," as reported by his wife, having three to four glasses of wine per week. Mr. Saunders was completely independent in all activities of daily living before this hospitalization. MMSE score on admission before surgery was 29. CAM-ICU (for delirium) on admission to the ICU was positive for delirium.

Psychosocial

Mr. Saunders was unable to focus attention for more than 5 seconds at a time and was intermittently agitated during the early stages of ICU stay. Delirium was treated with around-the-clock dosages of intravenous haldoperidol. He also received fentanyl patch (dose) for pain and lorazepam (dose and frequency taken) as needed for anxiety/sedation. Efforts were made to minimize and taper the use of the benzodiazepine (lorazepam) in an attempt to clear the delirium.

Anxiety and communication difficulties were identified by nurses as problems possibly influencing his "mental state" during ventilator weaning. Communication was inhibited by respiratory tract intubation, cognition problems, and lack of dentures. Because his thinking was unclear, nurses used visual cues in the form of written words, gestures, and pictures to augment their messages to Mr. Saunders. They cued him to use a simple communication board and asked yes/no questions by categories (e.g., family, your body, comfort needs) whenever possible. After the tracheostomy procedure was completed, his wife was advised to bring in his dentures to improve lip reading. He began using a tracheostomy speaking valve after 5-1/2 weeks of hospitalization.

The patient's wife was his sole support. They had no children or close relatives. A reserved woman, she remained positive when at the patient's bedside. Nurses coached her to use touch and encouragement at the bedside. Mrs. Saunders asked the therapists to teach her range of motion exercises and she performed these during afternoon visits. She provided calm and distracting talk during weaning trials, reading getwell cards from friends.

Cardiac

Mr. Saunders remained in a sinus tachycardia through most of the hospitalization with occasional PVCs. His hemoglobin and hematocrit dropped to 10/36 after the second back surgery. He received one unit of packed red blood cells and diuretics before weaning trials were resumed.

Respiratory

Mr. Saunders progressed from dependence on mechanical ventilation in assist control mode (FiO_2 = 40%, CPAP=5, PS=10) to tracheostomy mask oxygen at 50% FiO_2 over a 10-day period. Did he have pain that interfered with weaning?

GI

Nutritional balance was particularly challenging with Mr. Saunders due to the impaired absorption of nutrients during C. difficile infection. Nutrition/dietician consult should be obtained. The infection was treated with intravenous vancomycin. A jejunostomy tube was placed for continuous tube feeding and caloric requirements adjusted frequently with careful attention to blood albumin levels. Vancomycin drug levels must also be monitored.

Skin

Meticulous attention was given to wound healing at the back surgery site and fit of "turtle shell" to prevent friction or skin tears.

Rehabilitation

Mr. Saunders received early physical therapy, beginning as passive range during the most critical phase of his illness and progressing to active range of motion and chair sitting. His mobility was limited by the protective turtle-shell appliance required for healing of his spine during any out of bed activity. A daily chair sitting period was arranged, requiring coordination between physical therapy and nursing. The team initiated speech and swallowing rehabilitation (i.e., speech and swallowing evaluation) beginning with lollipops to reestablish swallowing.

Discharge Planning

Mr. Saunders's progress was slow and respiratory status still tenuous at the end of his ICU stay. He required significant physical rehabilitation following his critical illness. A long term acute care hospital (LTACH) was the best choice for continued care and rehabilitation. As Mr. Saunders's respiratory status and speaking ability improved, his anxiety diminished. Because Mr. Saunders had multiple risk factors for delirium, the exact cause of the delirium was unknown at discharge. Attention to normalizing the fluid and electrolyte balance, re-establishing and maintaining normal sleep–wake cycles, and gradually withdrawing the use of benzodiazepines continued as care was transferred to the LTACH. His mental status improved as evidenced by less frequent periods of inattention and confusion. Short term memory problems persisted and required frequent cueing and reminders from staff and his wife.

Conclusion

Nurses in the acute care setting must recognize and respond to the many factors that influence a critically ill older adult's ability to survive and rehabilitate from a catastrophic illness. To identify some of these risk factors, it is essential that nurses perform a comprehensive assessment of each older adult's preadmission health status, functional and cognitive ability, and social support systems. It is equally important that nurses understand the implications of common aging changes, co-morbidities, and acute pathology that interacts with and heightens the risk for adverse and often preventable medical outcomes. The application of evidence-based nursing interventions aimed at restoring physiologic stability, preventing complications, maintaining comfort and safety, and preserving pre-illness functional ability and quality of life are crucial components of caring for this extremely vulnerable population.

Acknowledgments

The authors would like to acknowledge the continual support and commitment to improving nursing care of older adults provided by The John A. Hartford

Foundation. Case study provided by the "Study of Ventilator Weaning: Care and Communication Processes" database using composite patient information and pseudonyms (R01-NR007973).

Resources

The Richmond Agitation and Sedation Scale (RASS) and The Confusion Assessment Method-ICU (CAM-ICU). Retrieved from http://www.icudelirium. org/delirium/training-pages/CAM-ICU%20trainingman.2005.pdf

Training manual includes information for administering both the RASS and the CAM-ICU. Copyright (c)2002, E. Wesley Ely and Vanderbilt University. Geriatric Protocols at http://www.ConsultGeriRN.org/

GNO *Geriatric Topics*

Topics relevant to this chapter include the following:

    Reducing Adverse Drug Events

    Falls

    Urinary Incontinence

    Atypical Presentation

    Delirium

    Pain

    Medications

Other topics relevant to the care of older adults are also available through this Web site. Hartford Institute for Geriatric Nursing http://www. ConsultGeriRN.org/index.html

Select *Try This Series*

Topics relevant to this chapter include the following:

- Brief Evaluation of Executive Dysfunction: An Essential Refinement in the Assessment of Cognitive Impairment
- Decision Making and Dementia
- Recognition of Dementia in the Hospitalized Older Adult
- Beers' Criteria for Potentially Inappropriate Medication Use in the Elderly Assessing Pain in Older Adults
- KATZ Index of Independence in ADL

Box 25.1

Nursing Standard of Practice Protocol: Comprehensive Assessment and Management of the Critically Ill

I. GOAL: To restore physiologic stability, prevent complications, maintain comfort and safety, and preserve pre-illness functional ability and quality of life (QOL) in older adults admitted to critical care units.

II. **OVERVIEW**: Caring for an older adult who is experiencing a serious or life-threatening illness often poses significant challenges for critical care nurses. Although older adults are an extremely heterogeneous group, they share some age-related characteristics that leave them susceptible to various geriatric syndromes and diseases. This vulnerability may influence both their intensive care unit (ICU) utilization rates and outcomes. Critical care nurses caring for this population must not only recognize the importance of performing ongoing, comprehensive physical, functional, and psychosocial assessments tailored to older ICU patients but also must be able to identify and implement evidence-based interventions designed to improve the care of this extremely vulnerable population.

III. BACKGROUND

    A. Definition

        Critically ill older adult: a person, age 65 or older, who is currently experiencing or at risk for some form of physiologic instability or alteration warranting urgent or emergent, advanced nursing/medical interventions and monitoring.

    B. Etiology/Epidemiology

        1. More than half (55.8%) of all ICU days are incurred by patients older than 65 (Angus et al., 2000 [Level IV]).

        2. Older adults are living longer, are more racially and ethnically diverse, often have multiple chronic conditions, and more than one-quarter report difficulty performing one or more activities of daily living (ADLs) (Administration on Aging, 2005 [Level IV]). These factors may affect both the course and outcome of critical illness.

        3. Once hospitalized for a life-threatening illness, older adults often:

            a. Experience high ICU, hospital, and long-term crude mortality rates.

            b. Are at risk for deterioration in functional ability and post-discharge institutional care (Chelluri et al., 1995 [Level V]).

            c. Older age is also a factor that may lead to:

                i. Physician bias in refusing ICU admission (Joynt et al., 2001; Mick & Ackerman, 2004 [both Level VI]).

                ii. The decision to withhold mechanical ventilation, surgery, or dialysis (Hamel et al., 1999 [Level III]).

                iii. An increased likelihood of an established resuscitation directive (Hakim et al., 1996 [Level III]).

            d. Most critically ill older adults:

                i. Demonstrate resiliency.

                ii. Report being satisfied with their QOL post-discharge.

                iii. Would reaccept ICU care and mechanical ventilation if needed. (Chelluri et al., 1995 [Level V]; Guentner et al., 2006 [Level IV]; Kleinpell & Ferrans, 2002 [Level IV]).

e. Chronologic age *alone* is not an acceptable or accurate predictor of poor outcomes after critical illness (Chelluri et al., 1995 [Level V]; Esteban et al., 2004 [Level IV]; Kleinpell, 2003 [Level IV]).
f. Factors that may influence an older adult's ability to survive a catastrophic illness include:
   i. Severity of illness
   ii. Nature and extent of co-morbidities
   iii. Diagnosis, reason for/duration of mechanical ventilation
   iv. Complications length of ICU/hospital stay
      - Preadmission nursing home residence
      - Pulmonary artery catheterization
      - Prehospitalization functional ability
      - Gender
      - Pre-existing cognitive impairment
      - Delirium
      - Ethnicity
      - Senescence
      - Ageism
      - Decreased social support
      - The critical care environment

Adnet et al., 2001 [Level IV]; Chelluri et al., 1993 [Level IV]; Chelluri et al., 1995 [Level V]; Djaiani & Ridley, 1997 [Level IV]; Esteban et al., 2004 [Level IV]; Hamel et al., 1999 [Level III]; Kass et al., 1992 [Level IV]; Knaus et al., 1991 [Level IV]; Mayer-Oakes et al., 1991 [Level IV]; Mick & Ackerman, 2004 [Level VI]; Nicolas et al., 1987 [Level IV]; Nierman et al., 2001 [Level IV]; Richmond et al., 2002 [Level IV]; Shapira et al., 1997 [Level IV]; Tullmann & Dracup, 2000 [Level VI]; Wu et al., 1990 [Level IV].

IV. PARAMETERS OF ASSESSMENT

A. Preadmission: Comprehensive assessment of a critically ill older adult's preadmission health status, cognitive and functional ability, and social support systems helps identify risk factors for cascade iatrogenesis, the development of life-threatening conditions, and frequently encountered geriatric syndromes. Factors that nurses need to consider when performing the admission assessment include the following:
1. Pre-existing cognitive impairment: Many older adults admitted to ICUs suffer from high rates of unrecognized, pre-existing cognitive impairment (Pisani, Inouye et al., 2003 [Level IV]; Pisani, Redlich, McNicoll, Ely, & Inouye, 2003 [Level IV]).
   a. Knowledge of preadmission cognitive ability could aid practitioners in:
      i. Assessing decision making capacity, informed consent issues, and evaluation of mental status changes throughout hospitalization (Pisani, Redlich et al., 2003 [Level IV])

      ii. Making anesthetic and analgesic choices

     iii. Considering one-to-one care options

     iv. Weaning from mechanical ventilation

      v. Assessing fall risk

     vi. Planning for discharge from the ICU

  b. Upon admission of an older adult to the ICU, nurses should ask relatives or other caregivers for baseline information about the older adult's:

      i. memory, executive function (e.g., fine motor coordination, planning, organization of information), and overall cognitive ability (Kane et al., 2004 [Level VI])

      ii. behavior on a typical day, how the patient interacts with others, their responsiveness to stimuli, how able they are to communicate (reading level, writing, and speech), and their memory, orientation, and perceptual patterns prior to their illness (Milisen, DeGeest, Abraham, & Delooz, 2001 [Level VI])

     iii. medication history to assess for potential withdrawal syndromes (Broyles, Happ, Tate, Swigart, & Hoffman, 2005 [Level IV])

  c. Developmental and Psychosocial Factors: Critical illness can render older adults unable to effectively communicate with the health care team, often related to physiologic instability, technology that leaves them voiceless, and sedative and narcotic use. Family members are therefore often a crucial source for obtaining important preadmission information. Upon ICU admission, nurses need to determine:

      i. What is the elder's past medical, surgical, and psychiatric history? What medications was the older adult taking before coming to the ICU? Does the elder regularly use illicit drugs, tobacco, or alcohol? Do they have a history of falls, physical abuse, or confusion?

      ii. What is the older adult's marital status? Who is the patient's significant other? Will this person be the one responsible to make decisions for the elder if they are unable to do so? Does the elder have an advanced directive for health care? Is the elder a primary caregiver to an aging spouse, child, grandchild, or other person?

     iii. How would the elder describe his/her ethnicity? Do they practice a particular religion or have spiritual needs that should be addressed? What was their quality of life like before becoming ill?

  d. Preadmission functional ability/nutritional status: Limited preadmission functional ability and poor nutritional status are associated with many negative outcomes for critically ill older adults (Mick & Ackerman, 2004 [Level VI]; Roche et al., 1999 [Level IV]; Rosenthal & Kavic, 2004 [Level VI]; Tullmann &

Dracup, 2000 [Level VI]). Therefore, nurses should assess the following:

i. Did the elder suffer any limitations in the ability to perform their ADLs preadmission? If so, what were these limitations?

ii. Does the elder use any assistive devices to perform their ADLs? If so, what type?

iii. Where did the patient live prior to admission? Did they live alone or with others? What was the elder's physical environment like (e.g., house, apartment, stairs, multiple levels)?

iv. What was the older adult's nutritional status like preadmission? Do they have enough money to buy food? Do they need assistance with making meals/obtaining food? Do they have any particular food restrictions/preferences? Were they using supplements/vitamins on a regular basis? Do they have any signs of malnutrition, including recent weight loss/gain, muscle wasting, hair loss, skin breakdown?

B. During ICU stay: There are many anatomic/physiologic changes that occur with aging (see Table 25.1). The interaction of these changes with the acute pathology of a critical illness, co-morbidities, and the ICU environment leads not only to atypical presentation of some of the most commonly encountered ICU diagnoses but may also elevate the older adult's risk for complications. The older adult must be systematically assessed for the following:

1. Co-morbidities/common ICU diagnoses

a. Respiratory: chronic obstructive pulmonary disease, pneumonia, acute respiratory failure, adult respiratory distress syndrome, rib fractures/flail chest

b. Cardiovascular: acute myocardial infarction, coronary artery disease, peripheral vascular disease, hypertension, coronary artery bypass grafting, valve replacements, abdominal aortic aneurysm, dysrhythmias

c. Neurologic: cerebral vascular accident, dementia, aneurysms, Alzheimer's disease, Parkinson's disease, closed head injury, transient ischemic attacks

d. Gastrointestinal: biliary tract disease, peptic ulcer disease, gastrointestinal cancers, liver failure, inflammatory bowel disease, pancreatitis, diarrhea, constipation, and aspiration

e. Genitourinary: renal cell cancer, chronic renal failure, acute renal failure, urosepsis, and incontinence

f. Immune/Hematopoietic: sepsis, anemia, neutropenia, and thrombocytopenia

g. Skin: necrotizing fasciitis, pressure ulcers

2. Acute Pathology: Thoracic or abdominal surgery, hypovolemia, hypervolemia, hypo/hyperthermia, electrolyte abnormalities,

hypoxia, arrhythmias, infection, hypo/hypertension, delirium, ischemia, bowel obstruction, ileus, blood loss, sepsis, disrupted skin integrity, multisystem organ failure.

3. ICU/Environmental Factors: Deconditioning, poor oral hygiene, sleep deprivation, pain, immobility, nutritional status, mechanical ventilation, hemodynamic monitoring devices, polypharmacy, high risk medications (e.g., narcotics, sedatives, hypnotics, nephrotoxins, vasopressors), lack of assistive devices (e.g., glasses, hearing aids, dentures), noise, tubes that bypass the oropharyngeal airway, poorly regulated glucose control, Foley catheter use, stress, invasive procedures, shear/friction, intravenous catheters

4. Atypical Presentation: Commonly seen in older adults experiencing the following: myocardial infarction, acute abdomen, infection, and hypoxia

V. NURSING CARE STRATEGIES

A. Preadmission: Based on their preadmission assessment findings, nurses should consider:
1. Obtaining appropriate consults (i.e., nutrition, physical/ occupational/speech therapist)
2. Implementing safety precautions
3. Using pressure-relieving devices
4. Organizing family meetings
5. Providing older adults with a consistent primary nurse

B. During ICU: Nursing interventions that may benefit:
1. Multiple organ systems:
   a. Encouraging early, frequent mobilization/ambulation
   b. Providing proper oral hygiene.
   c. Ensuring adequate pain control.
   d. Reviewing/assessing medication appropriateness.
   e. Avoiding polypharmacy/high risk medications (see Table 25.2).
   f. Securing and ensuring the proper functioning of tubes/ catheters.
   g. Actively taking measures to maintain normothermia.
   h. Closely monitoring fluid-volume status.
2. Respiratory
   a. Encourage and assist with coughing, deep breathing, incentive spirometer use; use alternative device when appropriate (e.g., PEP).
   b. Assess for signs of swallowing dysfunction and aspiration.
   c. Closely monitor pulse oximetry and arterial blood gas results.
   d. Consider the use of specialty beds.
   e. Advocate for early weaning trials and extubation as soon as possible.
   f. Exercise standard VAP precautions (Kunis & Puntillo, 2003 [Level VI]):

      1. Keep the head of the bed elevated to more than 30 degrees.

      2. Provide frequent oral care.

      3. Maintain adequate cuff pressures.

      4. Assess the need for stress ulcer prophylaxis.

      5. Turn the patient as tolerated.

      6. Maintain general hygiene practices.

3. Cardiovascular

  a. Carefully monitor the older adult's hemodynamic and electrolyte status.

  b. Closely monitor the older adult's EKG with an awareness of many conduction abnormalities seen in aging. Consult with physician regarding prophylaxis when appropriate.

  c. Advocate for the removal of invasive devices as soon as the patient's condition warrants. The least restrictive device may include long-term access.

  d. Recognize that both pre-existing pulmonary disease and manipulations of the abdominal and thoracic cavities may lead to unreliability of traditional values associated with central venous and pulmonary artery occlusion pressures (Rosenthal & Kavic, 2004 [Level VI]).

  e. Because of age-related changes to the CV system, the nurse should acknowledge (Rosenthal & Kavic, 2004 [Level VI]):

    i. Older adults often require higher filling pressures (i.e., CVPs in the 8 to 10 range, PAOPs in the 14 to18 range) to maintain adequate stroke volume and may be especially sensitive to hypovolemia.

    ii. Over-hydration of the older adult should also be avoided because it can lead to systolic failure, poor organ perfusion, and hypoxemia with subsequent diastolic dysfunction.

    iii. Certain drugs commonly used in the ICU setting may prove to be either not as effective (e.g., isoproterenol and dobutamine or more effective (e.g., afterload reducers).

4. Neurologic/Pain

  a. Closely monitor the older adult's neurologic/mental status.

  b. Screen for delirium and sedation level at least once per shift.

  c. Implement interventions to reduce delirium (Inouye et al., 1999 [Level II]; Jacobi et al., 2002 [Level V]; Milbrandt et al., 2005 [Level IV]; Tullmann & Dracup, 2000 [Level VI]; Yeh et al., 2004 [Level III]; Zeleznik, 2001 [Level VI]):

    i. Promote sleep, mobilize as early as possible, review medications that can lead to delirium, treat dehydration, reduce noise or provide "white noise," close doors/drapes to allow privacy, provide comfortable room temperature, encourage family and friends to visit, allow the older adult to assume the preferred sleeping positions, discontinue any unnecessary lines or tubes, and avoid the use of physical restraints using least restraint for minimum time only when absolutely necessary.

   ii. Maximize older adults' ability to communicate their needs effectively and interpret their environment.

      ▪ Promote the older adult wearing glasses, hearing aids, and other appropriate assistive devices.

      ▪ Face patients when speaking to them, get their attention before talking, speak clearly and loud enough for them to understand, allow them enough time (pause time) to respond to questions, provide them with a consistent provider (i.e., a primary nurse), use visual clues to remind them of the date and time, and provide written or visual input for a message (Garrett & Beukelman, 1995 [Level III]; Lasker, Hux, Garrett, Moncrief, & Eischeid, 1997 [Level III]).

      ▪ Provide older adults with alternate means of communication (e.g., providing a pen/paper; using nonverbal gestures; and/or using specially designed boards with alphabet letters, words, or pictures) (Connolly, 1995 [Level IV]; Patak, Gawlinski, Fung, & Berg, 2004 [Level IV]; Stovsky, Rudy, & Dragonette, 1988 [Level III]).

      ▪ Provide translators/interpreters as needed.

  d. Provide adequate pain control while avoiding over- or under-sedation. For a full discussion, see chapter 10, *Pain Management*.

5. Gastrointestinal

  a. Monitor for signs of GI bleeding and delayed gastric emptying/motility.

    i. Encourage adequate hydration, assess for signs of fecal impaction, and implement a bowel regimen.

    ii. Avoid use of rectal tubes.

  b. Advocate for stress ulcer prophylaxis.

  c. Provide dentures as soon as possible.

  d. Implement aspiration precautions.

    i. Keep the head of the bed elevated to a high Fowler's position, frequently suction copious oral secretions, bedside evaluate swallowing ability by a speech therapist, assess phonation and gag reflex, monitor for tachypnea.

  e. Advocate for early enteral/parental nutrition if consistent with advace directive.

  f. Ensure tight glucose control.

6. Genitourinary (GU)

  a. Assess any GU tubes to ensure patency and adequate urinary output. If an older adult should experience an acute decrease in urinary output, consider using bladder scanner (if available) rather than automatic straight catheterization to check for distension.

  b. Advocate for early removal of Foley catheters. Use other less invasive devices/methods to facilitate urine collection (i.e., external or condom catheters, offering the bedpan on a scheduled basis, and keeping the nurse's call bell/signal within the older adult's reach).

  c. Monitor blood levels of nephrotoxic medications as ordered.

 7. Immune/Hematopoietic

  a. Ensure the older adult is ordered appropriate DVT prophylaxis (i.e., heparin, sequential compression devices)

  b. Monitor laboratory results, assess for signs of anemia relative to patient's baseline

  c. Recognize early signs of infection: restlessness, agitation, delirium, hypotension, tachycardia, because older adults are less likely to develop fever as a first response to infection.

  d. Meticulously maintain infection control/prevention protocols.

 8. Skin

  a. Conduct thorough skin assessment.

  b. Vigilantly monitor room temperature, make every effort to prevent heat loss, and carefully use and monitor rewarming devices.

  c. Use methods known to reduce the friction and shear that often occurs with repositioning in bed.

  d. In severely compromised patients, the use of specialty beds may be appropriate.

  e. Techniques such as frequent turning, pressure-relieving devices, early nutritional support, as well as frequent ambulation may not only protect an older adult's skin but also promote the health of their cardiovascular, respiratory, and gastrointestinal systems.

  f. Closely monitor IV sites, frequently check for infiltrations and use of nonrestrictive dressings and paper tape.

VI. EVALUATION AND EXPECTED OUTCOMES

 A. Patient

  1. Hemodynamic stability will be restored.

  2. Complications will be avoided/minimized.

  3. Preadmission functional ability will be maintained/optimized.

  4. Pain/anxiety will be minimized.

  5. Communication with the health care team will be improved.

 B. Provider

  1. Employ consistent and accurate documentation of assessment relevant to older ICU patients.

  2. Provide consistent, accurate, and timely care in response to deviations identified through ongoing monitoring and assessment of older ICU patients.

3. Provide patient/caregiver with information and teaching related to their illness and regarding transfer of care and/or discharge.

C. Institution: include QA/QI
  1. Evaluate staff competence in the assessment of older critically ill patients.
  2. Utilize unit-specific, hospital-specific, and national standards of care to evaluate existing practice.
  3. Identify areas for improvement and work collaboratively across disciplines to develop strategies for improving critical care to older adults.

VII. Relevant Practice Guidelines

Jacobi et al. (2002). Clinical Practice Guidelines for the sustained use of sedatives and analgesics in the critically ill adult (Jacobi et al., 2002).Task Force of the American College of Critical Care Medicine (ACCM) of the Society of Critical Care Medicine (SCCM), American Society of Health-System Pharmacists (ASHP), and American College of Chest Physicians

ACC/AHA (2006). Guideline Update on perioperative cardiovascular evaluation for noncardiac surgery: Focused update on perioperative beta-blocker therapy. A report of the American College of Cardiology/American Heart Association Task Force on Practice Guidelines. Developed in collaboration with the American Society of Echocardiography, American Society of Nuclear Cardiology, Heart Rhythm Society, Society of Cardiovascular Anesthesiologists, Society for Cardiovascular Angiography and Interventions, and Society for Vascular Medicine and Biology.

References

Administration on Aging (2005). A profile of older Americans: 2005. Retrieved May 23, 2006, from http://www.aoa.gov/PROF/Statistics/profile/2005/2005profile.pdf. Evidence Level IV: Nonexperimental Study.

Adnet, F., Le Toumelin, P., Leberre, A., Minadeo, J., Lapostolle, F., Plaisance, P., et al. (2001). In-hospital and long-term prognosis of elderly patients requiring endotracheal intubation for life-threatening presentation of cardiogenic pulmonary edema. *Critical Care Medicine, 29*(4), 891–895. Evidence Level IV: Nonexperimental Study.

Aldemir, M., Ozen, S., Kara, I. H., Sir, A., & Bac, B. (2001). Predisposing factors for delirium in the surgical intensive care unit. *Critical care (London, England), 5*(5), 265–270. Evidence Level IV: Nonexperimental Study.

Angus, D. C., Kelley, M. A., Schmitz, R. J., White, A., Popovich, J. Jr., & Committee on Manpower for Pulmonary and Critical Care Societies (2000). Caring for the critically ill patient. Current and projected workforce requirements for care of the critically ill and patients with pulmonary disease: Can we meet the requirements of an aging population? *Journal of the American Medical Association, 284*(21), 2762–2770. Evidence Level IV: Nonexperimental Study.

Bates, B. (1995). *A guide to physical examination and history taking* (6th ed.). Philadelphia: J. B. Lippincott. Evidence Level VI: Expert Opinion.

Beers, M. H. (1997). Explicit criteria for determining potentially inappropriate medication use by the elderly: An update. *Archives of Internal Medicine, 157*(14), 1531–1536.

Bonk, M. E., Krown, H., Matuszewski, K., & Oinonen, M. (2006). Potentially inappropriate medications in hospitalized senior patients. *American Journal of Health System Pharmacists, 63*(12), 1161–1165. Evidence Level VI: Expert Opinion.

Broyles, L., Happ, M. B., Tate, J., Swigart, V., & Hoffman, L. (2005). Neurocognitive complexity, interpersonal conflict, and inconsistent care patterns in the case of an elderly ICU patient. *The Gerontologist, 45* (Special Issue II), 126. Evidence Level IV: Nonexperimental Study.

Chelluri, L., Grenvik, A., & Silverman, M. (1995). Intensive care for critically ill elderly: mortality, costs, and quality of life. Review of the literature. *Archives of Internal Medicine, 155*(10), 1013–1022. Evidence Level V: Literature Review.

Chelluri, L., Im, K. A., Belle, S. H., Schulz, R., Rotondi, A. J., Donahoe, M. P., et al. (2004). Long-term mortality and quality of life after prolonged mechanical ventilation. *Critical Care Medicine, 32*(1), 61–69. Evidence Level IV: Nonexperimental Study.

Chelluri, L., Pinsky, M. R., Donahoe, M. P., & Grenvik, A. (1993). Long-term outcome of critically ill elderly patients requiring intensive care. *Journal of the American Medical Association, 269*(24), 3119–3123. Evidence Level IV: Nonexperimental Study.

Connolly, M. A. (1995). Communicating with temporarily nonvocal patients. *Perspectives in Respiratory Nursing, 6*, 7–9. Evidence Level IV: Nonexperimental Study.

Creditor, M. C. (1993). Hazards of hospitalization of the elderly. *Annals of Internal Medicine, 118*(3), 219–223. Evidence Level VI: Expert Opinion.

Daly, B. J., Douglas, S. L., Kelley, C. G., O'Toole, E., & Montenegro, H. (2005). Trial of a disease-management program to reduce hospital readmissions of the chronically critically ill. *Chest, 128*(2), 507–517. Evidence Level II: Individual Experimental Study.

Djaiani, G., & Ridley, S. (1997). Outcome of intensive care in the elderly. *Anaesthesia, 52*(12), 1130–1136. Evidence Level IV: Nonexperimental Study.

Douglas, S. L., Daly, B. J., Brennan, P. F., Gordon, N. H., & Uthis, P. (2001). Hospital readmission among long-term ventilator patients. *Chest, 120*(4), 1278–1286. Evidence Level IV: Nonexperimental Study.

Douglas, S. L., Daly, B. J., Brennan, P. F., Harris, S., Nochomovitz, M., & Dyer, M. A. (1997). Outcomes of long-term ventilator patients: A descriptive study. *American Journal of Critical Care, 6*(2), 99–105. Evidence Level IV: Nonexperimental Study.

Douglas, S. L., Daly, B. J., Gordon, N., & Brennan, P. F. (2002). Survival and quality of life: Short-term versus long-term ventilator patients. *Critical Care Medicine, 30*(12), 2655–2662. Evidence Level IV: Nonexperimental Study.

Dubois, M. J., Bergeron, N., Dumont, M., Dial, S., & Skrobik, Y. (2001). Delirium in an intensive care unit: A study of risk factors. *Intensive Care Medicine, 27*(8), 1297–1304. Evidence Level IV: Nonexperimental Study.

Ely, E. W., Inouye, S. K., Bernard, G. R., Gordon, S., Francis, J., May, L., et al. (2001). Delirium in mechanically ventilated patients: Validity and reliability of the confusion assessment method for the intensive care unit (CAM-ICU). *Journal of the American Medical Association, 286*(21), 2703–2710. Evidence Level IV: Nonexperimental Study.

Esteban, A., Anzueto, A., Frutos-Vivar, F., Alia, I., Ely, E. W., Brochard, L., et al. (2004). Outcome of older patients receiving mechanical ventilation. *Intensive Care Medicine, 30*(4), 639–646. Evidence Level IV: Nonexperimental Study.

Fick, D. M., Cooper, J. W., Wade, W. E., Waller, J. L., Maclean, J. R., & Beers, M. H. (2003). Updating the Beers criteria for potentially inappropriate medication use in older adults: Results of a U.S. consensus panel of experts. *Archives of Internal Medicine, 163*(22), 2716–2724. Evidence Level VI: Expert opinion.

Fleisher, L. A., Beckman, J. A., Brown, K. A., Calkins, H., Chaikof, E., Fleischmann, K., et al. (2006). ACC/AHA 2006 Guideline update on perioperative cardiovascular evaluation for noncardiac surgery: Focused update on perioperative beta-blocker therapy: A report of the American College of Cardiology/American Heart Association Task Force on Practice Guidelines (Writing committee to update the 2002 guidelines on perioperative cardiovascular evaluation for noncardiac surgery.) *Journal of the American College of Cardiology, 47*(11), 2343–2355. Evidence Level I: Systematic Review.

Garrett, K., & Beukelman, D. R. (1995). Changes in the interaction patterns of an individual with severe aphasia given three types of partner support. *Clinical Aphasiology, 23*, 237–251. Evidence Level III: Quasi-experimental Study.

Graf, C., & Puntillo, K. (2003). Pain in the older adult in the intensive care unit. *Critical Care Clinics, 19*(4), 749–770. Evidence Level VI: Expert Opinion.

Guentner, K., Hoffman, L. A., Happ, M. B., Kim, Y., Dabbs, A. D., Mendelsohn, A. B., et al. (2006). Preferences for mechanical ventilation among survivors of prolonged mechanical ventilation and tracheostomy. *American Journal of Critical Care, 15*(1), 65–77. Evidence Level IV: Nonexperimental Study.

Hakim, R. B., Teno, J. M., Harrell, F. E., Jr., Knaus, W. A., Wenger, N., Phillips, R. S., et al. (1996). Factors associated with do-not-resuscitate orders: Patients' preferences, prognoses, and physicians' judgments. SUPPORT Investigators. Study to understand prognoses and preferences for outcomes and risks of treatment. *Annals of Internal Medicine, 125*(4), 284–293. Evidence Level III: Quasi-experimental Study.

Hamel, M. B., Teno, J. M., Goldman, L., Lynn, J., Davis, R. B., Galanos, A. N., et al. (1999). Patient age and decisions to withhold life-sustaining treatments from seriously ill, hospitalized adults. SUPPORT Investigators. Study to understand prognoses and preferences for outcomes and risks of treatment. *Annals of Internal Medicine, 130*(2), 116–125. Evidence Level III: Quasi-experimental Study.

Happ, M. B. (2000). Interpretation of nonvocal behavior and the meaning of voicelessness in critical care. *Social Science & Medicine, 50*(9), 1247–1255. Evidence Level IV: Nonexperimental Study.

Happ, M. B. (2001). Communicating with mechanically ventilated patients: State of the science. *AACN Clinical Issues, 12*(2), 247–258. Evidence Level IV: Nonexperimental Study.

Inouye, S. K., Bogardus, S. T., Charpentier, P. A., Leo-Summers, L., Acampora, D., Holford, T. R., et al. (1999). A multicomponent intervention to prevent delirium in hospitalized older patients. *The New England Journal of Medicine, 340*(9), 669–676. Evidence Level II: Individual Experimental Study.

Jacobi, J., Fraser, G. L., Coursin, D. B., Riker, R. R., Fontaine, D., Wittbrodt, E. T., et al. (2002). Clinical practice guidelines for the sustained use of sedatives and analgesics in the critically ill adult. *Critical Care Medicine, 30*(1), 119–141. Evidence Level V: Review.

Joynt, G. M., Gomersall, C. D., Tan, P., Lee, A., Cheng, C. A., & Wong, E. L. (2001). Prospective evaluation of patients refused admission to an intensive care unit: Triage, futility, and outcome. *Intensive Care Medicine, 27*(9), 1459–1465. Evidence Level IV: Nonexperimental Study.

Kane, R. L., Ouslander, J. G., & Abrass, I. B. (2004). *Essentials of clinical geriatrics* (5th ed.). New York: McGraw-Hill. Evidence Level VI: Expert Opinion.

Kass, J. E., Castriotta, R. J., & Malakoff, F. (1992). Intensive care unit outcome in the very elderly. *Critical Care Medicine, 20*(12), 1666–1671. Evidence Level IV: Nonexperimental Study.

Katz, S., Ford, A. B., Moskowitz, R. W., Jackson, B. A., & Jaffe, M. W. (1963). Studies of illness in the aged: The Index of ADL: A standardized measure of biological and psychosocial function. *Journal of the American Medical Association, 185*(12), 914–919.

Kidd, D., Stewart, G., Baldry, J., Johnson, J., Rossiter, D., Petruckevitch, A., et al. (1995). The Functional Independence Measure: A comparative validity and reliability study. *Disability & Rehabilitation, 17*(1), 10–14. Evidence Level III: Quasi-experimental Study.

Kleinhenz, M. E., & Lewis, C. Y. (2000). Chronic ventilator dependence in elderly patients. *Clinics in Geriatric Medicine, 16*(4), 735–756. Evidence Level VI: Expert Opinion.

Kleinpell, R. M. (2003). Exploring outcomes after critical illness in the elderly. *Outcomes Management, 7*(4), 159–169. Evidence Level IV: Nonexperimental Study.

Kleinpell, R. M., & Ferrans, C. E. (2002). Quality of life of elderly patients after treatment in the ICU. *Research in Nursing & Health, 25*(3), 212–221. Evidence Level IV: Nonexperimental Study.

Knaus, W. A., Wagner, D. P., Draper, E. A., Zimmerman, J. E., Bergner, M., Bastos, P. G., et al. (1991). The APACHE III prognostic system: Risk prediction of hospital mortality for critically ill hospitalized adults. *Chest, 100*(6), 1619–1636. Evidence Level IV: Nonexperimental Study.

Kresevic, D. M., & Mezey, M. (2003). Assessment of function. In M. Mezey, T. T. Fulmer, & I. L. Abraham (Eds.), *Geriatric nursing protocols for best practice* (2nd ed.). New York: Springer Publishing Company. Evidence Level VI: Expert Opinion.

Kunis, K. A., & Puntillo, K. A. (2003). Ventilator-associated pneumonia in the ICU: Its patho-physiology, risk factors, and prevention. *American Journal of Nursing*, *103*(8), 64AA–69AA. Evidence Level VI: Expert Opinion.

Lasker, J., Hux, K., Garrett, K. L., Moncrief, E. M., & Eischeid, T. J. (1997). Variations on the written choice communication strategy for individuals with severe aphasia. *Augmentative and Alternative Communication*, *13*, 108–116. Evidence Level III: Quasi-experimental Study.

Mangano, D. R., Layug, E. L., Wallace, A., & Tateo, I. (1996). Effect of atenolol on mortality and cardiovascular morbidity after noncardiac surgery. *New England Journal of Medicine*, *335*, 1713–1720. Evidence Level II: Individual Experimental Study.

Mayer-Oakes, S. A., Oye, R. K., & Leake, B. (1991). Predictors of mortality in older patients fol-lowing medical intensive care: The importance of functional status. *Journal of the American Geriatrics Society*, *39*(9), 862–868. Evidence Level IV: Nonexperimental Study.

McNicoll, L., Pisani, M. A., Zhang, Y., Ely, E. W., Siegel, M. D., & Inouye, S. K. (2003). Delirium in the intensive care unit: Occurrence and clinical course in older patients. *Journal of the American Geriatrics Society*, *51*(5), 591–598. Evidence Level IV: Nonexperimental Study.

Mick, D. J., & Ackerman, M. H. (2004). Critical care nursing for older adults: Pathophysiological and functional considerations. *Nursing Clinics of North America*, *39*(3), 473–493. Evidence Level VI: Expert Opinion.

Milbrandt, E. B., Kersten, A., Kong, L., Weissfeld, L. A., Clermont, G., Fink, M. P., et al. (2005). Haloperidol use is associated with lower hospital mortality in mechanically ventilated patients. *Critical Care Medicine*, *33*(1), 226–229. Evidence Level IV: Nonexperimental Study.

Milisen, K., DeGeest, S., Abraham, I. L., & Delooz, H. H. (2001). Delirium. In T. T. Fulmer, M. D. Foreman, & M. Walker (Eds.), *Critical care nursing of the elderly* (2nd ed.). New York: Springer Publishing Company. Evidence Level VI: Expert Opinion.

Miller, R. R., & Ely, E. W. (2006). Delirium and cognitive dysfunction in the intensive care unit. *Seminars in Respiratory & Critical Care Medicine*, *27*(3), 210–220. Evidence Level VI: Expert Opinion.

Nagappan, R., & Parkin, G. (2003). Geriatric critical care. *Critical Care Clinics*, *19*, 253–270. Evidence Level VI: Expert Opinion.

Nicolas, F., Le Gall, J. R., Alperovitch, A., Loirat, P., & Villers, D. (1987). Influence of patients' age on survival, level of therapy, and length of stay in intensive care units. *Intensive Care Medicine*, *13*(1), 9–13. Evidence Level IV: Nonexperimental Study.

Nierman, D. M., Schechter, C. B., Cannon, L. M., & Meier, D. E. (2001). Outcome prediction model for very elderly critically ill patients. *Critical Care Medicine*, *29*(10), 1853–1859. Evidence Level IV: Nonexperimental Study.

Patak, L., Gawlinski, A., Fung, N. I., Doering, L., & Berg, J. (2004). Patients' reports of health care practitioner interventions that are related to communication during mechanical ven-tilation. *Heart & Lung*, *33*(5), 308–320. Evidence Level IV: Nonexperimental Study.

Peterson, J. F., Pun, B. T., Dittus, R. S., Thomason, J. W. W., Jackson, J. C., Shintani, A. K., et al. (2006). Delirium and its motoric subtypes: A study of 614 critically ill patients. *Jour-nal of the American Geriatrics Society*, *54*(3), 479–484. Evidence Level IV: Nonexperimental Study.

Pisani, M. A., Inouye, S. K., McNicoll, L., & Redlich, C. A. (2003). Screening for preexisting cog-nitive impairment in older intensive care unit patients: Use of proxy assessment. *Journal of the American Geriatrics Society*, *51*(5), 689–693. Evidence Level IV: Nonexperimental Study.

Pisani, M. A., Redlich, C., McNicoll, L., Ely, E. W., & Inouye, S. K. (2003). Under-recognition of preexisting cognitive impairment by physicians in older ICU patients. *Chest*, *124*(6), 2267–2274. Evidence Level IV: Nonexperimental Study.

Poldermans, D., Boersma, E., Bax, J. J., Thomson, I. R., van de Ven, L. L., Blankensteijn, J. D., et al. (1999). The effects of bisoprolol on perioperative mortality and myocardial infarction in high risk patients undergoing vascular surgery. *New England Journal of Medicine*, *341*, 1789–1794. Evidence Level II: Individual Experimental Study.

Richards, C. L. (2003). Urinary tract infections in the frail elderly: Issues for diagnosis, treat-ment, and prevention. *International Urology and Nephrology*, *36*, 457–463. Evidence Level VI: Expert Opinion.

Richmond, T. S., Kauder, D., Strumpf, N., & Meredith, T. (2002). Characteristics and outcomes of serious traumatic injury in older adults. *Journal of the American Geriatrics Society*, *50*(2), 215–222. Evidence Level IV: Nonexperimental Study.

Roche, V. M., Kramer, A., Hester, E., & Welsh, C. H. (1999). Long-term functional outcome after intensive care. *Journal of the American Geriatrics Society, 47*(1), 18–24. Evidence Level IV: Nonexperimental Study.

Rosenthal, R. A. (2004). Nutritional concerns in the older surgical patient. *Journal of the American College of Surgeons, 199*(5), 785–791. Evidence Level VI: Expert Opinion.

Rosenthal, R. A., & Kavic, S. M. (2004). Assessment and management of the geriatric patient. *Critical Care Medicine, 32*(4 Suppl.), S92–S105. Evidence Level VI: Expert Opinion.

Sessler, C. N., Gosnell, M. S., Grap, M. J., Brophy, G. M., O'Neal, P. V., Keane, K. A., et al. (2002). The Richmond Agitation-Sedation Scale: Validity and reliability in adult intensive care unit patients. *American Journal of Respiratory & Critical Care Medicine, 166*(10), 1338–1344. Evidence Level IV: Nonexperimental Study.

Shapira, O. M., Kelleher, R. M., Zelingher, J., Whalen, D., Fitzgerald, C., Aldea, G. S., et al. (1997). Prognosis and quality of life after valve surgery in patients older than 75 years. *Chest, 112*(4), 885–894. Evidence Level IV: Nonexperimental Study.

Sheehy, C. M., Perry, P. A., & Cromwell, S. L. (1999). Dehydration: Biological considerations, age-related changes, and risk factors in older adults. *Biological Research for Nursing, 1*(1), 30–37. Evidence Level VI: Expert Opinion.

Stovsky, B., Rudy, E., & Dragonette, P. (1988). Comparison of two types of communication methods used after cardiac surgery with patients with endotracheal tubes. *Heart & Lung, 17*(3), 281–289. Evidence Level III: Quasi-experimental Study.

Sveinsson, I. S. (1975). Postoperative psychosis after heart surgery. *Journal of Thoracic & Cardiovascular Surgery, 70*(4), 717–726.

Tullmann, D. F., & Dracup, K. (2000). Creating a healing environment for elders. *AACN Clinical Issues, 11*(1), 34–50; quiz 153–154. Evidence Level VI: Expert Opinion.

Urden, L. D., Stacy, K. M., & Lough, M. E. (2002). Gerontological alterations and management. In *Thelan's critical care nursing: Diagnosis and management* (4th ed., pp. 199–220). St. Louis, MO: Mosby. Evidence Level VI: Expert Opinion.

Van Den Berghe, G., Wouters, P., Weekers, F., Verwaest, C., Bruyninckx, F., Schetz, M., et al. (2001). Intensive insulin therapy in the critically ill patients. *New England Journal of Medicine, 345*(19), 1359–1367. Evidence Level II: Individual Experimental Study.

Waldrop, J., & Stern, S. (2003). Disability: 2000. Retrieved May 16, 2006, from http://www.census.gov/prod/2003pubs/c2kbr-17.pdf. Evidence Level IV: Nonexperimental Study.

Wilson, L. M. (1972). Intensive care delirium: The effect of outside deprivation in a windowless unit. *Archives of Internal Medicine, 130*(2), 222–225. Evidence Level III: Quasi-experimental Study.

Wu, A. W., Rubin, H. R., & Rosen, M. J. (1990). Are elderly people less responsive to intensive care? *Journal of the American Geriatrics Society, 38*(6), 621–627. Evidence Level IV: Nonexperimental Study.

Zeleznik, J. (2001). Effectiveness of interventions to prevent delirium in hospitalized patients: A systematic review. *Journal of American Geriatrics Society, 49*(12), 1730–1732. Evidence Level VI: Expert Opinion.

Fluid Overload: Identifying and Managing Heart Failure Patients at Risk for Hospital Readmission

26

Jessica Coviello
Deborah A. Chyun

Educational Objectives

At the conclusion of this chapter, the reader will be able to:

1. describe the older adult with heart failure who is at risk for hospital readmission

2. conduct a comprehensive cardiac history

3. identify three physical findings that may be associated with fluid overload in an older adult patient with heart failure

4. name three key symptoms associated with fluid overload in the older adult patient with heart failure

5. define cardiovascular stability in relation to the five key indicators

6. plan monitoring strategies to reduce fluid overload in the older adult with heart failure

Overview

The most common cause of hospital admission in older adults is heart failure (Funk & Krumholtz, 1996 [Level IV]) and the most common cause for hospital readmission for the patient with heart failure is fluid overload. The evidence-based literature indicates that heart failure patients delay seeking medical

For a description of Evidence Levels cited in this chapter, see chapter 1, Developing and Evaluating Clinical Practice Guidelines, page 4.

Adapted from the American Association of Colleges of Nursing, "Preparing nursing students to care for older adults: Enhancing gerontology in senior-level undergraduate courses" curriculum module, Assessment and Management of Hypertension and Heart Failure, prepared by Deborah A. Chyun and Jessica Coviello.

advice despite progressive symptoms; the delay is, on average, anywhere from 12 hours to 14 days (Rich & Kitzman, 2005 [Level VI]). An important focus of research for the past several years has been to identify patients, particularly older patients, at risk for readmission. This chapter presents the complex nature of heart failure and fluid imbalance that places older adults at risk for hospital readmission due to fluid overload and nursing strategies to reduce hospital readmission rates. A detailed protocol for practice is presented highlighting the nursing assessment and management of heart failure.

Background

Cardiovascular disease (CVD), which includes hypertension (HTN) and heart failure (HF), along with stroke, arrhythmias, valvular heart disease, peripheral vascular disease (PVD), and coronary heart disease (CHD), are major contributors to mortality and co-morbidity in older adults, accounting for 40% of all deaths in those aged 75 to 85 and 48% of all deaths in those 85 and older (Thom et al., 2006 [Level VI]). Chronic heart failure is the leading cause of hospital admission in patients older than 65, and readmission rates to acute care facilities have averaged 17.2% nationally (Funk & Krumholtz, 1996 [Level IV]).

HF is a public health problem affecting more than 5 million Americans yearly (Thom et al., 2006 [Level VI]). The prevalence of HF increases with age, and more than 75% of those affected are older than 65. Development of HF is higher with male sex, lower level of education, low levels of physical activity, cigarette smoking, overweight, diabetes mellitus (DM), HTN, valvular heart disease, left ventricular hypertrophy (LVH) and CHD (Ho, Pinsky, Kannel, & Levy, 1993 [Level II]). The presence of HTN, as an antecedent, occurs in 75% of individuals with HF (Thom et al., 2006 [Level VI]). Both the incidence and prevalence of HF continues to increase as the population ages.

Hypertension is the most common cause of HF in patients without CHD, accounting for 24% of the cases of HF (Ho et al., 1993 [Level II]). HTN is also extremely common in Type II DM, occurring in 40% to 60% of older adults with Type II DM (Hypertension in Diabetes Study Group, 1993 [Level II]). Women with DM are at extremely high risk of developing HF (Levy, Larson, Vasan, Kannel, & Ho, 1996 [Level VI]. Individuals with HTN and DM often develop diastolic rather than systolic dysfunction (Piccini, Klein, Gheorghiade, & Bonow, 2004 [Level V]).

Risk Factors for Developing HF in Older Adults

Diabetes in particular is an important contributor to HF, with women and those individuals treated with insulin at the greatest risk. In a sample of older Medicare patients with Type II DM, 22% had a diagnosis of HF, and this prevalence increased with advancing age (Bertoni et al., 2004 [Level VI]). In addition, the presence of Type II DM is associated with higher HF-related morbidity and mortality. After myocardial infarction (MI) or coronary revascularization procedures, individuals with Type II DM also have a high morbidity and mortality due to a large extent to the development of HF. In a separate analysis of older adult patients receiving Medicare, the year following an MI, 11% of patients without DM, 17% of patients with DM on oral agents, and 25% of those treated with insulin were admitted for HF (Chyun, Vaccarino, Murillo, Young, & Krumholz, 2002 [Level VI]). Patients at risk for readmission after initial diagnosis for HF include the following (Chyun et al., 2002; Lewis et al., 2003; Rich & Kitzman, 2005 [all Level VI]):

- age >70 years
- newly diagnosed HF
- hospitalizations for any reason in the last 5 years
- social isolation
- HF related to acute MI or uncontrolled HTN
- history of alcohol abuse
- HF with acute infection
- HF with an exacerbation of a co-morbidity
- history of depression or anxiety
- noncompliance to diet, fluid intake, or medications

Pathophysiology of Heart Failure

Understanding the pathophysiology of HF provides insight into the rationale for treatment. Left ventricular (LV) remodeling is dependent on changes in the myocyte structure and function. These changes occur during compensated (asymptomatic) as well as decompensated (symptomatic) failure. The change in structure is dependent on several factors: over expression of neurohormones, peptides (norepinephrine, angiotensin II, cytokines, vasopressin, aldosterone) found in HF, which in turn produce increased hemodynamic stress on the left ventricle, sodium retention, and peripheral vasoconstriction, which then exert toxic effects on the myocyte leading to fibrosis. These factors are cyclical unless treated. Untreated, there is further disruption of LV architecture and performance. However, timing of treatment is important. Patients who have had HF for years prior to the aggressive treatment that is currently available will have high levels of neurohormone. Although treatment reduces these neurohormone levels, the danger is that without delicate titration of medications such as carvedilol (Coreg), a sudden disruption of long-standing compensatory mechanisms and a rebound episode of fluid overload can occur.

The standard American College of Cardiology/American Heart Association Task Force (ACC/AHA) guidelines classifies HF in four stages (Hunt et al., 2005 [Level VI]), as follows:

Stage A is considered a pre heart failure stage or an "at risk" stage. It includes patients with HTN, atherosclerotic disease, DM, obesity, metabolic syndrome, those using cardiotoxic substances (i.e., anthracyclines), or those with a family history of cardiomyopathy.

Stage B includes individuals with previous MI, LVH and low ejection fraction, and symptomatic valvular disease.

Stage C includes individuals with known heart disease and symptoms—shortness of breath and fatigue and reduced exercise tolerance—or those who are now asymptomatic due to treatment.

Stage D includes individuals with refractory HF requiring the use of specialized interventions and includes patients with marked symptoms at rest despite maximal medical therapy.

The symptoms of HF are related to impairment to fill the left ventricle (diastolic failure) or due to impairment of the left ventricle to empty (systolic failure). Atherosclerotic CHD is the most common etiology of HF in the United States, followed closely by HTN alone and valvular disease, although thyroid dysfunction and excessive alcohol intake may also lead to HF. In the absence of CVD, systolic function of the heart remains relatively unchanged in older adults, as does exercise tolerance. However, diastolic function is often impaired even in the absence of HTN or hypertrophic cardiomyopathy, which are known to contribute to diastolic failure. Diastolic dysfunction is characterized by an exaggerated heart rate (HR) with activity, which, clinically, is often one of the first signs.

Hypertension, CHD, and hypertrophic cardiomyopathy are all abnormalities that are exacerbated by tachycardia underscoring the importance of avoiding a high heart rate in all older individuals. Diastolic abnormalities caused by HTN, aortic stenosis (AS), or CHD may precipitate HF. Patients with either systolic or diastolic heart failure are at risk for fluid overload. Although discussed as two separate entities, many older adults have components of both systolic and diastolic dysfunction.

Assessment of Heart Failure

For older adults diagnosed with HF, the health history and physical assessment is directed at monitoring symptoms and assessing cardiovascular function. For nurses assessing and managing the patient with HF, the recognition of fluid overload is not always straightforward. Unlike the classic picture of HF observed in younger adults, the symptoms of fluid overload can be subtle and elusive in older adults. Once symptoms become pronounced in an older adult, nurses have a challenging task to resolve the HF, especially if it is of a long-standing duration. Monitoring parameters must be established in which the patient and nurse actively identify subtle changes and seek intervention as early as possible (Coviello, 2004 [Level VI]).

The Health History

HF has both a symptomatic and a nonsymptomatic phase. When symptoms occur, they are related to intravascular and interstitial fluid overload and/or inadequate tissue perfusion during exertion. HF in older adults is often inadequately recognized and treated. Both patients and providers frequently attribute symptoms of fluid overload to aging. Older adult responses to HF medications and treatment are variable. In addition, other drugs commonly used in this age group, such as nonsteroidal anti-inflammatory agents, can actually exacerbate fluid overload by increasing sodium retention.

HF is a pathophysiologic process in which left ventricular dysfunction occurs independently from symptom development. Symptom expression is dependent on compensatory mechanisms and the length of time HF has been present. Patients with acute HF, as seen with MI, may be more symptomatic because their compensatory mechanisms have not fully developed. In comparison, patients with long-standing HF may have severe dysfunction but may not become symptomatic at all until they eat a high sodium meal and develop fluid overload rapidly, oftentimes overnight. In this case, compensatory mechanisms are now exhausted and, as a result, fail. The window of opportunity to successfully intervene is narrow as is the margin of error. Treatment for fluid overload in this case must be swift and brisk but gentle enough to maintain blood pressure (Coviello, 2004 [Level VI]). Nurses need to be aware of the importance of both early recognition and early intervention in the patient with fluid overload. A few hour delay in providing treatment can mean the difference between successful management at home and hospital admission with variable outcomes.

Knowledge of the past medical history will help to anticipate problems related to other conditions, because their presence may complicate assessment and management of HF. Cardiac risk factors; levels of physical activity; and control of lipids, HTN, obesity, DM, and smoking need to be determined. Nurses should routinely ask questions related to activity-limiting dyspnea. A key indicator in establishing a baseline for functional capacity is to ask patients what their maximal asymptomatic activity is now, what it was 6 months ago, and what it was 1 year ago. Other important questions include "How far can you walk without getting short of breath?," "What is the activity that commonly produces shortness of breath?," and, "Do you experience shortness of breath at rest?" Repeating these questions in subsequent interviews will help monitor changes in activity associated with treatment or with suspected fluid gain. Is the patient physically capable of performing activities of daily living (ADLs)? Previous questions related to cardiovascular functional capacity may have already provided some information, but additional information on musculoskeletal and neurologic function is important.

Assessment of additional symptoms is also important. Orthopnea is the most sensitive and specific symptom of elevated filling pressures, and it tends to reliably parallel filling pressures in patients with this symptom (Grady et al., 2000 [Level VI]; Stevenson & Perloff, 1989 [Level II]). Nocturnal or exertional cough is often a dyspnea equivalent and should not be confused with the cough from an angiotensin converting enzyme (ACE) inhibitor, which is not associated with activity or position. Individual patients generally exhibit reproducible patterns of fluid overload. These should be documented, made available to all on the care team, and used in patient education and subsequent monitoring. Questions related to symptoms and function should be part of not only the initial assessment but also of subsequent visits as a means of surveillance (Grady et al., 2000 [Level VI]).

The clinical presentation of HF may include various symptoms reflective of pulmonary congestion and decreased cardiac output, which are important health history questions to include and/or observe during the health encounter. Although the presence of any one symptom is sufficient to warrant consideration of HF when they occur with other physical findings, orthopnea, paroxysmal nocturnal dyspnea, and progressive dyspnea on exertion are virtually diagnostic of fluid overload.

The presence of other co-morbidities among older adults, such as DM, renal dysfunction, and liver disease, along with systemic physiologic changes associated with aging, further complicate the assessment and management of HF in older adults. Co-morbidities should also be carefully assessed by reviewing laboratory data. DM may necessitate monitoring of blood glucose because wide variations in glucose can affect ischemic threshold. Renal and liver disease may affect pharmacodynamics of drugs used to treat HF. Anemia, a common medical condition in older adults, affects oxygenation, activity tolerance, and subsequent fluid balance. The presence of the co-morbidity chronic obstructive pulmonary disease (COPD) may necessitate special precautions when assessing and managing oxygen therapy and use of beta-blockers.

Because overuse of salt in the diet may precipitate fluid overload, a comprehensive dietary history is absolutely essential. Nurses should include specific questions concerning the additional use of salt or salt substitutes and review with older adult patients those foods high in sodium. For instance, important dietary questions related to use of canned products or deli meats that contain higher amounts of sodium should be included. A list of the sodium and potassium content of a variety of foods, including fruits and vegetables, can be helpful in providing the information necessary for a patient to make appropriate daily choices. Because assessment of nutritional status is critical to elicit accurate fluid and sodium intake, it is prudent in the acute care setting for older adults to have a dietary consultation. Additionally, because cachexia is a harbinger of a downward spiral in patients with HF, questions need to be included on the health history related to appetite and weight loss.

Current prescription and over-the-counter (OTC) medications should be assessed, along with any alternative therapies. Many older adults who are eligible for aspirin, beta-blockers, and ACE inhibitors do not receive these medications, despite the important role that these agents have in reducing CHD-related morbidity and mortality.

Included in the health history should be questions related to medication adherence and the patient's decision to either take or not take medications. Understanding a patient's rationale to selectively not take certain medications at certain times will help reveal ways for the nurse to intervene. Patients may wish to adjust their diuretic dose so that they can function socially during the day. This is not a compliance issue but rather a sound decision based on a patient's rationale as to how to fit the medication regimen into his or her lifestyle. The interview can reveal if "nonadherence" has a rationale or not. If a cause is not found, other issues need to be explored, such as cost, number of medications, and/or frequency of the doses. Ways to simplify the drug regimen should be explored.

Psychosocial factors, personal beliefs and behaviors, and environmental along with cultural influences all contribute to management of chronic disease. The importance of depression and social support has been well documented in older adults; therefore, all of these factors need to be assessed. The nursing assessment in individuals with HF should identify the individual's response to treatment, which can then be used to assist the individual in subsequent management of symptoms and the underlying condition, health-promotion and disease-prevention activities, and chronic disease management. Awareness of patients' own perception of why they sought medical care and a detailed analysis of the symptoms will assist in assessing individuals' or caregivers' ability to identify symptoms; their knowledge regarding their condition, its prognosis, general health beliefs; and their prior ability to manage this or other medical conditions.

The Physical Assessment of an Older Adult with Fluid Overload

Physical assessment of the patient with suspected fluid overload includes inspection, palpation, and auscultation of the peripheral vasculature, heart, lungs, and abdomen. Orientation, functional limitations, and mental status are examined as well as vital signs, including height and weight.

A patient's height and baseline weight are important indicators of both nutritional and fluid status. Weights should subsequently be taken daily by the patient, typically the first thing in the morning upon arising, before breakfast, and with no clothes or wearing light clothing to avoid false fluctuations. This provides the best baseline for the day. A 2-pound weight gain overnight or a 3-pound weight gain in a week is an indication that medical management must change. Measurement of an older adult's waist circumference is also important to determine at baseline because many times this is the location for fluid accumulation (Coviello, 2004 Level VI]). Once height and weight are measured, a body mass index (BMI) should be calculated. Research has shown that higher BMIs (25 to 30 kg/m^2) are associated with longer survival (Anker et al., 2003; Davos et al., 2003; Horwich et al., 2001; Lavie, Osman, Milani, & Mehra, 2003 [all Level VI]).

A thorough evaluation of the blood pressure (BP) should be performed. Various environmental factors can influence BP determination; therefore, the room should be of a comfortable temperature, the patient as relaxed as possible, and a 5-minute rest provided before taking the first reading. Clothing that covers the area where the cuff will be placed should be removed and the individual should be seated comfortably, with legs uncrossed and the back and arm supported. The middle of the cuff on the upper arm should be at a level of the right atrium (Pickering et al., 2005 [Level VI]). The initial BP reading should be taken in both arms. Proper cuff size is critical to obtaining an accurate measurement because many individuals are obese with large arm circumference; bladder length should be 80% of the arm circumference and width at least 40%. The midline of the bladder should be placed above the brachial artery, 2 to 3 cm above the antecubital fossa, where the artery should have first been palpated. When using the auscultatory method, which remains the "gold standard" for BP measurement, palpating the radial pulse first while inflating the cuff will identify the point at which the pulse disappears. For the subsequent auscultatory measurement, the cuff should then be inflated to at least 30 mm Hg above this point. The rate of deflation is also extremely important with a rate of 2 to 3 mm Hg per second recommended. The first and last audible sounds are the systolic BP (SBP) and diastolic BP (DBP), respectively. Two readings, taken 5 minutes apart, should be averaged and if there is a >5 mm Hg difference, additional readings should be obtained.

Pseudohypertension is a phenomenon resulting from noncompressibility of thickened arteries and, if not recognized, will result in the recording of falsely high BP when indirect methods are used. This tendency for peripheral arteries to become rigid with aging may result in a need to increase cuff pressure in order to compress the artery. This is common in older adults, particularly in men or those with HTN or stroke. If suspected, an intra-arterial reading must be obtained to avoid over-medication with antihypertensives. Older adults are also more likely to exhibit "white-coat" HTN, in which the BP may be elevated over 140/90 mm Hg in the presence of a health care worker and an actual reading at home is usually 135/85 mm Hg. Isolated systolic hypertension is also common in older adults and is defined by a SBP $\geq$ 140 and DBP < 90 mm Hg. Therefore, assessment of the BP not only requires careful attention to technique but also consideration of the physiologic abnormalities associated with aging.

In addition, the standing BP should be assessed because older adults have a tendency for postural hypotension. Orthostatic hypotension is diagnosed when the SBP falls by at least 20 mm Hg or the DBP by 10 mm Hg within 3 minutes. The presence of orthostatic hypotension may also reveal early dehydration in a patient who is usually otherwise stable (Sansevero, 1997 [Level VI]). Because dehydration is the second most common admission for an older adult with HF, standing BPs should be part of the routine assessment. In addition, patients should be assessed for dehydration whenever a condition exists in which fluid loss could occur. This includes not only with vomiting or diarrhea but also with diaphoresis due to extremes in temperature and humidity.

Inspection is the first step of the physical assessment. General inspection of the periphery includes the following:

- Observing color of the skin and mucous membranes.
- Inspecting the patient's nails, including nail beds, and the angle between the base of the nail and the skin of the cuticle (normally <160 degrees). An angle of 180 degrees is called "clubbing": the distal phalanx appears rounded. Clubbing is associated with chronic hemoglobin desaturation.
- If cachetic, check dependent areas for decubiti.

Palpation of the extremities occurs following inspection of the skin, color, and turgor as well as the color of the nail beds. Capillary refill of the nail should be assessed by compressing the nail for 2 to 3 seconds and then releasing. Note the time elapsed until the original color returns. Normally, the nail bed is pink and capillary refill occurs within 2 to 3 seconds. A pale or cyanotic nail with delayed capillary refill may indicate decreased peripheral perfusion. The peripheral pulses should be palpated bilaterally, including radial, femoral, pedal, and posterior tibial pulse. Note pulse rate, rhythm, and symmetry.

The presence of peripheral edema, a symptom that can be related to fluid overload from cardiac, renal, or peripheral vasculature disease, should be evaluated. Edema can also occur in response to calcium channel blockers. Dependent parts of the body such as the feet, the ankles, and the sacrum are the most likely locations to find edema. The presence and location of edema and whether it is pitting or nonpitting should be assessed. Depress an edematous area over a bony prominence for 5 to 15 seconds, then release. The grading scale for edema is as follows:

0 = no pitting
1+ = trace
2+ = moderate, disappears in 10 to 45 seconds
3+ = deep, disappears in 1 to 2 minutes
4+ = very deep, disappears in 3 to 5 minutes

Respiratory rate and effort should be assessed prior to auscultation of the lungs. If possible, oxygen saturation during rest and activity should be recorded. Patients whose oxygen levels desaturate during activity may require oxygen support at home. In addition, surveillance of oxygen saturation during sleep may be required if the patient or family reports difficulty with sleep at night. It is not uncommon to see sleep apnea in patients with HF (Arzt & Bradley, 2006 [Level III]; Cormican & Williams, 2005 [Level V]; Kaneko et al., 2003 [Level II]; Lanfranchi et al., 2003 [Level VI]; Mansfield et al., 2003 [Level III]). Use the diaphragm of the stethoscope to assess the lungs. Listen in all the lobes for diminished sounds, crackles, wheezes, or rhonchi. Lung sounds are an important part of the assessment, particularly in patients with a history of HF.

The cardiovascular assessment begins with checking the apical pulse location, pulse rate regularity, fullness, and amplitude noted. Heart sounds should be ascertained with both the diaphragm and the bell of the stethoscope. Note the presence of S1 and S2 and of extra sounds, S3, S4, murmurs, clicks, or rubs. If extra heart sounds are present, also examine the carotid arteries by listening on both sides of the neck with the bell. Bruits sound like murmurs so it is important to differentiate between the two. Some aortic murmurs will radiate into the neck. Always listen to the heart before listening for extra sounds in the neck. In addition, the carotids should not be palpated bilaterally because this can lead to dysrhythmias and decreased blood flow to the brain.

Jugular veins are assessed with the patient in supine, semi-Fowler's, and Fowler's position. With the patient's head in straight alignment, observe the jugular neck veins for the presence of distention. In the absence of pathology, the vein distention is not present. Jugular venous distention provides the most sensitive sign of elevated filling pressures and is present with fluid overload, cor pulmonale, or high venous pressure (Grady et al., 2000 [Level VI]).

The abdomen should then be examined. First, determine if the abdomen is soft and nontender. A protuberant abdomen with bulging flanks suggests the possibility of ascitic fluid. Because ascitic fluid characteristically sinks with gravity while gas-filled loops of bowel float to the top, percussion gives a dull note in dependent areas of the abdomen. Look for such a pattern by percussing outward in several directions from the central area of tympany. Map the area between tympany and dullness. To palpate the liver, place your hand behind the patient, parallel to and supporting the right 11th and 12th ribs and adjacent soft tissues below. Remind the patient to relax. By pressing your left hand forward, the patient's liver may be felt more easily by the other hand. Patients who are sensitive to palpation can rest their hand on your palpating hand. Note any tenderness. If at all palpable, the edge of the liver is soft, sharp, and regular. The liver can be enlarged with HF. To assess, place the patient in a semi-Fowler's position at the highest level at which the jugular neck pulsations remain visible. Firmly apply pressure with the palmar surface of the hand over the right upper quadrant of the patient's abdomen for 1 minute. A 1-cm rise in the jugular pressure confirms the presence of fluid overload. A hepatojugular reflux may be associated with or without tenderness. Patients may also complain of a feeling of fullness.

The neurological assessment is often overlooked; however, changes in heart rate and rhythm, a decrease in cardiac output, and side effects of cardiac medications may cause significant changes in mental status. Questions about the patient's mental status help assess orientation, mentation, and function. Because depression is common among both older adults and the chronically ill, signs of depression should be assessed. Examples include feelings of hopelessness and sadness (also see chapter 5, Depression). Nurses can observe and assess a patient's mood, thought processes, thought content, abnormal perceptions, insight, judgment, memory, and retention. The time, the day, and the year, as well as orientation to place, should be included. Memory of hospitalization, teaching that occurred while hospitalized, and subsequent events post-discharge can be addressed depending on whether a patient is hospitalized or being seen as an outpatient (Bennett & Sauve, 2003 [Level VI]; Coviello, 2004 [Level VI]).

To summarize, the physical examination findings consistent with HF include the following:

- Hepatomegaly/splenomegaly
- Jugular venous distention (JVD)
- Hepatojugular reflux
- Basilar crackles, bronchospasm, and wheezing
- Presence of S3 or S4; heart murmur
- Displaced apical impulse
- Elevated heart rate and BP
- Cool extremities

Laboratory and Diagnostic Studies

The initial laboratory evaluation of patients presenting with symptoms of HF should include complete blood count, urinalysis, serum electrolytes including calcium and magnesium, blood urea nitrogen, serum creatinine, fasting blood glucose, glycosylated hemoglobin A1c (HbA1c), lipid profile, liver function tests, and thyroid stimulating hormone. B-type natriuretic peptide (BNP) can be useful in the evaluation of symptomatic patients presenting in the urgent care setting in whom the clinical diagnosis of HF is uncertain. A baseline BNP in the patient with a confirmed diagnosis of HF can provide a yardstick to measure both the presence of fluid overload and response to therapy (Wang, Fitzgerald, Shulzer, Mak, & Nyas, 2005). Review of diagnostic tests results is important. Electrolyte abnormalities are common in older adults, particularly in individuals on chronic diuretic therapy. Renal function as well as electrolyte levels should remain current and repeated whenever a patient has to increase diuretic therapy for longer than 3 days due to fluid overload. Anemia is frequently observed and may contribute to hypoxia, myocardial ischemia, and fluid overload. Cardiac enzymes assist in determining the presence of acute MI when an acute fluid overload event occurs. This is not an uncommon occurrence in older adults who may have a MI in the total absence of symptoms or with atypical symptoms.

A 12-lead electrocardiogram (ECG) and chest x-ray (PA and lateral) should be performed initially in all patients presenting with symptoms of HF. A baseline ECG is vital so that ST and T waves, axis changes, prolongation in PR, and QRS and QT intervals can be assessed in response to medications and ongoing ischemia. A new-onset arrhythmia heralded by an episode of fluid overload is not uncommon. HF can cause a stretch of the atrium, which in turn can lead to atrial fibrillation, which is common in patients with CHF. Two-dimensional echocardiography with Doppler should be performed during the initial evaluation to assess left ventricular ejection fraction (LVEF), LV size, wall thickness, and valve function. Radionuclide ventriculography can be performed to assess ventricular volumes, LVEF, and myocardial perfusion abnormalities. Cardiac catheterization should be performed on patients presenting with symptoms of HF who have angina or significant ischemia or who have known, suspected, or are at high risk for CHD, unless the patient is not eligible for revascularization of any kind.

Holter monitoring may be considered in patients presenting with HF who have a history of MI and/or syncope and are being considered for an electrophysiology study to document inducibility of ventricular tachycardia. In addition, other candidates for electrophysiology include those with an LVEF of 30% or less with a QRS complex duration that exceeds 0.12 ms. Patients who meet the criteria may receive a dual chamber pacemaker in combination with an automatic implantable defibrillator in order to prevent sudden death from arrhythmia, as well as improve left ventricular function (Hunt et al., 2005 [Level VI]).

Interventions and Care Strategies

Initial goals in the acute management of HF are to alleviate symptoms and improve oxygenation, improve circulation, and correct the underlying causes of the HF. Longer term goals are to improve exercise tolerance and functional capacity, reduce readmission rates, and decrease mortality. The management of HF follows standard ACC/AHA Task Force expert consensus recommendations, including intensive treatment of coexistent hypertension, CHD, and renal disease (Hunt et al., 2005 [Level VI]). Importantly, optimal treatment of HTN is critical to both the prevention and treatment of HF. Although the level at which medication should be started is still debated (Chobanian et al., 2003 [Level VI]), the BP should be reduced to below 130/80 mm Hg.

There are key prognostic indicators of 4-year mortality for older adults diagnosed with HF. Patients with renal dysfunction, pulmonary disease, a BMI of $<25 \text{ kg/m}^2$, diabetes, hypertension, and cancer, as well as those who continue to smoke, have a greater risk of mortality. Those with a functional deficit in ADLs and IADLs (e.g., difficulty bathing, managing finances, walking several blocks, or pushing or pulling heavy objects) combined with one or more of these factors are at greater risk for mortality. A chart review and history during hospitalization should then include not only the standard accepted cardiac risk factors but also the key indicators as listed herein. Detecting these additional prognostic indicators can aid in developing interventions that can affect quality of life and survival (Lee, Lindquist, Segal, & Covinsky, 2006 [Level III]). Goals for therapy should include reaching goals for fasting blood sugar and HbA1c, BP, cholesterol, and HF therapy through the use of evidenced-based standards of care.

In *Stage A* HF, hypertension and lipid disorders are treated appropriately, and smoking cessation is encouraged, as is regular exercise. Metabolic syndrome is controlled and use of alcohol intake and illicit drug use is discouraged. ACE inhibitors or angiotensin receptor blockers (ARBs) are used to treat patients with vascular disease or in those with DM. In *Stage B*, these same measures are used, with ACE inhibitors, ARBs, and beta-blockers used in certain patients. In

Stage C, dietary sodium restriction is added to this regimen and diuretics are added to treat fluid retention, along with ACE inhibitors and beta-blockers. In certain patients, aldosterone antagonists, ARBs, digitalis, and hydralazines/nitrates are added. These patients my also require a pacemaker or implantable defibrillators to treat arrhythmias. In *Stage D,* end-of-life care/hospice care is initiated, and the use of extraordinary measures such as heart transplantation, chronic inotrope therapy, permanent mechanical support, and experimental drugs or surgery is considered. Nurses have an important role in assisting individuals and their caregivers in understanding the disease process and treatment options, including end of life care.

Open and honest discussion regarding the chronic, progressive nature of HF must begin early in the disease process because the natural history of HF involves declining physical as well as psychological functioning. Although depression is commonly seen in older adults, as well as individuals with CVD, there are few studies that have addressed this important problem in an older adult with HF (Lane, Chong & Lip, 2006 [Level I]). Because pharmacotherapy and behavioral interventions have demonstrated effectiveness, all older individuals should be screened for depression and treated appropriately. Early discussions related to the goals of care and advanced directives with frequent revisiting of patient understanding of the disease course and patient preferences as the illness progresses ensures patient participation in decision making. This is best done utilizing a multidisciplinary team approach where not only the caregivers and the patient/family unit are involved but there is also a spiritual and/or a psychological representative.

The benefits of the multidisciplinary team to provide care to HF patients have been discussed for the last several years. In most cases, they have been related to the use of the team approach to help keep patients stable in order to prevent hospital readmissions (Barrella & Monica, 1998 [Level V]; Naylor et al., 1994 [Level II]; Rich et al., 1995 [Level V]; Rich & Neese, 1999 [Level II]; Simon, Vandenbroek, Pearson, & Horowitz, 1999 [Level VI]). Comprehensive transitional care interventions have been shown not only to reduce costs and cardiac outcomes but also to have a beneficial effect on hospitalization for co-morbid conditions (Naylor et al., 2004 [Level II]). In the case of the patient in end-stage HF, a multidisciplinary team either for in-patient or outpatient management can provide cost effective service providing patients with their last wishes in the environment that they choose (Coviello, 2004; Coviello, Borges, & Masulli, 2002 [both Level VI]).

Once the initial history and physical assessment have been completed, an individualized care plan to monitor and treat fluid overload should be implemented. A 2-pound weight gain overnight or a 3-pound weight gain in the course of a week is reason to alter diuretic dosage for up to 3 days. If patients return to baseline weight before the 3-day period, they may reduce their dose back to the standard daily dose (Coviello, 2004 [Level VI]). Patients can be taught how to regulate their diuretic doses based on their symptoms and weight. The nurse and patient can construct a self-care algorithm that gives them a sound "recipe" to follow if fluid overload occurs. The important factor is early recognition and swift, brief action. Clear guidelines as to when to contact caregivers should also be provided. Consideration should be given to the patient's baseline functional capacity, as well as renal function. Diuretics are used in both systolic and diastolic HF to relieve congestive symptoms by promoting the excretion of sodium and water and by decreasing cardiac filling pressures, thereby decreasing preload. They should be used cautiously with diastolic dysfunction, where maintaining an adequate cardiac output is heavily preload dependent, to avoid syncope, falls, or confusion.

A double dose of oral diuretics for up to 3 days is usually well tolerated in both systolic and diastolic HF. When diuretics are used, serum-potassium levels should be monitored due to an increased risk of hyperkalemia with potassium-sparing agents and of hypokalemia with loop diuretics. Patients should be forewarned about signs of hypokalemia, such as profound weakness. Loop diuretics may be useful for patients who are volume sensitive or who have a tendency to retain fluid because of renal impairment. Aldosterone antagonists prevent hypokalemia resulting from loop diuretics; however, serum-potassium levels should be monitored due to an increased risk of hyperkalemia, as well as when ACE inhibitors are used. However, recent evidence suggests that many individuals, particularly African Americans, may still require potassium supplementation (Cavallari et al., 2004 [Level IV]). In addition, dehydration is a significant problem in older adults taking diuretics and appears to be an even greater concern in African Americans (Lancaster, Smiciklas-Wright, Heller, Ahern, & Jensen, 2003 [Level IV]), making assessment of hydration status an important nursing concern (Sansevero, 1997 [Level VI]).

Use of diuretic agents increases the risk for sudden loss of urinary control (i.e., urinary incontinence) in older adults, a very common, potentially reversible geriatric syndrome (for more information, visit www.ConsultGeriRN.org and select *Try This: Urinary Incontinence Assessment*). Practice with an older-adult population requires frequent monitoring and detection of symptoms related to the onset of urinary incontinence, which is often signaled by symptoms of urinary frequency, urgency, or nocturia. These symptoms may actually be present in an older adult from other coexisting problems. Nocturia is particularly evident in patients with heart disease, as when supine an increase in vascular return can precipitate a need to get up frequently at night to urinate. With nocturia comes the possibility of an older adult incurring a nighttime fall. Preexisting co-morbidities such as visual impairment or osteoarthritis of the hip and knees make timing to the bathroom facilities a factor in the prevention of such events. Overall, management considerations for older adults with heart disease and the new development of urinary incontinence or falls include reevaluation of medication regimen, activity considerations, and the use of additional adaptive aids to help ensure the avoidance of such preventable events. Use of a nighttime bedpan or urinal, frequent toileting rounds, and reduction of nighttime fluids all are possible worthwhile solutions.

Because of their negative chronotropic effect, beta-blockers are useful in the management of diastolic HF, thereby decreasing heart rate and increasing time for diastolic filling. More recently, beta-blockers have been shown to be beneficial in the treatment of systolic HF, where they are usually begun after symptoms have resolved; however, these agents should be initiated at low doses. Use of beta-blockers in combination with ACE inhibitors has demonstrated both an improvement in LVEF and functional capacity once titrated to tolerance. Although beta-blockers may potentially worsen insulin resistance, mask hypoglycemia, or aggravate orthostatic hypotension in older individuals with DM, these agents have been shown to contribute to improved outcomes. Therefore, careful monitoring and treatment for these effects are required.

Digoxin increases contractility and decreases heart rate. It is not used routinely with diastolic failure; however, it may be useful in those patients with persistent symptoms despite diuretic and ACE inhibitor therapy and in those who also have atrial fibrillation. Assessment should be made for digoxin toxicity as well as for interactions with quinidine, amiodarone, verapamil, and vasodilators; hypokalemia should be avoided. Other medications that have a positive inotropic effect are dopamine and dobutamine. Both of these drugs can improve contractility and subsequent cardiac output; however, they also increase myocardial oxygen demand. Amiodarone and milrinone are phosphodiesterase inhibitors that have been shown to be beneficial in the management of hospitalized patients with HF, providing a positive inotropic effect, as well as a vasodilation (see chapter 12, *Reducing Adverse Drug Events*, for potential sequelae to several CV medications).

Vasodilators are also useful in the treatment of systolic and diastolic failure through reduction in preload. As with diuretics, they should be used cautiously in those with diastolic HF. Hydralazine and isosorbide reduce both preload and afterload, relieving symptoms and improving exercise tolerance. This combination is commonly used when patients do not tolerate ACE therapy. In addition, recent studies have shown the combination is more effective in reducing morbidity and mortality in African Americans (Taylor et al., 2004 [Level II]). Morphine sulfate, often used in an emergent situation, also has a peripheral vasodilating effect and is useful with pulmonary edema or in patients with breathlessness at end of life.

With appropriate titration of these medications, an improvement in both left ventricular function and functional capacity can be achieved. Medications to treat HTN and lipid abnormalities may not be well tolerated and the potential for side effects and drug interactions is increased in the setting of polypharmacy. Both antihypertensive agents and lipid-lowering agents should be used in the lowest doses possible to bring about the desired goal for treatment.

Patients and caregivers need to understand the warning signs of HF and recurrent MI such as chest pain, pressure, shortness of breath, indigestion, nausea, dizziness, palpitations, confusion, weakness, and weight gain. A clear plan for obtaining immediate medical attention should be developed. This is especially important if an older person lives alone; some type of "medical alert" system may be needed. Understanding and the ability to follow the medication regimen is paramount; therefore, a thorough assessment of the patient and their caregivers is vital. The older individual may be on multiple medications and the schedule may be confusing. The need to maintain cardiac medications must be stressed and the risk of the patient abruptly discontinuing beta-blocker, nitrates, and antiarrhythmics must be assessed. All medications should be reviewed with patients and their caregivers, stressing desired effects, common side effects, and possible interactions with OTC medications (for more information, visit www.ConsultGeriRN.org and select Geriatric Topics "Medication"). Nurses should also review what to do if medications are accidentally omitted or become too costly to maintain. Long-term management of HF requires a multidisciplinary team approach (Phillips et al., 2004) and disease management programs have been effective in reducing readmission rates (Gonseth, Guallar-Castillon, Banegas, & Rodriguez-Artajo, 2004 [Level I]). Furthermore, even though many of these individuals are debilitated, exercise training has been shown to improve functional ability (McKelvie et al., 2002 [Level II]; Piepoli, Davos, Francis, Coats, & Collaborative, 2004 [Level I]; Rees, Taylor, Singh, Coats, & Ebrahim, 2006 [Level I]).

Medication titration for HF, coupled with activity progression, can enhance a patient's activity capacity. An active patient may notice early signs of fluid overload; therefore, questions related to activity tolerance can provide insight for nurses who monitor a patient. Patients with gradual fluid gain will first notice a change in their level of fatigue, which will translate into a change in their daily routine. Previous experience with fluid overload will also reveal to the nurse the patient's own unique signs and symptoms because not every patient has the same indicators. It is important to not only assess these factors directly with patients during the interview but also to reinforce that these symptoms are important for patients to monitor as well (Coviello, 2004 [Level VI]). In addition to changes in weight, deviation from the baseline functional ability may be an early clue, even before peripheral edema or lung congestion appears.

The prevention and treatment of HF in patients with DM requires optimal management of coexistent HTN, CHD, and left ventricular dysfunction. Additionally, control of hyperglycemia is an important issue because the presence of HF affects the choice of medications used to treat Type II DM. Although insulin and insulin secretagogues are considered safe for use in individuals with HF, metformin and thiazolidinediones (TZDs) are not recommended in individuals with moderate-to-severe HF, even though recent data suggest that they may lower the risk of death (Masoudi et al., 2005 [Level IV]). Decreased clearance of metformin in individuals with HF due to hypoperfusion or renal insufficiency can lead to potentially dangerous lactic acidosis. TZDs are sometimes associated with fluid retention, pedal edema, and weight gain, particularly when used in conjunction with insulin, and occasionally contribute to HF. However, this is relatively infrequent, usually occurring with higher doses, concomitant insulin treatment, or active HF (Nesto et al., 2004 [Level VI]); Tang, Francis, Hoogwerf, & Young, 2003 [Level IV]). Therefore, the use of these agents requires close monitoring for stages C and D heart failure. Careful clinical assessment prior to initiation of TZDs, lower doses with slow dose escalation, and careful ongoing monitoring should be implemented when these drugs are used in the presence of known structural heart disease or a prior history of HF.

Adequate control of BP is also essential in the management of HF. Treatment of older persons with HTN has been shown to reduce CVD morbidity and mortality (Mulrow, Lau, & Brand, 2006 [Level I]). An important nursing consideration is to monitor for adverse effects of medications used to manage HF, as well as HTN, along with patient and caregiver education. ACE inhibitors are important in the management of systolic HF and may also be helpful in diastolic failure. In the Heart Outcomes Prevention Evaluation (HOPE) Study, ACE inhibitors prevented cardiac events in high risk patients without HF or known low ejection fractions (HOPE Investigators, 2000 [Level II]).

In addition, ACE inhibitors have a renal protective benefit that is extremely important in preventing the development or worsening of HF, especially in patients with DM. Recent evidence suggests that use of ACE inhibitors is associated with a larger lower extremity muscle mass, which may have benefit in wasting syndromes and prevention of disability (Di Bari et al., 2004 [Level IV]) and that they are particularly efficacious in older adults (Wing et al., 2003 [Level II]).

ARBs are also used widely for the prevention and treatment of HF, particularly when patients are unable to use ACE inhibitors due to the development of cough (Brenner et al., 2001 [Level II]; Lindholm et al., 2002 [Level II]). Renal function and hyperkalemia should be assessed when using both classes of agents, especially in the presence of underlying renal dysfunction.

Case Study and Discussion

CTG is a 72-year-old woman with a history of diet-controlled glucose intolerance and HF with normal renal function who is seen in the geriatric clinic with a 3-day history of poor appetite, nausea, and occasional vomiting. She complains of a constant feeling of fullness. She was last hospitalized 3 months ago due to fluid overload related to newly diagnosed HF. Her diuretic was increased 6 weeks ago for mild ankle swelling. She denies recent lower extremity swelling, orthopnea, or paroxysmal nocturnal dyspnea. Her blood sugars have been well controlled in the 90 to 130 range without hypoglycemic episodes. She denies fever, chills, cough, or urinary symptoms. She says she never misses her medications. Until 5 days ago, she was able to walk 30 minutes a day without difficulty. She had noticed a gradual increase in fatigue during the last 10 days and found herself too tired to attend several social and church events in the evening. When asked what her daily weights have been, she confessed that because she had been feeling so good she had abandoned this as a daily practice. Concerned, however, about her recent symptoms, she weighed herself this morning and found that she had gained 6 pounds since she last weighed herself 2 weeks ago. However, she has been compliant to her medications for HF, which include:

> Coreg 6.25 mg twice a day
> Altace 5 mg daily
> Aldactone 12.5 mg daily
> Lasix 20 mg daily
> Imdur 15 mg daily

She has not taken a double dose of lasix with the additional weight gain as shown in her self-care action plan. She had been unaware of that weight gain because she had not been weighing herself. In addition, she had attended two social events 2 weekends ago that included eating out. Her self-care action plan had shown that she should increase her diuretic for 1 day following eating out the day before.

On physical examination, her blood pressure is 132/86 with a heart rate of 88 bpm. She is afebrile. She has fine crackles in the lower bases bilaterally. There is +1 edema. Heart sounds demonstrate S1, S2, and S3. Her apical impulse is displaced to the left. There is jugular neck vein distention. Her abdominal girth has increased 2 inches since her last visit.

Lasix was increased to 40 mg for a maximum of 3 days. If at any point during the 3 days her weight returned to baseline, she was instructed to return to her usual dose of lasix. She was advised of the importance of daily weighing to maintain her baseline weight. She was referred back to her self-care action plan for changes in diuretic depending on her daily weight and the maintenance of her low-sodium diet in light of her social schedule. She will return to the clinic in 1 week.

This patient exemplifies the need for educational reinforcement in a newly diagnosed HF patient who is just learning how to incorporate a self-care action plan. Like many patients who have had to take antibiotics in the past, compliance can wane when the patient feels well. It is important to make contact with a newly diagnosed HF patient fairly frequently to be available for questions that might influence the self-care decision making of the patient.

Summary

Hospital admissions can be reduced in older adults with HF:

- when care is spent in identifying the patient's own unique signs and symptoms of fluid overload.
- by creating monitoring parameters for the nurse in the form of the history and the physical assessment.
- by creating monitoring parameters for the patient in the form of a self-care algorithm with clear guidelines for self-care action.
- by achieving goals for clinical stability.

Resources

Relevant Practice Guidelines

ADA guidelines: Summary of Revisions for the 2007 Clinical Practice Recommendations *Diabetes Care* 2007, *30*, S3.

Chobanian, A. V., Bakris, G. L., Black, H. R., Cushman, W. C., Green, L. A., Izzo, J. L., et al. (2003). The seventh report of the Joint National Committee on Prevention, Detection, Evaluation and Treatment of High Blood Pressure. *Journal of the American Medical Association, 289*, 1560–1572.

Grady, K., Dracup, K., Kennedy, G., Moser, D., Piano, M., Stevenson, L., et al. (2000). Team anagement of patients with heart failure: A statement of healthcare professionals from the Cardiovascular Nursing Council of the American Health Association. *Circulation, 102*, 2443–2456.

Hunt, S. A., Abraham, W. T., Chin, M. H., Feldman, A. M., Francis, G. S., Ganiats, T. G., et al. (2005). ACC/AHA 2005 guideline update for the diagnosis and management of chronic heart failure in the adult [Electronic Version]. *Circulation*, e154–e235.

References

Anker, S., Negassa, A., Coats, A., Afzal, R., Poole-Wilson, P. A., Cohn, J. N., et al. (2003). Prognostic importance of weight loss in chronic heart failure and the effect of treatment with Angiotensin-converting-enzyme inhibitors: An observational study. *Lancet, 361*, 1077–1083. Evidence Level VI: Journal Article Expert Opinion.

Arzt, M., & Bradley, T. (2006). Treatment of sleep apnea in heart failure. *American Journal of Respiratory and Critical Care Medicine, 173*(12), 1300–1308. Evidence Level III: Quasi-experimental Study.

Barrella, P., & Monica, E. (1998). Managing congestive heart failure at home. *AACN Clinical Issues, 9*(2), 377–388. Evidence Level V: Review.

Bennett, S. J., & Sauve, M. J. (2003). Cognitive deficits in patients with heart failure: A review of the literature. *Journal of Cardiovascular Nursing, 18*(3), 219–242. Evidence Level VI: Journal Article Expert Opinion.

Bertoni, A. G., Bonds, D. E., Hundley, W. G., Burke, G. L., Massing, M. W., & Goff, D. C. (2004). Heart failure prevalence, incidence, and mortality in the elderly with diabetes. *Diabetes Care, 27*, 699–703. Evidence Level VI: Expert Opinion.

Brenner, B. M., Cooper, M. E., de Zeeuw, D., Keane, W. F., Mitch, W. E., Parving, H. H., et al. (2001). Effects of losartan on renal and cardiovascular outcomes in patients with type 2 diabetes and nephropathy. *New England Journal of Medicine, 345*(12), 861–869. Evidence Level II: RCT.

Cavallari, L. H., Fashingbauer, L. A., Beitelshees, A. L., Groo, V. L., Southworth, M. R., Viana, M. A. G., et al. (2004). Racial differences in patients' potassium concentrations during spironolactone therapy for heart failure. *Pharmacotherapy, 24*(6), 750–756. Evidence Level IV: Nonexperimental Study.

Chobanian, A. V., Bakris, G. L., Black, H. R., Cushman, W. C., Green, L. A., Izzo, J. L., et al. (2003). The seventh report of the Joint National Committee on Prevention, Detection, Evaluation and Treatment of High Blood Pressure. *Journal of the American Medical Association, 289*, 1560–1572. Evidence Level VI: Practice Guideline.

Chyun, D., Vaccarino, V., Murillo, J., Young, L., & Krumholz, H. (2002). Mortality, heart failure and recurrent myocardial infarction in the elderly with diabetes. *American Journal of Critical Care, 11*, 504–519. Evidence Level VI: Expert Opinion.

Cormican, L. J., & Williams, A. (2005). Sleep-disordered breathing in congestive heart failure: An opportunity missed? *British Journal of Cardiology, 12* (3), 171–172. Evidence Level V: Review.

Coviello, J. S. (2004). Cardiac Assessments 101: A new look at the guidelines for cardiac home-care patients. *Home Healthcare Nurse, 22*(2), 116–123. Evidence Level VI: Expert Opinion.

Coviello, J. S., Borges, L. H., & Masulli, P. S. (2002). Accomplishing quality of life in end-stage heart failure: A hospice multidisciplinary approach. *Home Healthcare Nurse, 20*(3), 193–198. Evidence Level VI: Expert Opinion.

Davos, C. H., Doehner, W., Rauchhaus, M., Cicoira, M., Francis, D. P., Coats, A. J., et al. (2003). Body mass and survival in patients with chronic heart failure without cachexia: The importance of obesity. *Journal of Cardiac Failure, 9*, 29–35. Evidence Level VI: Journal Article.

Di Bari, M., van de Poll-Franse, L. V., Onder, G., Kritchevsky, S. B., Newman, A., Harris, T. B., et al. (2004). Antihypertensive medications and differences in muscle mass in older persons: The Health, Aging and Body Composition Study. *Journal of the American Geriatrics Society, 52*(6), 961–966. Evidence Level IV: Nonexperimental Study.

Funk, M., & Krumholtz, H. (1996). Epidemiologic and economics impact of advance heart failure. *Journal of Cardiovascular Nursing, 10*(2), 1–10. Evidence Level IV: Nonexperimental Study.

Gonseth, J., Guallar-Castillon, P., Banegas, J. R., & Rodriguez-Artajo, F. (2004). The effectiveness of disease management programmes in reducing hospital readmission in older persons with heart failure: A systematic review and meta-analysis of published reports. *European Heart Journal, 25*(18), 1570–1595. Evidence Level I: Systematic Review.

Grady, K., Dracup, K., Kennedy, G., Moser, D., Piano, M., Stevenson, L., et al. (2000). Team Management of Patients with Heart Failure: A statement of healthcare professionals from the Cardio Vascular Nursing Council of the American Health Association. *Circulation, 102*, 2443–2456. Evidence Level VI: Expert Panel.

Ho, K. K., Pinsky, J. L., Kannel, W. B., & Levy, D. (1993). The epidemiology of heart failure: The Framingham Study. *Journal of the American College of Cardiology, 22*(4 Suppl. A), 6A–13A. Evidence Level II: Single RCT.

HOPE Investigators (2000). Effects of an angiotensin-converting enzyme inhibitor, ramipril, on cardiovascular events in high risk patients. *New England Journal of Medicine, 342*, 145–153. Evidence Level II: RCT.

Horwich, T., Fonorow, G., Hamilton, M., Maclellan, W., Woo, M., Tillisch, J. (2001). The relationship between obesity and mortality in patients with heart failure. *Journal of American College of Cardiology, 38*, 789–795. Evidence Level VI: Journal Article.

Hunt, S. A., Abraham, W. T., Chin, M. H., Feldman, A. M., Francis, G. S., Ganiats, T. G., et al. (2005). ACC/AHA 2005 guideline update for the diagnosis and management of chronic heart failure in the adult. *Circulation*, e154–e235. Retrieved March 16, 2007, at http://circ.ahajournals.org/cgi/reprint/112/12/e154. Evidence Level VI: Guideline, Expert Consensus.

Hypertension in Diabetes Study Group (1993). HDS 1: Prevalence of hypertension in newly presenting type 2 diabetic patients and the association with risk factors or cardiovascular disease. *Journal of Hypertension, 11*, 309–317. Evidence Level II: Surveillance Data.

Kaneko, Y., Floras, J. S., Usui, K., Plante, J., Tkacova, R., Kubo, T., et al. (2003). Cardiovascular effects of continuous positive airway pressure in patients with heart failure and obstructive sleep apnea. *New England Journal of Medicine. 348*(13), 1233–1241. Evidence Level II: Single Experimental Study.

Lancaster, K. J., Smiciklas-Wright, H., Heller, D. A., Ahern, F. M., & Jensen, G. (2003). Dehydration in black and white older adults using diuretics. *Annals of Epidemiology, 13*(7), 525–529. Evidence Level IV: Nonexperimental Study.

Lane, D. A., Chong, A. Y., & Lip, G. Y. H. (2006). Psychological interventions for depression in heart failure. *Cochrane Database of Systematic Reviews, 2*. Evidence Level I: Systematic Review.

Lanfranchi, P., Sommers, V., Braghiroli, A., Curra, U., Eleuteri, E., Gianuzzi, P., et al. (2003). Central sleep apnea in left ventricular dysfunction: Prevalence and implications for arrhythmic risk circulation. *Circulation 107*(5), 727–732. Evidence Level VI: Journal Article.

Lavie, C., Osman, A., Milani, R., & Mehra, M. (2003). Body composition and prognosis in chronic systolic heart failure: The obesity paradox. *American Journal of Cardiology, 91*, 891–894. Evidence Level VI: Journal Article.

Lee, S. J., Lindquist, K., Segal, M. R., & Covinsky, K. E. (2006). Development and validation of a prognostic index for 4-year mortality in older adults. *Journal of the American Medical Association, 295*(7), 801–807. Evidence Level III: Quasi-experimental Study.

Levy, D., Larson, M. G., Vasan, R. S., Kannel, W. B., & Ho, K. K. (1996). The progression from hypertension to congestive heart failure. *Journal of the American Medical Association, 275*(20), 1557–1562. Evidence Level VI: Journal Article.

Lewis, E. F., Moye, L. A., Rouleau, J. L., Sacks, F. M., Arnold, J. M., Warnica, J. W., et al.. (2003). Predictors of late development of heart failure in stable survivors of myocardial infarction: The CARE study. *Journal of the American College of Cardiology, 42*(8), 1446–1453. Evidence Level VI: Journal Article.

Lindholm, L. H., Ibsen, H., Borch-Johnsen, K., Olsen, M. H., Wachtell, K., Dahlof, B., et al. (2002). Risk of new-onset diabetes in the Losartan Intervention for Endpoint reduction in hypertension study. *Journal of Hypertension, 20*(9), 1879–1886. Evidence Level II: RCT.

Mansfield, D., Kaye, D., Brunner, L., Rocca, H., Solin, P., Murray, E., et al.. (2003). Raised sympathetic nerve activity in heart failure and central sleep apnea is due to heart failure severity. *Circulation, 107*(10), 1396–1400. Evidence Level III: Quasi-experimental Study.

Masoudi, F. A., Inzucchi, S. E., Wang, Y., Havranek, E. P., Foody, J. M., & Krumholz, H. (2005). Thiazolidinediones, metformin, and outcomes in older patients with diabetes and heart failure. *Circulation, 111*, 583–590. Evidence Level IV: Nonexperimental Study.

McKelvie, R. S., Teo, K. K., Roberts, R., McCartney, N., Humen, D., Montague, T., et al. (2002). Effects of exercise training in patients with heart failure: The exercise rehabilitation trial (EXERT). *American Heart Journal, 144*(1), 23–30. Evidence Level II: RCT.

Mulrow, C., Lau, J., & Brand, M. (2006). Pharmacotherapy for hypertension in the elderly. *Cochrane Database of Systematic Reviews*. Evidence Level I: Systematic Review.

Naylor, M., Brooten, D., Campbell, R. L., Maislin, G., McCauley, K. M., & Schwartz, J. S. (2004). Transitional care of older adults hospitalized with heart failure: A randomized, controlled trial. *Journal of the American Geriatrics Society, 52*, 675–684. Evidence Level II: RCT.

Naylor, M., Brooten, D., Jones, R., Lavizzo-Mourey, R., Mezey, M., & Pauly, M. (1994). Comprehensive discharge planning for the hospitalized elderly: A randomized clinical trial. *Annals of Internal Medicine, 120*, 999–1006. Evidence Level II: RCT.

Nesto, R. W., LeWinter, M., Bell, D., Bonow, R. O., Semenkovich, C. F., Fonseca, V., et al. (2004). Thiazolidinedione use, fluid retention, and congestive heart failure. *Diabetes Care, 27,* 256–263. Evidence Level VI: Consensus Review.

Phillips, C. O., Wright, S. M., Kern, D. E., Singa, R. M., Shepperd, S., & Rubin, H. R. (2004). Comprehensive discharge planning with postdischarge support for older persons with congestive heart failure. *Journal of the American Medical Association, 291*(11), 1358–1367.

Piccini, J. P., Klein, L., Gheorghiade, M., & Bonow, R. O. (2004). New insights into diastolic heart failure: Role of diabetes mellitus. *American Journal of Medicine Med, 116*(Suppl. 5A), 64S–75S. Evidence Level V: Review.

Pickering, T. G., Hall, J. E., Appel, L. J., Falkner, B. E., Graves, J., Hill, M. N., et al. (2005). Recommendations for blood pressures measurements in humans and experimental animals. *Circulation, 45,* 142–161. Evidence Level VI: Guideline Expert Opinion.

Piepoli, M. F., Davos, C., Francis, D. P., Coats, A., & Collaborative, E. (2004). Exercise training meta-analysis of trials in patients with chronic heart failure (ExTraMATCH). *British Medical Journal, 328*(7433), 189–192. Evidence Level I: Meta-analysis.

Rees, K., Taylor, R. S., Singh, S., Coats, A. J. S., & Ebrahim, S. (2006). Exercise-based rehabilitation for heart failure. *Cochrane Database of Systematic Reviews* (Vol. 1). Evidence Level I: Systematic Review.

Rich, M., Beckham, V., Wittenburg, C., Leven, C., Freedland, K., & Carney, R. (1995). A multidisciplinary intervention to prevent readmission of elderly patients with congestive heart failure. *New England Journal of Medicine, 33,* 1190–1195. Evidence Level V: Review.

Rich, M., & Kitzman, D. W. (2005). Third pivotal research in cardiology in the elderly (PRICE-III) symposium: Heart failure in the elderly: Mechanisms and management. *American Journal of Geriatric Cardiology, 14*(5), 250–261. Evidence Level VI: Expert Opinion.

Rich, M., & Neese, R. (1999). Cost-effectiveness analysis in clinical practice: The case of heart failure. *Archives of Internal Medicine, 159*(15), 1190–1195. Evidence Level II: RCT.

Sansevero, A. (1997). Dehydration in the elderly: Strategies for prevention and management. *Nurse Practitioner, 22*(4), 41–42, 51–52, 54–57. Evidence Level VI: Journal Article.

Simon, S., Vandenbroek, A., Pearson, S., & Horowitz, J. (1999). Prolonged beneficial effects of a home-based intervention on unplanned readmissions and mortality among patients with congestive heart failure. *Archives of Internal Medicine, 159*(3), 257–261. Level VI: Expert Opinion.

Stevenson, L., & Perloff, J. (1989). The limited reliability of physical signs for estimating hemodynamics in chronic heart failure. *Journal of American Medical Association, 288*(8), 973–979. Evidence Level II: RCT.

Tang, W. H., Francis, G. S., Hoogwerf, B. J., & Young, J. B. (2003). Fluid retention after initiation of thiazolidinedione therapy in diabetic patients with established chronic heart failure. *Journal of the American College of Cardiology, 41*(8), 1394–1398. Evidence Level IV: Nonexperimental Study.

Taylor, A. L., Ziesche, S., Yancy, C., Carson, P., D'Agostino, R., Ferdinand, K., et al. (2004). Combination of isosorbide dinitrate and hydralazine in Blacks with heart failure. *New England Journal of Medicine, 352,* 2049–2057. Evidence Level II: RCT.

Thom, T., Haase, N., Rosamond, W., Howard, V. J., Rumsfeld, J., Manolio, T., et al. (2006). Heart disease and stroke statistics – 2006 update: A report from the American Heart Association Statistics Committee and Stroke Statistics Subcommittee [Electronic Version]. *Circulation, 113,* e85–e151. Retrieved June 16, 2006, from http://circ.ahajournals.org. Evidence Level VI: Expert Opinion.

Wang, C., Fitzgerald, J., Schulzer, M., Mak, E., & Nyas, N. (2005). Does this dyspneic patient in the emergency department have congestive heart failure? *Journal of the American Medical Association, 294*(15), 1944–1956.

Wing, L. M., Reid, C. M., Ryan, P., Beilin, L. J., Brown, M. A., Jennings, G. L., et al. (2003). A comparison of outcomes with angiotensin-converting-enzyme inhibitors and diuretics for hypertension in the elderly. *New England Journal of Medicine, 348,* 583–592. Evidence Level II: RCT.

Cancer Assessment and Intervention Strategies

27

Janine Overcash

Educational Objectives

At the conclusion of this chapter, the reader will be able to:

1. recognize the incidence and prevalence of U.S. statistics on malignancy in older adults

2. identify three common malignancies in older adults

3. recognize three common co-morbidities in older adults with cancer

4. identify three common cancer-related emergencies in older adults

5. identify three instruments useful in the assessment of older adults

6. identify three important elements of a health history specific to an older cancer patient

7. identify three important elements of a physical examination specific to an older cancer patient

8. define clinical parameters of frailty of an older adult with cancer

OVERVIEW

The probability of developing a malignancy increases with age. In the years between 1998 and 2002, the National Cancer Institute Surveillance, Epidemiology, and End Results Program (SEER) found that 56% of all cancers were diagnosed in adults 65 years and older (Ries et al., 2007). Cancer is often one of many diagnoses (or co-morbidities) found in the medical history of an adult 65 or older (Extermann, Overcash, Lyman, Parr, & Balducci, 1998 [Level IV]). Acute care nurses must appreciate that cancer is common in older adult patients and be aware of potential health limitations and emergencies associated with the

For a description of Evidence Levels cited in this chapter, see chapter 1,
Developing and Evaluating Clinical Practice Guidelines, page 4.

615

diagnosis and treatment of malignancy. This chapter presents the incidence and prevalence of cancers more common in adults aged 65 and older. Assessment strategies and instruments are identified and potential medical emergencies associated with the cancer-disease process and treatment are discussed.

Incidence and Prevalence of Malignancies Common in Older Patients

The National Cancer Institute suggests that in 2002, there were approximately 10.1 million cancer survivors in the United States, and most (61%) were older than 65 (National Center for Health Statistics, 2002). The median age at the time of diagnosis is 67 years and the median age at death due to malignancy is 73 years (Ries et al., 2007). The leading cancer diagnosis in women living in the United States is breast cancer; for men, it is prostate cancer (American Cancer Society, 2007). According to the SEER data, the median age at diagnosis of colorectal cancer is 71; of lung cancer, the median age at diagnosis is 69; of breast cancer, the median age is 61; of prostate cancer, the median age is 68; and of bladder cancer, the median age is 73 (Ries et al., 2007). The leading cause of cancer-related death in the United States is from lung and bronchus malignancy (American Cancer Society, 2007).

Assessment of the Older Cancer Patient

A person aged 70 and older has, on average, 5.6 diagnoses (Fried et al., 2001 [Level II]). Common nonmalignant co-morbidities in the United States are hypertension, osteoarthritis, and coronary heart disease (National Center for Health Statistics, 2002 [Level I]). A diagnosis of cancer may be only one of several co-morbidities and it is important to understand how the malignant and nonmalignant conditions affect an older adult's health. An acute health crisis may be the result of the culmination of several co-morbidities interacting with the cancer diagnosis and treatment (Reiner & Lacasse, 2006 [Level II]). Older adults with cancer, those with multiple co-morbidities, and those who are hospitalized more than 120 days are more likely to die in the hospital (Kozyrskyi, Black, Chateau, & Steinbach, 2005[Level II]). It is therefore vital to conduct an assessment that considers multiple diagnoses as well as the emotional and social components of daily living in the acute care setting. Nurses are in a primary role to gather the panorama of health care information with the intention of providing a basis of quality care (Overcash, 2004a [Level IV]; Overcash, 2004b [Level III]; Sinding, Wiernikowski, & Aronson, 2005 [Level II]).

Caring for an older adult is complicated due in part to factors such as health care access and insurance concerns that may impede adequate medical and nursing attention. Further, an older adult who lives alone is less likely to receive adequate health care (Goodwin, Hunt, Key, & Samet, 1987 [Level IV]). Conversely, older men who are married tend to have better cancer survival outcomes (Goodwin et al., 1987 [Level IV]; Vercelli et al., 2006 [Level II]. Understanding access to regular health care and caregivers will help the construction of realistic discharge plans (Bindman, Chattopadhyay, Osmond, Huen, & Bacchetti, 2005 [Level III]).

Caregiver coping strategies are important to understand in order to provide the necessary support in an effort to enhance the quality of life of the patient/family/caregiver triad (McMillan et al., 2006 [Level II]). Caregivers report the most stress with managing medications, recognizing significant signs and symptoms, and maintaining a level of pain control for the patient (Haley, 2003 [Level III]). Receiving adequate information in the management of an older person with cancer has been found to be considered very important to caregivers (Hudson, 2006 [Level III]); however, despite the evidence, many caregivers report a lack of sufficient support and education (Akechi et al., 2006 [Level III]). Integrating the caregiver, support person, and/or spouse into the patient assessment may reveal limitations that occur in the home and impact health care. Understanding such limitations that occur outside the hospital is critical in developing a reasonable discharge plan and reducing the incidence of return emergency room visits after discharge home (Guttman et al., 2004 [Level III]).

Geriatric syndromes are health problems that are multifaceted and can be caused by several synergistic factors (Flood et al., 2006 [Level III]). Examples of geriatric syndromes are incontinence, pain, dementia falls, and weight loss. Acute care nurses must consider the presence of geriatric syndromes on assessment to reduce the opportunity of harmful complications caused by cancer and cancer treatment (Naeim & Reuben, 2001 [Level V]).

Due to the complexity of care in an older cancer patient, it is essential to conduct a complete assessment. The comprehensive geriatric assessment (CGA) can be helpful in identifying many of the actual and potential health concerns that may affect the health of an older person (Balducci & Yates, 2000 [Level IV]). The premise for conducting a CGA in an older cancer patient is to cast a wide assessment net around issues that contribute to the spectrum of health in order to determine actual and potential limitations and to develop reasonable intervention strategies.

Comprehensive Geriatric Assessment (CGA)

A CGA is an assessment designed to consider physical, emotional, functional, and social elements that comprise health and quality of life of older patients (Pfeiffer, 1991 [Level IV]; Rubenstein, Siu, & Wieland, 1989 [Level IV]). A CGA for an older person with cancer is particularly important in the detection of limitations that can potentially go unnoticed until signs and symptoms become magnified and cause alteration in independence or interfere with daily living (Burns, Nichols, Martindale-Adams, & Graney, 2000 [Level II]; Extermann et al., 1998 [Level IV]). Be careful and do not assume that an older adult who appears independent is without limitations (Extermann et al., 1998 [Level IV]). A 76-year-old woman may look healthy and active; however, upon screening with a CGA, signs of dementia, potential for falls, and/or other limitations may be found. A CGA early in the hospital admission and after discharge home has been found to be important in the care, and often survival, of an older person (Sinoff, Clarfield, Bergman, & Beaudet, 1998 [Level III]).

No one definition of a CGA exists. A CGA can be developed to include screening instruments necessary to meet the needs of a particular older-patient population. The instruments that commonly comprise the CGA and that guide screening practices in many health care domains are all found on www.ConsultGeriRN.org and other chapters in this text. Whereas a CGA may be more relevant to primary-care settings, understanding such issues as medication history and polypharmancy, caregiver situation, and emotional condition is also important to an acute assessment.

Prescreening older cancer patients to target those who would be most likely to benefit from the entire CGA may be helpful to acute care nurses (Applebaum & Wilson, 1987 [Level IV]). The CGA often requires a reasonable length of time to administer and acute care nurses are often limited by time constraints. The abbreviated comprehensive geriatric assessment (aCGA) can be used to target older cancer patients in need of further screening with the more time-consuming CGA (Extermann et al., 1998 [Level IV]). The aCGA is not used in lieu of the full CGA but rather is intended to save clinician time by identifying patients who need more in-depth screening (Overcash, Beckstead, Moody, Extermann, & Cobb, 2006 [Level II]).

The following instruments can identify functional, physical, emotional, and medication history as well as cognitive impairment in acute care patients and are generally included in a CGA (see related chapters):

A. Assess for emotional distress.
   1. The Geriatric Depression Scale (Yesavage et al., 1982 [Level II]).
   2. The SF-12 Tool (Ware, Kosinski, & Keller, 1996 [Level II]). The SF-12 is a general health-related quality-of-life instrument widely used in research and clinical assessment. Two summary scores are the culmination of the measures from the mental health aspect and the physical health domain. The SF-12 is simple to administer and provides the clinician with a measure of emotional and physical health.
B. Assessment for cognitive limitations.
   1. Mini-Mental State Exam (MMSE) (Folstein, Folstein, & McHugh, 1983 [Level II]).
C. Assess the number and indications of medications. Look for medications with the same indications and potential harmful interactions, and consider any difficulty with cancer-treatment agents. For more information on polypharmacy screening, visit www.ConsultGeriRN.org and select "Try This: The Beers Medication Screen, Criteria for Potentially Inappropriate Medication Use in the Elderly").
D. Assess for geriatric syndromes such as urinary incontinence, falls, or depression (for more information, visit www.HarfordIGN.org and select "Try This: "Urinary Incontinence Assessment, Fall Risk Assessment, or The Geriatric Depression Scale").
E. Assess prior fall history (American Geriatrics Society, 2001 [Level VI]).
   1. If a patient has fallen in the last year, then further screening is recommended.
      a. The Physical Performance Test Battery (Simmonds, 2002 [Level II]) has age-related norms and is a valid and reliable tool used with cancer patients.
      b. The 6-Minute Walk assesses the speed and ability to ambulate for the entire time (Enright et al., 2003 [Level II]).

    c. The timed Get Up & Go Test includes rising from a chair, walking 3 meters, and returning to the chair in a sitting position (Podsiadlo & Richardson, 1991 [Level II]).

    d. Assessment of physical status can take place on observation of gait (Tinetti, 1986 [Level II]) using the Gait Assessment Scale (Tinetti, Mendes de Leon, Doucette, & Baker, 1994 [Level II]).

F. Assess the ability to perform self-care activities.

  1. Activities of Daily Living Scale (Katz, Downs, Cash, & Grotz, 1970 [Level II])

  2. Instrumental Activities of Daily Living Scale (Lawton & Brody, 1969 [Level II])

Health History

The subjective information obtained from an older adult is a critical factor in the development of the plan of care. Respect and confidence are not only prudent but also standard practice for acute care nurses and can set the stage for a productive health centered dialogue. Nurses should assess the reason(s) for seeking care (i.e., chief complaint) and include the family and support person(s). The following issues should be considered when conducting a health history of an older adult with cancer:

A. Assess history of present illness in regard to cancer diagnosis, cancer stage at diagnosis, cancer stage currently, and cancer treatment (i.e., surgical, chemotherapy, radiation therapy, hormonal therapy).

B. Assess past medical history as related to a diagnosis of cancer (include dates of diagnosis and treatments and regular oncological assessment continue).

C. Assess family medical history of malignancy and ages on diagnosis (i.e., some families have strong familial histories of malignancy and younger generations should consider genetic counseling).

D. Assess regular cancer-screening examinations.

E. Assess for common geriatric syndromes (i.e., issues such as incontinence or falls).

Physical Examination

Conducting a physical examination of an older adult must orchestrate an understanding of normative aging changes and knowledge of likely pathology. The physical examination is also an opportunity to teach about the importance of self examination (i.e., breast and skin exams) and provides relevant health information. When older adults perceive the physical examination as informative and understandable, they are more likely to be more satisfied with their health care encounter (Foxall, Barron, & Houfek, 2003 [Level II]).

Physical examination provides objective information to nurses that is synergistic to self report measures. Self report measures are instruments such as the Instrumental Activities of Daily Living (IADLs) assessment (Lawton & Brody, 1969 [Level II]) and Activities of Daily Living (ADLs) (Katz et al., 1970 [Level II]), which focus on tasks vital to independent living. It has been shown that self-report instruments tend to over-estimate abilities (Kuriansky, Gurland, & Fleiss, 1976 [Level IV]; Naeim & Reuben, 2001 [Level V]) and objective assessments (e.g., observing gait or balance) may produce more realistic data.

Functional status, and not chronological age, is an important indicator of cancer treatment tolerance (Balducci & Yates, 2000 [Level IV]; Garman & Cohen, 2002 [Level III]). Changes in functional status may help determine cancer-treatment tolerance or disease progression (Chen et al., 2003 [Level II]; Given, Given, Azzouz, & Stommel, 2001 [Level II]; Reiner & Lacasse, 2006 [Level II]). Assessment of physical function and recognition of patients with physical deficiency can also identify those patients who have an increased risk of hospitalization (Wyrwich & Wolinsky, 2000 [Level III]). It is important to conduct a functional assessment at regular intervals while the patient is receiving acute care to look at trends throughout the cancer-treatment process. Patients may show functional compromise during periods following cancer therapy and become more functionally apt when not receiving treatment.

Physical examination and functional-status assessment can help reveal a clinical presentation of frailty. Fried et al. (2001 [Level II]) suggest that *frail* in part can be defined as follows:

- older than age 85
- dependent in one or more ADLs
- the presence of one or more geriatric syndromes

Older adults who are considered frail are more likely to receive palliative cancer treatment as compared to those not considered frail and who receive curative therapy (Balducci & Yates, 2000 [Level IV]).

A complete head-to-toe assessment including the general elements of a subjective and objective physical exam, accompanied with the CGA assessment instruments and performance evaluations, provides the infrastructure to develop a reasonable treatment plan. Assessment of an older adult with cancer is a vital, dynamic component of care for the interdisciplinary health care team.

Medical Emergencies Associated With Cancer and Cancer Treatment

A diagnosis of cancer can lead to medical emergencies such as electrolyte imbalances, unstable fractures, and neutropenia (i.e., low white cell counts) leading to infection. It is important to obtain cancer-related history and physical information concerning the type of treatment and the exact diagnosis with metastasis (i.e., spread of the malignancy from the original site). It is also important for acute care nurses to know the cycle of chemotherapy administration for a particular patient. Chemotherapy such as doxorubicin and cyclophamide often are given 4 times, 3 weeks apart. As the chemotherapy proceeds, various issues such as nausea and vomiting, neutropenia, and mouth sores may occur and be present upon acute evaluation. The following are considered oncological emergencies and require acute care.

Hypercalcemia

Hypercalcemia is a reasonably common complication associated with multiple myeloma, breast, and lung cancers. The most common cause of hypercalcemia is malignancy (Fisken, Heath, Somers, & Bold, 1981 [Level IV]) and generally found in 3% to 5% of emergency admission patients (Lee et al., 2006 [Level II]). Nonmalignant causes are hyperparathyroidism and renal failure. When hyperthyroidism is associated with hyperparathyroidism and malignancy, survival is much greater as compared to hypercalcemia due to malignancy alone (Hutchesson, Bundred, & Ratcliffe, 1995 [Level III]). It is important to measure parathyroid hormones in patients with hypercalcemia in order to predict time of survival (Hutchesson et al., 1995 [Level III]).

Hypercalcemia is defined as calcium concentration of greater than 10.2 mg/dL (Lee et al., 2006 [Level II]). Signs and symptoms of hypercalcemia are often not evident in patients with mild or moderate hypercalcemia (i.e., calcium levels of 10.3 to 14.0 mg/dL). Gastrointestinal discomfort, changes in level of consciousness, and general nonspecific discomfort can be experienced in cases of moderate hypercalcemia. Other signs and symptoms are lethargy, confusion, anorexia, nausea, constipation, polyuria, and polydipsia (Halfdanarson, Hogan, & Moynihan, 2006 [Level II]).

Treatment of hypercalcemia depends on the severity. Thiazide diuretics should be discontinued. Hydration must be maintained to diminish risk of exacerbation of hypercalcemia (Bushinsky & Monk, 1998 [Level V]). Severe hypercalcemia should be considered a medical emergency. Intravenous normal saline and loop diuretics should be implemented but will only last as long as the treatments are infusing. Bisphosphonates can help reduce bone reabsorption resulting in reduced serum calcium levels (Budayr, Nissenson, & Klien, 1989 [Level I]). Calcitonin also can be administered subcutaneously or intramuscularly and can also reduce calcium levels (Halfdanarson et al., 2006 [Level II]).

Tumor Lysis Syndrome

Tumor Lysis Syndrome (TLS) is caused when a tumor breaks down and "intercellular ions, nucleic acids, proteins and their metabolites" release into the extracellular space (Del Toro, Morris, & Cairo, 2005, p. 3 [Level IV]). The syndrome develops when chemotherapy or radiation therapy causes hyperkalemia, hyperuricemia, and hyperphosphatemia, which can increase the risk for renal failure and reduced cardiac function (Cantril & Haylock, 2004 [Level V]). As chemotherapy agents become more effective, the risks increase for TLS. Agents including "cisplatin, etoposide, flurarabine, intrathecal methotrexate, paclitaxel, rituximab, radiation therapy, interferon alpha, corticosteroids and tamoxifen" can cause TLS (Davidson et al., 2004, p. 546 [Level IV]; Lin, Lucas, & Byrd, 2003 [Level II]).

Hyperphosphatemia and hypocalcemia can occur about 24 to 48 hours following the first chemotherapy administration. Signs and symptoms such as muscle cramps, anxiety, depression, confusion, hallucinations, cardiac arrhythmia, and seizures can result (Cantril & Haylock, 2004 [Level V]). Untreated TLS can lead to renal failure (Davidson et al., 2004 [Level IV]).

Hyperkalaemia is created by a release of potassium from the debilitation of the tumor cells. High serum potassium levels can cause severe arrhythmias and sudden death (Cairo & Bishop, 2004 [Level IV]).

Hyperuricemia (i.e., uric acid >10 mg/dl) can result in acute obstruction uropathy and cause hematuria, flank pain, hypertension, edema, lethargy, and restlessness (Cairo & Bishop, 2004 [Level IV]; Cantril & Haylock, 2004 [Level V]). Hydration, administration of allupurinol, and diuresis generally comprise the first-line treatment (Cantril & Haylock, 2004 [Level V]). Treatment with rasburicase has been found to be effective in the treatment and prevention of hyperuricemia and TLS (Annemans et al., 2003 [Level I]).

The signs and symptoms associated with TLS include decreased urine output, seizures, and arrhythmias. Electrolytes must be assessed to determine the presence of hyperkalemia, hyperuricemia, and hyperphosphatemia. Electrocardiograms should be obtained to assess arrhythmia.

Spinal Cord Compression

Spinal cord compression is not uncommon and can occur when metastasis spreads to the vertebral bodies and invades the spinal cord. The spinal column in the thoracic area is the most common location and must be recognized immediately to prevent critical, irreversible damage (Halfdanarson et al., 2006 [Level II]). Spinal cord compression can lead to paraplegia and long-term neurological deficits (Hirschfeld, Beutler, Seigle, & Manz, 1988 [Level IV]).

Signs and symptoms are numbness and tingling in the extremities and upper thorax and back pain (Lowey, 2006 [Level IV]). Pain can radiate or localize and may seem chronic, which may disguise the emergent spinal cord compression and delay critical treatment. Bowel and bladder dysfunction can also result.

Diagnosis is often made with magnetic resonance imaging (MRI), computed tomography (CT), and sometimes plain radiographic films of the affected area. Treatment is often initiated with glucocortocoids followed by radiation therapy and/or surgery. Surgery has been debated, but many agree it is reasonable in conjunction with radiation therapy and sometimes chemotherapy (McLain & Bell, 1998 [Level IV]; Schmidt, Klimo, & Vrionis, 2005 [Level IV]). Nurses have the ability to recognize the signs and symptoms of this debilitating and often lethal oncological emergency (Bucholtz, 1999 [Level II]).

Neutropenic Fever

Neutropenic fever is an oncological medical emergency caused by the diminishment of neutrophils by various chemotherapeutic agents. Neutropenia is considered present when the neutrophil count is less than 1.0×10^9/L; severe neutropenia is neutrophil counts less than 0.5×10^9/L (Halfdanarson et al., 2006 [Level II]).

Generally fever is the presenting sign; however, skin rashes and mucositis may also be present. For some patients, neutropenic fever can occur after the first cycle of chemotherapy; patients who have undergone aggressive surgery with bowel resections are at increased risk (Sharma, Rezai, Driscoll, Odunsi, & Lele, 2006 [Level II]).

An instrument has been developed to help screen for the likelihood of neutropenia and the identification of patients who are likely to benefit from prophylaxis granulocyte-colony–stimulating factors (G-CSFs) (Donohue, 2006[Level III]). G-CSF works to elevate white blood cell counts necessary in fighting infection. A great amount of nursing literature exists on the definition, prevention, and management of neutropenic fever. Prevention of neutropenia and neutropenic fever should be proactive in the administration of G-CSFs in patients who are considered at high risk for neutropenia (Krol et al., 2006 [Level IV]). An older cancer patient receiving myelotoxic chemotherapy (i.e., cyclophosphamide, doxorubicin, vincristine, and prednisolone) is considered high risk and should receive prophylactic G-CSF administration (Repetto et al., 2003 [Level I]).

Case Study and Discussion

A 76-year-old White woman presents to the emergency department with delirium and trauma to her left hip. The patient's daughter reports that the patient fell in the bathroom several hours earlier. She has a diagnosis of breast cancer and is currently undergoing chemotherapy and has received four cycles of Adriamycian and Cyclophospimide. She also has a history of osteoarthritis, hypertension, and gastric reflux disease. Presenting signs and symptoms are delirium, cracked mucus membranes, low B/P at 88/42, and tachycardia.

Situations such as dehydration are not uncommon in an older person undergoing chemotherapy. Patients may have vomiting or diarrhea and become dehydrated as a result. Seniors have less functional reserve and are therefore more likely to suffer from complications of cancer treatment (Balducci, 2006 [Level V]). Older adults require careful examination and intervention in order to maintain and enhance health and independence.

1. In this clinical scenario, which geriatric syndromes are present?
   Answer: Falls, delirium, pain associated with trauma, functional-status limitations, and ambulatory difficulty.
   Rationale: This patient has multiple geriatric syndromes and is at risk for further deconditioning. It is important to recognize the geriatric syndromes present and anticipate any additional injuries. Ensure caregiver support and help facilitate a plan for care while at home.
2. In this clinical scenario, which oncological emergency is this patient at greatest risk to develop?
   Rationale: Based on the signs and symptoms of dehydration, hypercalcemia is of concern. Hydrate to prevent hypercalcemia and to reduce signs and symptoms of dementia. Falls are also of concern because the risk of future falls is associated with prior falls. Dehydration in an older adult cancer patient can be associated with many problematic health and functional limitations.

Conclusion

Acute care of an older patient requires nurses' health assessment skills to be proactive in detecting and addressing limitations that can result from a cancer diagnosis and treatment. Nonmalignant co-morbidities and geriatric syndromes play a role in the diagnosis and treatment of cancer and should be assimilated into the critical thinking involved in developing the nursing plan of care. Careful health assessment and evaluation are critical to acute care nurses in understanding the disease progress, treatment tolerance, and presence of oncological emergencies. Nurses working in acute settings must be acquainted with principles of geriatric care that should be applied to patients with any type of diagnosis and not limited to malignancy. Understanding normative aging changes versus pathology can help facilitate a specialized plan of care with enhanced health and independence as the intended patient outcomes.

Resources

The National Comprehensive Cancer Network offers Clinical Practice Guidelines, including Senior Adult Oncology. http://www.nccn.org/professionals/physician'gls/default.asp

The American Geriatrics Society offers clinical guidelines in using the CGA in the older person. http://www.americangeriatrics.org

The Oncology Nursing Society offers recommendations for practice of the oncology patient. www.ons.org

References

Akechi, T., Akizuki, N., Okamura, M., Shimizu, K., Oba, A., Ito, T., et al. (2006). Psychological distress experienced by families of cancer patients: Preliminary findings from psychiatric consultation of a cancer center hospital. *Japanese Journal of Clinical Oncology*, *36*(5), 329–332. Evidence Level III: Quasi-experimental Study.

American Cancer Society (2007). *Cancer facts & figures 2007*. Atlanta: American Cancer Society. Retrieved May 4, 2007, from. http://www.cancer.org/downloads/STT/CAFF2007PWSecured.pdf.

American Geriatrics Society, British Geriatric Society, & American Academy of Orthopaedic Surgeons Panel on Falls Prevention (2001). Guideline for the prevention of falls in older persons. *Journal of the American Geriatrics Society*, *49*(5), 664–672. Evidence Level VI: Expert Opinion.

Annemans, L., Moeremans, K., Lamotte, M., Garcia Conde, J., Van Den Berg, H., Myint, H., et al. (2003). Pan-European multicentre economic evaluation of recombinant urate oxidase (rasburicase) in prevention and treatment of hyperuricaemia and tumour lysis syndrome in haematological cancer patients. *Support Care Cancer*, *11*(4), 249–257. Evidence Level I: Systematic Review.

Applebaum, R. A., & Wilson, N. L. (1987). Prescreening at-risk elders for entry into a community-based long term care program. *Home Health Care Services Quarterly*, *8*(1), 75–86. Evidence Level IV: Nonexperimental Study.

Balducci, L. (2006). Management of cancer in the elderly. *Oncology (Williston Park)*, *20*(2), 135–143; discussion 144, 146, 151–132. Level V: Literature Review.

Balducci, L., & Yates, J. (2000). General guidelines for the management of older patients with cancer. *Oncology (Williston Park)*, *14*(11A), 221–227. Evidence Level IV: Nonexperimental Study.

Bindman, A. B., Chattopadhyay, A., Osmond, D. H., Huen, W., & Bacchetti, P. (2005). The impact of Medicaid managed care on hospitalizations for ambulatory care sensitive conditions. *Health Services Research, 40*(1), 19–38. Evidence Level III: Quasi-experimental Study.

Bucholtz, J. D. (1999). Metastatic epidural spinal cord compression. *Seminars in Oncology Nursing, 15*(3), 150–159. Evidence Level II: Single Experimental Study.

Budayr, A. A., Nissenson, R. A., & Klien, R. F. (1989). Increased serum levels of a parathyroid-like protein malignancy-associated hypercalcemia. *Annals of Internal Medicine, 111,* 807–812. Evidence Level I: Systematic Review.

Burns, R., Nichols, L. O., Martindale-Adams, J., & Graney, M. J. (2000). Interdisciplinary geriatric primary care evaluation and management: Two-year outcomes. *Journal of the American Geriatrics Society, 48,* 8–13. Evidence Level II: Single Experimental Study.

Bushinsky, D. A., & Monk, R. D. (1998). Calcium: Electrolyte quintet. *Lancet, 352*(9124), 306–311. Evidence Level V: Literature Review.

Cairo, M. S., & Bishop, M. (2004). Tumour lysis syndrome: New therapeutic strategies and classification. *British Journal of Haematology, 127*(1), 3–11. Evidence Level IV: Nonexperimental Study.

Cantril, C. A., & Haylock, P. J. (2004). Emergency: Tumor lysis syndrome. *American Journal of Nursing, 104*(4), 49–52; quiz 52–43. Evidence Level V: Review.

Chen, H., Cantor, A., Meyer, J., Corcoran, M. B., Grendys, E., Cavanaugh, D., et al. (2003). Can older cancer patients tolerate chemotherapy? A prospective pilot study. *Cancer, 97*(4), 1107–1114. Evidence Level II: Single Experimental Study.

Davidson, M. B., Thakkar, S., Hix, J. K., Bhandarkar, N. D., Wong, A., & Schreiber, M. J. (2004). Pathophysiology, clinical consequences, and treatment of tumor lysis syndrome. *American Journal of Medicine, 116*(8), 546–554. Evidence Level IV: Nonexperimental Study.

Del Toro, G., Morris, E., & Cairo, M. S. (2005). Tumor lysis syndrome: Pathophysiology, definition, and alternative treatment approaches. *Clinical Advances in Hematology and Oncology, 3*(1), 54–61. Evidence Level IV: Nonexperimental Study.

Donohue, R. (2006). Development and implementation of a risk assessment tool for chemotherapy-induced neutropenia. *Oncology Nursing Forum, 33*(2), 347–352. Evidence Level III: Quasi-experimental Study.

Enright, P. L., McBurnie, M. A., Bittner, V., Tracy, R. P., McNamara, R., Arnold, A., et al. (2003). The 6-minute walk test: A quick measure of functional status in elderly adults. *Chest, 123*(2), 387–398. Evidence Level II: Single Experimental Study.

Extermann, M., Overcash, J., Lyman, G. H., Parr, J., & Balducci, L. (1998). Co-morbidity and functional status are independent in older cancer patients. *Journal of Clinical Oncology, 16*(4), 1582–1587. Evidence Level IV: Nonexperimental Study.

Fisken, R. A., Heath, D. A., Somers, S., & Bold, A. M. (1981). Hypercalcaemia in hospital patients. Clinical and diagnostic aspects. *Lancet, 1*(8213), 202–207. Evidence Level IV: Nonexperimental Study.

Flood, K. L., Carroll, M. B., Le, C. V., Ball, L., Esker, D. A., & Carr, D. B. (2006). Geriatric syndromes in elderly patients admitted to an oncology-acute care for elders unit. *Journal of Clinical Oncology, 24*(15), 2298–2303. Evidence Level III: Quasi-experimental Study.

Folstein, M., Folstein, S., & McHugh, P. (1983). Mini-mental state: A practical method for grading the cognitive state of patient for the clinic. *Journal of Psychiatric Research, 12,* 189–198. Evidence Level II: Single Experimental Study.

Foxall, M. J., Barron, C. R., & Houfek, J. (2003). Women's satisfaction with breast and gynecological cancer screening. *Women Health, 38*(1), 21–36. Evidence Level II: Single Experimental Study.

Fried, L. P., Tangen, C. M., Walston, J., Newman, A. B., Hirsch, C., Gottdiener, J., et al. (2001). Frailty in older adults: Evidence for a phenotype. *Journals of Gerontology Series A: Biological Sciences and Medical Sciences, 56*(3), M146–M156. Evidence Level II: Single Experimental Study.

Garman, K. S., & Cohen, H. J. (2002). Functional status and the elderly cancer patient. *Critical Reviews in Oncology/Hematology, 43*(3), 191–208. Evidence Level III: Quasi-experimental Study.

Given, B., Given, C., Azzouz, F., & Stommel, M. (2001). Physical functioning of elderly cancer patients prior to diagnosis and following initial treatment. *Nursing Research, 50*(4), 222–232. Evidence Level II: Single Experimental Study.

Goodwin, J. S., Hunt, W. C., Key, C. R., & Samet, J. M. (1987). The effect of marital status on stage, treatment, and survival of cancer patients. *Journal of the American Medical Association, 258*(21), 3125–3130. Evidence Level IV: Nonexperimental Study.

Guttman, A., Afilalo, M., Guttman, R., Colacone, A., Robitaille, C., Lang, E., et al. (2004). An emergency-department–based nurse discharge coordinator for elder patients: Does it make a difference? *Academic Emergency Medicine, 11*(12), 1318–1327. Evidence Level III: Quasi-experimental Study.

Haley, W. E. (2003). Family caregivers of elderly patients with cancer: Understanding and minimizing the burden of care. *Journal of Supportive Oncology, 1*(4 Suppl. 2), 25–29. Evidence Level III: Quasi-experimental Study.

Halfdanarson, T. R., Hogan, W. J., & Moynihan, T. J. (2006). Oncologic emergencies: Diagnosis and treatment. *Mayo Clinic Proceedings, 81*(6), 835–848. Evidence Level II: Single Experimental Study.

Hirschfeld, A., Beutler, W., Seigle, J., & Manz, H. (1988). Spinal epidural compression secondary to osteoblastic metastatic vertebral expansion. *Neurosurgery, 23*(5), 662–665. Evidence Level IV: Nonexperimental Study.

Hudson, P. L. (2006). How well do family caregivers cope after caring for a relative with advanced disease and how can health professionals enhance their support? *Journal of Palliative Medicine, 9*(3), 694–703. Evidence Level III: Quasi-experimental Study.

Hutchesson, A. C., Bundred, N. J., & Ratcliffe, W. A. (1995). Survival in hypercalcaemic patients with cancer and coexisting primary hyperparathyroidism. *Postgraduate Medical Journal, 71*(831), 28–31. Evidence Level III: Quasi-experimental Study.

Katz, S., Downs, T. D., Cash, H. R., & Grotz, R. C. (1970). Progress in development of the index of ADL. *Gerontologist, 10*(1), 20–30. Evidence Level II: Single Experimental Study.

Kozyrskyi, A. L., Black, C., Chateau, D., & Steinbach, C. (2005). Discharge outcomes in seniors hospitalized for more than 30 days. *Canadian Journal on Aging, 24*(Suppl. 1), 107–119. Evidence Level II: Single Experimental Study.

Krol, J., Paepke, S., Jacobs, V. R., Paepke, D., Euler, U., Kiechle, M., et al. (2006). G-CSF in the prevention of febrile neutropenia in chemotherapy in breast cancer patients. *Onkologie, 29*(4), 171–178. Evidence Level IV: Nonexperimental Study.

Kuriansky, J. B., Gurland, B. J., & Fleiss, J. L. (1976). The assessment of self-care capacity in geriatric psychiatric patients by objective and subjective methods. *Journal of Clinical Psychology, 32*(1), 95–102. Evidence Level IV: Nonexperimental Study.

Lawton, M. P., & Brody, E. M. (1969). Assessment of older people: Self-maintaining and instrumental activities of daily living. *Gerontologist, 9*(3), 179–186. Evidence Level II: Single Experimental Study.

Lee, C. T., Yang, C. C., Lam, K. K., Kung, C. T., Tsai, C. J., & Chen, H. C. (2006). Hypercalcemia in the emergency department. *American Journal of the Medical Sciences, 331*(3), 119–123. Evidence Level II: Single Experimental Study.

Lin, T. S., Lucas, M. S., & Byrd, J. C. (2003). Rituximab in B-cell chronic lymphocytic leukemia. *Seminars in Oncology, 30*(4), 483–492. Evidence Level II: Single Experimental Study.

Lowey, S. E. (2006). Spinal cord compression: An oncologic emergency associated with metastatic cancer: Evaluation and management for the home health clinician. *Home Healthcare Nurse, 24*(7), 439–446; quiz 447–438. Evidence Level IV: Nonexperimental Study.

McLain, R. F., & Bell, G. R. (1998). Newer management options in patients with spinal metastasis. *Cleveland Clinic Journal of Medicine, 65*(7), 359–356. Evidence Level IV: Nonexperimental Study.

McMillan, S. C., Small, B. J., Weitzner, M., Schonwetter, R., Tittle, M., Moody, L., et al. (2006). Impact of coping skills intervention with family caregivers of hospice patients with cancer: A randomized clinical trial. *Cancer, 106*(1), 214–222. Evidence Level II: Single Experimental Study.

Naeim, A., & Reuben, D. (2001). Geriatric syndromes and assessment in older cancer patients. *Oncology (Williston Park), 15*(12), 1567–1577, 1580; discussion 1581, 1586, 1591. Evidence Level V: Literature Review.

National Center for Health Statistics. (2002). Leading causes of health for all males and females in the United States. *Centers for Disease Control.* Evidence Level I: Systematic Review.

National Center for Health Statistics. (2006). Trends in Health and Aging. *US Department of Health and Human Services Centers for Disease Control and Prevention.*

Overcash, J. A. (2004a). Narrative research: A viable methodology for clinical nursing. *Nursing Forum, 39*(1), 15–22. Evidence Level IV: Nonexperimental Study.

Overcash, J. A. (2004b). Using narrative research to understand the quality of life of older women with breast cancer. *Oncology Nursing Forum, 31*(6), 1153–1159. Evidence Level III: Quasi-experimental Study.

Overcash, J. A., Beckstead, J., Moody, L., Extermann, M., & Cobb, S. (2006). The Abbreviated Comprehensive Geriatric Assessment (aCGA) for use in the older cancer patient as a prescreen: Scoring and interpretation. *Critical Reviews in Oncology/Hematology, 59*(3), 205–210. Evidence Level II: Single Experimental Study.

Pfeiffer, E. (1991). Comprehensive geriatric assessment. *Southern Medical Journal, 84*(5 Suppl. 1), S6–S10. Evidence Level IV: Nonexperimental Study.

Podsiadlo, D., & Richardson, S. (1991). The timed "Get Up & Go": A test of basic functional mobility for frail elderly persons. *Journal of the American Geriatrics Society, 39*(2), 142–148. Evidence Level II: Single Experimental Study.

Reiner, A., & Lacasse, C. (2006). Symptom correlates in the gero-oncology population. *Seminars in Oncology Nursing, 22*(1), 20–30. Evidence Level II: Single Experimental Study.

Repetto, L., Biganzoli, L., Koehne, C. H., Luebbe, A. S., Soubeyran, P., Tjan-Heijnen, V. C., et al. (2003). EORTC cancer in the Elderly Task Force guidelines for the use of colony-stimulating factors in elderly patients with cancer. *European Journal of Cancer, 39*(16), 2264–2272. Evidence Level I: Systematic Review.

Ries, L. A. G., Melbert, D., Krapcho, M., Mariotto, A., Miller, B. A., Feuer E. J., et al. (Eds). SEER Cancer Statistics Review, 1975–2004, National Cancer Institute. Bethesda, MD. Retreived May 4, 2007, from http://seer.cancer.gov/csr/1975_2004/, based on November 2006SEER data submission, posted to the SEER Web site, 2007.

Rubenstein, L. Z., Siu, A. L., & Wieland, D. (1989). Comprehensive geriatric assessment: Toward understanding its efficacy. *Aging (Milano), 1*(2), 87–98. Evidence Level IV: Nonexperimental Study.

Schmidt, M. H., Klimo, P., Jr., & Vrionis, F. D. (2005). Metastatic spinal cord compression. *Journal of the National Comprehensive Cancer Network, 3*(5), 711–719. Evidence Level IV: Nonexperimental Study.

Sharma, S., Rezai, K., Driscoll, D., Odunsi, K., & Lele, S. (2006). Characterization of neutropenic fever in patients receiving first-line adjuvant chemotherapy for epithelial ovarian cancer. *Gynecologic Oncology, 103*(1), 181–185. Evidence Level II: Single Experimental Study.

Simmonds, M. J. (2002). Physical function in patients with cancer: Psychometric characteristics and clinical usefulness of a physical performance test battery. *Journal of Pain and Symptom Management, 24*(4), 404–414. Evidence Level II: Single Experimental Study.

Sinding, C., Wiernikowski, J., & Aronson, J. (2005). Cancer care from the perspectives of older women. *Oncology Nursing Forum, 32*(6), 1169–1175. Evidence Level II: Single Experimental Study.

Sinoff, G., Clarfield, A. M., Bergman, H., & Beaudet, M. (1998). A two-year follow-up of geriatric consults in the emergency department. *Journal of the American Geriatrics Society, 46*(6), 716–720. Evidence Level III: Quasi-experimental Study.

Tinetti, M. E. (1986). Performance-oriented assessment of mobility problems in elderly patients. *Journal of the American Geriatrics Society, 34*(2), 119–126. Evidence Level II: Single Experimental Study.

Tinetti, M. E., Mendes de Leon, C. F., Doucette, J. T., & Baker, D. I. (1994). Fear of falling and fall-related efficacy in relationship to functioning among community-living elders. *Journals of Gerontology, 49*(3), M140–M147. Evidence Level II: Single Experimental Study.

Vercelli, M., Lillini, R., Capocaccia, R., Micheli, A., Coebergh, J. W., Quinn, M., et al. (2006). Cancer survival in the elderly: Effects of socio-economic factors and health care system features (ELDCARE project). *European Journal of Cancer, 42*(2), 234–242. Evidence Level II: Single Experimental Study.

Ware, J., Jr., Kosinski, M., & Keller, S. D. (1996). A 12-item short-form health survey: Construction of scales and preliminary tests of reliability and validity. *Medical Care, 34*(3), 220–233. Evidence Level II: Single Experimental Study.

Wyrwich, K. W., & Wolinsky, F. D. (2000). Physical activity, disability, and the risk of hospital-ization for breast cancer among older women. *Journals of Gerontology Series A: Biological Sciences and Medical Sciences, 55*(7), M418–M421. Evidence Level III: Quasi-experimental Study.

Yesavage, J. A., Brink, T. L., Rose, T. L., Lum, O., Huang, V., Adey, M., et al. (1982). Development and validation of a geriatric depression screening scale: A preliminary report. *Journal of Psychiatric Research, 17*(1), 37–49. Evidence Level II: Single Experimental Study.

Issues Regarding Sexuality

28

Jacqueline M. Arena
Meredith Wallace

Educational Objectives

On completion of this chapter, the reader should be able to:

1. describe an older adult's interest in sexuality

2. identify barriers and challenges to sexual health among older adults

3. discuss normal and pathological changes of aging and their influence on sexual health

4. identify interventions that may help older adults achieve sexual health

Overview

Sexuality is an innate quality present in all human beings and is extremely important to an individual's self-identity and general well-being (Wallace, 2003 [Level V]). Sexuality is defined as "a central aspect of being human throughout life and encompasses sex, gender identities and roles, sexual orientation, eroticism, pleasure, intimacy and reproduction" (World Health Organization, 2004 [Level VI]). Sexual health as a manifestation of sexuality is "a state of physical, emotional, mental and social well-being related to sexuality" (World Health Organization, 2004 [Level VI]). Sexual health contributes to the satisfaction of

For a description of Evidence Levels cited in this chapter, see chapter 1, Developing and Evaluating Clinical Practice Guidelines, page 4

physical needs; however, it is often not as apparent that sexual contact fulfills many social, emotional, and psychological components of life as well. This is evidenced by the fact that human touch and a healthy sex life may evoke sentiments of joy, romance, affection, passion, and intimacy, whereas despondency and depression often result from an inability to express one's sexuality (Kamel & Hajjar, 2003 [Level V]). When this occurs, sexual dysfunction, defined as impairment in normal sexual functioning, may result (American Psychiatric Association, 1994 [Level VI]).

It is frequently assumed that sexual desires and the frequency of sexual encounters begin to diminish later in life. Moreover, the notion of older adults engaging in sexual activities has become taboo in today's youth-loving society (Kamel & Hajjar, 2003 [Level V]). Despite this stereotype, sexual identity and the need for intimacy do not disappear with increasing age, and older adults do not morph into celibate, asexual beings. Current research conducted by the AARP (1999 [Level IV]) found that in a study of 1,709 older adults, 38.4% had intercourse once a week or more. A study of 179 residents of subsidized independent-living facilities revealed that the majority had physical and sexual experiences in the past year (Ginsberg, Pomerantz, & Kramer-Feeley, 2005 [Level IV]).

Background and Statement of the Problem

Despite the persistence of sexual patterns throughout the lifespan, there is limited research and information to assist nurses to assess and intervene to promote sexual health among older adults. Lack of research literature and insufficient clinical resources are a product of the lack of societal recognition of sexuality as a continuing human need and a factor that perpetuates lack of sexual assessment and intervention among the older population. In addition to the lack of literature, there are several factors that further impact the sexual health of older adults. Zeiss and Kasl-Godley (2001 [Level V]) stress that although sexuality remains rather central and complex throughout the lifespan, many physical, psychosocial, and environmental changes contribute to decreased sexuality in older adults. Evidence suggests that despite older adults' continued sexual interest and desires, many barriers may prevent them from engaging in fulfilling sexual health. These barriers include the presence of normal and pathological aging changes, environmental barriers to sexual health, and special problems of the elderly that interfere with sexual fulfillment, such as cognitive impairment.

Health Providers' Views Toward Sexuality and Aging

Nurses' hesitancy to discuss sexuality with older adults has a significant impact on the sexual health of this population. Gott, Hincliff, and Galena (2004 [Level IV]) report that general practitioners do not discuss sexual health frequently in providing primary care to older adults. Their study of 55 older men and women resulted in the finding that a major factor affecting sexual discussion between patients and their physicians included the hesitancy of discussing sexuality with a health care provider who was not the patient's age or sex. In this qualitative study, clients stated that sexuality discussions would be more comfortable and forthcoming with health care providers who matched their sex and age. Moreover, attitudes toward sexuality later in life, making jokes about sexuality, shame/embarrassment and fear, perception of sexual problems as not serious, and lack of knowledge regarding available interventions were also seen as barriers to sexual discussion between older clients and health care providers (Gott & Hinchliff, 2003 [Level IV]).

General discomfort with discussing sexuality among nurses and lack of experience in assessment and management of sexual dysfunction among older adults often prevent nurses from addressing the sexual needs of this population. Moreover, the sexuality of older adults is generally excluded from sparse gerontological curricula. Without education and experience in managing sensitive issues around sexuality, health professionals are often not comfortable discussing sexual issues with older adults. Peck (2001 [Level V]) reports that creating a trusting and comfortable environment and increasing familiarity with diverse sexual issues may enhance the assessment of sexual health among older adults.

Nurses' understanding of sexuality should be broadened beyond that of a relationship between just men and women. Many clients within various health care systems are gay or lesbian, bisexual, and transgender (GLBT) adults, and these alternative sexual preferences require respect and consideration. In a focus-group study, older gay and lesbians reported extensive discrimination in accessing health care services by excluding them from program planning (Brotman, Ryan, & Cormier, 2003 [Level IV]). Discrimination among GLBT older adults is especially seen in the development of residential services to meet the needs of older adults. In a qualitative analysis of geriatric health care providers to gay and lesbian older adults, providers demonstrated open attitudes but lacked commitment in planning services to meet the needs of older lesbians (Chamberland, 2003 [Level IV]). In a larger study of 400,000 GLBT adults, discrimination was seen among administrators, care providers, and other residents of a retirement-care community (Johnson, Jackson, Arnette, & Koffman, 2005 [Level IV]).

Normal and Pathological Aging Changes

The "sexual response cycle," or the organized pattern of physical response to sexual stimulation, changes with age in both women and men. After menopause, a loss of estrogen in women results in significant sexual changes. This deficiency frequently results in the thinning of the vaginal walls and decreased or delayed vaginal lubrication, which may lead to pain during intercourse (Harvard Medical School, 2003 [Level VI]). Additionally, the labia atrophy, the vagina shortens, and the cervix may descend downward into the vagina, causing further pain and discomfort. Moreover, vaginal contractions are fewer and weaker during orgasm, and after sexual intercourse is completed, women return to the prearoused stage faster than they would at an earlier age (Harvard Medical School, 2003 [Level VI]). The result of these physiological age-related changes in women is the potential for significant alterations in sexual health that have traditionally received little attention from research or individual health care providers. The pain resulting from anatomical changes and vaginal dryness may result in the avoidance of sexual relationships in order to prevent painful intercourse.

Men also experience decreased hormone levels, mainly testosterone, yet this seems to have a limited impact on sexual functioning due to the fact that only a minimal amount of testosterone is needed for the purposes of sex. This reduction in testosterone, which has been controversially labeled viropause or andropause and male menopause, generally begins between the ages of 46 and 52 and is characterized by a gradual decrease in the amount of testosterone (Kessenich & Cichon, 2001 [Level V]). The loss of testosterone is not pathological and does not result in sexual dysfunction. However, men may experience fatigue, loss of muscle mass, depression, and a decline in libido (Kessenich & Cichon, 2001 [Level V]). As a result of normal aging changes, older men require more direct stimulation of the penis to experience a somewhat weaker erection (Araujo, Mohr, & McKinlay, 2004 [Level IV]). As with postmenopausal women, orgasms are fewer and weaker in older men, the force and amount of ejaculation is reduced, and the refractory period after ejaculation is significantly increased from that of younger men (Araujo et al., 2004 [Level IV]). The Massachusetts male aging study of 1,085 older men indicated that age was identified as an independent risk factor for decreased sexual function in older men (Araujo et al., 2004 [Level IV]).

Bodily changes, such as wrinkles and sagging skin, may cause both older women and men to feel insecure about initiating a sexual encounter and maintaining emotionally secure relationships. In addition, lack of knowledge and understanding among older adults about sexuality is common because sexual education was rarely provided in formal educational systems as the older adults developed and was rarely discussed informally. Strict beliefs and values are likely to impact sexual action, freedom, and desires and may result in sexual frustration and conflict. Physical changes in the sexual response cycle that occur with increasing age do not completely explain the extensive changes in sexuality that occur among older adults. Many individual psychosocial and cultural factors play a role in how older adults perceive themselves as sexual beings. Zeiss and Kasl-Godley (2001 [Level V]) emphasize that liberal and positive attitudes toward sexuality, greater sexual knowledge, satisfaction with intimate relationships, good social lives, general psychological health, and a sense of self-worth and self-efficacy are associated with greater sexual interest, activity, and satisfaction.

Although sexual disorders have not been well addressed among the older population, they have been defined and fall into four categories: hypoactive sexual desire disorder, sexual arousal disorder, orgasmic disorder, and sexual pain disorders (Walsh & Berman, 2004 [Level V]). With improved assessment and diagnosis of these sexual disorders, older adults may benefit from limited research supporting the efficacy of sildenafil citrate for the treatment of some sexual disorders among women, including female sexual arousal disorder (FSAD), and for men with erectile dysfunctions (see nursing care strategies, Box 28.1).

In addition to normal aging changes and pathological sexual disorders, there are a number of medical conditions that have been associated with poor sexual health and functioning in the older population (Morley & Tariq, 2003 [Level V]). Rosen (2006 [Level V]) reports that the main predictors of sexual dysfunction are age, cardiovascular diseases, and diabetes. One of the most frequently occurring medical conditions among older adults is cardiovascular disease. In a study of 2,763 postmenopausal women, the presence of coronary heart disease was associated with lack of interest, inability to relax, arousal and orgasmic disorders, and general discomfort with sex (Addis, Ireland, Vittinghoff, Lin, Stuenkel, & Hulley, 2005 [Level II]). Diabetes is a large problem among older adults, effecting approximately 14.7 million individuals in the United States each year. Approximately 40% of those with diabetes are 65 or older (CDC, 2007 [Level IV]. In a study of eight women aged 24 to 83, older women with diabetes reported lower sexual function, desire, and enjoyment than their younger counterparts (Rockcliffe-Fidler & Kiemle, 2003 [Level IV]). The presence of depression among older adults impacts sexual health, in that depression often causes a decline in desire and ability to perform with this disease and treatment. The presence of loss and depression should be assessed among older adults and considered for the impact of these emotional and psychological factors on sexual health (see chapter 5, *Depression*).

Other medical conditions occurring among older adults also have the potential to impact sexual health. Older adults who have experienced strokes and subsequent aphasias reported alterations in sexual health (Lemieux, Cohen-Schneider, & Holzapfel, 2001 [Level IV]). In this study, difficulties in communication were major contributors to the sexual dysfunction. Parkinson's disease (PD) is predominantly an older-adult disease with the potential for impact on sexual health. In a study of 444 older adults with PD, sexual limitations were reported in 73.5% of the sample as a product of difficulty in movement (Mott, Kenrick, Dixon, & Bird, 2005 [Level IV]). Benign prostatic hypertrophy (BPH) in older men may result in altered circulation to the penis affecting erectile function and sexual arousal. Rosen (2006 [Level V]) reports that in conjunction with other predictors of poor sexual health, BPH further impacts erectile function and may contribute to ejaculatory dysfunction.

Medications used to treat commonly occurring medical illnesses among older adults also impact sexuality. Two of the major groups of medications are antidepressants and antihypertensives. Causative antidepressants include the commonly used selective serotonin reuptake inhibitors (SSRI). Montejo, Llorca, Izquierdo, and Rico-Villademoros (2001 [Level IV]) report in a study of 610 women and 412 men that 59.1% of the individuals taking SSRI antidepressant medications reported sexual dysfunction. Although the use of MAO inhibitors and tricylic antidepressants has decreased in favor of the SSRIs with lower side-effect profiles, these medications also impact sexual function by reducing sexual drive and causing impotence and erectile and orgasmic disorders. Antihypertensives, ACE inhibitors, and alpha and beta cell blockers also result in impotence and ejaculatory disturbances among older adults (Girerd et al., 2003 [Level IV]). Antipsychotics, commonly used statin medications, and H2 blockers also impact the sexual health of older adults.

Special Issues Related to Older Adults and Sexuality

Cognitively impaired older adults continue to have sexual needs and desires (Alagiakrishnan et al., 2005 [Level IV]) that present a challenge to nurses. These continuing sexual needs often manifest in inappropriate sexual behavior. Sexual behaviors common to cognitively impaired older adults may include cuddling, touching of the genitals, sexual remarks, propositioning, grabbing and groping, use of obscene language, masturbating without shame, aggression, and irritability (Nagaratnam & Gayagay, 2002 [Level IV]). In a study by Alagiakrish-nan and colleagues (2005 [Level IV]), of 41 cognitively impaired older adults, 1.8% had sexually inappropriate behavior manifesting in verbal and physical problems. In a study that used computed tomography (CT) of the head to scan 10 patients with these problematic sexual behaviors, cerebral infarction was seen in 6 of them, and severe disease in 2 others, supporting the organic basis for these symptoms (Nagaratnam & Gayagay, 2002 [Level IV]).

Masturbation is a method in which cognitively impaired men and women may become sexually fulfilled. Nurses in long term care facilities may assist older adults to improve sexual health by providing an environment in which an older adult may masturbate in private. Alkhalil and colleagues (2004 [Level V]) report that the use of Gabapentin to decrease sexual behavior problems (e.g., inappropriate sexual overtures and public masturbation) has demonstrated ef-fectiveness anecdotally. Accurate assessment and documentation of the ability of cognitively impaired older adults to make competent decisions regarding sex-ual relationships with others while in long term care is essential. If it has been determined that a resident is incapable of decision making, then the health care staff must prevent the cognitively impaired resident from unsolicited sexual advances by a spouse, partner, or other residents.

Environmental settings may also influence sexuality among older adults. Normally, engaging in sexual intercourse occurs within the privacy of one's bed-room; however, for some older adults, extended-care facilities are the substitute for what one called home. Kamel & Hajjar (2003 [Level V]) are of the opinion that a large proportion of long term care residents are sexually inactive, yet say they would like to be sexually active. These residents state that many of the obstacles they face regarding their sexuality include lack of opportunity, lack of available partner, poor health, feeling sexually undesirable, and guilt for having sexual feelings. Furthermore, negative staff attitudes and beliefs regarding res-idents' sexual activity bar the expression of sexuality in long term care settings (Hajjar & Kamel, 2004 [Level V]).

Of all AIDS cases, 11% are developed in adults older than 50, underscoring the significant risk of HIV transmission in the older age group. Older adults with HIV are more likely to be diagnosed late in the disease, progress more quickly, and have a shorter survival (Goodroad, 2003 [Level V]). Falvo and Nor-man (2004 [Level IV]) conducted a sex education workshop for older adults that supported the acquisition and retention of HIV prevention knowledge 3 months after workshop completion. Goodroad (2003 [Level V]) states that nurses are in a unique position to assess and manage HIV among the older population, but greater education regarding the risk for HIV in the older population is needed.

Assessment

A model to guide sexual assessment and intervention is available and has been well used among younger populations since the 1970s. The PLISSIT model (An-non, 1976 [Level VI]) begins by first seeking permission (P) to discuss sex-uality with the older adult. Because many sexual disorders originate in feel-ings of anxiety or guilt, asking permission may put the client in control of the discussion and facilitate communication with the health care provider. This permission may be gained by asking general questions, such as "I would like to begin to discuss your sexual health; what concerns would you like to share with me about this area of function?" Questions to guide the sexual assessment of older adults are available on many health care assessment forms. The next step of the model affords an opportunity for the health care provider to share limited information (LI) with the older adult. In the case of older adults, this part of the model gives health care providers the opportunity to dispel myths of aging and sexuality and to discuss the impact of normal and pathological aging changes, as well as medications for sexual health. The next part of the model guides the health care provider to provide specific suggestions (SS) to improve sexual health. In so doing, nurses may implement several of the interventions recommended for improved sexual health, such as safe sex practices, more effective management of acute and chronic diseases, removal or substitution of causative medications, environmental adaptations, and need for discussions with partners and families. The final part of the model calls for intensive therapy (IT) when needed for clients whose sexual dysfunction goes beyond the scope of nursing management. In these cases, referral to a sexual therapist is appropriate.

Sexual assessments will be most effective using open-ended questions, such as, "Can you tell me how you express your sexuality?," "What concerns you about your sexuality?," "How has your sexuality changed as you have aged?," "What changes have you noticed in your sexuality since you have been diagnosed or treated for disease?," and "What thoughts have you had about ways in which you would like to enhance your sexual health?" The loss of relationships with significant, intimate partners is unfortunately common among older adults and often ends communication about the importance of self to the person experiencing the loss. This greatly impacts an older adult's sexual health. Asking an older adult about past and present relationships in his or her life will help to aid this assessment.

Barriers to sexual health should be assessed, including normal and pathological changes of aging, medications, and psychological problems, such as depression. Moreover, lack of knowledge and understanding about sexuality, loss of partners, and family influence on sexual practice often present substantial barriers to sexual health among older adults. Nurses should assess for the presence of physiological changes through a health history, review of systems, and physical examination for the presence of normal and aging changes that impact sexual health. Older adults may view the normal changes of aging and their subsequent impact on appearance as embarrassing or indicative of illness. This may result in a negative body image and a reluctance to pursue sexual health. It is important for nurses to consider the impact of normal and pathological changes of aging on body image and assess their impact frequently.

As discussed previously, there are a number of medical conditions that have been associated with poor sexual health and functioning (Morley & Tariq, 2003 [Level V]), including depression, cardiac disease (Addis et al., 2005 [Level II]), diabetes (Rockliffe-Fidler & Kiemle, 2003 [Level IV]), stroke and aphasia (Lemieux et al., 2001 [Level IV]), Parkinson's disease (Mott, Kenrick, Dixon, & Bird, 2005 [Level IV]), and BPH (Rosen, 2006 [Level V]). Effective assessment of these illnesses using open-ended health history questions, review of systems, physical examination, and appropriate lab testing will provide necessary information for appropriate disease management and improved sexual function.

Assess the impact of medications among older adults, especially those commonly used to treat medical illnesses among older adults such as antidepressants (Montejo et al., 2001 [Level IV]) and antihypertensives (Girerd et al., 2003 [Level IV]). Potential medications should be identified by reviewing a client's medication bottles and the client should be questioned about the potential impact of these medications on sexual health. If the medication is found to impact sexual health, alternative medications should be considered. Older adults should also be questioned regarding the use of alcohol because this substance also has a potential impact on sexual response.

Intervention and Care Strategies

Following a thorough assessment of normal and pathological aging changes, as well as environmental factors, a number of interventions may be implemented to promote the sexual health of older adults. These interventions fall into several broad categories, including (1) education regarding age-associated change in sexual function; (2) compensation for normal aging changes; (3) effective management of acute and chronic illness effecting sexual function; (4) removal of barriers associated with difficulty in fulfilling sexual needs; and (5) special interventions to promote sexual health in cognitively impaired older adults.

Client Education

The most important intervention to improving sexuality among the older population is education. It is important to remember that sexuality was likely not addressed in formal educational systems as the older adults developed and was rarely discussed informally. Older adults may possess dated values that impact sexual action, freedom, and desires, leading to both sexual frustration and conflict. Masters reported in his seminal work on the sexuality of older adults (1986 [Level VI]) that older women were raised to believe that when menstruation ceased, they would cease to be feminine. Knowledge is essential to the successful fulfillment of sexuality for all people.

The incidence of HIV and AIDS infection is rising among older adults, with 11% of all AIDS cases resulting in adults older than 50. This underscores the significant risk of HIV transmission in the older age group and the need for effective teaching regarding safe sex practices. Teaching about the use of condoms to prevent the transmission of sexually transmitted diseases is essential. In response to this rise in HIV cases and the presence of other sexually transmitted diseases, it is essential to provide older adults with safe sex information provided by the Centers for Disease Control.

Compensating for Normal Aging Changes

Assisting older adults to compensate for normal aging changes related to sexual dysfunction will greatly lessen the impact of these changes on sexual health. Among women, the discussion of anatomical changes in sexual anatomy will help them to anticipate these changes. For example, the decreases in the size of the vagina and increased vaginal dryness among women may require the use of artificial water-based lubricants (Araujo et al., 2004 [Level IV]). In men, delayed response and the increased length of time needed for erections and ejaculation are among normal changes of aging, of which older adults may not be aware. When older adults understand the impact of normal aging changes, they then understand the need to plan for more time and direct stimulation to become aroused.

One of the most important preventive measures older adults may undertake to reduce the impact of normal aging changes on sexual health is to continue to engage in sexual activity. Planning for more time during sexual activities; being sensitive to changes in one another's bodies; the use of aids to increase stimulation and lubrication; the exploration of foreplay, masturbation, sensual touch, and different sexual positions; along with education about these common changes associated with sex and aging may help immensely. By doing so, changes in sexual response patterns are less likely to occur. Eating healthy foods, getting adequate amounts of sleep, exercising, stress-management techniques, and not smoking are also important to sexual health.

Effective Management of Acute and Chronic Illness

Effective management of both acute and chronic illnesses that impair sexual health is also important. Interventions that improve sexual health are frameworked within the current interventions to treat disease. In other words, effective disease management using primary, secondary, and tertiary interventions will not only effectively treat the disease but also result in improved sexual health. Consequently, better glucose control among diabetics enhances circulation and may increase arousal and sexual response, whereas appropriate treatment of depression with medication and psychotherapy will enhance desire and sexual response (Beutel et al., 2005; Girerd et al., 2003 [Level IV]); Morley & Tariq, 2003 [Level V]; Rockliffe-Fidler & Kiemle, 2003 [Level IV]; Walsh & Berman, 2004 [Level V]).

Sparse research is available to guide the treatment of sexual disorders among older adults. New research has demonstrated the efficacy of sildenafil citrate for the treatment of some sexual disorders among women, including FSAD. In a double-blind randomized controlled trial of this medication in a study of 202 postmenopausal women with FSAD, significant improvements were noted in the control group who received the medication compared with the placebo group (Berman et al., 2003 [Level II]). Walsh and Berman (2004 [Level V]) report that centrally acting serotonin agonists and vasodilating creams are also undergoing investigation and may result in more effective treatment for age-related FSAD. The emergence of sildenafil for erectile dysfunction in men has also been demonstrated in multiple clinical trials to be a generally well-tolerated treatment for erectile dysfunction in older men (Fink, MacDonald, Rutks, Nelson, & Wilt, 2002 [Level I]).

Medications used to treat diseases may result in sexual dysfunction among older adults (see http://www.netdoctor.co.uk/menshealth/feature/medicinessex.htm for a list of these medications). There are many medications that may result in decreased sexual drive and impotence as well as orgasmic and ejaculatory disorders. These medications are widely prescribed for many chronic illnesses among older adults, including psychological disorders such as depression, hypertension, elevated cholesterol, sleep disorders, and peptic ul-cer diseases. Moreover, because of the hesitancy among older adults and nurses to discuss sexual problems, the effect of these medications on sexual function is often not discussed in clinical settings. This may result in either prolonged sexual dysfunction among older adults or a noncompliance with the medica-tion. Recognition of the continuing sexual needs of older adults among nurses is essential to beginning a dialogue about sexual problems. Effective assessment will uncover medications affecting an older adult's sexual function and lead to the consideration of stopping the medication in favor of alternative disease-management strategies or substituting the medication causing the dysfunction with another one with fewer sexual side effects.

Removal of Barriers to Sexual Health

One of the greatest barriers to sexual health among older adults lies within nurses' persistent beliefs that older adults are not sexual beings. Nurses should be encouraged to open lines of communication in order to effectively assess and manage the sexual health needs of aging individuals with the same consistency as other bodily systems and treat alterations in sexual health with available evidence-based strategies.

An essential intervention to promoting sexual health in this population is to attempt to educate nurses regarding the continuing sexual needs and desires persisting throughout the lifespan. Education regarding older adult sexuality as a continuing human need should be included in multidisciplinary education and staff-development programs. Educational sessions may begin by discussing prevalent societal myths around older adult sexuality. Nurses should be encour-aged to discuss their own feelings about sexuality and its role in the life of older adults. Moreover, the development of policies and procedures to manage sexual issues of older adults is important throughout environments of care.

Environmental adaptations to ensure privacy and safety among long term care and community-dwelling residents are essential. Arrangements for privacy must be made so the dignity of older adults is protected during sexual activity. For example, nurses may assist in finding other activities for the resident's roommate so that privacy may be obtained or in securing a common room that may be used by older adults for private visits. Call lights or telephones should be kept within reach during sexual activity and adaptive equipment such as hospital beds, side rails, and trapezes may need to be obtained. Interventions such as providing rooms for privacy and offering consultations for residents regarding evaluation and treatment of their sexual problems are a few of the many ways this may be accomplished (Wallace, 2003 [Level V]). Roach (2004 [Level IV]) suggests that nursing home staff and administration work to develop environments that are supportive and respectful of older residents' continuing sexual rights and that promote sexual health.

Families are an integral part of the interdisciplinary team. However, for older couples, especially those in relationships with new partners, it is often difficult for families to understand that their older relative may have a sexual relationship with anyone other than the person they are accustomed to them being with. A family meeting, with a counselor if needed, is appropriate to help the family understand and accept the older adult's decisions about the relationship.

Special Interventions to Promote the Sexual Health of Cognitively Impaired Older Adults

Cognitively impaired older adults continue to have sexual needs and desires but may lack the capacity to make appropriate decisions regarding sexual relationships. Accurate assessment and documentation of ability to make informed decisions regarding sexual relationships must be conducted by an interdisciplinary team. If an older adult is not capable of making competent decisions, participation in sexual relationships may be considered abusive and must be prevented. On the other end of the spectrum, nurses should not attempt to prevent sexual relationships and may play an important role in promoting sexual health among older adults who are cognitively competent to make decisions regarding sexual relationships. In these cases, nurses should implement all necessary interventions to promote the sexual health of older adults.

Inappropriate sexual behavior such as public masturbation, disrobing, or making sexually explicit remarks to other patients or health care professionals may be a warning sign of unmet sexual needs among older adults. A full sexual assessment should be conducted using clear communication and limit-setting in these situations. Following this, a plan should be developed to manage this behavior while providing the utmost respect for and preserving the dignity of the older adult. Providing an environment in which older adults may pursue their sexuality in private may be a simple solution to a difficult problem. Medication management for hypersexual behavior may be considered. Pathological hypersexuality is usually related to the presence of cognitive disorders in older adults (Levitsky and Owens, 1999 [Level V]). Antipsychotic medications have traditionally been used to treat hypersexuality. However, Levitsky and Owens (1999 [Level V]) report that antiandrogens, estrogens, Gonadotropin-releasing hormone analogues, and serotonergic medications may be successful when other methods are ineffective.

Case Study and Discussion

Mrs. Jones is a highly functioning 79-year-old widow, recently admitted to a nursing home with mild cognitive impairment (MCI). Mrs. Jones began a friendship with Mr. Carl, who is cognitively intact and wheelchair bound. Mr. Carl is married to a woman who resides outside the facility. The nursing staff has noticed more and more intimate touches among the two residents and is concerned about Mrs. Jones's competency to make the decision to participate in this increasingly intimate relationship. Moreover, general concern about the sexual relationship within a long term care setting prevails among the nursing staff.

The first step in this situation is to conduct a full assessment to determine Mrs. Jones's capacity to participate in this intimate relationship. The right to Mrs. Jones's autonomy is complicated by the presence of MCI and must be explored further. The question remains, does Mrs. Jones have the decisional capacity to participate in an intimate relationship?

The actual and projected outcomes of the intimate relationship would require assessment to determine what nursing actions are required regarding this relationship. If an assessment of Mrs. Jones finds that she is incapable of understanding the consequences of her relationship with Mr. Carl, then she must be protected from unsolicited sexual advances by a spouse, partner, or other residents. However, if the assessment leads nurses to believe that Mrs. Jones and Mr. Carl understand the risks and consequences of their relationship, then the right to autonomy prevails.

If clinicians determine that older adults have the decisional capacity to consent to a sexual relationship, then a comprehensive health history, review of systems, and physical examination to determine normal and pathological changes of aging that may play a role in this sexual relationship must be conducted. Appropriate lab work for the potential presence of sexually transmitted diseases should be included. A care plan focusing the need to promote sexual health for this couple should be developed. Teaching about normal and pathological aging changes and the impact of these changes, as well as medications on sexual function, should be conducted. Normal changes of aging must be compensated for and diseases affecting sexual response should be treated with medications that will not impact sexual health. Safety regarding sexually transmitted diseases and privacy should be provided for the residents, ensuring that their dignity is respected at all times.

Summary and Conclusions

One of the most prevalent myths of aging is that older adults are no longer interested in sex. It is commonly believed that older adults no longer have any interest or desire to participate in sexual relationships. Because sexuality is mainly considered a young person's activity, often associated with reproduction, society does not usually associate older adults with sex. Furthermore, most of the current information society has regarding sexuality in older adults is from young, Caucasian, healthy, and educated individuals (Zeiss & Kasl-Godley, 2001 [Level V]). In the youth-oriented society of today, many consider sexuality among older adults to be distasteful and prefer to assume it does not exist. However, despite popular belief, sexuality continues to be important, even in the lives of older adults.

Whereas the sexual health of older adults has been largely ignored in past decades, evolving images of older adults as healthy and vibrant members of society may result in a decrease in the prevalence of myths of this population as nonsexual beings. Changes in the societal image of older adults as asexual celibate beings will greatly enhance removal of barriers to sexual health in the older population. Improved assessment and management of normal and pathological changes of aging and appropriate environmental adaptations and management of special issues of sexuality and aging will also result in improved sexual health in the older population. Moreover, the development of new interventions including oral erectile agents may also play a role in enhanced sexual health among older adults.

The fulfillment of sexual needs may be just as satisfying for older adults as it is for younger people. However, several normal and pathological changes of aging complicate sexuality among older adults. Environmental changes may create further barriers to sexual expression among older adults. Despite the many barriers to achieving sexual health among an aging population, nurses are in a critical position to understand sexual needs and capabilities in later life and to assist older adults in developing compensatory strategies for improving sexual health in order to have the best possible sexual life. If these strategies and interventions are undertaken, increased awareness and acceptance of elderly sexuality will ultimately take place, and the concept of sex in old age will no longer be such a shocking topic.

Resources

World Health Organization (2004). Sexual Health: A New Focus for WHO. Progress. *Reproductive Health Research, 67*,1–8. http://www.who.int/reproductive-health/gender/sexual_health.html

MedlinePlus http://www.nlm.nih.gov/medlineplus/sexualhealthissues.html

National Institutes on Aging http://www.niapublications.org/engagepages/sexuality.asp

American Foundation for Urological Disease, Inc. http://www.impotence.org

Prentiss Care Networks Project (Care Networks for Formal and Informal Caregivers of Older Adults) http://caregiving.case.edu

Geriatric Video Productions http://www.geriatricvideo.com/

Nursing Spectrum Education/CE: Self-Study Modules http://www.nursingspectrum.com/ContinuingEducation/NSSelfStudy/index.cfm

Hartford Institute for Geriatric Nursing (2003). Partners for dissemination of best nursing practices in care of older adults. http://www.ConsultGeriRN.org/resources/education/bsnPartners.html

Videos

A Rose by Any Other Name (1976). Post Perfect Productions, Backseat Bingo Films

Freedom of Sexual Expression: Dementia and Resident Rights in Long Term Care Facilities. Terra Nova Films

The Heart Has No Wrinkles. Terra Nova Films

Box 28.1

Nursing Standard of Practice Protocol: Sexuality in Older Adults

I. GOAL: To enhance the sexual health of older adults.

II. OVERVIEW: Although it is generally believed that sexual desires decrease with age, several researchers have identified that sexual desires, thoughts, and actions continue throughout all decades of life. Human touch and a healthy sex lives evoke sentiments of joy, romance, affection, passion, and intimacy, whereas despondency and depression often result from an inability to express one's sexuality. Health care providers play an important role in assessing and managing normal and pathological aging changes in order to improve the sexual health of older adults.

III. BACKGROUND AND STATEMENT OF PROBLEM

A. Definitions
   1. *Sexuality*: a central aspect of being human throughout life and encompasses sex, gender identities and roles, sexual orientation, eroticism, pleasure, intimacy, and reproduction (World Health Organization, 2004)
   2. *Sexual health*: a state of physical, emotional, mental, and social well-being related to sexuality (World Health Organization, 2004)
   3. *Sexual dysfunction*: impairment in normal sexual functioning (American Psychiatric Association, 1994)
B. Etiology and/or Epidemiology
   1. Despite the continuing sexual needs of older adults, many barriers prevent sexual health among older adults (Zeiss and Kasl-Godley, 2001 [Level V])
   2. Health care providers often lack knowledge and comfort in discussing sexual issues with older adults (Gott, Hincliff, & Galena, 2004 [Level IV])
   3. The older population is more susceptible to many disabling medical conditions; a number of medical conditions are associated with poor sexual health and functioning (Morley & Tariq, 2003 [Level V]) including cardiac disease (Addis et al., 2005 [Level II]); stroke and aphasia (Lemieux, Cohen-Schneider, & Holzapfel, 2001[Level IV]); Parkinson's disease (Mott, Kenrick, Dixon, & Bird, 2005 [Level IV]); diabetes (Rockliffe-Fidler & Kiemle, 2003 [Level IV]); BPHy (Rosen, 2006 [Level V]); and dental problems (Heydecke, Thomason, Lund, & Feine, 2005) that make sexuality difficult.
   4. Medications among older adults, especially those commonly used to treat medical illnesses, also impact sexuality, such as antidepressants (Montejo, Llorca, Izquierdo, & Rico-Villademoros, 2001[Level IV]) and antihypertensives (Girerd et al., 2003 [Level IV]).
   5. Normal aging changes, such as a higher frequency of vaginal dryness in women and erectile dysfunction in men, make sexual health difficult to achieve (Harvard Medical School, 2003; Araujo, Mohr, & McKinlay, 2004 [Level IV]).
   6. Environmental barriers also present barriers to sexual health among older adults (Hajjar & Kamel; 2003 [Level V]).

IV. ASSESSMENT

A. The PLISSIT model (Annon, 1976 [Level VI]) begins by first seeking permission (P) to discuss sexuality with an older adult. The next step of the model affords an opportunity for the health care provider to share limited information (LI) with the older adult. The next step guides the health care provider to provide specific suggestions (SS) to improve sexual health. The Final part calls for intensive therapy (IT) when needed for clients whose sexual dysfunction goes beyond the scape of nursing management.

B. Ask open-ended questions such as "Can you tell me how you express your sexuality," "What concerns you about your sexuality?," and "How has your sexuality changed as you have aged?"

C. Assess for presence of physiological changes through a health history, review of systems, and physical examination for the presence of normal and aging changes that impact sexual health.

D. Review medications among older adults, especially those commonly used to treat medical illnesses that also impact sexuality, such as antidepressants (Montejo, Llorca, Izquierdo, & Rico-Villademoros, 2001[Level IV]) and antihypertensives (Girerd et al., 2003 [Level IV]).

E. Assess medical conditions that have been associated with poor sexual health and functioning (Morley & Tariq, 2003 [Level V]) including cardiac disease (Addis et al., 2005 [Level II]); stroke and aphasia (Lemieux et al., 2001 [Level IV]); Parkinson's disease (Mott et al., 2005 [Level IV]); diabetes (Rockliffe-Fidler & Kiemle, 2003 [Level IV]); BPH (Rosen, 2006); and dental problems (Heydecke et al., 2005).

V. NURSING CARE STRATEGIES

A. Communication and Education
   1. Discuss normal age-related physiological changes.
   2. Address how the effects of medications/medical conditions may affect one's sexual function.
   3. Facilitate communication with older adults and their families regarding sexual health as desired, including:
      a. Encourage family meetings with open discussion of issues if desired.
      b. Teach about safe sex practices.
      c. Discuss use of condoms to prevent transmission of STDs and HIV.

B. Health Management
   1. Perform a thorough patient assessment.
   2. Conduct a health history, review of systems, and physical examination.
   3. Effectively manage chronic illness.

4. Improve glucose monitoring and control among diabetics.
5. Ensure appropriate treatment of depression and screening for depression (see chapter 5, *Depression*).
6. Discontinue/substitute medications that may result in sexual dysfunction (e.g., hypertension or depression medications).
7. Accurately assess and document older adults' ability to make informed decisions (see chapter 23, *Health Care Decision Making*).
8. Participation in sexual relationships may be considered abusive if an older adult is not capable of making decisions.

C. Sexual Enhancement
1. Compensate for normal changes of aging
   a. Females:
      i. Use of artificial water-based lubricants
      ii. Treatment of FSAD with sildenafil citrate (Viagra) (Berman et al., 2003)
      iii. Use of centrally acting serotonin agonists and vasodilating creams (Walsh & Berman, 2004)
   b. Males:
      i. Recognizing the possibility for more time and direct stimulation for arousal due to aging changes
      ii. Use of sildenafil citrate (Viagra) for erectile dysfunction (Fink et al., 2002)
2. Environmental Adaptations
   a. Ensure privacy and safety among long term care and community-dwelling residents (Wallace, 2003)

VI. EXPECTED OUTCOMES

A. Patients will:
1. Report high quality of life as measured by a standardized quality of life assessment.
2. Be provided with privacy, dignity, and respect surrounding their sexuality.
3. Receive communication and education regarding sexual health as desired.
4. Be able to pursue sexual health free of pathological and problematic sexual behaviors.

B. Health care providers will:
1. Include sexual health questions in their routine history and physical.
2. Frequently reassess patients for changes in sexual health.

C. Institutions will:
1. Include sexual health questions on intake and reassessment measures.
2. Provide education on the ongoing sexual needs of older adults and appropriate interventions to manage these needs with dignity and respect.

3. Provide needed privacy for individuals to maintain intimacy and sexual health (e.g., in long term care).

VII. FOLLOW-UP MONITORING OF CONDITION

Sexual outcomes are difficult to directly assess and measure. However, with the illustrated link between sexual health and quality of life, quality of life measures such as the SF-36 Health Survey may be used to determine the effectiveness of interventions to promote sexual health. Retrieved March 7, 2007, at http://www.rand.org/health/surveys/sf36item/question.html.

Content for this protocol was adapted from geronurseonline.org (protocol now available at www.ConsultGeriRN.org).

References

AARP Modern Maturity Sexuality Study. NFO Research: Atlanta. Retrieved May 1, 2005, from http://assets.aarp.org/rgcenter/health/mmsexsurvey.pdf. Evidence Level IV: Nonexperimental Study.

Addis, I. B., Ireland, C. C., Vittinghoff, E., Lin, F., Stuenkel, C. A., & Hulley, S. (2005). Sexual activity and function in postmenopausal women with heart disease. *Obstetrics and Gynecology, 106,*121–127. Evidence Level II: Single Experimental Study.

Alagiakrishnan, K., Lim, D., Brahim, A., Wong, A., Wood, A., Senthilselvan, A., et al. (2005). Sexually inappropriate behavior in demented elderly people. *Postgraduate Medical Journal, 81*(957), 463–466. Evidence Level IV: Nonexperimental Study.

Alkhalil, C., Tanvir, F., Alkhalil, B., & Lowenthal, D. T. (2004). Treatment of sexual disinhibition in dementia: Case reports and review of the literature. *American Journal of Therapeutics, 11*(3), 231–235. Evidence Level V: Review.

American Psychiatric Association (1994). *Diagnostic and statistical manual of mental disorders* (4th ed.). Washington, DC: Author. Evidence Level VI: Respected Opinion.

Annon, J. (1976). The PLISSIT model: A proposed conceptual scheme for behavioral treatment of sexual problems. *Journal of Sex Education Therapy, 2*(2), 1–15. Evidence Level VI: Respected Opinion.

Araujo, A. B., Mohr, B. A., & McKinlay, J. B. (2004). Changes in sexual function in middle-aged and older men: Longitudinal data from the Massachusetts male aging study. *Journal of the American Geriatrics Society, 52*(9), 1502–1509. Evidence Level IV: Nonexperimental Study.

Bergström-Walan, M., & Nielsen, H. H. (1990). Sexual expression among 60 80-year-old men and women: A sample from Stockholm, Sweden. *The Journal of Sex Research, 27*(2) 289–295.

Berman, J. R., Berman, L. A., Toler, S. M., Gill, J., Haughie, S., & Sildenafil Study Group. (2003). Safety and efficacy of sildenafil citrate for the treatment of female sexual arousal disorder: A double-blind, placebo-controlled study. *The Journal of Urology, 170*(6 Pt 1), 2333–2338. Evidence Level II: Single Experimental Study.

Beutel, M. E., Wiltink, J., Hauck, E. W, Auch, D., Behre, H. M., Brahler, E., et al. (2005). Correlations between hormones, physical, and affective parameters in aging urologic outpatients. *European Urology, 47,* 749–755.

Brotman, S., Ryan, B., & Cormier, R. (2003). The health and social service needs of gay and lesbian elders and their families in Canada. *The Gerontologist, 43*(2), 192–202. Evidence Level IV: Nonexperimental Study.

Centers for Disease Control (2007). Data & trends: National diabetes surveillance system. Retrieved March 2, 2007, from http://www.cdc.gov/diabetes/statistics/prev/national/figpersons.htm.

Chamberland, L. (2003). Elderly women, invisible lesbians. *Canadian Journal of Community Mental Health (Revue Canadienne De Sante Mentale Communautaire)*, *22*(2), 85–103. Evidence Level IV: Nonexperimental Study.

Cooper, A., & Scherer, C. (1998). Questions & answers: Sex and lust: Sexual peaks. Retrieved July 14, 2006, from http://www.selfhelpmagazine.com/ qa/qasexpeak.html.

Falvo, N., & Norman, S. (2004). Never too old to learn: The impact of an HIV/AIDS education program on older adults' knowledge. *Clinical Gerontologist*, *27*(1/2), 103–117. Evidence Level IV: Nonexperimental Study.

Fink, H. A., MacDonald, R., Rutks, I. R., Nelson, D. B., & Wilt, T. J. (2002). Sildenafil for male erectile dysfunction: A systematic review and meta-analysis. *Archives of Internal Medicine*, *162*(12), 1349–1360. Evidence Level I: Systematic Review.

Ginsberg, T. B., Pomerantz, S. C., & Kramer-Feeley, V. (2005). Sexuality in older adults: Behaviours and preferences. *Age and Ageing*, *34*(5), 475–480. Evidence Level IV: Nonexperimental Study.

Girerd, X., Mounier-Vehier, C., Fauvel, J. P., Marquand, A., Babici, D., & Hanon, O. (2003). Medical management of libido disturbances in treated hypertensive patients: Differences between men and women. *Arch Mal Coeur Vaiss*, *96*(7–8), 758–762. Evidence Level IV: Nonexperimental Study.

Goodroad, B. K. (2003). HIV and AIDS in people older than 50. *A continuing concern. Journal of Gerontological Nursing*, *29*(4), 18–24. Evidence Level V: Review.

Gott, M., & Hinchliff, S. (2003). How important is sex in later life? The views of older people. *Social Science & Medicine*, *56*(8), 1617–1628. Evidence Level IV: Nonexperimental Study.

Gott, M., Hinchliff, S., & Galena, E. (2004). General practitioner attitudes to discussing sexual health issues with older people. *Social Science & Medicine*, *58*(11), 2093–2103. Evidence Level IV: Nonexperimental Study.

Hajjar, R. R., & Kamel, H. K. (2004). Sexuality in the nursing home, part 1: Attitudes and barriers to sexual expression. *Journal of the American Medical Directors Association*, *5*(2 Suppl.), S42–S47. Evidence Level V: Review.

Harvard Medical School (2003). *Sexuality in midlife and beyond: A special report from Harvard Medical School*. Boston: Harvard Health Publications. Evidence Level VI: Respected Opinion.

Heydecke, G., Thomason, J. M., Lund, J. P., & Feine, J. S. (2005). The impact of conventional and implant supported prostheses on social and sexual activities in edentulous adults results from a randomized trial 2 months after treatment. *Journal of Dentistry*, *33*(8), 649–657.

Johnson, M. J., Jackson, N. C., Arnette, J. K., & Koffman, S. D. (2005). Gay and lesbian perceptions of discrimination in retirement care facilities. *Journal of Homosexuality*, *49*(2), 83–102. Evidence Level IV: Nonexperimental Study.

Kamel, H. K., & Hajjar, R. R. (2003). Sexuality in the nursing home, part 2: Managing abnormal behavior: Legal and ethical issues. *Journal of the American Medical Directors Association*, *4*(4), 203–206. Evidence Level V: Review.

Kessenich, C. R., & Cichon, M. J. (2001). Hormonal decline in elderly men and male menopause. *Geriatric Nursing*, *22*, 24–27. Evidence Level V: Review.

Lemieux, L., Cohen-Schneider, R., & Holzapfel, S. (2001). Aphasia and sexuality. *Sexuality and Disability*, *19*(4), 253–266. Evidence Level IV: Nonexperimental Study.

Levitsky, A. M., & Owens, N. J. (1999). Pharmacologic treatment of hypersexuality and paraphilias in nursing home residents. *Journal of the American Geriatrics Society*, *47*, 231–234. Evidence Level V: Review.

Masters, W. H. (1986). Sex and aging: Expectations and reality. *Hospital Practice, August 15*, 175–198. Evidence Level VI: Expert Opinion.

Montejo, A. L., Llorca, G., Izquierdo, J. A., & Rico-Villademoros, F. (2001). Incidence of sexual dysfunction associated with antidepressant agents: A prospective multicenter study of 1,022 outpatients. Spanish working group for the study of psychotropic-related sexual dysfunction. *The Journal of Clinical Psychiatry*, *62* (Suppl. 3), 10–21. Evidence Level IV: Nonexperimental Study.

Morley, J. E., & Tariq, S. H. (2003). Sexuality and disease. *Clinics in Geriatric Medicine*, *19*(3), 563–573. Evidence Level V: Review.

Mott, S., Kenrick, M., Dixon, M., & Bird, G. (2005). Sexual limitations in people living with Parkinson's disease. *Australian Journal on Ageing*, *24*(4), 196–202. Evidence Level IV: Nonexperimental Study.

Nagaratnam, N., & Gayagay, G. (2002). Hypersexuality in nursing home facilities: A descriptive study. *Archives in Gerontology and Geriatrics, 35*(3), 195–203. Evidence Level IV: Nonexperimental Study.

Peck, S. A. (2001). The importance of the sexual health history in the primary care setting. *Journal of Obstetric, Gynecologic, and Neonatal Nursing: JOGNN / NAACOG, 30*(3), 269–274. Evidence Level V: Review.

Roach, S. M. (2004). Sexual behaviour of nursing home residents: Staff perceptions and responses. *Journal of Advanced Nursing, 48*(4), 371–379. Evidence Level IV: Nonexperimental Study.

Rockliffe-Fidler, C., & Kiemle, G. (2003). Sexual function in diabetic women: A psychological perspective. *Sexual and Relationship Therapy, 18*(2), 143–159. Evidence Level IV: Nonexperimental Study.

Rosen, R. C. (2006). Assessment of sexual dysfunction in patients with benign prostatic hyperplasia. *BJU International, 97* (Suppl. 2), 29–33; discussion 44–45. Evidence Level V: Review.

Wallace, M. (2003). Sexuality in long term care. *Annals of Long Term Care, 11*(2), 53–59. Evidence Level V: Review.

Walsh, K. E., & Berman, J. R. (2004). Sexual dysfunction in the older woman: An overview of the current understanding and management. *Drugs & Aging, 21*(10), 655–675. Evidence Level V: Review.

World Health Organization (2004). Sexual Health: A New Focus for WHO. Progress in Reproductive Health Research. Retrieved May 10, 2005. Evidence Level VI: Respected Opinion.

Zeiss, A. M., & Kasl-Godley, J. (2001). Sexuality in older adults' relationships. *Generations, 25*(2), 18–25. Evidence Level V: Review.

Substance Misuse and Alcohol Use Disorders

29

Madeline Naegle

Educational Objectives

On completion of this chapter, the reader will be able to:

1. describe common substance-related disorders diagnosed in people older than 55

2. outline screening steps for substance-use disorders in people 55 and older

3. discuss the rationale and steps of assessment of an identified substance-use disorder

4. describe intervention strategies for substance-related disorders in people 55 and older

5. list potential referral resources for older adults (and their families) experiencing substance-related disorders

Overview

Alcohol dependence and drug use among people 55 and older is changing as a function of an aging population anticipated to live longer and more active lives. The projected increase from 33 million to approximately 80 million older adults by 2050 predicts that the frequency of substance-related problems among elders will increase, and nurses must be prepared to identify and intervene with them (U.S. Bureau of Census, 1996). In addition, because the area of drug use among ethnic minorities is grossly understudied, suggestions for nursing interventions

For a description of Evidence Levels cited in this chapter, see chapter 1, Developing and Evaluating Clinical Practice Guidelines, page 4

must be interpreted in a culturally competent way and individualized to the primary membership group for an older adult (Grant et al., 2004).

Background and Significance

Substance-use problems are costly to society with direct and indirect economic costs of alcohol abuse and dependence, including costs of illness and crime, estimated at $184 billion in 1998 (NIAAA, 2000). Another $143.4 billion in costs is attributed to illicit and prescription drugs (NIAAA, 2000). In older adults, the misuse of medications in people older than 60 costs the United States $60 billion annually. Nearly 22% of community-dwelling older adults use potentially addictive prescription medications; risks of psychological and/or physical dependence associated with this phenomenon are considerable (Simoni-Wastila, Zuckerman, Singhai, Briesacher, & Hsu, 2005 [Level III]). Although the rate of alcohol dependence in the general population remains somewhat stable at 6% for men and 2% for women, the rates of heavy alcohol use among older people are emerging as a new area of study. Among people older than 60 seen in primary care, 15% of men and 12% of women regularly drank in excess of the NIAAA recommended levels (i.e., one drink per day and no more than three drinks on any one occasion) (Fink, Elliott, Tsai, & Beck, 2005 [Level III]; NIAAA, 1995). The burden of disease associated with smoking continues to be heaviest among older individuals, who have smoked the longest and manifest the most health problems. In 2004, 18.5 million Americans older than 45 smoked (about 42% of all adult smokers) and 9% of older Americans were smokers in 2000 (National Center for Health Statistics, 2007), for whom health risks are greater than for younger smokers (Rimer, Orleans, Reintz, Critinzia, & Fleisher, 1990 [Level III]). As baby-boomers age, their lifetime illicit drug use is anticipated to continue at the levels of their younger years, contributing to the number of people older than 55 using illicit drugs (i.e., marijuana and cocaine) (SAMHSA, 2000). Using survey research and modeling methods to project trends, the number of people 50 and older who use marijuana is projected to increase from 1.0% in 1999 to 2.9% (3.3 million users) by 2020. Use of many illicit drugs is expected to increase from 2.2% (1.6 million) to 3.1% (3.5 million), and nonmedical use of psychotherapeutic drugs is projected to increase from 1.2% to 2.4% (Colliver, Compton, Gfroerer, & Condon, 2006 [Level III]). If borne out, these projections represent significant changes in drug use by older individuals and emphasize the need for both education and improved proactive treatment planning.

Growing numbers of older people, coupled with their reluctance to seek assistance for mental health problems (i.e., fewer than 3% of older people visit a mental health professional), suggest that nurses and health professionals caring for older adults in all settings need to be knowledgeable about substance use, abuse, and dependence (Bartels et al., 2004 [Level III]). Psychiatric disorders often co-occur with alcohol abuse in older adults with a prevalence ranging from 12% to 30% (Koenig & Blazer, 1996; Oslin, 2005 [Level III]), and depression is both a cause and a consequence of excessive drinking. The Prism study, a randomized trial of 23,828 participants, found that 14% of older adults had positive assessments for depressive or anxiety disorders and 6% were consuming alcohol at levels that placed them at risk for health problems (Levkoff et al., 2004 [Level IV]).

Health problems related to drug and alcohol use are influenced by metabolic changes that increase morbidity in advancing age. Older people respond differently to alcohol because of decreased total body water, decreased rates of alcohol metabolism in the gastrointestinal tract, and increased sensitivity to alcohol combined with decreased tolerance (USDHHS, 2004b [Level VI]). Consequently, more dramatic behavioral changes occur at lower doses in older adults, and social and legal problems are more frequent and more pronounced than in younger people (USDHHS, 2004b [Level VI]).

Assessment of Substance Use Disorders

Substance use and related disorders in older adults are classified in the categories of use, abuse, and dependence. In reference to older adults, however, the category of misuse is most often applicable. Older people tend to use alcohol and other drugs in response to physical and psychological symptoms they experience as they age. Classification categories are linked to the particular substance used; the length of time of use, misuse, abuse, or dependence; and the social, legal, and health consequences for the individual. For example, people who drink four or fewer drinks per year are considered *abstinent* and *low-risk drinkers*, which for an older adult is no more than one drink daily and is not considered problematic (USDHHS, 2005). Most individuals who are users of and/or dependent on alcohol, nicotine, and illicit drugs have developed these disorders before the age of 60, and one-half to two-thirds of elderly alcoholics are believed to have developed the disease early in life. "Late-onset alcoholism" or patterns of prescription drug abuse, marked by increased use of alcohol or over-reliance on prescription drugs, appears to be more closely associated with the losses, chronic illness, psychological traumas, and other stresses of advancing age. A common example of this is the change from social use to risky drinking or drug misuse by people who have lost a spouse, partner, or job; are estranged from family or are facing serious illness; or any combination of situations mentioned (USDHHS, 2004b [Level VI]).

Alcohol Use Disorders

The most common substance-abuse problems among older adults stem from alcohol consumption, including interactions of alcohol with prescribed and over-the-counter (OTC) drugs (USDHHS, 2004b [Level VI]).

At-Risk or Problem Drinking

At-risk drinking is a pattern, which, while not appearing to cause usual alcohol-related problems, may bring about harmful consequences to the user or others, including accidents, health and/or mental health problems, or social and legal problems. For people older than 60, consumption of amounts of alcohol that caused no problems earlier in life may result in social, legal, or medical problems. This is linked to sensitivity, the frequency of use of prescribed drugs (i.e., alcohol interacts with at least 50% of prescription drugs), and the frequent co-occurrence of other chronic illnesses. Similarly, a decline in visual, hearing, or other perceptual capacities make alcohol consumption hazardous. Heavy drinking is associated with ulcers, respiratory disease, stroke, and myocardial infarction. Most adults decrease alcohol consumption with age but significant numbers (5% to 16%) continue heavy consumption at age 60 and older (Blow et al., 2000 [Level III]).

A recent New York City study found that 7% of individuals 65+ in all ethnic groups are drinking excessively (NYC DH&MH, 2005). Approximately 11% of men and 9% of women 75 years and older report heavy use, placing them at risk for a range of problems (Lyness, Canine, King, Cox, & Yoedino, 1997 [Level III]).

Abuse

Abuse of a substance is characterized by a maladaptive pattern of use, leading to impairment or distress (legal, interpersonal, emotional/mental) such as failing to fulfill role obligations, use in physically hazardous situations, occurring in a 12-month period (modified from American Psychiatric Association, 2000). Even when an individual does not meet the *DSM-TR-IV* criteria for abuse or dependence, alcohol consumption at levels of more than seven drinks per week for people older than 65 is linked to health consequences. Excessive alcohol consumption may place an older individual at risk for falls(Kursthaler, et al. 2005 [Level III]), self-neglect, diminished cognitive capacity, and long-term alcohol use is related to the development of common medical problems such as sleep complaints, restlessness and agitation, liver-function abnormalities, pneumonia, pancreatitis, gastrointestinal bleeding, and trauma, as well as chronic diseases, particularly neuropsychiatric and digestive disorders, diabetes, cardiovascular disease, and pancreatic or head and neck cancer (Blow, 1998; US-DHHS, 2004b [Level IV]). Because of the high co-morbid occurrence of alcohol and nicotine dependence, chronic obstructive pulmonary disease (COPD) and cancer of the mouth often co-occur, as do esophageal and laryngeal cancer (US-DHHS, 2004b). Excess alcohol use also impacts health by interfering with the absorption and utilization of prescribed drugs and nutrients.

Drug Dependence (Addiction)

Drug dependence is a maladaptive pattern of substance use that leads to impairment or distress (i.e., legal, interpersonal, emotional/mental occurring in a 12-month period (American Psychiatric Association, 2000). Addiction is a chronic illness characterized by brief "slips" from sobriety and "relapse," a return to regular use of the substance. It has two components: (1) physiological dependence, which occurs with alcohol, tobacco, benzodiazepines, barbiturates, amphetamines, and opioids; involves "tolerance," the need for increasing amounts of a substance to achieve the desired effect; and "withdrawal," manifested in a characteristic pattern of symptoms when the substance is suddenly terminated, including craving; and (2) psychological dependence, which is the perceived need to use the drug. Psychological dependence occurs with abuse, and is the more difficult dependence to resolve.

Illicit Drug Use

Illicit drug use in late adulthood is less prevalent than alcohol abuse or prescription-drug misuse. Recent trends associated with the baby-boomer generation, however, suggest that this may be changing. Marijuana use, for example, is now more prevalent among persons 55+ than among adolescents and, in 2000, more than one-half million persons 55+ reported illicit drug use (CSAT, 2000). Two recent studies indicate, however, that among people older than 50 reporting illicit drug use, toxicology screens on small samples as seen in urban emergency departments were positive for cocaine (63%), opiates (16%), and marijuana (14%) (Rivers et al., 2004 [Level III]; Schlaerth, Splawn, Ong, & Smith, 2004 [Level III]).

Many older persons are in recovery from the use of alcohol, cocaine, heroin, or other drugs. Changes associated with aging, such as the number of losses that increase with age, and the onset of chronic illness may be perceived as stressors and become "triggers," placing the individual at risk for relapse. Nurses should be aware of situations and stressors that may predispose an individual to relapse. In this discussion, the term drug encompasses OTC medications, prescription medications, nicotine, alcohol, and illicit drugs. Herbs and food supplements are also being used frequently, especially by older adults. Whereas the chemical composition of drugs of abuse is essential to understanding their effects of mind and body, this chapter focuses primarily on drug misuse and the effects and consequences of excessive use for health, as well as appropriate nursing assessment and intervention strategies. Please reference www.nih.nida.gov for a full listing of drugs of abuse and their chemical attributes.

Drug Misuse

Drug misuse, defined as use of a drug for reasons other than for which it was prescribed, occurs with increasing frequency with advancing age because (1) prescriptions for multiple medications and cognitive changes, ranging from "benign senile forgetting" to early signs of dementia, can lead to medication misuse; (2) failure to discard expired medications; (3) trading medications with friends and companions; and (4) combinations of medication and alcohol. The most common resulting problems are related to overdose, additive effects, and adverse reactions to drugs used or drug interactions, especially with alcohol. Although people older than 65 comprise only 13% of the population, they are prescribed more than 33% of all prescription drugs, and the nonmedical use of prescription drugs is increasing in persons older than 60 (NIDA, 2007 [Level V]). Among older women who misuse medications and alcohol, as high as 30% developed such habits after age 60 (CASA, 1998 [Level IV]).

Taking numerous drugs for multiple medical conditions (i.e., polypharmacy) may be complicated by an older person's use of alcohol or illicit drugs (Lang, 2001 [Level VI]). Prescription drug use/misuse contributes to falls, the second most common cause of death and cognitive impairment in American adults (NIDA, 2007 [Level V]). In people age 18 to 70 treated for falls, 40% of men and 8% of women tested positive for alcohol, benzodiazepines (9% vs 3%), or both (3% vs 0.3%) (Kursthaler et al., 2005 [Level IV]).

Smoking and Nicotine Dependence

Today's older Americans have smoked at rates among the highest of any U.S. generation (American Lung Association, 2006 [Level IV]), resulting in many health problems and contributing to the estimated 438,000 American deaths annually caused by smoking (CDC, 2005 [Level V]). An older adult's vulnerability to the effects of smoking varies by gender with men being more than twice as likely as women to die of stroke secondary to smoking (American Lung Association, 2003 [Level IV]). The risk of dying of a heart attack for men 65 and older is twice that for women smokers and 60% higher than for nonsmoking men of the same age. Smokers also have higher risk than nonsmokers for Alzheimer's disease or other types of dementia, as well as visual problems (CDC, 2005 [Level V]).

Polysubstance Abuse

Polysubstance abuse, the misuse, abuse, or dependence of three or more drugs, is not uncommon in older adults. In older people, prescription analgesics are frequently used for chronic pain and can induce dependence, depending on the class of drug being used. Pain is a common complaint in older people; older problem drinkers report more severe pain, greater disruption of activities due to pain, and the frequent use of alcohol to manage pain (Brennan, Schutte, & Moos, 2005 [Level III]). These findings underscore the importance of monitoring the drinking behavior of patients who present with pain complaints, especially those with a history of alcohol abuse or dependence. Examples of substances that older adults often self-administer are alcohol, tobacco, benzodiazepines, marijuana, and analgesic opioids.

Assessment of Substance-Use Problems

History

Nurses should review data obtained on the most recent nursing and medical histories and findings of the most recent physical examination. When patients are using excess alcohol, there will be deviations in standard liver-function tests (LFTs) and elevations in gamma glutamyltransferase (GGT) and carbohydrate deficient transferrin (CDT) levels (Godsell, Whitfield, Conigrave, Hanratty, & Saunders, 1995 [Level III]). Patients who report use of marijuana and/or other drugs should have toxicology tests to establish baseline use level. Findings should be the basis for brief interventions and counseling.

Nurses in clinical practice need to note frequent changes in habits of drug use and note these in substance-use histories, dating from first use to the current situation. Nurses should ask if an individual ever experienced problems related to drug or alcohol use, spontaneously stopped using a drug or alcohol, or is in recovery and participating in self-help programs, such as Alcoholics Anonymous or Narcotics Anonymous.

In taking the patient history, it is important that the nurse ask the patient about a history of smoking, alcohol use, OTC medications, prescription and recreational drugs, and herbal and food/drink supplement use. The

Quantity-Frequency Index (described herein) should be used to record such information. Another helpful technique in assessing drug use is the Brown Bag technique (see chapter 12, *Reducing Adverse Drug Events*). Ask patients to bring in a brown bag containing all of the prescribed, OTC, food supplements, and other legal/illicit drugs that they consume weekly. Use this material to develop the history and to discuss the implications of the drug use with patients. Be sure to talk with patients about what the use of any drug means to them—that is, if the drug is used to relieve pain, feelings of loneliness, or anxiety (Brennan et al., 2005 [Level III]).

Screening

Screening for alcohol and/or other drug-related problems by nurses, physicians, and other care providers is infrequent in primary and secondary care settings as well as on admission to hospitals or long-term-care facilities (McGlynn et al., 2003 [Level III]). Health providers, family members, and friends may overlook substance-related problems in older persons because they do not disrupt their lives or are not clearly linked to physical disorders. Because health professionals are often pessimistic that older persons can change long-standing behaviors, they do not raise questions about drug and alcohol use; therefore, drug-using patterns are not clearly linked to health problems such as COPD, stroke, or depression. Evidence suggests that many health professionals doubt the effectiveness of alcohol or drug treatment (Vastag, 2002 [Level V]).

Now, however, alcohol and other drug disorders are more often recognized as chronic conditions, characterized by slips and relapses, which respond to treatment (McLellan, Lewis, O'Brien, & Kleber, 2000 [Level VI]). Interventions and treatment must be matched to exacerbations of the disease and stages of recovery. Screening identifies risky drug use or heavy drinking and abuse and dependence (i.e., addiction).

Screening Tools for Alcohol and Drug Use

A Quantity-Frequency Index such as the Khavari Alcohol Test (described next) asks respondents to report their *usual frequency* of drinking, *the usual amount* consumed per occasion, the *maximum amount consumed* on any one occasion, and the *frequency of the maximum amount* (NIAAA, 2003 [Level VI]).

The Khavari Alcohol Test (KAT)

The KAT (Khavari & Farmer, 1978 [Level VI]) consists of the four questions noted previously that are asked for each type of beverage (beer, wine, spirits, liqueurs) and can be administered in 6 to 8 minutes. The amounts can then be compared with NIAAA norms for persons older than 65, which are one drink per day for men and women and no more than three drinks per occasion (USDHHS, 2005 [Level VI]).

Additional questions, such as (1) "Did you ever feel you had a problem related to alcohol or other drug use?," and (2) "Have you ever been treated for an alcohol or drug problem?," can also reveal personal information about problems and treatment related to drug use.

The Michigan Alcohol Screening Test-Geriatric Version (MAST-G)

The MAST-G is an effective tool for screening elders in all settings. The complete drug-use history should be used in comprehensive assessment. The original instrument from which this was derived has a sensitivity of 93.9% and a specificity of 78.1% (Blow et al., 1992 [Level III]).

Alcohol Use Disorders Identification Test (AUDIT)

This 10-item questionnaire has good validity in ethnically mixed groups and scores classify alcohol use as hazardous, harmful, or dependent. Administration: 2 minutes (Saunders, Aasland, Babor, de la Fuente, & Grant, 1993 [Level III]). The AUDIT has been found to have high specificity in adults older than 65 (Babor, Biddle, Saunders, & Monteiro, 2001 [Level IV]).

Fagerstrom Test for Nicotine Dependence (FTND) (revised)

This six-question scale provides an indicator of the severity of nicotine dependence (Scores of 0–2, Very Low, to 8–10, Very High). The questions inquire as to first use early in the day, amount and frequency, inability to refrain, and smoking despite illness. This instrument has good internal consistency and reliability in culturally diverse, mixed-gender samples (Pomerleau, Carton, Lutzke, Flessland, & Pomerleau, 1994 [Level V]).

Intervention and Care Strategies

Because drug and alcohol use affects physical, mental, spiritual, and emotional health, interdisciplinary collaboration is essential to the success of all treatment modalities used for substance-use disorders and related problems. Primary-care providers, psychologists, dentists, nurses, and social workers should all be equipped to detect and refer a problem, and all dimensions of health should be addressed during treatment and aftercare. This is especially true for older persons who are disinclined to seek or continue care with mental health or addictions specialists. Interventions with older adults need to be flexible, individualized, and implemented over time. Brief interventions, such as Frames, and motivational interviewing have been found to be equally effective in producing short-term reduction in alcohol consumption for older as well as younger persons and for both men and women (Ballesteros, Gonzalez-Pinto, Querejeta, & Arino, 2004; Wutzke, Conigrave, Saunders, & Hall, 2002 [Level I]).

Research findings suggest that once enrolled in treatment for alcohol dependence, however, older people treated in chemical-dependency programs with Naltrexone and individualized, supportive, medically based psychosocial interventions have better outcomes than younger patients (Oslin, Pettinati, & Volpolicelli, 2002; Satre, Arean, & Weisner, 2004 [both Level III]).

Inpatient Hospitalization

An older adult who suddenly stops consuming more than 10 ounces of alcohol a day for a week experiences symptoms of withdrawal and has a greater duration of symptoms than younger people. Onset of withdrawal may be as early as 4 to 8 hours after the last drink and can persist up to 72 hours. A key determination is whether the patient requires detoxification. This clinical judgment is made following a history, including history of drug and alcohol use, and physical and mental-status assessments.

A 10- to 28-day period of acute-care hospitalization in a mental health unit or alcohol and drug treatment center is indicated for an older person addicted to alcohol, benzodiazepines, heroin, amphetamines, or cocaine when (1) the living situation and access to the drug makes abstinence unlikely, (2) a likelihood of severe withdrawal symptoms, (3) co-morbid physical or psychiatric diagnoses such as depression and accompanying suicidal ideation are present, (4) daily ingestion of alcohol or a sedative hypnotic has been above the recommended doses for 4 weeks or more, and (5) mixed addiction, as in alcohol and benzodiazepines or cocaine and alcohol. It is helpful if programs specifically designed to meet the needs of older persons are available (USDHHS, 2004a [Level VI]).

Ambulatory Care

People dependent on alcohol, tobacco, and heroin can be successfully withdrawn in community-based care through the collaboration of a medical doctor or nurse practitioner and family members and friends. Specialists in addiction should be sought as supervisors/collaborators in the process. Older persons drinking at risky levels or abusing alcohol or other drugs are generally treated in the community. Tobacco cessation protocols are now available directly to consumers as well as to primary-care providers and mental health professionals.

Residential Treatment

Residential treatment is available in specialty care centers, therapeutic communities, and some long term care facilities. Programs designed specifically for the older person, although not numerous, are beneficial in their focus on the specific challenges to abstinence that an older person faces, such as the long-standing nature of the habits of use, a diminished social network, and challenges to financial and health resources.

Therapeutic Communities

Therapeutic communities provide long-term (up to 18 months) treatment and are abstinence-oriented programs. They use 12-Step Models of individual and group counseling, as well as participation in a social community, to address drug-related problems. For the isolated, older drug user with a history of frequent relapse, these are good treatment options.

Pharmacological Treatment

Agents for pharmacological treatment of substance abuse and dependence are more numerous than previously but not all are appropriate for use with elders. The best outcomes of pharmacological interventions occur when they are used with individual and/or group counseling. Attendance at 12-step programs also enhances adherence to treatment regimens.

Alcohol Abuse/Dependence Pharmacological Treatment

Alcohol Dependence: Naltrexone, in the form of Revia, is used to decrease cravings in heavy drinkers and is now available in injectable form, Vivitrex. Vivitrex is an extended-release formulation of naltrexone that acts up to 28 days to decrease the euphoric effects of and craving for alcohol (Bartus et al., 2003). Evidence suggests that it is well tolerated by older people who do not have renal problems. Study findings stress the importance of psychosocial interventions to improve adherence to pharmacologic interventions for alcohol dependence, a finding similar to those regarding smoking cessation (Reid, Teeson, Sannibale, Matsuda, & Haber, 2005 [Level III]). Acamprosate (Campral), a recent addition to prescription drug choices, has appeared promising but outcomes in reducing the craving and consumption of alcohol are variable. Antabuse or Disulfiram to deter alcohol consumption produce an elevation in vital signs and severe gastrointestinal symptoms if alcohol is ingested and is poorly tolerated by an alcoholic older than 55. In addition, it must be taken every day if aversive effects on consumption are to occur.

Opioid Dependence: The use of methadone, an opioid agonist, assists the opioid-dependent person to focus on psychological and life problems. The drug Buprenorphine, both an opioid antagonist and agonist, is longer acting and now available. Involvement in psychosocial treatment may assist in patient adherence to pharmacologic treatment (Mayer, Farrell, Ferri, Amato, & Davoli, 2005 [Level I]).

Smoking: Buproprion in doses of 75 mg with administration begun 2 weeks before the smoker intends to quit has proved a helpful adjunct to smoking cessation (NYC DH&MH, 2002 [Level III]). Nicorette transdermal patches and nicotine gum are now available OTC and there is research support for their pharmacological contribution to smoking cessation. The best outcomes with smoking cessation are a combination of individual or group psychosocial support and the medications described herein (NYC DH&MH, 2002 [Level III]).

Individualized Plan of Care

Individualized care plans should be developed for elders at risk for substance abuse or dependence in accord with the classes of drugs used and the severity of the disorders. Guidelines for all interventions should include the following:

- A nonjudgmental, health-oriented approach to substance-related problems. Drug/alcohol use and abuse are highly stigmatized in American society, particularly in minority communities, leading to denial and/or rejection by family members. When nurses and other health professionals understand addiction as a disease, approaches similar to care for other chronic illness can be planned.

- A supportive, encouraging approach to the possibilities of changing use habits. Using the Stages of Change Model helps the patient/client understand that change occurs in stages and that support and assistance are available at each stage (Prochaska & Di Clemente, 1992 [Level II]).
- Education of patient and family on the risks associated with drug misuse in older people. Because older persons use so many medications, the potential health consequences may be minimized in the eyes of others.
- Assessment of substance use in relation to lifestyle, existing chronic illnesses, nutritional patterns, sleep, exercise, sexual patterns, and recreation. Counsel the patient and/or family about the effects of substances used in these areas of the patient's life.
- Set the goal of "Harm Reduction" in the forms of decreased use and supervised use if abstinence is not imperative or achievable.
- Monitor substance-use patterns at each encounter or visit, documenting changes and providing reinforcement of positive changes and/or movement toward treatment.
- Enhance the involvement of members of the patient's support system, including family and friends identified by the patient, community-based groups, support groups, appropriate clergy, or organizational groups such as senior centers.
- Support the development of coping mechanisms, including modifications in social, housing, and recreational environments, to minimize associations with settings and groups in which substance use and abuse are common (USDHHS, 2004a [Level VI]).

Counseling and Psychotherapy

Older people tend to seek care from their primary care, medical specialist, or nurse/nurse practitioner provider even in regard to assistance with mental health and substance-related problems. This practice relates to old beliefs about depression or anxiety being manifestations of weakness or lack of character.

Excess use of alcohol or use of an illicit drug or misuse of prescriptions drugs remain socially stigmatized, especially among older persons. Counseling done by the nurse using a brief intervention model or supportive counseling is more readily acceptable to older patients than referral to mental health or substance-abuse clinics.

Optimally, short-term psychotherapy by a practitioner knowledgeable in substances and their problematic use is extremely helpful. The model of cognitive behavioral therapy, in particular, has demonstrated good outcomes with excessive drinking and marijuana use (Project Match, 1997 [Level III]). These approaches assist an older person to modify behavior and to deal with negative feelings and/or chronic pain that often motivate use.

Treatment Outcomes

Health care providers and older persons may feel pessimistic about the possibilities of changing their substance-use behavior. Health providers often do not intervene because they believe that older people cannot change. Treatment outcomes for older persons with substance-use problems, however, have been shown to be as good as or better than those for younger people (Atkinson & Ganzini, 1994 [Level VI]; Oslin, Liberto, O'Brien, Krois, & Norbeck, 1997 [Level III]). A compromising factor to good treatment outcomes is the inconsistency with which aftercare is available to older adults by community and specific to the needs of older adults.

Case Study and Discussion

Joseph and Mary P., both 71, reside in a small rural community where Mr. P. owned the only pharmacy. Retired 5 years, Mr. P. suffers from arthritis and Mrs. P. has mitral valve insufficiency, which frequently results in cardiac symptoms that are frightening but readily managed. She has also been treated for generalized anxiety disorder for which she has been prescribed Paxil. The couple enjoys a nightly cocktail hour at which Mr. P. consumes two scotch whiskies and Mrs. P. has "wine." Recently, the visiting nurse who has been monitoring Mrs. P.'s recovery from a recent episode of congestive heart failure, received a phone call from their daughter who stated that on her last three evening phone calls to her parents, Mrs. P. sounded somewhat confused and her speech was slurred. When the daughter questioned Mr. P. about their drinking, he became irritable and defensive.

The visiting nurse made it a point to visit the P.'s in the early evening on her way home. She found them enjoying their cocktails and took the opportunity to conduct a drug and alcohol assessment, including making a list of all of their medications. The nurse diagnosed "drug misuse" because it appears that neither of them considered how their continued alcohol use was affecting their bodies in older age. She conducted a brief intervention, giving them feedback about their respective illnesses, pointed out the pros and cons of modifying their drinking, such as decreasing the gastric distress Mr. P. experiences, and the benefits of limited wine intake while taking Paxil. The nurse educated them (building on autonomy and responsibility) about the relationship between bodily changes and the increased effects of alcohol on their sleep patterns, mood, and balance. She also pointed out that both were consuming alcohol above one daily drink and recommended that they cut down to one standard drink per day. At first, they seemed unhappy about the recommendation but both committed to attempting to do so. When she visited 2 weeks later, they had begun to journal their drinking and both were recording consistent declines in the amount of alcohol consumed.

Summary and Conclusions

Two current trends are predicted to result in an increase in the already significant number of men and women older than 55 who experience various substance-use–related disorders: the growing numbers of older persons in America, and the continuation of drug and alcohol use patterns established earlier in life. Although most people decrease the amount of alcohol and kinds of drugs they use with age, anywhere from 10% to 24% of older persons do not (US-DHHS, 2004b [Level VI]). The most common type of substance-use disorders is heavy drinking, especially by Caucasian men older than 65 and living alone (US-DHHS, 2004b [Level VI]). The high numbers of prescription drugs used by elders also pose serious problems related to misuse and drug interactions. Health professionals are disinclined to query elders about substance use, with the result that problems become known in the context of the care of other medical disorders. Nurses in daily contact with institutionalized and community-dwelling elders must be skilled in screening for and counseling about the use of nicotine, alcohol, and prescription, illicit, and OTC drugs. Educating patient and family about health risks and referring patients to specialists and community resources are essential "best practices."

Resources

Web sites

AHCPR Guidelines: AHCPR Clinical Practice Guidelines are available to download.
http://www.ahcpr.gov

American Nurses' Association
http://www.ana.org

American Psychiatric Association
http://www.apa.org

American Psychiatric Nursing Association
http://www.apna.org

Center for Disease Control and Prevention
www.cdc.gov/tobacco/how2quit.htm

National Institute of Mental Health: Download patient teaching materials for Panic Disorders, Obsessive Compulsive Disorder, Posttraumatic Stress, Acute Stress, and General Anxiety Disorders
http://www.nih.nimh.gov

National Institute of Alcohol and Alcohol Abuse (NIAAA)
http://www.nih.niaaa.gov
National Institute of Drug Abuse (NIDA)
http://www.nih.nida.gov

Centers for Disease Control and Prevention (CDC)
http://www.cdc.gov/tobacco/how2quit.html

NYC Department of Health
http://www.nyc.gov/htm/doh/html

International Nurses' Society on Addictions
http://www.intnsa.org/

American Lung Association
http://www.ffsonline.org

Assessment Tools

Clinical Guidelines for the Use of Buprenorphine in the Treatment of Opioid Dependence. Download from http://www.guideline.gov/summary/summary. aspx?ss=15&doc-id=5887&nbr=3873

See GeroNurseOnline, topic Substance Abuse, for assessment tools and other important resources at http://www.ConsultGeriRN.org

Alcohol Use Disorders Identification Test (AUDIT Tool) AUDIT: Saunders, J. B., Asland, O. G., Babor, T. F., et al. 1993 [Level III]). WHO collaborative project on early detection of persons with harmful alcohol consumption II. Development of the screening instrument AUDIT. *Addiction, 88,* 79–804.

Clinical Institute Withdrawal Assessment of Alcohol Scale, Revised (CIWA-AR). (Sullivan, Sykora, Schneiderman, Naranjo, & Sellers, 1989 [Level III]). Downloaded from http://209.85.165.104/search?q=cache:ypb-pA96p3EJ: images2.clinical tools.com/images/pd.

Quantity-Frequency Index: *The Khavari Alcohol Test* (KAT) (Khavari & Farmer, 1978)

Fagerstrom Test for Nicotine Dependence (FTND) (revised 1991). Access online at American Psychiatric Association PsychNET 2002 at http://www.apa.org/ videos/fagerstrom.html

FRAMES: Dyehouse, J., Howe, S., & Ball, S. (1996 [Level VI]). FRAMES model in the Training Manual for Nursing Using Brief Intervention for Alcohol Problems. U.S. Department of Health and Human Services: Rockville, MD. Access online at SAMHA (Substance Abuse and Mental Health Association) Pathways Courses: Silence Hurts. http://pathwayscourses.samhsa.gov/ vawp/vawp_supps_pg20.htm

SMAST: Naegle, M.A. (2003).Try This: Best practices in nursing care of older adults: Alcohol use screening and assessment, Issue # 17. A series provided by The Hartford Institute for Geriatric Nursing. New York University College of Nursing. http://www.ConsultGeriRN.org/publications/trythis/issue17.pdf

Guidelines

The National Quality Forum is completing review for "Evidence-based practices to treat substance use disorders." These guidelines are inclusive of primary care, the settings in which most elders seek treatment. Accessed March 29, 2007, from http://www.qualityforum.org/projects/completed/substance_ abuse.asp

The following guidelines were accessed March 29, 2007, from AHRQ/NGC Web site at www.guideline.gov:

■ Elder abuse prevention. University of Iowa Gerontological Nursing Interventions Research Center, Research Translation and Dissemination Core– Academic Institution. 2004 Dec. 68 pages. NGC:004196 or access hardcopy from Gerontological Nursing Interventions Research Center

(GNRIC) at University of Iowa. Accessed March 29, 2007, from http://www.nursing.uiowa.edu/centers/gnirc/rtdcore.htm

- Screening and ongoing assessment for substance use. New York State Department of Health—State/Local Government Agency (U.S.). 2005 Mar. 11 pages. NGC:004202. Accessed May 3, 2007, from http://www.guideline.gov/summary/summary.aspx?doc_id=6848&nbr=004202&string=alcohol+AND+abuse

- Management of alcohol withdrawal delirium. An evidence-based practice guideline. American Society of Addiction Medicine—Medical Specialty Society. 2004 Jul 12. 8 pages. NGC:004109. Accessed May 3, 2007, from http://www.guideline.gov/summary/summary.aspx?doc_id=6543&nbr=004109&string=alcohol+AND+abuse

- Detoxification and substance abuse treatment: An overview of the psychosocial and biomedical issues during detoxification. Substance Abuse and Mental Health Services Administration (U.S.)—Federal Government Agency (U.S.). 2006. 23 pages. NGC:004931. Accessed May 3, 2007, from http://www.guideline.gov/summary/summary.aspx?doc_id=9117&nbr=004931&string=alcohol+AND+abuse

- Screening and management of substance use disorders. Michigan Quality Improvement Consortium. 2003 Aug. (revised 2005 Aug.). 1 page. NGC:004548. Accessed May 3, 2007, from http://www.guideline.gov/summary/summary.aspx?doc_id=8161&nbr=004548&string=alcohol+AND+abuse

- Medication-assisted treatment for opioid addiction in opioid treatment programs: Clinical pharmacotherapy. Substance Abuse and Mental Health Services Administration (U.S.)—Federal Government Agency (U.S.). 2005. 23 pages. NGC:004672. Accessed May 3, 2007, from http://www.guideline.gov/summary/summary.aspx?doc_id=8349&nbr=004672&string=alcohol+AND+abuse

- Medication-assisted treatment for opioid addiction in opioid treatment programs: Phases of treatment. Substance Abuse and Mental Health Services Administration (U.S.)—Federal Government Agency (U.S.). 2005. 20 pages. NGC:004674. Accessed May 3, 2007, from http://www.guideline.gov/summary/summary.aspx?doc_id=8351&nbr=004674&string=alcohol+AND+abuse

- Medication-assisted treatment for opioid addiction in opioid treatment programs: Drug testing as a tool. Substance Abuse and Mental Health Services Administration (U.S.)—Federal Government Agency (U.S.). 2005. 17 pages. NGC:004676. Accessed May 3, 2007, from http://www.guideline.gov/summary/summary.aspx?doc_id=8353&nbr=004676&string=alcohol+AND+abuse

- Detoxification and substance abuse treatment: Settings, levels of care, and patient placement. Substance Abuse and Mental Health Services Administration (U.S.)—Federal Government Agency (U.S.). 2006. 10 pages. NGC:004930. Accessed May 3, 2007, from http://www.guideline.gov/summary/summary.aspx?doc_id=9116&nbr=004930&string=alcohol+AND+abuse

- Medication-assisted treatment for opioid addiction in opioid treatment programs: Approaches to providing comprehensive care and maximizing patient retention. Substance Abuse and Mental Health Services Administration (U.S.)—Federal Government Agency (U.S.). 2005. 22 pages. NGC:004675. Accessed May 3, 2007, from http://www.guideline.gov/summary/summary.aspx?doc_id=8352&nbr=004675&string=alcohol+AND+abuse

- Substance abuse treatment and family therapy. Substance Abuse and Mental Health Services Administration (U.S.)—Federal Government Agency (U.S.). 2004. 232 pages. NGC:003872. Accessed May 3, 2007, from http://www.guideline.gov/summary/summary.aspx?doc_id=5886&nbr=003872&string=alcohol+AND+abuse

Older Americans Substance Abuse and Mental Health Technical Assistance Center

Evidence-Based Practices for Preventing Substance Abuse and Mental Health Problems in Older Adults
http://www.samhsa.gov/OlderAdultsTAC/EBPLiteratureReviewFINAL.pdf

Box 29.1

Nursing Standard of Practice Protocol: Substance Abuse in Older Adults

I. **GOAL:** Implement best nursing practices to care for older persons with drug, alcohol, tobacco, or other drug abuse or dependencies.

II. OVERVIEW

A. Several factors increase the risks associated with alcohol and drug use for an older individual, making any drug use in circumstances that, earlier in life were commonplace, potentially harmful. Constitutional risk factors include changes in body composition like decreased muscle mass, decreased organ efficiency (especially kidney and liver), and increased vulnerability of the central nervous system (Lang, 2001 [Level VI]; Kennedy, 2000 [Level IV]).

B. The consequences of alcohol use in combination with other drugs and excessive use include falls, impaired cognition, malnourishment, and decreased resistance to disease, interpersonal, and legal problems (Kennedy, 2000 [Level IV]).

C. At-risk drinking for older adults increases the likelihood of negative health consequences and is defined as more than one drink per day, 7 days a week, or more than three drinks on any one occasion (USDHHS, 2004 [Level V]).

D. Any amount of smoking places older persons at risk for negative health consequences, and advancing age increases the likelihood of the emergence of respiratory and cardiovascular illnesses.

III. BACKGROUND/STATEMENT OF PROBLEM

A. Definitions
1. *Substance Use Disorders*: A broad category of disorders that include a continuum of use or misuse of alcohol, tobacco, prescription or illicit drugs, and the abuse or dependence on these drugs (modified from APA, 2000).
2. *Substance Abuse*: A maladaptive pattern of substance use evidenced in recurrent and significant adverse consequences related to the repeated use of substances. It is associated with repeated failure to fulfill role obligations, use in situations where use is physically hazardous, and/or when it results in legal and/or interpersonal problems (modified from APA, 2000).
3. *Substance Dependence*: A pattern of self-administration of a drug that is maladaptive and results in the development of tolerance, withdrawal, and compulsive drug-taking behavior. Dependence is both physiologic and psychological (modified from APA, 2000).
4. *Drug Misuse*: Use of a drug for purposes other than that for which it was intended.
5. *Polysubstance-Related Disorder*: Misuse, abuse, or dependence on three or more drugs (modified from APA, 2000).
6. *Tolerance*: (1) A need for markedly increased amounts of a substance to achieve intoxication or the desired effects, or (2) a markedly diminished effects with the continued use of the same amount of a substance (APA, 2000).
7. *Withdrawal*: A characteristic group of signs and symptoms that has its onset following the sudden cessation of consumption of a drug (including alcohol and nicotine) that induces physiologic dependence (APA, 2000).
8. *At-Risk Drinking*: Defined as more than one drink per day, 7 days a week, or more than three drinks on any one occasion. For elders, at-risk drinking increases the likelihood of negative health consequences (Fleming, Manwell, Barry, & Johnson, 1998 [Level III]).

B. Etiology and/or Epidemiology
1. In 1998, the prevalence of alcoholism, alcohol abuse, or problem drinking in persons aged 60+ was estimated at 5% to 10% in community studies. Approximately 11% of men and 9% of women 75 years and older report heavy use, placing them "at risk" for a range of problems (Fleming et al., 1998 [Level III]).
2. Excessive drinking among individuals of all ethnic groups 65+ years is approximately 7%, down from 12% in persons ages 55 to 64 (NYC DH&MH, 2005).
3. 500,000 persons ages 55 and older reported monthly use of illicit drugs in the National Household Survey of Drug Use National Institute of Drug Abuse (NIDA, 2001).
4. Approximately 11% of women older than 59 misuse psychoactive drugs (Fingeld-Connett, 2004 [Level IV]).

C. Risk Factors (USDHHS, 2004b [Level VI])
1. Family history of dependence on alcohol, tobacco, prescription or illicit drugs
2. Co-occurrence of addiction with dependency or abuse of another substance dependence (i.e., alcohol and tobacco)
3. Lifelong pattern of substance use, including heavy drinking
4. Male gender
5. Social isolation
6. Recent and multiple losses
7. Chronic pain
8. Co-occurrence with depression
9. Unmarried and/or living alone

IV. PARAMETERS OF ASSESSMENT

A. Screening for alcohol, tobacco, and other drug use is recommended for all community-dwelling and hospitalized older adults. It is essential that the nurse:
1. state the purpose of questions about substances used and link them to health and safety
2. be empathic and nonjudgmental
3. ask the questions when the patient is alcohol- and drug-free
4. inquire re: patient's understanding of the question (Aalto, Pekuri, & Seppa, 2003 [Level III])

B. Assessment/Screening Tools
1. The Quantity-Frequency Index (Khavari & Farber, 1978 [Level VI]): Review all classes of drugs: alcohol, nicotine, illicit drugs, prescription drugs, OTC drugs and vitamin supplements, for each drug used. *Record the Types* of drugs, including types of beverages; *Frequency*: the number of occasions on which the drug is consumed (daily, weekly, monthly); *Amount of drug consumed* on each occasion during the last 30 days. The psychological function that the substance serves for the individual is also important to identify. The Quantity-Frequency Index tool should be part of the intake nursing history. The Brown Bag approach is useful. The patient is asked to bring all drugs and supplements listed herein to the interview with the provider (Armor, Polish, & Stambul, 1978 [Level VI]).
2. Short Michigan Alcohol Screening Test-Geriatric Version (SMAST-G):
Highly valid and reliable, this is a 10-item tool that can be used in all settings. Three minutes for administration. This instrument is derived from the MAST-G with a sensitivity of 93.6% and positive predictive values of 87.2% (Blow et al., 1992 [Level III]).
3. Alcohol Use Disorders Identification Test (AUDIT):
This 10-item questionnaire has good validity in ethnically mixed groups and scores classify alcohol use as hazardous, harmful, or

dependent. Administration: 2 minutes. Sensitivity scores range from 0.74% to 0.84% and specificity around 0.90% in mixed age and ethnic groups (Allen, Fertig, Litten, & Babor, 1997 [Level III]). This instrument is highly effective for use with elders as well (Roberts, Marshall, & MacDonald, 2005 [Level III]).

    4. Fagerstrom Test for Nicotine Dependence (Pomerleau, et al., 1994 [Level V]):

    This six-question scale provides an indicator of the severity of nicotine dependence (Scores of 0–2, Very low, to 8–10, Very High). The questions inquire as to first use early in the day, amount and frequency, inability to refrain, and smoking despite illness. This instrument has good internal consistency and reliability in culturally diverse, mixed-gender samples (Pomerleau et al., 1994 [Level V]).

C. Atypical Presentation:

Men and women older than 65 may have substance-use and dependence problems even though the signs and symptoms may not correspond to those listed in the *DSM-IV TR*.

D. Signs of CNS Intoxication (i.e., slurred speech, drowsiness, unsteady gait, decreased reaction time, impaired judgment, disinhibition, ataxia):

    1. Assess in individual or collateral (speaking with family members) data collection, consumption of amount and type of depressant medications including alcohol, sedatives, hypnotics, and opioid or synthetic opioid analgesics.

    2. Assess vital signs and determine respiratory, cardiac, or neurological depression.

    3. Assess for treatable existing medical conditions, including depression.

    4. Arrange for emergency room/hospitalization treatment as necessary.

    5. Obtain urine for toxicology, if possible.

E. At-risk Drinking Consumption of alcohol in excess of one drink per day for seven days a week or more than three drinks on any one occasion (USDHHS, 2005 [Level VI]).

    1. Assess for readiness to change behavior using Stages of Change Model (Prochaska & Di Clemente, 1992 [Level II]).

    2. Is drinker concerned about amount or consequences of the drinking? Has she/he contemplated cutting down?

    3. Does she/he have a plan for cutting down/stopping consumption?

    4. Has he/she previously stopped but then resumed risky drinking?

    5. Personalized feedback and education and education on at-risk drinking results in a reduction in at-risk drinking among older primary-care patients (Fink et al., 2005 [Level III]).

F. Signs of Withdrawal of CNS Depressant Drugs (including alcohol such as tremors, disorientation, tachycardia, irritability, anxiety, insomnia, moderate diaphoresis):
   1. May develop extreme CNS stimulation and progress to seizures, hallucinosis, withdrawal delirium, extreme hypertension, profuse diarrhea, from 4 to 8 hours and for up to 72 hours following cessation of alcohol intake (Delirium Tremens/DTs).
   2. Assess for risk factors: (a) previous episodes of detoxification, (b) recent heavy drinking, (c) medical co-morbidities including liver disease, pneumonia, anemia, (d) previous history of seizures or delirium (Wetterling, Weber, Depfenhart, Schneider, & Junghanns, 2006 [Level III]).
   3. Assess neurological signs using the *CIWA-AR*. This Clinical Institute Withdrawal Assessment of Alcohol Scale, revised (CIWA-Ar), is a 10-item rating scale that delineates symptoms of gastric distress, perceptual distortions, cognitive impairment, anxiety, agitation, and headache (Sullivan, Sykora, Schneiderman, Naranjo, & Sellers, 1989 [Level III]).
   4. Medicate with a short-acting benzodiazepine (Lorazepam or Oxazepam) in doses titrated to patient's score on the CIWA, patient's age and weight (Sullivan et al., 1989 [Level III]).
G. Reported Sleep Disturbance, Anxiety, Depression, Problems with Attention and Concentration (Acute Care):
   1. Assess for neuropsychiatric conditions using the Mental Status exam, Geriatric Depression Scale, or Hamilton Anxiety Scale.
   2. Obtain sleep history because drugs disrupt already altered sleep patterns in older persons.
   3. Assess intake of all drugs, including alcohol, OTC, prescription, herbal and food supplements, and nicotine. Use Brown Bag strategy.
   4. If positive for alcohol use, assess for last time of use and amount used.
   5. Assess for alcohol or sedative drug withdrawal as indicated.
H. Smoking Cigarettes or Using Smokeless Tobacco:
   1. Assess for level of dependence using the Fagerstrom Test (See tool above).

V. NURSING-CARE STRATEGIES

A. At-risk Drinking (consumption of alcohol in excess of one drink per day for seven days a week or more than three drinks on any one occasion.):
   1. Hydrate with clear fluid p.o. as indicated. Limit use of intravenous fluid except as necessary. Hospitalize if:
      a. Blood alcohol level (BAL) >100 mg/dL
      b. Severe withdrawal symptoms
      c. Suicidal ideation or attempts

      d. Co-morbid conditions that compromise treatment

      e. Polysubstance dependence

  2. Conduct Brief Intervention (FRAMES) (Dyehouse, Howe, & Ball, 1996 [Level VI]):

      a. Feedback information to patients about current health problems or potential problems associated with their level of consumption.

      b. Responsible choice about how to respond to the information provided to the patients is their choice.

      c. Advice must be clear about drinking their amounts and recommended moderate levels of drinking.

      d. Menu of choices is provided by the nurse to the patient/client regarding future drinking behaviors.

      e. Empathy is essential to the exchange. Offer information based on scientific evidence, acknowledge the difficulty of change, avoid confrontation.

      f. Self-efficacy of the individual is supported and the nurse helps patient explore options for change.

B. Smoking cigarettes or using smokeless tobacco.

  1. Apply the Five A's Intervention (AHCPR Guidelines):

      a. Ask: Identify and document tobacco use.

      b. Advise: Urge the user to quit in a strong personalized manner.

      c. Assess: Is the tobacco user willing to make a quit attempt at this time?

      d. Assist: If user is willing to attempt, refer for individual or group counseling and pharmacotherapy.

      e. Arrange: Referrals to providers, agencies, and self-help groups. Monitor pharmacotherapy once quit date is established. FDA-approved pharmacotherapies for smoking cessation are:

        ■ Bupropion SR (Zyban) and nicotine replacement products such as nicotine gum, nicotine inhalers, nicotine nasal spray, and nicotine patch. Psychoeducation about these medications is essential.

        ■ Zyban, for example, should not be combined with alcohol. Nurses working with in-patients in a case-management model were found to produce outcomes in smoking cessation (Smith, Reilly, Houston-Miller, DeBusk, & Taylor, 2002; Daniel, Cropley, Usher, & West, 2004 [both Level II]).

  2. Communicate Caring and Concern:

      a. Encourage moderate intensity exercise as a means of reducing cravings for nicotine because 5 minutes of such exercises is associated with short-term reduction in the desire to smoke and tobacco withdrawal symptoms (Daniel et al., 2004 [Level II]).

      b. Arrange: Schedule follow-up contact in person or by telephone within 1 week after planned quit date. Continue telephone counseling for those using nicotine patches (Cooper et al., 2004; Boyle et al., 2005 [Level III]).

C. Smoking Marijuana: Little research regarding effective intervention for psychological dependence on marijuana is available. Some guidance can be found in smoking cessation and self-help approaches.

1. Refer to Steps for Smoking Cessation.
2. Refer patient to addiction specialist for counseling for psychological dependence and/or cognitive-behavioral therapy.
3. Refer to community-based self-help groups such as Narcotics Anonymous, Alcoholics Anonymous, and Al-Anon.
4. Encourage development or expansion of patient's social support system.

D. Heroin or Opioid Dependence

1. Older long-term opioid users may relapse and require treatment. Methadone or Buprenorphine are current pharmacological treatment options, effective in conjunction with self-help programs and/or psychosocial interventions (Clinical Guidelines for the use of Buprenorphine in the treatment of opioid addiction, 2006 [Level IV]).
2. Treatment with methadone, a synthetic narcotic agonist, suppresses withdrawal symptoms and drug cravings associated with opioid dependence but requires daily dosing of 60 mg, minimum. It is dispensed only in specially licensed clinics.
3. Buprenorphine (Subutex or Suboxone), recently approved for use in office practice by trained physicians, is an opioid partial agonist-antagonist. Alone and in combination with Naloxone (Suboxone), it can prevent withdrawal when someone ceases use of an opioid drug and can be used for long-term treatment. Naloxone is an opioid antagonist used to reverse depressant symptoms in opiate overdose and at different dosages to treat dependence.
   ■ Close collaboration with the prescriber is required because these drugs should not be abruptly terminated, used with antidepressants, and interact negatively with many prescription medications.
4. Naltrexone, a long-acting opioid antagonist, blocks opioid effects and is most effective with those who are no longer opioid-dependent but are at high risk for relapse (Srisurapanont & Jarusuraisin, 2005 [Level III]).
5. Treatment of an older patient who has become addicted to oxycontin or other opioids should be done in consultation with an addictions specialist nurse or physician.
   a. It is recommended that the prescriber avoid opioids and the synthetic opioids Demerol, Dilaudid, and Oxycontin. The opioids have high potential for addiction and Demerol has been associated with delirium in elders (Collins & Kleber, 2004 [Level VI].

      b. Barbiturates should be avoided for use as hypnotics and the use of benzodiazepines for anxiety should be limited to 4 months (USDHHS, 2004b [Level VI]).

  E. Relapse Prevention

    1. Monitor pharmacologic treatment such as Naltrexone as short-term treatment for alcohol dependence. The benefits of this treatment are dependent on adherence, and psychosocial treatment should accompany its use (WHO, 2000 [Level I]). Methadone or Buprenorphine should be used for long-term treatment of opioid dependence.

    2. Refer to community-based Alcoholics Anonymous, Narcotics Anonymous, Al-Anon groups, and encourage attendance.

    3. Educate family and patient regarding signs of risky use or relapse to heavy or alcohol-dependent behavior.

    4. Counsel patient to reduce drug use (Harm Reduction) and engage in relationship healing/building, community or intellectually rewarding activities, spiritual growth, which increase valued nondrinking rewards.

    5. Counsel in the development of coping skills:

      a. Anticipate and avoid temptation.

      b. Learn cognitive strategies to avoid negative moods.

      c. Make lifestyle changes to reduce stress, improve the quality of life, and increase pleasure.

      d. Learn cognitive and behavioral activities to cope with cravings and urges to use.

      e. Encourage development or expansion of patient's social support system.

VI. EVALUATION/EXPECTED OUTCOMES

  A. Patient will have:

    1. Improved physical health and function.

    2. Improved quality of life, sense of well-being and mental health.

    3. More satisfying interpersonal relationships.

    4. Enhanced productivity and mental alertness.

    5. Decreased likelihood of falls and other accidents.

  B. Nurses will have:

    1. Increased accuracy in detecting patient problems related to use/misuse of substances.

    2. Interventions will be more evidence-based resulting in better outcomes.

  C. Institution will have:

    1. Increased number of referrals to ambulatory substance-abuse/mental health treatment programs.

    2. Improved links with community-based organizations engaged in prevention, education, and treatment of elders with substance-related disorders.

VII. FOLLOW-UP MONITORING OF CONDITION

    A. Evaluate for increase in substance use/misuse associated with growing numbers of aging adults.

    B. Increase outreach to targeted vulnerable populations.

    C. Document chronic care needs of elders diagnosed with substance-related disorders.

    D. Monitor alcohol use among older adults with chronic pain (Brennan, Schutte, & Moos, 2005 [Level III]).

    E. Communicate findings to all members of the involved caregiver team.

VIII. GUIDELINES

The National Quality Forum is completing review for "Evidence-based practices to treat substance use disorders." These guidelines are inclusive of primary care, the settings in which most elders seek treatment.

References

Aalto, M., Pekuri, P., & Seppa, K. (2003). Primary health care professionals' activity in intervening in patients' alcohol drinking during a 3-year brief intervention implementation project. *Drug and Alcohol Dependence, 69*(1), 9–14. Evidence Level III: Quasi-experimental Study.

Allen, J. P., Litten, R. Z., Fertig, J. B., & Babor, T. (1997). A review of research on the Alcohol Use Disorders Identification Test (AUDIT). *Alcohol, Clinical and Experimental Research, 21*(4), 613–619. Evidence Level III: Quasi-experimental Study.

American Lung Association (2003). Smoking. Downloaded from http://www.lungusa.org/site/apps/s. Evidence Level IV: Nonexperimental Study.

American Lung Association (2006). Smoking among older adults. http://www.lungusa.org/site/apps/s. Evidence Level IV: Nonexperimental Study.

American Psychiatric Association (2000). *Diagnostic and statistical manual of mental disorders-IV-TR* (4th ed.). Washington, DC: American Psychiatric Association: Author.

Armor, D. J., Polish, M., & Stambul, H. B. (1978). *Alcoholism and treatment.* New York: Plenum Press. Evidence Level VI: Expert Opinion.

Atkinson, R. M., & Ganzini, L. (1994). Substance abuse. In Coffey, C. E., & Cummings, J. L. (Eds), *Textbook of geriatric neuropsychiatry.* Washington, DC: American Psychiatric Press. Evidence Level VI: Expert Opinion.

Babor, T. F., Biddle, J. H., Saunders, J. B., & Monteiro, M. G. (2001). *AUDIT, The alcohol use disorders identification test: Guidelines for use in primary care.* Geneva, Switzerland: The World Health Organization. Evidence Level IV: Nonexperimental Study.

Ballesteros, J., Gonzalez-Pinto, A., Querejeta, I., & Arino, J. (2004). Brief interventions for hazardous drinkers delivered in primary care are equally effective in men and women. *Addiction, 9*(9), 103–108.

Bartels, S. J., Coakley, E. H., Zubritsky, C., Ware, J. H., Miles, K. M., Arean, P. A., et al. (2004). Improving access to geriatric mental health services: A randomized trial comparing treatment engagement with integrated versus enhanced referral care for depression, anxiety, and at risk alcohol use. *American Journal of Psychiatry, 16*(8), 1455–1456. Evidence Level III: Quasi-experimental Study.

Bartus, R. T., Emerich, D. F., Hotz, J., Blaustein, M., Dean, R. L., Perdodmo, B., et al. (2003). Vivitrex, an injectable, extended release formulation of naltrexone, provides pharmokinetic and pharmacodynamic evidence of efficacy for 1 month in rats. *Neuropsychopharmacology, 28*(11):1973–1982.

Blow, F. (1998). *Substance abuse among older adults consensus panel for the treatment improvement protocol (TIP) Series 26*. Retrieved March 22, 2007, from http://www.ncbi.nlm.nih.gov/books/bv.fcgi?rid=hstat5.chapter.48302.

Blow, F. C., Brower, K. J., Schulenberg, J. E., Demo-Danenberg, L. M., Young, J. P., & Beresford, T. P. (1992). Michigan Alcoholism Screening Test-Geriatric Version: A new elderly specific screening instrument. *Alcoholism, Clinical and Experimental Research, 16*(2), 372. Evidence Level III: Quasi-experimental Study.

Blow, F. C., Walton, M. A., Barry, K. L., Coyne, L. C., Mudd, J., & Copeland, L. A. (2000). The relationship between alcohol problems and health functioning of older adults in primary care settings. *Journal of the American Geriatrics Society, 48*, 769–774. Evidence Level III: Quasi-experimental Study.

Boyle, R. G., Solberg, L. I., Asche, S. E., Boucher, J. L., Pronk, N. P., & Jensen, D. J. (2005). Offering telephone counseling to smokers using pharmacotherapy. *Nicotine & Tobacco Research, 7*(Suppl. 1), S19–S27. Evidence Level III: Quasi-experimental Study.

Brennan, P. L., Schutte, K. K., & Moos, R. H. (2005). Pain and use of alcohol to manage pain: Prevalence and 3-year outcomes among older problem and non-problem drinkers. *Society for the Study of Addiction, 100*, 777–786. Evidence Level III: Quasi-experimental Study.

Center for Alcohol and Substance Abuse (CASA) (1998). *Under the rug: Substance abuse and the mature woman*. New York: Columbia University. Evidence Level IV: Nonexperimental Study.

Centers for Disease Control (CDC) (2005). Annual smoking attributable mortality, years of potential life lost, and productivity losses: United States, 1997–2001. *Morbidity and Mortality Weekly Report, 54*(25), 625–628. Evidence Level V: Review.

Collins, E. D., & Kleber, H. D. (2004). Opioids. In M. Galanter & H. D. Kleber (Eds.), *Textbook of substance abuse treatment*. Washington, DC: American Psychiatric Association. Level VI: Expert Opinion.

Colliver, J. D., Compton, W. M., Gfroerer, J. C., & Condon, T. (2002). Projecting drug use among aging baby boomers by 2020. *Annals of Epidemiology, 16*(4), 257–265. Evidence Level III: Quasi-experimental Study.

Cooper, T. V., DeBon, M. W., Stockton, M., Kleges, R. C., Steenbergh, T. A., & Sherrill-Mittleman, D., et al. (2004). Correlates of adherence to transdermal nicotine. *Addictive Behaviors, 29*(8), 1565–1578.

Daniel, J., Cropley, M., Usher, M., & West, R. (2004). Acute effects of a short bout of moderate versus light intensity exercise versus inactivity on tobacco withdrawal symptoms in sedentary smokers. *Psychopharmacology, 174*(3), 320–326. Evidence Level II: Individual Experimental Study.

Dyehouse, J., Howe, S., & Ball, S. (1996). *FRAMES model in training manual for nursing using brief intervention for alcohol problems*. Retrieved March 22, 2007, from http://pathwayscourses.samhsa.gov/vawp/vawp_supps_pg20.htm. Evidence Level VI: Expert Opinion.

Fingeld-Connett, D. (2004). Treatment of substance misuse in older women using a Brief Intervention Model. *Journal of Gerontological Nursing*, 31–37. Evidence Level IV: Nonexperimental Study.

Fink, A., Eliott, M. N., Tsia, M., & Beck, J. C. (2005). An evaluation of an intervention to assist primary care physicians in screening and educating older patients who use alcohol. *Journal of the American Geriatrics Society, 53*(11), 1937–1943. Evidence Level III: Quasi-experimental Study.

Fleming, M. F., Manwell, L. B., Barry, K. L., & Johnson, K. (1998). At-risk drinking in an HMO primary care sample. Prevalence and health policy implications. *American Journal of Public Health, 88*(1), 90–93. Evidence Level III: Quasi-experimental Study.

Godsell, P. A., Whitfield, J. B., Conigrave, K. M., Hanratty, S. R., & Saunders, J. B. (1995). Carbohydrate deficient transferring levels in hazardous alcohol consumption. *Alcohol and Alcoholism, 30*(1), 61–66. Evidence Level III: Quasi-experimental Study.

Grant, B. F., Dawson, D. A., Stinson, F. S., Chou, S. P., Dufour, M. C., & Pickering, R. P. (2004). The 12-month prevalence and trends in DSM-IV alcohol abuse and dependence: United States, 1991–1992 and 2001–2002. *Drug and Alcohol Dependence, 74*(3), 223–234.

Kennedy, G. J. (2000). *Geriatric mental health care: A treatment guide for health professionals*. New York: The Guilford Press. Evidence Level IV: Nonexperimental Study.

Khavari, K. A., & Farber, P. D. (1978). A profile instrument for the quantification and assessment of alcohol consumption: The Khavari Alcohol Test. *Journal of Studies on Alcohol Abuse, 39*, 1525. Evidence Level VI: Expert Opinion.

Koenig, H. G., & Blazer, D. G. (1996). Depression. In Birren, J. E. (Ed.), *Encyclopedia of Gerontology, Age, Aging and the Aged,, Vol. I.* (pp. 425–428). San Diego: Academic Press.

Kurtsthaler, I., Wambacher, M., Golser, K., Sperner, G., Sperner-Unterweger, B., Haidekker, A., et al. (2005). Alcohol and benzodiazepines in falls: An epidemiological view. *Drug & Alcohol Dependence, 79*(2), 225–230. Evidence Level III: Quasi-experimental Study.

Lang, M. M. (2001). Screening for cognitive impairment in the older adult. *Nurse Practitioner, 26*(11), 26, 32–34, 36–37, 41–43. Evidence Level VI: Expert Opinion.

Levkoff, S. E., Chen, H., Coakley, E., Herr, E. C., Oslin, D. W., & Katz, I. (2004). Design and sample characteristics of the PRISM-E multi-site randomized trial to improve behavioral health care for the elderly. *Journal of Aging and Health, 16*(1), 3–27. Evidence Level IV: Nonexperimental Study.

Lyness, J. M., Canine, E. D., King, D. A., Cox, C., & Yoedino, Z. (1997). Psychiatric disorders in older primary care patients. *Journal of General Internal Medicine, 14*, 249–254. Evidence Level III: Quasi-experimental Study.

Mayer, S., Farrell, M., Ferri, M., Amato, L., & Davoli, M. (2005). Psychosocial treatment for opiate abuse and dependence (Review). The Cochrane Collaboration. Downloaded from www.thecochranelibrary.com. Evidence Level I: Systematic Review.

McGlynn, E. A., Asch, S. M., Adams, J., Kessey, J., Hicks, J., DeCristofaro, A., et al. (2003). The quality of health care delivered to adults in the United States. *New England Journal of Medicine, 348*(26), 2635–2645. Evidence Level III: Quasi-experimental Study.

McLellan, A. T., Lewis, D. C., O'Brien, C. P., & Kleber, H. D. (2000). Drug dependence, a chronic medical illness (2000). *Journal of the American Medical Association, 284*(13), 1689–1695. Evidence Level VI: Expert Opinion.

National Center for Health Statistics (2007). Raw data from the *National Health Interview Survey*, Available March 22, 2007, from http://www.cdc.gov/nchs/nhis.htm.

National Institute of Alcohol Abuse and Alcoholism (NIAAA) Q/F Index (2003). In Allen, J. P. & Wilson, V. (Eds.), *Assessing alcohol problems: A guide for clinicians and researcher* (pp. 667–671). Bethesda, MD: U.S. Department of Health and Human Services. Evidence Level VI: Expert Opinion.

National Institute of Alcohol Abuse and Alcoholism (NIAAA) (2000). Economic costs alcohol abuse United States (December 2000). Downloaded from http://pubs.niaaa.nih.gov/publications/economic-2000/index.htm.

National Institute of Alcohol Abuse and Alcoholism (NIAAA) (1995). *The physician's guide to helping patients with alcohol problems.* NIH Pub. No. 95-3769. Bethesda, MD: Author.

National Institute of Drug Abuse (NIDA) (2001). *The economic costs of drug abuse in the United States, 1992–1998.* Retrieved August 1, 2005, from http://www.nida.nih.gov.

National Institute of Drug Abuse (NIDA) (2007). Trends in prescriptions drug abuse: Research report series. Retrieved from www.http.drugabuse.gov/ResearchReports/Prescription/prescriptions5.html. Evidence Level V: Review.

New York City Department of Health and Mental Hygiene (2005). Alcohol use in New York City. *NYC Vital Signs, 4*(1), 1–4.

New York City Department of Health and Mental Hygiene (2002). Treating nicotine addiction. *City Health Information, 21*(6). New York: New York City Department of Health and Mental Hygiene. Evidence Level III: Quasi-experimental Study.

Oslin, D. W. (2005). Treatment of late-life depression complicated by alcohol dependence. *The American Journal of Geriatric Psychiatry, 13*(6), 419–500. Evidence Level III.

Oslin, D. W., Liberto, J. G., O'Brien, J., Krois, S., & Norbeck, J. (1997). Naltrexone as an adjunctive treatment for older patients with alcohol dependence. *American Journal of Geriatric Psychiatry, 5*, 324–332. Evidence Level III. Quasi-experimental study.

Oslin, D. W., Pettinati, H., & Volpolicelli, J. R. (2002). Alcohol treatment adherence: Older age predicts better adherence and drinking outcomes. *The American Journal of Geriatric Psychiatry, 10*(6), 740–747. Evidence Level III. Quasi-experimental study.

Pomerleau, C. S., Carton, S. M., Lutzke, M. L., Flessland, K. A., & Pomerleau, O. F. (1994). Reliability of the Fagerstrom Tolerance Questionnaire and Fagerstrom Test for Nicotine Dependence. *Addictive Behavior, 19*(1), 33–39. Evidence Level V: Program Evaluation.

Prochaska, J. O., & Di Clemente, C. C. (1992). Stages of change in the modification of problem behaviors. *Progress in Behavior Modification, 28,* 183–218. Evidence Level II: Individual Experimental Study.

Project MATCH (1997). Matching alcoholism treatments to client heterogeneity: Project MATCH post-treatment drinking outcomes. *Journal of Studies on Alcohol, 58,* 7–29. Evidence Level III: Quasi-experimental Study.

Reid, S. C., Teeson, M., Sannibale, C., Matsuda, M., & Haber, P. S. (2005). The efficacy of compliance therapy in pharmacotherapy for alcohol dependence: A randomized controlled study. *Journal of Studies on Alcohol, 66*(6), 833–841. Evidence Level III: Quasi-experimental Study.

Rimer, B. K., Orleans, C. T., Keintz, M., Cristinzia, S., & Fleisher, L. (1990). The older smoker: Status, challenges and opportunities for intervention. *Chest, 97,* 547–553. Evidence Level III: Quasi-experimental Study.

Rivers, E., Shirazi, E., Aurora, T., Mullen, M., Gunnerson, K., Sheridan, B., et al. (2004). Cocaine use in elder patients presenting to an inner city emergency department. *Academic Emergency Medicine, 11*(8), 874–877. Evidence Level III: Quasi-experimental Study.

Roberts, A. M., Marshall, E. J., & MacDonald, A. J. (2005). Which screening test for alcohol consumption is best associated with "at risk" drinking in older primary care attenders? *Primary Care Mental Health, 3*(2), 131–138. Evidence Level III: Quasi-experimental Study.

Satre, J. R., Arean, P. A., & Weisner, C. (2004) Five-year alcohol and drug treatment outcomes of older adults versus middle-aged and younger adults in a managed care program. *Addiction, 99*(10), 1286–1297. Evidence Level III: Quasi-experimental Study.

Saunders, J. B., Aasland, O. G., Babor, T. F., de la Fuente, J. R., & Grant, M. (1993). Development of the Alcohol Use Disorders Identification Test (AUDIT): WHO collaborative project on early detection of persons with harmful alcohol consumption II. *Addiction, 88*(6), 791–804. Evidence Level III: Quasi-experimental Study.

Schlaerth, K. R., Splawn, R. G., Ong, J., & Smith, S. D. (2004). Change in patterns of illegal drug use in an inner city population over 50: An observational study. *Journal of Addictive Diseases, 23*(2), 95–107. Evidence Level III: Quasi-experimental Study.

Simoni-Wastila, L., Zuckerman, I. H., Singhai, P. K., Briesacher, B., & Hsu, V. D. (2005). National estimates of exposure to prescription drugs with addiction potential in community-dwelling elders. *Substance Abuse, 20*(1), 33–42. Evidence Level III: Quasi-experimental Study.

Smith, P. M., Reilly, K. R., Houston-Miller, N., DeBusk, R. F., & Taylor, C. B. (2002). Application of a nurse-managed inpatient smoking cessation program. *Nicotine and Tobacco Research, 4*(2), 211–222.

Srisurapanont, M., & Jarusuraisin, N. (2005). Naltrexone for the treatment of alcoholism: A meta-analysis of randomized controlled trials. *The International Journal of Neuropsychopharmacology, 8,* 267–280. Evidence Level III: Quasi-experimental Study.

Sullivan, J. T., Sykora, K., Schneiderman, J., Naranjo, C. A., & Sellers, E. M. (1989). Assessment of alcohol withdrawal: The revised Clinical Institute Withdrawal Assessment for Alcohol scale (CIWA-AR). *British Journal of Addictions, 84,* 1353–1357. Evidence Level III: Quasi-experimental Study.

U.S. Bureau of the Census (1996). 65+ in the United States. *Current Population Reports, Special Studies, P23–P190.* Washington, DC: U.S. Government Printing Office.

U.S. Department of Health and Human Services, National Institute of Alcohol Abuse and Alcoholism (2005). *Helping patients who drink too much: A clinician's guide.* Rockville, MD: USDHHS. Evidence Level VI: Expert Opinion.

U.S. Department of Health and Human Services (2004a). *Substance abuse among older adults: A guide for social service providers* (DHHS Publication No. SMA 00-3393). Rockville, MD: USDHHS, Substance Abuse and Mental Health Services Administration, Center for Substance Abuse Treatment. Evidence Level VI: Expert Opinion.

U.S. Department of Health and Human Services (2004b). *Substance abuse among older adults: A guide for physicians* (DHHS Publication No. SMA 00-3394). Rockville, MD: USDHHS, Substance Abuse and Mental Health Services Administration, Center for Substance Abuse Treatment. Evidence Level VI: Expert Opinion.

Vastag, B. (2003). Addiction poorly understood by clinicians. *Journal of the American Medical Association, 290* (10),1299–1303.

Wetterling, T., Weber, B., Depfenhart, M., Schneider, B., & Junghanns, K. (2006). Development of a rating scale to predict the severity of alcohol withdrawal syndrome. *Alcohol and Alcoholism, 41*(6), 611–615. Evidence Level III: Quasi-experimental Study.

World Health Organization (2000). A systematic review of opioid antagonists for alcohol dependence. *Management of Substance Dependence Review Series*. Downloaded from www.who.int.org. Evidence Level I: Systematic Review.

Wutzke, S. E., Conigrave, K. M., Saunders, J. B., & Hall, W. D. (2002). The long-term effectiveness of brief interventions for unsafe alcohol consumption: A 10-year follow-up. *Addictions, 97*(6), 665–675. Evidence Level I: Systematic Review.

Appendix

National Geriatric Websites Links

Aging Institutions and Associations

Administration on Aging	http://www.aoa.gov
Alzheimer's Association	http://www.alz.org
American Association of Homes and Services for the Aging	http://www.aahsa.org
American Association of Retired Persons	http://www.aarp.org
American Geriatrics Society	http://www.americangeriatrics.org
Geriatrics at Your Fingertips Online Edition	http://www.geriatricsatyourfingertips.org
American Healthcare Association	http://www.ahca.org
American Medical Directors Association Resources in Long-term Care	http://www.amda.com/resources
American Nurses Association	http://www.nursingworld.org
The American Society of Consultant Pharmacists	http://www.ascp.com/resources
American Society on Aging	http://www.asaging.org
Building Academic Geriatric Nursing Capacity	http://www.geriatricnursing.org
Centers for Medicare & Medicaid Services	http://www.cms.hhs.gov
Gerontological Society of America	http://www.geron.org
Hartford Geriatric Nursing Initiative	http://www.HGNI.org
Hospice and Palliative Nurses Association	http://www.hpna.org
Institute for Healthcare Improvement	http://www.ihi.org/ihi
The John A. Hartford Foundation	http://www.jhartfound.org

The John A. Hartford Foundation
Centers of Geriatric Nursing
Excellence:

Oregon Health Sciences
University School of Nursing

http://www.ohsu.edu/hartfordcgne

University of Arkansas for
Medical Sciences College of
Nursing

http://hartfordcenter.uams.edu/

University of California San
Francisco

http://nurseweb.ucsf.edu/www/resrch4
.htm

University of Iowa College of
Nursing

http://www.nursing.uiowa.edu/hartford

University of Pennsylvania
School of Nursing

http://www.nursing.upenn.edu/centers/
hcgne

Nursing Gero TIPS

http://www.nursing.upen.edu/center/
hcgne/ gero_tips

National Chronic Care Consortium

http://www.nccconline.org

National Citizen's Coalition for
Nursing Home Reform

http://www.nccnhr.org

National Conference of
Gerontological Nurse
Practitioners

http://www.ncgnp.org

National Council on Aging

http://www.ncoa.org

National Gerontological Nursing
Assciation

http://www.ngna.org

National Institute on Aging

http://www.nia.nih.gov

On-line Resources for Geriatric
Healthcare Providers

https://www.geriatricvideo.com

Journals/Magazines/Educational/Resources/Statistics

Hartford Institute for Geriatric
Nursing:
research, resources and links

http://www.hartfordIGN.org

GeroNurseOnline:
geriatric nursing protocols,
continuing education,resources,
advocacy information, and
affiliated National Nursing
Organizations

http://www.hartfordIGN.org

American Association of Colleges
of Nursing

http://www.aacn.nche.edu/Education/
Hartford

American Journal of Nursing:
New Look at the Old series,
cutting- Edge research/best
practices, in print/video
How to Try This series, geriatric
nursing assessment tools,
articles, demonstrations, videos.

http://www.NursingCenter.com/
AJNolderadults

Careplans	http://www.careplans.com
Centers for Disease Control and Prevention Department of Health and Human Services	http://www.cdc.gov
Clinical Geriatrics	http://www.clinicalgeriatrics.com
ElderWeb	http://www.elderweb.com/home
Geriatric Nursing	http://journals.elsevierhealth.com/periodicals/ymgn
The Gerontlogist	http://gerontologist.gerontologyjournals.org
Journal of the American Geriatrics Society	http://www.blackwellpublishing.com/journal.asp?ref=0002-8614&site=1
The Joint Commission (JCAHO): sentinel events, patient safety, performance measures	http://www.jointcommission.org
Journal of Gerontological Nursing	http://www.jognonline.com
The Merck Manual Online	http://www.merck.com
Geriatric Merck Manual	http://www.merck.com/mmpe/sec22/ch337
National Guideline Clearinghouse/ Agency for Healthcare Research and Quality (AHRQ): evidence based guidelines	http://www.guideline.gov
Registered Nurses Association of Ontario Nursing Best Practice Guidelines Project	www.rnao.org/bestpractices
Terra Nova Films: videos on aging	http://www.terranova.org
US Department of Health and Human Services	http://www.hhs.gov
U.S. Food and Drug Administration	http://www.fda.gov

Curriculum Guides

Hartford Institute for Geriatric Nursing	http://www.hartfordign.org/resources/education/bsnPartners.html
Long-Term Care Nursing Leadership and Management	http://www.nursing.umn.edu/CGN/LTCNurseLeader
Teaching Gerontology Newsletter	http://www.brookdale.org

Gerontology Centers/Education Centers

Andrus Gerontology Center	http://www.usc.edu/dept/gero
Brookdale Center on Aging	http://brookdale.org
Gerontological Nursing Interventions Research Center	http://www.nursing.uiowa.edu/centers/gnirc
National Association of Geriatric Education Centers	http://www.nagec.org

Practicing Physicians Education in Geriatrics: geriatric toolkits	http://www.gericareonline.net
Stanford Geriatric Education Center Ethnogeriatric Education	http://sgec.stanford.edu
UAMS Reynolds Center on Aging	http://centeronaging.uams.edu
University of Iowa Geriatric Education lecture series, assessment tools, E-Learning	http://www.medicine.uiowa.edu/igec/index.html
University of Iowa Geriatric Mental Health Training Series	http://www.nursing.uiowa.edu/hartford/nurse/training.htm
Wayne State University Institute of Gerontology	http://www.iog.wayne.edu/agingandhealthresources

Websites Retrieved July 19, 2007

Index